Essentials of Human Disease in Dentistry

Essentials series

The *Essentials* are an international, best-selling series of textbooks, all of which are designed to support lecture series or themes on core topics within the health sciences.

Roitt's Essential Immunology, 13th Edition
by Peter J. Delves, Seamus J. Martin, Dennis R. Burton, Ivan M. Roitt
November 2016

Essential Practical Prescribing
by Georgia Woodfield, Benedict Lyle Phillips, Victoria Taylor, Amy Hawkins, Andrew Stanton
April 2016

Essential Primary Care
by Andrew Blythe (Editor), Jessica Buchan (Editor)
March 2016

Hoffbrand's Essential Haematology, 7th Edition
by A. Victor Hoffbrand, Paul A. H. Moss
September 2015

Essentials of Human Disease in Dentistry

Second Edition

**Mark Greenwood BDS, MDS,
PhD, FDSRCS, MB ChB, FRCS (Eng. and Ed.),
FRCS (OMFS), FHEA**

NHS Consultant, Oral and Maxillofacial Surgery
Honorary Clinical Professor of Medical Education
Dentistry at the School of Dental Sciences
Newcastle University
Newcastle upon Tyne, UK

WILEY Blackwell

This edition first published 2018
© 2018 John Wiley & Sons Ltd

Edition History
John Wiley & Sons (1e, 2009)

Registered Offices
John Wiley & Sons, Inc., 111 River Street, Hoboken, NJ 07030, USA
John Wiley & Sons Ltd, The Atrium, Southern Gate, Chichester, West Sussex, PO19 8SQ, UK

Editorial Office
9600 Garsington Road, Oxford, OX4 2DQ, UK

For details of our global editorial offices, customer services, and more information about Wiley
products visit us at www.wiley.com.

Wiley also publishes its books in a variety of electronic formats and by print-on-demand. Some content
that appears in standard print versions of this book may not be available in other formats.

Library of Congress Cataloging-in-Publication Data

Names: Greenwood, M. (Mark), author.
Title: Essentials of human disease in dentistry / by Mark Greenwood.
Other titles: Textbook of human disease in dentistry
Description: Second edition. | Hoboken, NJ : Wiley, 2018. | Preceded by Textbook of human
    disease in dentistry / Mark Greenwood, Robin A. Seymour, and John G. Meechan. 2009. |
    Includes bibliographical references and index. |
Identifiers: LCCN 2017040601 (print) | LCCN 2017041146 (ebook) | ISBN 9781119251828 (pdf) |
    ISBN 9781119251859 (epub) | ISBN 9781119251842 (pbk.)
Subjects: | MESH: Dental Care–methods | Clinical Medicine–methods | Disease | Comprehensive
    Dental Care | Handbooks
Classification: LCC RK305 (ebook) | LCC RK305 (print) | NLM WU 49 | DDC 617.6/3–dc23
LC record available at https://lccn.loc.gov/2017040601

Cover Design: Wiley
Cover Image: © MedicalRF.com/Gettyimages

Set in 10/12pt Adobe Garamond by SPi Global, Pondicherry, India
Printed and bound in Singapore by Markono Print Media Pte Ltd

10 9 8 7 6 5 4 3 2 1

Contents

Contributors

JR Adams BDS, MB BS, FDS, FRCS (OMFS)
Consultant in Oral and Maxillofacial Surgery, Royal Victoria Infirmary
Newcastle upon Tyne, UK

N Ali MA, MRCOphth
Specialist Registrar in Ophthalmology, Royal Victoria Infirmary
Newcastle upon Tyne, UK

A Balakrishnan MB BS, AFRCS (Ed.)
Senior Clinical Fellow in Vascular Surgery, Freeman Hospital
Newcastle upon Tyne, UK

RJ Banks BDS, MB BS, FDS, FRCS (OMFS)
Consultant, Oral and Maxillofacial Surgery, Sunderland Royal Hospital
Sunderland, UK

T Barakat MB BS, FRCS, FEBVS
Vascular Fellow, Freeman Hospital
Newcastle upon Tyne, UK

F Birrell MA, MB BChir, FRCP, DipClinEd
Consultant Physician, Wansbeck General Hospital
Northumberland, UK

SJ Bourke MD, FRCP, FRCPI, DCH
Consultant Physician, Royal Victoria Infirmary
Newcastle upon Tyne, UK

H Bourne MB ChB, FRCPath
Consultant, Department of Immunology, Royal Victoria Infirmary
Newcastle upon Tyne, UK

AL Brown MA, MD, FRCP
Consultant Nephrologist/Honorary Senior Clinical Lecturer, Freeman Hospital
Newcastle upon Tyne, UK

SJ Brown MB BS, BSc (Hons), MRCPsych
Formerly Specialist Registrar in Psychiatry
Newcastle upon Tyne, UK

S Clark BDS, MB ChB, FDS, FRCS (Ed.), FRCS (OMFS), FFST (Ed.), PGDipClinEd
Consultant in Oral and Maxillofacial Surgery, Manchester Royal Infirmary
Manchester, UK

CC Currie BDS, MRes, MFDS
Clinical Fellow in Oral Surgery, School of Dental Sciences, Newcastle University
Newcastle upon Tyne, UK

J Durham BDS, PhD, FDS(OS)RCS
Professor/Consultant in Oral Surgery, School of Dental Sciences, Newcastle University
Newcastle upon Tyne, UK

M Greenwood BDS, MDS, PhD, FDSRCS, MB ChB, FRCS (Eng. and Ed.), FRCS (OMFS), FHEA
Consultant/Clinical Professor, Oral and Maxillofacial Surgery Unit
Newcastle Dental Hospital/Royal Victoria Infirmary
Newcastle upon Tyne, UK

P Griffiths FRCS, FRCOphth
Consultant/Senior Lecturer in Ophthalmology, Royal Victoria Infirmary
Newcastle upon Tyne, UK

J Hanley MB ChB, MD, FRCP, FRCPath
Consultant Haematologist, Royal Victoria Infirmary
Newcastle upon Tyne, UK

FE Hogg BDS, MFDS, MPaedDent, Med, FHEA
Specialist Registrar in Paediatric Dentistry
Glasgow Dental Hospital/Royal Hospital for Children
Glasgow, UK

S Hogg BSc, PhD, FHEA
Formerly Senior Lecturer, School of Dental Sciences, Newcastle University
Newcastle upon Tyne, UK

RH Jay MA, MD, FRCP, DipClinEd
Consultant Physician, Royal Victoria Infirmary
Newcastle upon Tyne, UK

A Lennard MB BS (Hons), FRCP, FRCPath
Consultant Haematologist/Honorary Senior Lecturer, Royal Victoria Infirmary
Newcastle upon Tyne, UK

RI Macleod BDS, PhD, FDSRCSE, DDRRCR
Consultant in Oral and Maxillofacial Radiology (retired), School of Dental Sciences
Newcastle University
Newcastle upon Tyne, UK

S Mathia MB BS, MRCP (UK)
Specialist Registrar in Haematology, Royal Victoria Infirmary
Newcastle upon Tyne, UK

JG Meechan BDS, BSc, PhD, FDSRCPS, FDSRCS (Ed.)
Honorary Consultant/Senior Lecturer (retired), School of Dental Sciences
Newcastle University
Newcastle upon Tyne, UK

EK Montgomery MB BS, MRCP, Nephrol
Consultant Nephrologist, Newcastle Hospitals NHS Foundation Trust
Newcastle upon Tyne, UK

E Ong MB BS, MSc, FRCP, FRCPI, DTM&H
Consultant Physician/Honorary Senior Lecturer in Medicine
Department of Infectious Diseases and Tropical Medicine, Royal Victoria Infirmary
Newcastle upon Tyne, UK

CM Robinson BDS, MSc, PhD, FDSRCS, FRCPath
Senior Lecturer in Oral Pathology/Honorary Consultant, School of Dental Sciences
Newcastle University
Newcastle upon Tyne, UK

JA Sayer MB ChB FRCP PhD FHEA
Professor of Renal Medicine, Institute of Genetic Medicine, Newcastle University
Newcastle upon Tyne, UK

RA Seymour BDS, PhD, FDSRCS (Ed. and Eng.)
Emeritus Professor, School of Dental Sciences, Newcastle University
Newcastle upon Tyne, UK

K Staines BChD, FDSRCS, MOMRCS Ed.
Consultant/Honorary Senior Clinical Lecturer in Oral Medicine
School of Oral and Dental Science, University of Bristol
Bristol, UK

G Stansby MA, MB, MChir, FRCS (Eng.)
Professor of Vascular Surgery, Newcastle University
Newcastle upon Tyne, UK

C Stroud MB ChB, FRCPath
Consultant Immunologist, Department of Immunology, Royal Victoria Infirmary
Newcastle upon Tyne, UK

C Taylor BSc (Hons), PhD, FRCPath (Deceased)
Consultant Clinical Scientist (Virology)
Health Protection Agency, UK

PJ Thomson BDS, MSc, PhD, MD, DDSc, FDSRCS, FFDRCSI, FRCS (Ed.)
Professor, School of Dental Sciences, University of Queensland
Australia

G Toms BSc, PhD
Professor of Applied Virology (retired), Newcastle University
Newcastle upon Tyne, UK

S Waugh MB ChB, BSc, PhD, MRCPCH, FRCPath
Consultant Medical Virologist, Royal Victoria Infirmary
Newcastle upon Tyne, UK

RR Welbury BDS, MB BS, FDSRCS, FDSRCPS, FRCPCH, FFGDP
Professor, School of Dentistry, University of Central Lancashire
Preston, UK

Preface to the first edition

The concept of human disease teaching in dentistry arose out of General Dental Council recommendations in their report 'The First Five Years', published in 2002 and currently under revision. This suggested an integrated approach to the teaching of general medicine and surgery, and the related disciplines. There are slight variations in the subjects incorporated into human disease teaching across UK dental schools, but general medicine and surgery teaching is common to all. Pharmacology, pathology and microbiology are also included in the course at Newcastle University, and the material in this book forms the basis of the theoretical elements of that course.

A dentist should have a firm grounding in all these disciplines to facilitate a broader knowledge and understanding of human disease, which can then be focused on issues of direct relevance to dentistry. This approach enables informed dialogue with colleagues in other healthcare professions, including general medical practitioners.

It is hoped that this book will prove useful to dental undergraduates studying human disease, and that it will also be of use to candidates preparing for the membership examinations of the Royal Colleges of Surgeons.

M Greenwood
RA Seymour
JG Meechan
Newcastle upon Tyne, UK
January 2009

Preface to the second edition

This second edition of *Textbook of Human Disease in Dentistry*, now called *Essentials of Human Disease in Dentistry*, aims to build on the strengths of the first edition, but has been updated in several key areas. The underlying principle remains the same – to provide the dental student/dental practitioner with a firm background knowledge of the relevant aspects of general medicine and surgery, pharmacology, pathology and microbiology. New additions to this edition include multiple choice–style questions at the end of each chapter, together with relevant references.

It is hoped that this edition will continue to be of value to undergraduate students of dentistry and those preparing for their postgraduate dental examinations.

M Greenwood
Newcastle upon Tyne, UK
August 2017

Acknowledgements

I would like to acknowledge the contributing authors of this book, both for this text and the first edition, and for the invaluable help they give to the smooth running of the undergraduate course in Newcastle.

Acknowledgement is also due to Iain Macleod for his help with some of the illustrations, David Sales for many of the line drawings, and Beryl Leggatt and S Wilkinson for the secretarial help.

Where illustrations have been imported from other publications, due acknowledgement has been given.

About the companion website

Don't forget to visit the companion website for this book:

 www.wiley.com/go/greenwood/human-disease-in-dentistry

The companion website provides all the figures from the book in PowerPoint for download.

Scan this QR code to visit the companion website:

CHAPTER 1
Clinical examination and history taking

M Greenwood

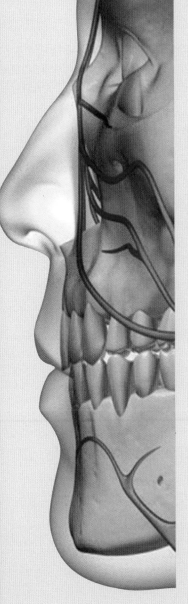

Key topics

- Essential components of a medical history
- Key issues that may arise from the medical history

Learning objectives

- To be familiar with the main components of a medical history.
- To be aware of the medical terms used in taking a medical history, and their meaning.
- To be aware of the normal vital signs.

Essentials of Human Disease in Dentistry, Second Edition. Mark Greenwood.
© 2018 John Wiley & Sons Ltd. Published 2018 by John Wiley & Sons Ltd.
Companion website: www.wiley.com/go/greenwood/human-disease-in-dentistry

Components of a medical history

The medical history aims to:
- Enable the formulation of a differential diagnosis or diagnosis
- Put the patient's disease process into the correct medical and social context.
- Establish a rapport with the patient.

Clinicians engaged in obtaining medical histories should introduce themselves to the patients and give their designations. The taking of the history may then commence and should follow a scheme similar to that shown in Table 1.1.

Presenting complaint

The presenting complaint can be recorded in medical terms, but often is better expressed in the patient's own words. When recording the history in writing, quotation marks should be placed around the patient's words. In a verbal case presentation, it should be stated that the patient's own words are being used. It is important to avoid presumptive diagnoses in the presenting complaint. For example, patients do not *present* with iron deficiency anaemia; they may present with symptoms that arise *from* it. It should be remembered that symptoms are the features of the illness that the patient describes; signs are physical findings obtained by the clinician.

History of the presenting complaint

The history of the presenting complaint should be a chronological but succinct account of the patient's problem. It is important to start at the onset of the problem and describe its progression. Symptoms should be similarly described.

Points to include when asking patients about pain are as follows:
- Site
- Character – for example, tight/band-like (in the chest, suggestive of cardiac origin)
- Does the pain radiate anywhere?
- Onset – sudden or gradual

Table 1.1 Areas to be covered in a medical history.
Presenting complaint
History of presenting complaint
Past medical history
Allergies
Past dental history
Drugs
Social history
Family history
Psychiatric history

- Severity (ask the patient to rate on a scale of 1–10, with 10 being the most severe)
- Duration
- Exacerbating/relieving factors (including the use and efficacy of medication)
- Preceding events or associated features
- Has the pain occurred before? / Is it getting better or worse?

Past medical history

It is worth asking a generic set of opening questions – for example, 'Do you have any heart or chest problems?' Questioning should then focus on specific disorders – for example, asthma, diabetes, epilepsy, hypertension, hepatitis, jaundice or tuberculosis. It is also worth specifically asking about any previous problems with the arrest of haemorrhage. Past problems with intravenous sedation or general anaesthesia should be noted. It is worth asking about any previous history of rheumatic fever, which may have led to cardiac valve damage. In 2008, the National Institute for Health and Care Excellence (NICE) discontinued the regular use of antibiotic prophylaxis for bacteraemia-producing dental procedures in patients with cardiac damage. There were some concerns about this, however, such as the lack of an evidence base for prophylaxis and the fact that Europe and the USA differed in their practices.

Before 2008, a consistent upward trend was apparent in the population-corrected incidence of infective endocarditis in England. Soon after the implementation of the NICE guidelines, the slope of the trend line increased further, although there is no direct evidence that this was due to the discontinuation of antibiotic prophylaxis in dentistry. In 2016, NICE modified the guidance slightly to state that: 'Antibiotic prophylaxis against infective endocarditis is not recommended *routinely* [my emphasis] for people undergoing dental procedures'. This addition emphasises NICE's standard advice on healthcare professionals' responsibilities. Doctors and dentists should offer the most appropriate treatment options, in consultation with their patients and/or their carers or guardians. In doing so, they should take into account the recommendations of NICE guidance and the values and preferences of patients, and also apply their clinical judgement.

To guide decision-making, NICE has provided information regarding which might be considered high-risk and moderate-risk groups for the development of infective endocarditis – see Table 1.2.

It is clearly important that positive findings be recorded. Some important negative findings too are worth recording.

Allergies

Any known allergies should be recorded. This is one aspect of the medical history that should be recorded even if there are no known allergies. Any allergies that are identified should be highlighted in the clinical record.

Table 1.2 Stratification of the risk of infective endocarditis.

High-risk categories
- Patients with a previous history of infective endocarditis
- Patients with any form of prosthetic heart valves (including a transcatheter valves)
- Those in whom prosthetic material was used for cardiac valve repair
- Patients with any type of cyanotic congenital heart disease
- Patients with any type of congenital heart disease repaired with prosthetic material, whether placed surgically or by percutaneous techniques, for the first 6 months after the procedure or lifelong if a residual shunt or valvular regurgitation remains

Moderate-risk categories
- Patients with a previous history of rheumatic fever
- Patients with any other form of native valve disease (including the most commonly identified conditions: bicuspid aortic valve, mitral valve prolapse or calcific aortic stenosis)
- Patients with unrepaired congenital anomalies of the heart valves

Past dental history

In a general history, the dental history should be relatively brief. It can include details of the regularity or otherwise of dental attendance and the use of local anaesthesia or sedation. Any adverse events, including post-extraction haemorrhage, could also be included here.

Drugs

Any medication taken by the patient should be recorded. The use of recreational drugs can be included in this section or in the social history.

'Recreational' drugs

Dentists should have a working knowledge about the implications of patients using recreational drugs, as the use of such drugs is relatively common. Cannabis has a sympathomimetic action that could potentially exacerbate the systemic effects of adrenaline in dental local anaesthetics. Heroin and methadone are both opioid drugs, with methadone being used in drug rehabilitation programmes. Oral methadone has a high sugar content and can lead to rampant caries. Heroin can lead to addicts having a low threshold for pain and can cause thrombocytopaenia, in addition to interfering with drugs that dentists may prescribe. Other details regarding recreational drugs are given in Chapter 19 (titled 'Psychiatric disorders').

Complementary therapies

Complementary therapies are often used by patients. Many patients do not deem it important to tell dental practitioners that they are using such preparations, as they do not feel that it may be of any relevance. It is important to remember, however, that some of the drugs that dental practitioners prescribe can be affected by some complementary therapies. A summary of some of the more common potential interactions is given in Table 1.3.

Table 1.3 Complementary medicines and their interactions with conventional medicines with potential consequences.

Herb	Conventional drug	Potential problem
St. John's wort	Monoamine oxidase inhibitors and serotonin reuptake inhibitors Antidepressants Iron	Mechanism of herbal effect uncertain Insufficient evidence of safety with concomitant use – therefore not advised May limit iron absorption
Karela, ginseng	Insulin, sulfonylureas, biguanides	Altered glucose concentrations
Feverfew, garlic ginseng, ginger	Warfarin	Altered prothrombin time/INR
Echinacea used for >8 weeks	Anabolic steroids, methotrexate, amiodarone, ketoconazole	Hepatotoxicity
Feverfew	Non-steroidal anti-inflammatory drugs (NSAID)	Inhibition of herbal effects
Ginseng	Oestrogens, corticosteroids	Additive effects
Evening primrose oil	Anticonvulsants	Lowered seizure threshold
Kava	Benzodiazepines	Additive sedative effects, coma
Echinacea, zinc (immunostimulants)	Immunosuppressants (such as corticosteroids, cyclosporine)	Antagonistic effects

Implanted cardiac devices

Some ultrasonic scalers and ultrasonic baths produce electromagnetic interference and may therefore be a risk to patients with implanted cardiac devices such as pacemakers and implanted defibrillators. Other such devices include electronic apex locators and electrocautery devices. There is a degree of confusion in the current literature regarding what devices are and are not considered safe to use, and consultation with the appropriate authorities is therefore important.

Social history

This should be a succinct but comprehensive assessment of the patient's social circumstances. It should include the following details:

- Smoking behaviour
- Alcohol consumption – type and quantity – recommended not to exceed 14 units per week (female) and 21 units per week (male)
- Occupation (or previous occupation if retired)
- Home circumstances – a brief description of the residence – for example, a house, flat or sheltered accommodation. Who else lives in the household?

Family history

Any disorders with a genetic origin should be recorded.

Psychiatric history

This will only need to be included in specific cases. More detail is given in Chapter 18 (titled 'Medicine for the elderly').

In hospital practice, after the history comes the systems review. Specific questions are asked to further refine the available knowledge on the patient's overall medical condition. Many schemes are described, and the following scheme has been adapted for the dental clinician.

General questions

As with the history, a series of general questions can help to encompass the wide-ranging possibilities in terms of the underlying medical problems. Questions cover the following topics:

- Appetite
- Weight loss
- Fevers
- The presence of lumps or bumps
- Any rashes or itchy rashes
- Lethargy or fatigue

Cardiovascular system

- Chest pain (a differential diagnosis is given in Chapter 21, titled 'Medical emergencies')
- Dyspnoea – difficult or disordered breathing (beware of co-existing/alternative respiratory causes)
- If dyspnoea on exertion, try and quantify in terms of metres walked or number of stairs climbed before dyspnoea occurs
- Paroxysmal nocturnal dyspnoea (waking up in the night feeling breathless – see Chapter 5, titled 'Cardiovascular disorders')
- Orthopnoea (breathlessness on lying flat – see Chapter 5)
- Ankle oedema – beware of other possible causes of lower limb swelling
- Palpitations (awareness of the beating of the heart)
- Calf claudication (distance walked until pain occurs in the 'calf' muscles of the leg, referred to as the 'claudication distance')

Respiratory system

- The presence of cough, and its duration
- Whether the cough produces sputum
- Haemoptysis (coughing up blood)
- Wheezing

Gastrointestinal system

- Indigestion
- Nausea or vomiting
- Dysphagia (difficulty swallowing)
- Odynophagia (pain on swallowing)
- Haematemesis (vomiting of blood), described as looking like 'coffee grounds'
- Change in bowel habits
- Change in bowel motion – for example, pale stool and dark urine is virtually pathognomonic of obstructive jaundice (see Chapter 7, titled 'Gastrointestinal disorders')
- Melaena is the production of black stool containing blood altered by gastric acid; fresh blood indicates bleeding from further down the gastrointestinal tract

Neurological system

A brief overview is required, in particular:
- Any history of fits or faints
- Disturbance in sensation – particularly in the orofacial region
- Headache or facial pain

Musculoskeletal system

- Gait (overlaps with neurological system)
- Pain/swelling/stiffness of joints
- Impairment of function

Genitourinary system

This is usually of little relevance to the dental practitioner. Repeated urinary tract infections may be relevant insofar as the patient may be undergoing antibiotic treatment – of which the dental practitioner should be aware. For dental patients in general hospital settings, enquiry is useful regarding symptoms of prostatism. Some patients who require significant surgical procedures may require catheterisation, and an enlarged prostate gland can lead to difficulties with catheter insertion. 'Hesitancy' is the term that is used to describe difficulty in initiating the urine stream, and 'terminal dribbling' is difficulty in stopping. Frequency of urination and nocturia (passing urine at night) should all be included.

Clinical observations in the clothed patient

While it is evident that clinical examination is important, much of the background to a patient's medical condition is gained from the history. Physical examination often serves to confirm what is suspected from the history.

Overall view of the patient

Does the patient look generally well? Is the patient of normal weight, or is he or she cachectic or obese? It is important to note whether the patient is alert or appears to be confused (Table 1.4 lists potential causes of confusion in a patient). As soon as the patient enters the surgery, note should be taken of the gait. Is the patient pale or flushed or of normal complexion? Is he or she breathless?

Not all the preceding observations are necessarily diagnostic of the precise nature of disease. However, if something does not look normal, then it probably is not, and an explanation needs to be found.

In hospitalised patients, it is important that the vital signs be recorded (Table 1.5). This is discussed further in a following section (titled 'Vital signs').

Examination of the hands

In the hands, there are several observable signs that can be of interest to a dental practitioner. The overall appearance of the hands should be noted, together with any abnormalities of the nails, skin and muscles.

Palmar erythema can be seen in pregnancy, rheumatoid arthritis and patients with liver problems. Swollen proximal interphalangeal (PIP) joints suggest rheumatoid arthritis together with ulnar deviation of the hands (Figure 1.1). Swollen distal interphalangeal (DIP) joints suggests osteoarthritis. Gout and the skin condition psoriasis can also cause DIP joint swelling. In psoriasis, there may be the additional feature of finger nail pitting.

Dupuytren's contracture may also be seen. In this condition, the palmar fascia contracts, leading to the little finger (particularly of the right hand) being held passively in a flexed position. There is usually a palpable nodular thickening of the connective tissue overlying the ring and little fingers. The aetiology is often unknown, but can be associated with alcoholism.

Table 1.4 Potential causes of confusion in a patient.
Hypoxia
Infection
Epilepsy
Hypoglycaemia
Drug or alcohol withdrawal
Stroke, myocardial infarction (MI)
Raised intracranial pressure

Table 1.5 The vital signs.
Pulse rate
Blood pressure
Temperature
Respiratory rate

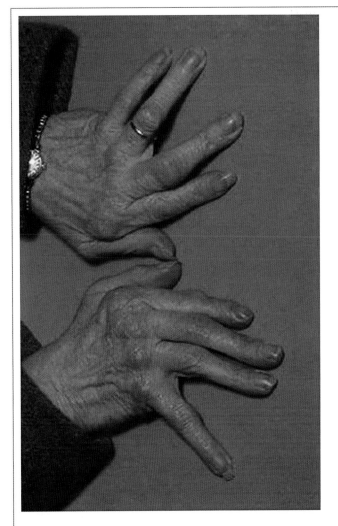

Figure 1.1 Rheumatoid hands. Note the ulnar deviation, which can cause significant limitations in activities of daily living.

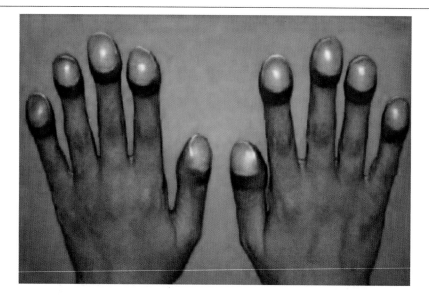

Figure 1.2 Finger clubbing. There is a loss of angle between the nail surface and the skin of the finger, and the nail bed is 'boggy' to pressure.

Clubbing of the fingers should always be looked for and can represent disease processes in diverse systems (Figure 1.2). There is a loss of the angle between the nail and nail bed, and the fingernail has an exaggerated curvature in the longitudinal plane. The area around the nail fold feels boggy to palpation. Potential causes of finger clubbing are given in Table 1.6.

The fingernails may also show splinter haemorrhages that can result from mild trauma, but these may also be a sign of endocarditis (see Chapter 5, titled 'Cardiovascular disorders'). Leukonychia (white fingernails) may be seen in patients with liver disease. Koilonychia (spoon-shaped fingernails) can be seen in patients with chronic iron deficiency anaemia.

The face

If the patient's complexion is examined, it may display evidence of jaundice. This is rather subjective and unreliable. The best area to look for jaundice is the sclera of the eyes. The clinical and metabolic syndrome seen in chronic kidney disease known as 'uraemia' may also impart a yellowish tinge to the skin. The eyelids may exhibit xanthelasma – deposits in the eyelids, signifying hyperlipidaemia (Figure 1.3). Corneal arcus (Figure 1.4) can be seen in some patients. It is sometimes associated with an increased risk of coronary artery disease. There may also be the malar flush of mitral stenosis or the butterfly rash seen in systemic lupus erythematosus (SLE; see Chapter 11, titled 'Musculoskeletal disorders').

Central cyanosis may be seen by asking the patient to protrude the tongue – a bluish hue is indicative of this. Peripheral cyanosis (seen in the nail beds) is caused by peripheral vasoconstriction, which may be normal, seen in cold conditions or in shock, but may also signify peripheral vascular insufficiency.

Table 1.6 Causes of finger clubbing.

Cardiothoracic causes
- Infective endocarditis
- Cyanotic congenital cardiac disease
- Intrathoracic pus – for example, lung abscess, bronchiectasis
- Bronchial carcinoma
- Fibrosing alveolitis

Gastrointestinal causes
- Inflammatory bowel disease
- Cirrhosis of the liver

Other causes
- Familial
- Secondary to thyrotoxicosis
- Idiopathic

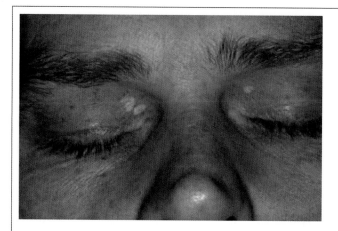

Figure 1.3 Xanthelasma.

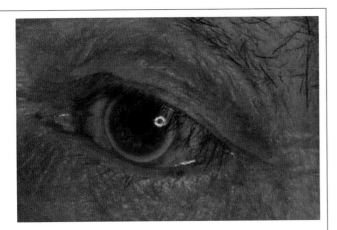

Figure 1.4 A patient with corneal arcus (also sometimes called 'arcus senilis').

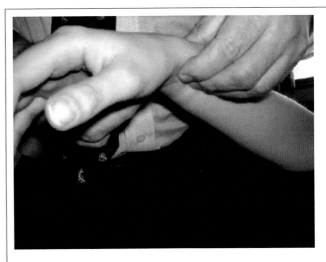

Figure 1.5 Taking the radial pulse. The radial artery is passing roughly along a straight line in this area, and two or three examining fingers can therefore be used for palpation.

Examination of the cardiovascular system in the clothed patient

All clinical examinations should follow the following scheme: inspection, palpation, percussion and auscultation.

Dyspnoea (difficult or disordered breathing) should be noted. It should be borne in mind that there may be a respiratory cause. Is the patient short of breath at rest (SOBAR), or only short of breath on exertion (SOBOE)? If the upper part of the thorax is exposed, there may be evidence of the upper end of a median thoracotomy scar. This will most commonly have facilitated access for a coronary artery bypass graft (CABG) or valve replacement procedure.

In the hands, splinter haemorrhages should be looked for together with finger clubbing and signs of anaemia. Osler's nodes and Janeway lesions may be evident (see Chapter 5, titled 'Cardiovascular disorders').

The radial pulse (thumb side of the wrist) should be taken (Figure 1.5). This is discussed further in a following section (titled 'Vital signs'). Some dental practitioners are proficient in palpating a central pulse in addition to the radial pulse (which is a peripheral pulse). The carotid pulse (a central pulse) is palpated in the neck, along the anterior border of the sternocleidomastoid muscle.

The blood pressure should be taken. The blood pressure cuff is placed around the upper arm, which is placed at rest (see Chapter 5E, titled 'Hypertension').

Jugular venous pressure

Jugular venous pressure (JVP) is a difficult thing to assess. The internal jugular vein acts as a manometer that reflects the right atrial pressure. JVP is measured with the patient sitting at 45° with the head turned slightly to the left. JVP is the vertical height of the column of blood visible in the right internal jugular vein, measured in centimetres from the sternal angle. It is raised if it is >3 cm.

Oedema can be seen in some cardiac patients. Pulmonary oedema reflects left ventricular failure, whereas peripheral oedema reflects right ventricular failure. Left- and right-sided failure together constitutes congestive cardiac failure. Due to gravitational effects, peripheral oedema is seen most commonly in the ankles, but it may be seen in the sacral region in bedridden patients.

Respiratory system

On inspection, the patient may demonstrate breathlessness, cyanosis or finger clubbing (Table 1.6). There may be tar stains on the fingers from smoking – often incorrectly regarded as nicotine stains. In the clothed patient, it may be difficult to assess the thoracic shape, but symmetry should be looked for in respiratory movements, together with use of accessory muscles of respiration. Chest deformities may lead to difficulties in respiration either in isolation or together with spinal deformities. 'Kyphosis' refers to increased forward spinal curvature, and 'scoliosis' refers to increased lateral spinal curvature. On palpation, the trachea should be central in the sternal notch.

Gastrointestinal system

On inspection, the patient may show signs of purpura or spider naevi. Spider naevi can be emptied by pressing on the centre, and they refill from this point. They are only seen in the distribution of the superior vena cava. Leukonychia may be seen (a sign of hypoalbuminaemia). Finger clubbing may also be seen. In cases of marked hepatic dysfunction, a liver flap may be observed – when the hands are held outstretched, they demonstrate a marked flapping movement.

A jaundiced patient may show scratch marks on the skin due to the intense itchiness arising from the bile salts deposited within the skin. Palmar erythema may also be noted, signifying an underlying liver disorder.

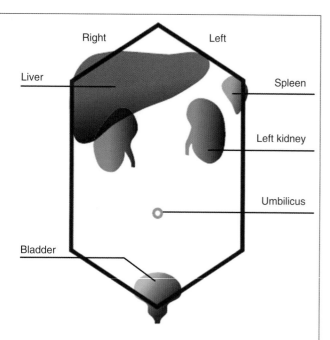

Figure 1.6 A schematic diagram of the abdomen (not to scale).

Table 1.7 Causes of tachycardia and bradycardia.
Tachycardia (pulse rate >100 beats/min)
• Physiological – for example, exercise, emotion • Related to fever • Secondary to drugs – for example, adrenaline, atropine • Hyperthyroidism • Smoking • Excess caffeine
Bradycardia (pulse rate <60 beats/min)
• Physiological – for example, in athletes • Immediately post-vaso-vagal attack • Sick sinus syndrome • Hypothyroidism

Table 1.8 Commonly seen abnormalities of the radial pulse.
Sinus tachycardia – pulse >100 beats/min
Sinus bradycardia – pulse <60 beats/min
Atrial fibrillation – irregularly irregular pulse
Ventricular extrasystole – 'missed beats'

It is unusual for a dental practitioner to be called upon to examine other systems. A diagram of the abdomen is shown in Figure 1.6.

Vital signs

All hospital patients should have their vital signs measured. Vital signs are summarised in Table 1.5.

In contemporary hospital practice, vital signs are reviewed as part of the National Early Warning Score (NEWS). Any changes (normal score being zero) should prompt a review of the patient.

Pulse

The pulse is usually taken from the radial artery. In very small children and babies, the brachial pulse may be palpated in the antecubital fossa. The pulse should be assessed for its rate (in beats per minute), rhythm and volume. The rhythm of the pulse may be regular or irregular. If the pulse is irregular, this may be in a predictable pattern, in which case it is described as 'regularly irregular'. If the pulse is completely disordered, it is described as 'irregularly irregular'. The most common example of the latter is in patients with atrial fibrillation (see Chapter 5, titled 'Cardiovascular disorders'). It should be ascertained whether the pulse is strong, or weak and 'thready'. A bounding pulse can be a sign of carbon dioxide retention in patients with chronic obstructive pulmonary disease (COPD).

A pulse rate of >100 beats/min is described as 'tachycardia', and a pulse rate of <60 beats/min is described as 'bradycardia' (causes given in Table 1.7). Other abnormalities of the pulse are listed in Table 1.8.

Blood pressure

The method for measuring blood pressure is given in Chapter 5E (titled 'Hypertension'). The figures quoted are given in millimetres of mercury. The upper figure is the systolic blood pressure (120–140 mmHg), and the lower figure the diastolic blood pressure (60–90 mmHg). Pathological changes in blood pressure are discussed in Chapter 5 (titled 'Cardiovascular disorders').

Temperature

The normal body temperature, measured orally, is 35.5–37.5°C. Many automated digital devices are now available for measuring body temperature, often in the form of a probe inserted into the external auditory meatus. In infants, the thermometer may be inserted into the armpit (axilla).

Respiratory rate

Several disease processes may be manifest by alterations in the respiratory rate and are discussed in the relevant chapters. The normal respiratory rate in a resting adult who is fit and well is 12–18 breaths/min.

Specific lesions

It is useful to have a standard set of parameters to be used in the assessment of lumps and ulcers. These can be applied to any clinical situation with minor modifications if required. These are summarised in Table 1.9 (lumps) and Table 1.10 (ulcers).

Table 1.9 Generic features to be considered in the assessment of lumps.

History

When/how was the lump first noticed?

Are there any symptoms?

Has the lump changed since it was noticed?

Does the lump ever disappear?

Are there any other lumps?

Examination

Site

Size

Shape

Surface – smooth or not – fixed to skin/deep structures

Colour of overlying skin/mucosa

Is it tender?

Edge – indistinct or well defined

Consistency – soft, fluctuant, rubbery or hard

Is it compressible?

Is it pulsatile?

Does it transilluminate when the light from a torch is shone through it?

Enlargement of local lymph nodes?

Consider blood and nerve supply to surrounding area

Is this a localised lump, or part of an associated generalised condition?

Table 1.10 Features to be considered in the assessment of ulcers.

History

Where/how was it noticed?

Symptoms

Changes since noticed

Any previous history of similar ulcers?

Examination

Site

Size

Shape

Base – slough, granulation tissue, deeper anatomy visible

Edge – sloping, suggesting healing

Punched out (square edge)

Undermined edge – for example, TB

Rolled – basal cell cancer (see Chapter 11, titled 'Musculoskeletal disorders')

Everted – squamous cell cancer (Chapter 11)

Depth

Discharge – swab for microbiological analysis

Enlargement of local lymph nodes?

Consider blood and nerve supply to surrounding area

Is this a localised ulcer, or part of an associated generalised condition?

SUMMARY

Most of the assessments of any patient's medical condition is made on the basis of a thorough history.

Examination findings usually serve to confirm suspicions and refine findings.

FURTHER READING

Oxford Handbook of Clinical Medicine. Oxford: Oxford University Press; 2014.

Scully's Medical Problems in Dentistry. London: Churchill Livingstone; 2014.

Antibiotic prophylaxis. Available from: https://www.nice.org/guidance/cg64 (last update 2016).

General Dental Council. Maintaining Standards: Guidance to Dentists on Professional and Personal Conduct. Available from: http://www.gdc-uk.org/Newsandpublications// Publications/ Publications/MaintainingStandards.

Resuscitation Council (UK). Available from: http://www.resusc.org.uk/pages/medental.htm.

MULTIPLE CHOICE QUESTIONS

1. Orthopnoea is a possible symptom of:

   a) Indigestion
   b) Seizures
   c) Productive cough
   d) Left-sided heart failure
   e) Bowel cancer
   Answer = D

2. Which of the following are *not* likely causes of confusion in a patient?

   a) Hypoxia
   b) Infection
   c) Epilepsy
   d) Prescription of a non-steroidal anti-inflammatory drug (NSAID)
   e) Raised intracranial pressure
   Answer = D

3. Koilonychia (spoon-shaped fingernails) is a potential sign of:

   a) Vitamin K deficiency
   b) Albumin deficiency
   c) Chronic iron deficiency anaemia
   d) Infective endocarditis
   e) Patients with liver disease
   Answer = C

4. A facially visible sign of hypercholesterolaemia is:

   a) Malar flush
   b) Xanthelasma
   c) Cyanosis
   d) Jaundice
   e) Ptosis
   Answer = B

5. Which of the following signs is *not* a potential feature of rheumatoid arthritis?

   a) Dupuytren's contracture
   b) Ulnar deviation of the hands
   c) Elbow nodules
   d) Pulmonary fibrosis
   e) Enlarged spleen
   Answer = A

6. The stated alcohol consumption limit per week for females is:

   a) 2 units per week
   b) 6 units per week
   c) 10 units per week
   d) 14 units per week
   e) 20 units per week
   Answer = D

7. Which of the following is *not* a recognised cause of finger clubbing?

   a) Cyanotic congenital heart disease
   b) Bronchial carcinoma
   c) Inflammatory bowel disease
   d) Fibrosing alveolitis
   e) Myocardial infarction
   Answer = E

8. The artery used to take the pulse at the wrist in a patient is the:

   a) Brachial artery
   b) Ulnar artery
   c) Radial artery
   d) Popliteal artery
   e) Dorsalis pedis artery
   Answer = C

9. 'Tachycardia' is defined as:

   a) A pulse rate of more than 100 beats per minute
   b) Another word to describe ventricular extrasystole
   c) A pulse rate of more than 90 beats per minute
   d) A pulse rate of more than 110 beats per minute
   e) A pulse rate of more than 120 beats per minute
   Answer = A

10. 'Bradycardia' is defined as:

    a) A pulse rate of less than 100 beats per minute
    b) A pulse rate of less than 90 beats per minute
    c) A pulse rate of less than 80 beats per minute
    d) A pulse rate of less than 70 beats per minute
    e) A pulse rate of less than 60 beats per minute
    Answer = E

CHAPTER 2
Inflammation and anti-inflammatory drugs

CM Robinson and RA Seymour

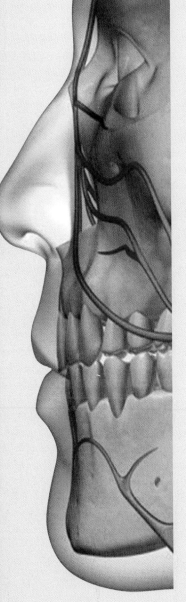

Key topics

- Overview of the pathology and clinical features of wound healing and inflammation
- Descriptive terms used in the clinicopathology of inflammatory disorders

Learning objectives

- To be familiar with the main pathological processes involved in wound healing and inflammation.
- To be familiar with some of the drugs commonly used in the treatment of inflammatory conditions.

Essentials of Human Disease in Dentistry, Second Edition. Mark Greenwood.
© 2018 John Wiley & Sons Ltd. Published 2018 by John Wiley & Sons Ltd.
Companion website: www.wiley.com/go/greenwood/human-disease-in-dentistry

Cell and tissue injury – Introduction

Cells are under constant threat of injury as a consequence of changes in their local environment. There are numerous potentially injurious agents that a cell may encounter. The type of mediator depends on the location of the cell within the body. There are agents that cause physical damage to cell integrity – for example, mechanical trauma, thermal injury and chemical damage. Cellular viability is affected by the deleterious effects of microorganisms. Cells are also prone to damage following reductions in oxygen and nutrient supply. Cell injury may be induced by DNA-damaging agents, such as ionising radiation.

Cell injury may be reversible or irreversible. This depends on the type of injurious agent, the duration of the adverse conditions and the ability of the cell to adapt to the changes. If the cell is unable to adapt and survive, there are two distinct pathways leading to cell death – necrosis and apoptosis (programmed cell death). Consequences of tissue injury are shown in Table 2.1 and described in the following text.

Necrosis

Necrosis is the death of groups of cells. It has profound consequences on tissue integrity and function. In some circumstances, for example, in the heart, ischaemic necrosis of the myocardium can result in complete organ failure and death of the individual. Various types of necrosis are described, depending on the microscopic appearances observed within tissues when stained with haematoxylin and eosin (H&E). Haematoxylin stains cell nuclei dark blue, whereas eosin stains the cytoplasm and the connective tissue proteins a reddish pink colour.

Coagulative necrosis

Coagulative necrosis is the most common type of necrosis and can occur in most organs and tissues. Immediately following cell death, the architecture of the tissue is retained. The cell outlines are discernible along with tissue architecture. There is progressive loss of nuclear staining, and there is a loss of cytoplasmic detail, with condensation and breakdown of intracellular proteins. Eventually, all that remains are the 'ghost'

Table 2.1 Potential consequences of tissue injury.

Inflammation
Coagulative necrosis
Colliquative necrosis
Caseous necrosis
Fibrinoid necrosis
Fat necrosis
Gangrene

outlines of cells embedded in the extracellular matrix that comprises the tissue. Accompanying necrosis is an ensuing inflammatory reaction, which results in progressive dissolution of the damaged tissue with variable attempts at regeneration and repair, depending on the affected tissue.

Colliquative necrosis

Colliquative necrosis is observed in the brain following cerebral infarction. The brain has little in terms of robust collagenous supporting tissues, and the necrotic neurons and glial tissue break down to form a liquid material (liquefactive degeneration). The latter is progressively removed by microglia (macrophages/histiocytes), leaving a fluid-filled cavity.

Caseous necrosis

Caseous necrosis is characterised by structureless necrotic tissue, which has the textural quality of crumbly cheese. It is typically seen in the context of granulomatous inflammation caused by *Mycobacterium tuberculosis*.

Fibrinoid necrosis

Fibrinoid necrosis is seen in malignant hypertension and diseases characterised by vasculitis. Necrosis of smooth muscle cells in the arterial wall causes plasma to leak into the tunica media with deposition of fibrin. Fibrin takes on a distinct bright red colour when stained with H&E.

Fat necrosis

Damage to adipose tissue and the release of stored intracellular fat elicits an intense acute inflammatory response, which is typically followed by a dense fibrotic repair reaction.

Gangrene

Gangrene is necrosis with accompanying putrefaction (breakdown) of the tissues. Gangrene is typically seen in the lower extremities (legs and toes), and is usually the result of supervening infection of the necrotic tissue with bacteria, particularly *Clostridium*.

Apoptosis

Apoptosis is the process whereby cells can be removed in a controlled manner, without disrupting the integrity of the organ or tissue. Apoptosis is also called 'programmed cell death', which emphasises that it is a cellular process induced and executed by specific biochemical pathways. Apoptosis has a pivotal role in development, and controls organ size and tissue morphogenesis. In the adult, apoptosis counterbalances cellular proliferation, helping to maintain optimal cell numbers and cell types within a particular tissue. Apoptosis is also essential for the establishment of a functional immune system, through deletion of unwanted lymphocyte clones. Apoptosis is considered to play an important role in ageing, and deregulated apoptosis is involved in the pathogenesis of neoplasia.

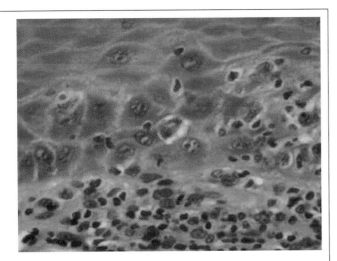

Figure 2.1 The histopathological appearance of an apoptotic keratinocyte (centre of photomicrograph). H&E stain. (See text for details.)

Table 2.2 Wound healing.
Soft tissue
• Healing by primary intention
• Healing by secondary intention
Bone
• Haematoma formation in fracture line
• Formation of granulation tissue and osteoclastic activity
• Woven bone forms a fracture callus
• Remodelling of woven bone to form lamellar bone

Cells undergoing apoptosis show distinct morphological characteristics when viewed by light microscopy in H&E-stained tissue sections (Figure 2.1). The dying cell shrinks, and there is a loss of cellular adhesion. The chromatin of the nucleus condenses and fragments, producing the appearance of 'nuclear dust'. The dead cell is phagocytosed by adjacent cells or histiocytes. There is no induction of the inflammatory cascade that typically accompanies cell death by necrosis.

Wound healing

Wound healing describes the processes that take place, following tissue injury, which are required to restore or replace damaged tissue. The effectiveness of the healing process is dependent on the ability of the constituent cells to regenerate, reorganise and recreate the original tissue architecture.

Cells in the adult can be classified by their potential to regenerate. Labile cells are continuously being lost and replaced. They include haematopoietic cells of the bone marrow and epithelial cells that constitute the epidermis and line the mucous membranes. Stable cells are not continuously replaced, but can be induced to regenerate in certain conditions; examples include hepatocytes of the liver and the renal tubular cells that make up the kidney. Non-dividing cells cannot be stimulated to proliferate and therefore have no capacity for regeneration; examples include cardiac myocytes and neurons. Labile cells that make up simple tissue structures such as the skin and the mucous membranes are the most effective at restoring tissue architecture following injury (regeneration). Stable cells can be induced to proliferate; however, in the liver and kidney, the complexity of the organ structure precludes successful regeneration and the establishment of physiological function. Damaged tissue composed of non-dividing cells is either removed to leave a tissue defect (e.g. colliquative necrosis following cerebral infarct) or repaired by fibrous tissue to produce a scar (e.g. fibrosis following a myocardial infarct).

Skin is used as a model for studying wound healing. Healing of skin is usually described as occurring by primary intention when the wound edges are approximated, and by secondary intention when there is a tissue defect that prevents closure of the wound (Table 2.2).

A surgical incision that has been closed by sutures heals by primary intention. In these circumstances, the apposed wound edges are stuck together by fibrin, which forms a scab at the skin surface. Below the scab, within the damaged epidermis, the basal keratinocytes proliferate and migrate across the narrow defect, and the epithelium completely regenerates within 5–7 days. The fibrin that sticks the incised edges of the dermis together is gradually replaced by cellular fibrovascular tissue. Small capillary buds grow into the wound, providing oxygen and nutrients, and fibroblasts migrate into the area, producing collagen and other extracellular matrix proteins. Gradually, the fibrovascular tissue becomes less vascular and matures to form fibrous scar tissue.

On occasions, it is not possible to appose the edges of a wound, and the tissue defect heals by secondary intention. Initially, the tissue defect is composed of necrotic tissue admixed with clotted blood (haematoma). The necrotic tissue is removed by histiocytes, and the clotted blood is gradually replaced by highly cellular fibrovascular tissue, called 'granulation tissue' (referring to the visual appearance of the tissue in the base of a wound, which is bright red and has a rather granular appearance). It is important to point out here that granulation tissue is distinct from 'granulomatous inflammation', which is discussed in the following text.

Granulation tissue is composed of proliferating endothelial cells that form rudimentary imperforate capillaries, small capillary buds and loops. As the granulation tissue matures, the capillaries become dilated and engorged with blood. There are fibroblasts producing collagen and extracellular matrix proteins that progressively fill the tissue defect. In addition, there are myofibroblasts, which are specialised fibroblasts that contain contractile smooth muscle filaments. Myofibroblasts are thought to play an important role in wound contraction, which facilitates closure of the tissue defect. In some circumstances, this causes marked tissue distortion with attendant cosmetic and functional problems. Towards the skin surface, the epidermal keratinocytes at the margins of the defect divide and migrate below the scab to form a thin sheet of epithelial cells. Gradually, the tissue defect is completely covered by

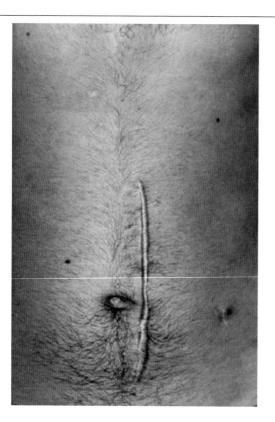

Figure 2.2 A hypertrophic scar. Keloid scars extend beyond the wound margins.

full-thickness epidermis, and the scab is exfoliated. Sometimes, the production of fibrous repair tissue is excessive, and the dermis becomes bulky and lumpy – this is referred to as a 'hypertrophic' or 'keloid' scar (Figure 2.2).

Wound healing proceeds in a similar manner following bone injury (Table 2.2). For example, following the fracture of a limb bone, a haematoma forms at the site of injury and invests dead pieces of soft tissue and devitalised fragments of bone. The soft tissue is removed by histiocytes, and the bone is removed by osteoclasts. Granulation tissue gradually replaces the haematoma, and woven bone is laid down to form a fracture callus. The woven bone of the callus is eventually remodelled to lamellar bone and, consequently, within 6–8 weeks, there is very little evidence of the injury; this is known as 'regeneration'. Healing of long bones is dependent, however, on close apposition of the broken ends of the bone and immobilisation of the fracture site. Failure to ensure the latter may result in failure of bone regeneration and the production of a fibrous union (pseudarthrosis; false joint).

The liver has a complex architecture, with hepatocytes arranged in a lobular configuration around hepatic vessels and bile ducts. Hepatocytes are stable cells that can be induced to proliferate, and small groups of cells are capable of regenerating and recreating the lobular architecture following injury. However, following extensive damage to the liver – for example, owing to long-standing alcohol abuse – there is disorganised nodular regeneration of hepatocytes, as opposed to lobular regeneration, and there is also extensive fibrosis, which results in liver cirrhosis. The kidney is similar, in that the tubular cells are capable of regeneration, but the complex microanatomy of the organ is difficult to recreate, and organ damage usually heals by fibrosis.

Inflammation – Introduction

Inflammation is a protective response, the goal of which is to eliminate the injurious agent and the consequences of tissue damage. Ideally, the inflammatory process facilitates repair of damaged tissue; however, in some circumstances, inflammation can have harmful effects on the tissues and compromise the well-being of the individual.

Inflammation is a complex reaction that occurs in vascularised tissue and comprises changes in blood vessels, which lead to the accumulation of fluid that contains leukocytes, the inflammatory exudate. Inflammation is classified into *acute* and *chronic* phases. Acute inflammation is usually of relatively short duration, lasting minutes, hours or a few days. It is characterised by the accumulation of tissue fluid, plasma proteins and the emigration of leukocytes, principally neutrophils.

Chronic inflammation is of longer duration, and is characterised by the accumulation of specialised immune cells – for example, lymphocytes, plasma cells and macrophages. Long-standing inflammation may cause further tissue damage, which is termed 'bystander damage'. After neutralisation/elimination of the cause of inflammation, there follows attempts at repair. The process of repair is characterised by the proliferation of blood vessels producing richly vascular granulation tissue, and there is usually attendant fibrosis. The inflammatory cascade is orchestrated by chemical mediators triggered by the inflammatory stimulus. The chemical mediators are derived from the plasma, and are released by a variety of cells involved in inflammation.

Conventionally, the process of inflammation is described by the suffix '-itis', preceded by the organ and/or tissues affected (Table 2.3).

Inflammation is caused by:

- Microorganisms: bacteria, viruses, fungi, parasites.
- Physical agents: mechanical trauma, thermal injury, chemical damage, exposure to radiation.
- Tissue necrosis.
- Hypersensitivity reactions.

The clinical signs of inflammation, called the 'cardinal signs', are redness, heat, swelling, pain and loss of function (Table 2.4). Redness is a consequence of increased blood flow to the inflamed tissue, and is called 'hyperaemia'. In peripheral tissues, for example, the skin, the increased blood flow causes the skin surface to feel warmer. In addition, inflammatory chemical mediators contribute to a rise in body temperature, called 'pyrexia'. The development of swelling is mainly a consequence of accumulating tissue fluid, called 'oedema'. Progression of the inflammatory response produces symptoms of pain; there is distortion and stretching of the tissues, and inflammatory chemical mediators

Table 2.3 Inflammation of different body organs.

Organ/tissue	Tissues	Inflammation
Brain	Meninges	Meningitis
Heart	Endocardium	Endocarditis
	Myocardium	Myocarditis
	Pericardium	Pericarditis
Large bowel	Colon	Colitis
	Peritoneum	Peritonitis
Liver	Liver parenchyma	Hepatitis
Lungs	Lung parenchyma	Pneumonitis
	Alveoli	Alveolitis
	Bronchi	Bronchitis
Tooth	Dental pulp	Pulpitis
	Periodontal ligament	Periodontitis

Table 2.4 Cardinal signs of acute inflammation.

Redness – *rubor*
Heat – *calor*
Swelling – *tumor*
Pain – *dolor*
Loss of function – *functio laesa*

sensitise pain receptors in the affected tissues. Loss of function is a consequence of increased pain and swelling.

Pathogenesis of acute inflammation

The acute inflammatory response involves three main processes:
- Vascular response – changes in vessel calibre and blood flow.
- Humoral response – increased vascular permeability and fluid exudation.
- Cellular response – formation of a cellular exudate.

Changes in vessel calibre and blood flow occur at the onset of inflammation. Initially, there is transient vasoconstriction of arterioles that lasts a few seconds, which is followed by prolonged vasodilation and opening of capillary beds, which increases the blood flow to the area (hyperaemia). Physiological fluid exchange within a capillary network is governed by the principles described by Starling, which depends on an intact endothelium.

In inflammation, the capillaries become leaky, and there is escape of protein-rich fluid into the tissues (fluid exudate). Vascular leakage is mainly caused by the formation of gaps between the endothelial cells, and is mediated by a variety of different chemical mediators, which include histamine, bradykinin and leukotrienes. The gaps form by endothelial contraction following remodelling of the intracellular actin cytoskeleton.

Vascular permeability is also caused by direct injury to endothelial cells. The loss of protein from the plasma reduces the intravascular osmotic pressure and, coupled with the increase in hydrostatic pressure due to vasodilation, there is a net outflow of fluid into the tissues. Consequently, blood viscosity increases and capillary blood flow becomes slow. These changes precede and facilitate the development of the cellular exudate.

Normally, blood flow through vessels is axial; plasma flows adjacent to the vessel wall, and the cellular component of blood travels as a column in the central part of the vessel lumen, away from the vessel wall. In inflammation, as the blood viscosity increases and the blood flow slows down, leukocytes drop out of axial flow and come in close proximity to the endothelial cells that line the blood vessel; this process is called 'margination'. Following margination, leukocytes, principally neutrophils, adhere to the endothelial cells. Initially, the adhesion is transient and the neutrophils roll along the endothelium, finally coming to rest under the influence of strong intercellular binding.

Over time, the neutrophils almost entirely line the vessel – a process called 'pavementation'. The adherence of leukocytes to the endothelium is mediated by specific cell adhesion molecules (CAMs). Four groups of CAMs are involved: selectins, immunoglobulins, integrins and mucin-like glycoproteins that are under the influence of chemoattractants (bacterial products, components of the complement pathway particularly C5a, leukotrienes and chemokines). The leukocytes insert pseudopodia between the endothelial cells and start the process of emigration into the extravascular compartment. Extravasated neutrophils bind to microorganisms by opsonisation and are capable of phagocytosis and intracellular killing.

Sequelae of acute inflammation

Resolution

Resolution is defined as the complete restoration of normal tissue architecture following inflammation (Table 2.5). Resolution proceeds if there is minimal tissue damage and the tissue has the capacity to regenerate. Resolution is characterised by the restitution of physiological vascular permeability and drainage of excess tissue fluid via the lymphatics. Macrophages play a pivotal role in removing necrotic debris, which facilitates

Table 2.5 Sequelae of acute inflammation.

Resolution
Organisation
Suppuration
Fibrinous inflammation
Serous inflammation
Ulceration

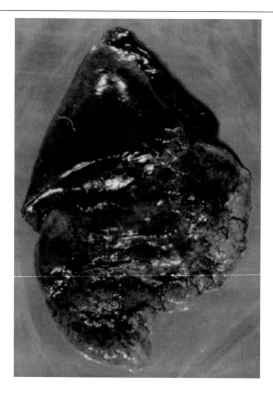

Figure 2.3 Acute lobar pneumonia showing consolidation in the upper lobe.

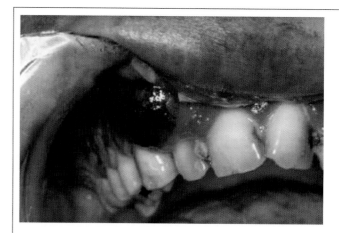

Figure 2.4 An acute dental abscess.

regeneration of the tissue architecture. The best example of an acute inflammatory condition that resolves completely is acute lobar pneumonia (pneumonitis) (Figure 2.3).

Organisation

In situations where there is extensive tissue damage or there is no capacity for resolution, the affected tissue heals by organisation. Organisation is characterised by the production of granulation tissue. Macrophages clear the dead necrotic material, and new capillary buds grow into the area of inflamed tissue. Migrating and proliferating fibroblasts produce extracellular matrix rich in collagen, causing fibrosis. Healing by organisation often results in distortion of the affected tissues, producing a scar. In some circumstances, scarring may adversely affect organ function – for example, inflammation of the bowel wall with ensuing fibrosis may cause a stricture and obstruction.

Suppuration

Suppuration is the formation of pus, composed of dead and dying neutrophils, bacteria and degenerating cellular debris. Suppuration is usually caused by a persistent bacterial infection. Some species of bacteria are invariably associated with the formation of pus and are called 'pyogenic bacteria' (e.g. *Staphylococcus aureus* and *Streptococcus pyogenes*). Pus is usually contained within

a cavity lined by inflamed granulation tissue and fibrous tissue, called an 'abscess' (Figure 2.4). A hollow body cavity filled with pus is called an 'empyema' (e.g. empyema of the gallbladder).

Fibrinous inflammation

Fibrinous inflammation develops when the inflammatory exudate is rich in fibrin. The fibrin cross-links to form a thick coating. This appearance is typified by the post-mortem description of 'bread and butter' pericarditis, in which the visceral and parietal surfaces of the inflamed pericardium resemble those of two pieces of buttered bread that have been pressed together and then pulled apart.

Serous inflammation

Serous inflammation is characterised by the accumulation of a watery fluid exudate that contains relatively few inflammatory cells. Serous inflammation occurs on the serosal surfaces of the gastrointestinal tract (peritonitis). The watery content of a blister on the skin surface is a consequence of serous inflammation.

Ulceration

An ulcer is a defect of the tissue surface produced by the sloughing of inflamed necrotic tissue. Inflammation of the skin and mucous membranes may typically lead to the development of ulceration (Figure 2.5).

Pathogenesis of chronic inflammation

Chronic inflammation takes time to develop, and is characterised by the accumulation of lymphocytes, plasma cells and macrophages. There is a complex interplay between the various cell types involved in chronic inflammation. The macrophage, derived from the mononuclear phagocyte system, is considered to play a central role in coordinating the chronic inflammatory response. The bone marrow harbours the

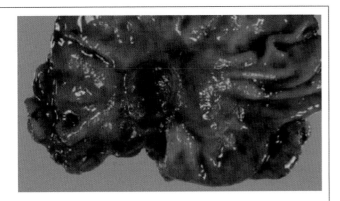

Figure 2.5 A gastric ulcer.

precursor cells, which are released into the blood as monocytes. Monocytes enter the tissues by the same process described for emigrating neutrophils, and they are then termed 'macrophages'. Macrophages scattered throughout the parenchymal connective tissues are termed 'histiocytes'. In some organs and locations, macrophages have different names – liver, 'Kupffer cells'; lungs, 'alveolar macrophages'; central nervous system (CNS), 'microglia'; and lymph nodes, 'sinus histiocytes'. Nevertheless, activated macrophages at all sites have the same role, and are involved in both phagocytosis and the recruitment of other chronic inflammatory cells via the secretion of an array of cytokines, chemotactic factors and growth factors. In addition to the accumulation of specific immune cells, the affected tissues also show attempts at repair, and there is production of granulation tissue and progressive fibrosis (organisation).

Chronic inflammation is usually seen in patients with prolonged exposure to toxic agents, persistent infection or autoimmune disease. Chronic inflammation may follow the acute inflammatory response, particularly if there is suppuration and abscess formation. In these circumstances, failure in draining pus leads to the development of chronic inflammation. For example, in the transition of acute suppurative osteomyelitis to chronic osteomyelitis, fragments of dead bone bathed in pus act as a stimulus for the accumulation of a chronic inflammatory cell infiltrate. In some instances, chronic inflammation develops insidiously, and is not preceded by any significant acute inflammatory response; such cases may be referred to as having primary chronic inflammation.

Primary chronic inflammation

Persistent infection

Microorganisms that resist phagocytosis and intracellular killing induce a chronic inflammatory response. Examples include viral infections and bacterial infections such as *Mycobacterium tuberculosis*.

Foreign body reactions

Foreign body reactions may be induced by either endogenous or exogenous material. Typical examples of endogenous toxins include dead bone in chronic osteomyelitis, degenerate adipose tissue in fat necrosis, and keratin debris from a ruptured epidermoid cyst. Exogenous materials include surgical sutures (stitches), silica particles and asbestos fibres, the latter two causing lung fibrosis.

In the mouth, amalgam debris from restorative procedures can be displaced into soft tissue and taken up by macrophages. This can impart tattooing to the mucosa – an 'amalgam tattoo'.

Autoimmune disease

In this group of diseases, the immune system is inappropriately activated against 'self'-antigens. The generation of autoantibodies and the associated hypersensitivity reactions result in sustained chronic inflammation. An example is autoimmune (Hashimoto's) thyroiditis.

Granulomatous inflammation

Granulomatous inflammation is a distinct type of chronic inflammation characterised by the accumulation of activated macrophages, which superficially have an epithelial-like appearance and are termed 'epithelioid macrophages'. A granuloma is a focal aggregate of epithelioid macrophages that is usually surrounded by a rim of lymphocytes and plasma cells. In addition, some of the macrophages fuse to form giant cells. The giant cells comprise a large amount of cytoplasm with multiple nuclei, sometimes up to 20 per cell. Morphologically distinct types are recognised: cells with haphazardly arranged nuclei are termed 'foreign body giant cells'; cells with nuclei arranged in a horseshoe configuration are termed 'Langerhans giant cells'; and those with a peripheral ring of nuclei and central clear cytoplasm due to lipid accumulation are called 'Touton giant cells'.

The presence of granulomatous inflammation in biopsy material leads to a restricted list of diagnostic possibilities that may be distinguished by additional clinical information or further investigations. Granulomatous disorders can be broadly divided into three groups: those caused by microorganisms (tuberculosis, syphilis, deep mycoses); those associated with foreign body implantation; and, finally, idiopathic diseases (Crohn's disease, sarcoidosis, granulomatosis with polyangiitis, giant cell arteritis) (Table 2.6).

Systemic effects of inflammation

Inflammation may also be accompanied by profound systemic effects. These include pyrexia. In addition, there may be feelings of malaise, anorexia and nausea, with accompanying weight loss. The inflammatory reaction may cause enlargement of regional lymph nodes (lymphadenitis) and, in some instances, enlargement of the spleen (splenomegaly). There are also changes in the

Table 2.6 Causes of granulomatous inflammation.

Diagnosis	Histopathology tests	Clinical tests
Infective causes		
Tuberculosis	ZN stain	Chest X-ray
	Modified ZN stain	Sputum culture
		Tuberculin test
		Heaf test
		Mantoux test
Syphilis	Warthin–Starry stain	Serology – antibodies
		TPIT
		VDRL
		Wassermann reaction
Deep mycoses	PAS and DPAS stain	Check immune status
	Grocott stain	Culture fresh tissue for microbiology
Foreign body implantation		
Foreign body reactions	Birefringent material on cross-polarisation	History of foreign body implantation
	X-ray diffraction studies	
Idiopathic diseases		
Crohn's disease		Barium enema
		Endoscopy
Sarcoidosis		SACE
		Serum calcium
		Liver function tests
		Chest X-ray
		Liver ultrasound
Granulomatosis with polyangiitis (GPA)		cANCA
Giant cell arteritis		ESR/PV
		Angiography

cANCA: cytoplasmic antineutrophil cytoplasmic antibody; DPAS: diastase PAS; ESR: erythrocyte sedimentation rate; PAS: periodic acid–Schiff reagent; PV: plasma viscosity; SACE: serum angiotensin-converting enzyme; TPIT: *Treponema pallidum* immobilisation test; VDRL: venereal disease research laboratory test; ZN: Ziehl–Neelsen.

blood, which can be used as clinical indicators of inflammatory disease – for example, the erythrocyte sedimentation rate and plasma viscosity increase as a consequence of the production of acute phase proteins and immunoglobulins.

Increasing serum levels of C-reactive protein (CRP) is used as an indicator of inflammatory disease. In long-standing chronic inflammation – for example, rheumatoid arthritis – elevated serum amyloid A protein may result in the deposition of amyloid in a variety of organs and tissues (secondary/reactive amyloidosis). There may be increased numbers of circulating leukocytes (leukocytosis). Neutrophilia is characteristic of pyogenic inflammation, whereas eosinophilia is often a consequence of allergic disease or parasitic infection. Lymphocytosis is typically seen in chronic inflammatory diseases. Mononucleosis is associated with Epstein–Barr virus infection (infectious mononucleosis/glandular fever). Anaemia may also be a feature of prolonged inflammatory disease, as a consequence of chronic blood loss or toxic bone marrow suppression.

Anti-inflammatory drugs

Anti-inflammatory drugs block or target various aspects of the inflammatory response. Examples include antihistamines, corticosteroids and non-steroidal anti-inflammatory drugs

(NSAIDs). The latter are dealt with in Chapter 14 (titled 'Pain and anxiety control').

Antihistamines

This is a collective group of drugs that antagonise histamine at receptor sites. They do not alter the formation or release of histamine from tissues or mast cells. Antihistamines are classified according to the histamine (H) receptors that they block (H_1, H_2, H_3). H_1 receptor antagonists are often referred to as the 'classic' antihistamines. H_2 receptor antagonists are used in the management of peptic ulceration, and are considered in Chapter 7 (titled 'Gastrointestinal disorders'). H_3 receptor blockers have been synthesised, but their clinical use and value have yet to be determined.

H_1 receptor antagonists

Examples of this category of antihistamines include chlorphenamine (chlorpheniramine), promethazine and loratadine.

H_1 blockers are competitive antagonists as they interact with H_1 receptors on cell membranes, which results in a decrease in the availability of these receptors for the actions of histamine. Hence, H_1 blockers antagonise the action of histamine on smooth muscles, and thus reduce histamine-induced vasodilation, capillary permeability, and the flare and itch components of the triple response of Lewis. The full description of this physiological response is given in standard texts of physiology. Some H_1 receptor antagonists also have central effects, including sedation and the reduction of nausea and vomiting. These actions are not related to the antagonism of histamine.

Most H_1 receptor antagonists are taken orally; they are well absorbed from the gastrointestinal tract, metabolised in the liver and excreted via the kidneys. Therapeutic effects can be observed 15–30 min after dosage.

Uses

H_1 blockers are widely used in the treatment and prevention of a variety of allergic conditions – for example, rhinitis, hay fever and certain allergic dermatoses such as acute urticaria. Topical preparations may be useful in relieving the itching associated with insect bites. The drugs are also widely used in common cold remedies, usually combined with a decongestant. (While such constituents reduce symptoms, they do not prevent or shorten the duration of the common cold.) The central effects of H_1 blockers make them useful in the prophylaxis of motion sickness and as a sedative, especially in children.

Unwanted effects

Sedation is the main unwanted effect associated with certain H_1 receptor blockers, but the extent and severity of this unwanted effect vary between preparations. Alcohol should be avoided in patients taking antihistamines, as it can enhance the sedative effect. The so-called second generation of antihistamines (cetirizine and loratadine) do not cause sedation, since they are unable to cross the blood–brain barrier.

Topical antihistamine creams are readily available to the public to relieve skin itching and also for insect bites. Such preparations may cause hypersensitivity reactions, and should be avoided in patients with a history of eczema and other allergic-based skin disorders. Their use should be limited to 3 days.

Dental uses of antihistamines

Only H_1 receptor blockers have any dental application. Chlorphenamine 10–20 mg, given by intramuscular or subcutaneous injection, is a useful adjunctive treatment in the management of anaphylaxis (see Chapter 20, titled 'Haematology'). Chlorphenamine must be administered after adrenaline. Promethazine has both sedative and weak atropine-like properties and may be useful as a preoperative sedative agent, particularly in children (see Chapter 14, titled 'Pain and anxiety control').

Corticosteroids

Corticosteroids are naturally occurring substances produced by the adrenal cortex (see Chapter 12, titled 'Dermatology and mucosal lesions'). Synthetic corticosteroids are used extensively in all aspects of clinical medicine as they possess potent anti-inflammatory and immunosuppressive properties. In this section, only the anti-inflammatory properties will be considered. Immunosuppressive actions of corticosteroids are dealt with in Chapter 4 (titled 'Immunological disease').

Anti-inflammatory action of corticosteroids

Corticosteroids inhibit many of the processes associated with inflammation, which include decreased production of prostanoids owing to decreased expression of cyclo-oxygenase-2; decreased generation of cytokines (interleukin (IL)-1 to IL-8 and tumour necrosis factor-α (TNF-α)); reduction in the concentration of complement proteins in the plasma; decreased generation of nitric oxide; and decreased histamine release from mast cells. At the cellular level, corticosteroids reduce polymorphonuclear leukocyte (PMN) chemotaxis and phagocytosis.

These various actions are mediated by corticosteroids binding with glucocorticoid receptors in the cytoplasm of various cells. Such binding then brings about either suppression or induction of various transcription factors, which switch on the genes for the various cytokines listed earlier.

Anti-inflammatory actions of corticosteroids applicable to dentistry

Oral ulceration and oral mucosal lesions

Corticosteroids are widely used in the treatment of recurrent aphthous ulceration and other oral mucosal lesions such as lichen planus, mucous membrane pemphigoid and pemphigus. Many of these conditions are treated by topical applications, and examples of such preparations include hydrocortisone sodium succinate oromucosal tablets (2.5 mg), beclomethasone spray (50–100 µg) and betamethasone soluble tablets (500 µg) dissolved in water and used as a mouthwash. Applying any topical medication to the oral mucosa is difficult, and often the best results are achieved when there is maximal contact time between the lesion and the medication. For severe cases of oral ulceration, systemic corticosteroids may be necessary, and the drug of choice is prednisolone.

Pulpal inflammation

Corticosteroids can be applied over a carious exposure of the dental pulp to try and reduce pulpal inflammation and pain. One such preparation, Ledermix®, contains triamcinolone and tetracycline (demeclocycline hydrochloride). The efficacy of Ledermix® remains equivocal.

Bell's palsy

This is a unilateral facial paralysis affecting one or more branches of the facial nerve (see Chapter 9, titled 'Neurology and special senses'). Bell's palsy is of unknown aetiology, but may be subsequent to a viral infection. Systemic prednisolone is the treatment of choice, and therapy must be started within 5–6 days of the onset of paralysis. It is usual to start off treatment with prednisolone at a high dose, reducing this over a period of 10 days.

Postoperative pain and swelling after dental surgery

There has been much interest in the use of systemic corticosteroids to reduce pain and swelling after the removal of impacted lower third molars and after orthognathic surgery. For such purposes, a course of corticosteroids is usually short, so unwanted effects are few. Methylprednisolone and betamethasone are the corticosteroids used for this purpose, usually administered intramuscularly just before surgery, or dexamethasone intravenously. The efficacy of corticosteroids for reducing postoperative pain after dental surgical procedures remains uncertain, and such pain may respond better to an NSAID (see Chapter 14, titled 'Pain and anxiety control').

FURTHER READING

Cross S. *Underwood's Pathology: A Clinical Approach*, sixth edition. London: Churchill Livingstone; 2013.

MULTIPLE CHOICE QUESTIONS

1. At post-mortem examination, a patient who died of myocardial infarction would show evidence of:
   a) Fibrinoid necrosis
   b) Gangrene
   c) Colliquative necrosis
   d) Coagulative necrosis
   e) Apoptosis
   Answer = D

2. At post-mortem examination, a patient who died of cerebral infarction would show evidence of:
   a) Gangrene
   b) Colliquative necrosis
   c) Coagulative necrosis
   d) Apoptosis
   e) Fibrinoid necrosis
   Answer = B

3. The skin has the potential to regenerate because:
   a) It has an excellent blood supply
   b) The injury is usually superficial
   c) The majority of cells are stable
   d) Healing is by primary intention
   e) The majority of cells are labile
   Answer = E

4. Granulation tissue contains:
   a) Pyogenic bacteria
   b) Langerhans giant cells
   c) Epithelioid macrophages
   d) Fibrovascular tissue
   e) Well-formed granulomas
   Answer = D

5. Granulomas contain:
   a) Endothelial cells
   b) Macrophages
   c) Epithelial cells
   d) Myofibroblasts
   e) Fibroblasts
   Answer = B

6. H_1 receptor antagonists are prescribed to patients with:
   a) Peptic ulceration
   b) A previous episode of anaphylaxis
   c) Hay fever
   d) Acute glomerulonephritis
   e) Rheumatic fever
   Answer = C

CHAPTER 3
Principles of infection and infection control

S Waugh, E Ong, S Hogg, JG Meechan, RA Seymour, M Greenwood, C Taylor[†] and G Toms

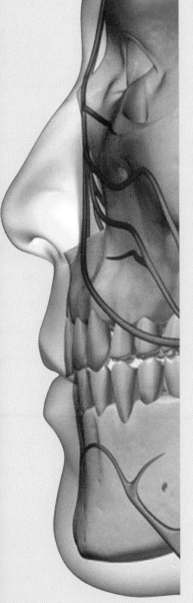

Key topics

- An overview of infection and infection control
- Methods of infection control
- Clinical examples of bacterial, viral and fungal infections and their management

Learning objectives

- To be familiar with the common methods of infection transmission and control
- To be aware of some of the common bacterial, viral and fungal infections and outlines of their management

[†]Deceased

Essentials of Human Disease in Dentistry, Second Edition. Mark Greenwood.
© 2018 John Wiley & Sons Ltd. Published 2018 by John Wiley & Sons Ltd.
Companion website: www.wiley.com/go/greenwood/human-disease-in-dentistry

3A STERILISATION, DISINFECTION AND ANTISEPTICS

Sterilisation and disinfection

Sterilisation has been defined as the killing or removal of all viable organisms. Concern about transmissible spongiform encephalopathies such as Creutzfeldt–Jakob disease (CJD) and particularly variant-CJD (vCJD) has generated research that has resulted in a much greater understanding of prions, the transmissible agents of the disease. The debate about whether prions are organisms probably reflects similar discussions decades ago regarding the nature of viruses, but the absence of even nucleic acid puts prions in a class apart, at least for now. The fact that prions have been identified as a transmissible agent of disease means that any definition of sterilisation should take them into account. *Sterilisation* is therefore more accurately defined as 'the inactivation or removal of all self-propagating biological entities'.

Disinfection is a less precise concept and has been variously defined, the best definition being that it is 'the reduction in viable organisms to the point where risk of infection is acceptable'.

A related term that is in common use is *antisepsis*, which is usefully defined as 'the disinfection of skin or wounds'.

General principles

The efficacy of a sterilisation or disinfection method is described by the relationship

$$N = k/CT$$

where N is the number of surviving organisms, C is the concentration of the sterilising agent (temperature in the case of heat) and T is the time for which the agent is applied. The constant k depends on many factors, including the species of organism present, its physiological state and many other environmental variables – not least among which is the presence of contaminating organic material such as blood or saliva.

For a given value of C, a graph of Log_{10} viable count versus time can be useful to predict when sterility will be achieved (Figure 3A.1). The slope of the curve is known as the 'death rate', and D is the time taken to achieve a 90% reduction in viable organisms. Survival curves such as the one shown may have a shoulder, a tail or both, signifying that individual cells respond differently to the sterilising agent. In practice, this means that absolute sterility cannot be guaranteed. Therefore, by convention, an instrument is considered sterile if there is less than a one-in-a-million chance of there being one viable organism present.

What should be sterilised?

Ideally, everything in a surgery should be sterile, but this is not practicably possible. The aim is to prevent infection and, importantly, cross-infection. Therefore, anything coming into direct contact with the surgical site should be sterile, and everything else should be disinfected.

Decontamination and pre-cleaning

The presence of contaminating material – especially organic matter such as saliva, blood, faeces and tissue – can significantly degrade the sterilisation or disinfection process by either physically preventing access of the agent or chemical inactivation. In order to ensure proper sterilisation, instruments should therefore be pre-cleaned. If the instruments have been in contact with infectious material, the pre-cleaning should include adequate disinfection to render them safe before they are packaged for sterilisation.

Sterilisation and disinfection methods

Methods of sterilisation and disinfection include dry or moist heat, a wide variety of liquid or gaseous chemicals, β- or γ-emitting ionising radiation and filtration (Table 3A.1). The choice of method depends on the nature of the material being treated, the contaminating organisms and the degree of inactivation required. For example, it is possible to sterilise milk, but this effectively changes its character. On the other hand, it is possible to retain milk's character and reduce its microbial load to a level that increases the shelf-life of milk appreciably by raising its temperature for a period of time (the pasteurisation process).

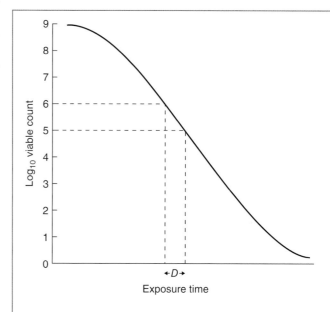

Figure 3A.1 A graphical demonstration of viable organism reduction with time (see text).

Table 3A.1 Methods of sterilisation.
<ul><li>Heat – dry, moist</li><li>Irradiation</li><li>Filtration</li><li>Chemicals</li></ul>
Gases Alcohols Aldehydes Bisbiguanides Chlorine compounds Iodophores Strong oxidising agents Phenols Quaternary ammonium compounds

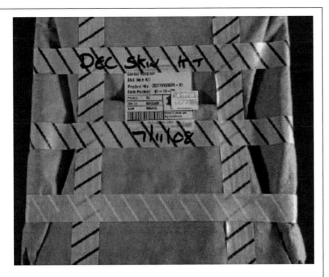

Figure 3A.2 Bowie–Dick tapes on a surgical pack. The brown cross-hatchings demonstrate that the autoclaving process has been carried out. The lower horizontal tape shows a tape that has not been successfully subjected to the autoclaving process.

Monitoring efficacy

It used to be the practice to include test organisms in every batch of material being sterilised; however, this results in a delay before sterility can be confirmed, which is often unacceptable. In modern practice, procedures are followed that are known to result in sterility for different materials and batch sizes, and the performance of the equipment in terms of the temperature and holding time is carefully monitored.

The Bowie–Dick tape is a method of ensuring that an autoclave has been functioning appropriately (Figure 3A.2). When the cross-hatchings on the tape turn brown, the sterilisation process has been effective.

Heat

Heat is the most familiar of methods used, because it is versatile, reliable, easy to control, cheap and efficient. It works by transferring energy to the organism and, depending on the conditions chosen, it can be used to sterilise or disinfect.

Dry heat

Dry heat sterilisation refers to conditions in which there is an absence of water in the environment being heated, but this does not include any water present in the object being sterilised. Dry heat sterilisation therefore includes a wide variety of conditions in which the level of moisture present in the system as a whole varies between complete dryness and almost complete saturation. This relative humidity affects the efficiency of the process in a complex manner. For example, the time required to effect a 99.99% reduction in the viability of *Bacillus stearothermophilus* spores at 120°C is approximately 6 min in the absence of any moisture, rising to a maximum of approximately 9 hours at a relative humidity of 30% and then dropping to 35 min near saturation. Moreover, different organisms vary in their susceptibility to dry heat. There are significant practical consequences of this relationship because, in a closed system, there may be pockets of air trapped in the material being sterilised. This will become more or less saturated with water vapour, depending on a variety of conditions in the immediate vicinity, such as the porosity of the material, the overall amount of air and water present and the volume of the container. It is, therefore, imperative that these and other factors be taken into account if sterility has to be guaranteed.

Dry heat sterilisation is used to sterilise solid material such as glassware and some instruments that are susceptible to corrosion, non-aqueous liquids and heat-stable powders such as drugs.

Moist heat

Sterilisation by moist heat depends on the use of saturated water vapour (steam) usually at a temperature between 121°C and 134°C for various periods. Typical conditions are 15 min at 121°C; 10 min at 126°C; and 3 min at 134°C. Steam can only be heated above 100°C by increasing the pressure above normal atmospheric pressure. It is imperative that the system be fully saturated with water vapour; hence, the equipment used to perform moist heat sterilisation (autoclave) is designed such that, when operated properly, all other gases are excluded. This is achieved either by downward displacement by the steam (which forces the less dense air out through a drain), by vacuum pumps or by steam pulsing.

Moist heat sterilisation is much more efficient than dry heat for two reasons. First, it takes less heat to denature fully hydrated proteins; and, second, during the process, moist heat releases its latent heat of vaporisation, which transfers considerably more energy than dry heat.

Irradiation

Ionising radiation is commonly used to sterilise large numbers of small items such as syringes, needles, catheters and gloves. However, because of the associated hazards, it is only suitable for use in specially constructed commercial environments. γ-Rays, X-rays and accelerated electrons (β-rays) are all commonly used at a dose in the region of 2.5 Mrad. Irradiation is a very effective means of achieving sterilisation; however, there is inevitable damage to the material being irradiated, so it is mostly used for single-use items. If an item is to be repeatedly irradiated, then a careful log must be kept to ensure that the damage is kept within known limits.

Radiation of each type works by producing radicals that damage cellular DNA. Common sources of radicals are water (OH· and H·), usually intracellular water, and oxygen (O·). Radiation is, therefore, normally carried out in an aerobic atmosphere. In the absence of oxygen, the dose must be increased.

Filtration

Filtration is different from other methods of sterilisation or disinfection because it works by physically removing microorganisms, rather than killing or inhibiting them. It is used when heat, irradiation or chemical treatment would result in damage to the substance being sterilised. It is also used to sterilise products such as intravenous fluids when heat treatment would release breakdown products of microorganisms that, because they cause fever, are known as 'pyrogens'.

Filtration is remarkably versatile and is widely used throughout the pharmaceutical and water industries. It also has wide application in scientific work as the pore sizes of membranes can be controlled with such precision as to allow the separation of macromolecules.

Chemicals

Gases

The gas most commonly used to sterilise medical equipment is ethylene oxide. In some cases, formaldehyde gas is used, but this is less efficient, and is only used when ethylene oxide is not available. Formaldehyde is more commonly used as a fumigant to disinfect rooms or equipment such as workstations that pose a biohazard threat.

Ethylene oxide is used to sterilise items that are sensitive to moisture or heat above 60°C. It works by alkylating microbial proteins and nucleic acids and must come into direct contact with the object being sterilised, so any packaging must be porous. After contact, sufficient time must elapse to allow removal of gas residue.

Antiseptics

Terminology

Antiseptics are substances used to destroy microorganisms on living tissues, such as the dentist's hands. Disinfectants are used to destroy microorganisms on inanimate objects such as work surfaces. Thus, an antiseptic has to be more selective in its action.

Antiseptics have several uses in dentistry, which include disinfecting surfaces for cross-infection control, skin preparations prior to surgery and the control of bacterial plaque. This section will focus on skin preparations and antiseptic mouthwashes.

Skin preparations

A variety of antiseptics are used to cleanse the skin prior to puncture wounds or surgical incisions. Preparations include alcohol, chlorhexidine, cetrimide, povidone-iodine and triclosan. Hydrogen peroxide and potassium permanganate solutions are also used for wound debridement. Some patients may be allergic to chlorhexidine or povidone-iodine, and this should be identified at an early stage, so that use can be avoided.

Antiseptic mouthwashes (antiplaque agents, plaque-inhibitory agents)

Antiseptics are used extensively in dentistry for the control of bacterial plaque and the subsequent effects on caries and periodontal disease. The ideal properties of an antiplaque agent are listed in Table 3A.2. A large number of agents have been used as antiseptic mouthwashes, and these are classified in Table 3A.3.

The most widely used mouthwashes contain as their active ingredient either chlorhexidine, phenols or quaternary ammonium compounds (QACs). Only these agents will be considered in this section.

Chlorhexidine

Chlorhexidine is a cationic chlorophenyl bisbiguanide with outstanding bacteriostatic properties. It remains the number one antiplaque agent. Chlorhexidine is mainly used as a mouthrinse, and several proprietary brands are now available to the public. The concentration of chlorhexidine varies from mouthwash to mouthwash, but the usual levels range from

Table 3A.2 Ideal properties of antiplaque agents.

Eliminate pathogenic bacteria only

Prevent the development of resistant bacteria

Exhibit substantivity

Be safe to oral tissues at the concentrations and dosages recommended

Significantly reduce plaque and gingivitis

Inhibit the calcification of plaque to calculus

Not stain teeth or alter taste

Have no adverse effects on the teeth or dental materials

Be easy to use

Be inexpensive

Table 3A.3 Classification of antiplaque agents.

Cationic surfactants
- Bisbiguanides – for example, chlorhexidine digluconate, alexidine
- Quaternary ammonium compounds – for example, cetylpyridinium chloride, benzethonium chloride, benzalkonium chloride, domiphen bromide
- Pyrimidine derivatives – for example, hexetidine
- Bispyridine derivatives – for example, octenidine hydrochloride

Phenolic compounds
- Listerine® (thymol 0.06%, eucalyptol 0.09%, methyl salicylate 0.06%, methanol 0.04%)
- Triclosan

Herbal extracts
- Sanguinarine

Heavy metal salts
- Zinc chloride and citrate
- Stannous fluoride
- Copper sulphate

Enzymes
- Mucinase
- Mutanase
- Dextranase
- Amyloglucosidase/glucose oxidase

Anionic surfactants
- Aminoalcohols – for example, Octapinol, Decapinol
- Plax®
- Sodium dodecyl sulphate
- Sodium lauryl sulphate

0.12 to 0.2% w/v. Chlorhexidine is also incorporated into dental gel (0.5–1% w/v), varnish (40%) and local delivery devices (gelatine chips – e.g. Periochip®) for placement into periodontal pockets.

Pharmacological properties of chlorhexidine

Chlorhexidine's mode of action is purely topical, and the bactericidal action is mediated via the bacterial cell wall. Contact with the cell wall is therefore essential, and this is facilitated by electrostatic forces between the negatively charged bacterial cell and the net positively charged chlorhexidine molecule. Having gained access to the cell membrane, chlorhexidine disorientates its lipoprotein structure, destroying the osmotic barrier of the bacteria. Cell permeability increases, and intracellular components such as potassium ions leak through the damaged membrane.

The short-term use of chlorhexidine causes a striking reduction in the number of bacteria in saliva – by 85% – after only 24 hours. A maximum reduction of 95% occurs after around 5 days. Cessation of chlorhexidine mouthrinse results in the rapid return of normal salivary bacterial counts. Long-term use of chlorhexidine has been associated with increased microbial resistance and reduced sensitivity.

Other properties of chlorhexidine as an antiplaque agent

1. *Substantivity.* This is defined as the ability of a compound to bind to surfaces (molecules) and then be released from such surfaces over time. When a compound is bound to such a surface, then it is inactive. Activity is restored when the compound is in the free (unbound) form. Chlorhexidine exhibits excellent substantivity. After rinsing with 10 ml of a 0.2% aqueous solution of chlorhexidine for 1 min, approximately 30% of the drug is retained in the mouth. The drug is bound by electrostatic forces to acidic protein groups such as phosphates and sulphates. Calcium ions in saliva are able to displace chlorhexidine from the acidic binding sites. This displacement is comparatively slow and may help to explain the prolonged bacteriostatic effect of the drug in the mouth. Free calcium ions also reduce the oral binding of chlorhexidine and increase its release from protein-binding sites. This finding has important implications with respect to the use of chlorhexidine mouthrinses and the use of toothpastes. Many proprietary toothpastes contain calcium salts as filler agents. Thus, if chlorhexidine is used soon after toothbrushing, there will be a high concentration of calcium ions present in the mouth. This will affect the binding of chlorhexidine and reduce its substantivity. Patients should be advised to use chlorhexidine at least 30 min after toothbrushing to avoid the interaction between calcium ions in the toothpaste and the mouthwash.

2. *Reduced pellicle formation.* The pellicle is derived from salivary glycoproteins and forms readily on clean tooth surfaces. This structure is also the substrate for early bacterial colonisation and hence the precursor to plaque formation. Chlorhexidine blocks the acidic groups of salivary glycoproteins and hence reduces their adsorption to hydroxyapatite and the formation of the acquired pellicle. The reduced pellicle formation may impact upon bacterial colonisation and hence the early stages of plaque formation.

3. *Plaque growth.* An important feature of plaque growth (and hence the impact upon gingival tissues) is the ability of other bacteria to bind to existing bacteria that have previously colonised the surface (acquired pellicle). Chlorhexidine binds the extracellular polysaccharides of bacterial capsules, and such binding prevents other bacteria from being incorporated into the developing plaque mass.

4. *Reduces plaque adhesiveness.* Several properties and components contribute to the ability of bacterial plaque to adhere to the tooth surface. One such constituent is acidic agglutination factor. Calcium ions are essential for the properties of this factor, and chlorhexidine will compete with the calcium ions. This could reduce the adhesive properties of plaque.

Unwanted effects of chlorhexidine

Brown staining of teeth, restorations and the oral mucosa are the main unwanted effects of chlorhexidine. Dietary factors also enhance chlorhexidine's staining potential, especially if mouthwash is used when there is a high intake of food/beverages rich in tannins. These include tea, coffee and red wine. Staining is also related to the concentration of chlorhexidine in the mouthwash. Chlorhexidine-induced staining requires professional removal.

Many patients find the taste of chlorhexidine unpleasant, and prolonged use blunts further the taste acuity for sweet and salt. Chlorhexidine binds to the proteins on the taste buds, blunting their activity.

Regular use of chlorhexidine is also associated with increased supragingival calculus formation. The mechanism of this unwanted effect is uncertain, but may relate to chlorhexidine's effect on the pellicle and/or calcium ions.

Rare unwanted effects of chlorhexidine include parotid swelling and hypersensitivity reactions. Parotid swelling may be due to over-vigorous rinsing, resulting in negative pressure in the gland and aspiration of the mouthwash into the parotid.

The efficacy of chlorhexidine appears to be less in the presence of blood. The compound binds to various proteins found in blood, and such binding renders chlorhexidine inactive. There are obvious implications with the use of chlorhexidine in the subgingival environment, where the tissues are often inflamed and blood may be present. The use of chlorhexidine in these circumstances will be more beneficial once the inflammation is brought under control. If a chlorhexidine chip is being used to supplement root surface instrumentation, then the chip should be placed some 7 days later when the risk of bleeding is significantly reduced.

Phenols

These are a group of antiseptic compounds that have been used in medicine for over 100 years. Preparations of phenols and their derivatives have widespread application as disinfectants and antiseptics. Most phenols exert a non-specific antibacterial action, which is dependent on the ability of the non-ionised form of the drug to penetrate the lipid component of the cell walls of Gram-negative organisms. The resulting structural damage affects the permeability control of the bacteria. Phenolic compounds also exhibit anti-inflammatory properties. This may result from their ability to inhibit neutrophil chemotaxis, neutrophil superoxide ion generation and prostaglandin synthetase production. All these functions are important in the inflammatory response. Phenolic compounds are found in the proprietary mouthwash Listerine®. Triclosan is another phenolic compound that is incorporated into mouthwashes and toothpastes.

Quaternary ammonium compounds (QACs)

QACs are also cationic antiseptics and surface-acting agents. Thus, the molecules have a net positive charge and react with the negatively charged bacterial cell wall. QACs tend to be more effective against Gram-positive than Gram-negative microorganisms. This may suggest that these agents would be more beneficial as antiplaque agents when used against early developing bacterial plaque. Examples of QACs include benzethonium chloride, benzalkonium chloride and cetylpyridinium chloride. QACs are mainly used as pre-brushing rinses. Despite many claims, the efficacy of such rinses is questionable.

3B PRINCIPLES OF INFECTION AND INFECTION CONTROL, DIAGNOSIS AND TREATMENT OF BACTERIAL INFECTIONS

Introduction

There are three main stages involved in establishing a diagnosis: history, examination and special investigations. Certain simple infections may be diagnosed clinically and managed empirically, but microbiological studies may be helpful in some infections and essential in others. In order to select the most appropriate management for a clinical infection, it is important to understand the nature of the disease and the pathogenic organism involved. If antimicrobial agents are indicated for the treatment of an infection, then the microbiology laboratory can play a pivotal role in helping with their selection. Antimicrobial resistance, infections with multiresistant isolates and antibiotic-associated complications such as *Clostridium difficile*–associated diarrhoea are some developing problems and major causes of public concern. The principles of judicious prescribing are therefore of fundamental importance to safe clinical practice.

When deciding on the optimal management for a particular condition, healthcare professionals need to be able to balance the potential benefits of antimicrobial agents against the potential risks to the individual and to public health from unnecessary prescribing. This section will concentrate on the role of the microbiology laboratory in aiding the diagnosis and treatment of bacterial infections.

Use of the laboratory in the diagnosis of bacterial infections

The main goals of a diagnostic microbiology laboratory are to provide guidance to clinicians about the prevention, diagnosis, management and control of infection. In order to do this, the laboratory must be able to identify the presence of potentially pathogenic organisms and provide guidance on appropriate therapy. Reliable identification of an organism is important for a number of reasons. It may help to confirm a clinical diagnosis, give some indication of the likely prognosis and guide appropriate management. Accurate identification is also essential for epidemiological purposes, including the recognition and control of outbreaks of infection.

Taxonomy is the systematic classification, naming and identification of living organisms. Systematic naming of an individual organism involves its classification into successively smaller groups, starting with a specific 'kingdom', followed by a 'division', 'family', 'genus' and, finally, the 'species' – for example, *Staphylococcus aureus* (Table 3B.1). In practice, this identification may be made at the molecular level using an organism's genetic make-up (genotype), or by its physical characteristics – that is, the way in which it physically expresses its genes (phenotype). Although molecular techniques are

Table 3B.1 Classification of *Staphylococcus aureus*.

Kingdom	Prokaryota
Division	Eubacteria
Family	Micrococcaceae
Genus	*Staphylococcus*
Species	*Staphylococcus aureus*

becoming more widely available in routine microbiology, many of the standard methods still rely on recognising the phenotypic characteristics of organisms.

Bacteria belong to the kingdom 'prokaryota'. They are simple, unicellular microorganisms, usually <5 micrometres (μm) in size. They form a major part of the normal human flora, but may also act as pathogens or opportunistic pathogens under certain circumstances. Therefore, the routine diagnostic laboratory tests must be able to identify the presence of potential bacterial pathogens, often from within mixtures of normal flora (commensal organisms). To do this, the laboratory will employ a number of different techniques, capitalising on the different phenotypic or genotypic characteristics of the organisms that are sought. Important phenotypic features of bacteria include their shape, size and appearance; staining characteristics; nutritional requirements; growth rate; enzymes and antigenic determinants.

Diagnostic microbiological techniques can be broadly classified into (1) microscopy; (2) culture; and (3) non-cultural methods that include molecular techniques and serology.

Microscopy

The discovery of optics in the 1500s paved the way for the visualisation of bacteria in the following century. Anton von Loewenhoek, a Dutch scientist, examined a variety of materials using a simple microscope based on a design by Robert Hooke. Studying the microscopic appearance of dental plaque, Loewenhoek described small motile particles, which he called 'animalcules'. These later proved to be bacteria. Microscopy was first adopted in pathology laboratories in the 1800s and has remained a fundamental diagnostic method in microbiology ever since. There are now much more sophisticated techniques available.

Light microscopy

Specimens are commonly examined by light microscopy; they may be examined directly, or stained preparations may first be made from the samples. Liquid specimens such as urine samples and cerebrospinal fluid (CSF) may be examined directly for the presence of inflammatory cells. For example, in CSF samples, the number and type of white blood cells are used as important diagnostic pointers. In cases of bacterial meningitis, such as meningococcal meningitis, the inflammatory cells are predominantly neutrophils, while in viral meningitis, such as enteroviral meningitis, the majority of the leukocytes present in the CSF will be lymphocytes. The ratio of the number of white blood cells to the number of red blood cells present is also important, as CSF samples may sometimes be contaminated by blood during collection and, unless the red blood cells are also enumerated, the CSF might be mistaken as having elevated white cell counts. A white blood cell–red blood cell ratio of >1:500 is suggestive of infection or inflammation. Direct microscopy is also used in the diagnosis of parasitic infections: emulsified faecal samples can be examined for the presence of the ova, cysts or trophozoites of intestinal parasites such as *Giardia lamblia* or *Ascaris lumbricoides*.

Phase contrast microscopy

Phase contrast microscopes may be used to improve the visualisation of transparent microorganisms suspended in fluids. They are set up such that particles present in the examined fluid scatter the transmitted light, which becomes out of phase and thereby interferes with the light waves that have simply passed through the clear fluid. This makes the microorganisms or particles and their structures stand out in contrast to their fluid background. Phase contrast microscopy can be used to perform white and red blood cell counts on urine samples.

Dark ground microscopy

Certain very fine bacteria may be more readily visualised when brightly lit against a dark background, using a dark field microscope. For example, this method may be used to provide a rapid presumptive diagnosis of syphilis. A freshly collected swab taken from a lesion of suspected primary or secondary syphilis, when smeared on a slide and examined by dark ground microscopy, may reveal the presence of fine, motile spirochaetes characteristic of *Treponema pallidum*. If oral lesions are suspected to be syphilitic, however, direct microscopy should not be used, as it may give misleading results owing to the presence of other spirochaetes in the mouth as part of the normal flora.

Fluorescent microscopy

The detection of certain microorganisms can be enhanced by staining samples directly with fluorescent dyes such as acridine orange, auramine or fluorescein, or with specific antibodies labelled with fluorescent markers. These stains or fluorochromes transform ultraviolet (UV) light into visible light. Using this technique, target organisms such as the *Mycobacterium* or *Legionella* species can be seen glowing against a dark background when stained specimens are examined with a fluorescent microscope.

Table 3B.2 Gram stain method.
1. Spread aliquot of sample thinly on clean glass slide. Heat-fix.
2. Stain with crystal violet for 1 min. Rinse with sterile water.
3. Decolourise with acetone or ethanol for a few seconds. Rinse with sterile water.
4. Counterstain with carbol fuchsin or safranin for 1 min. Rinse with sterile water.
5. Allow to dry and examine under a light microscope.

Electron microscopy

Developed in the 1950s, the electron microscope's increased resolution allowed the visualisation of viruses. This technique, however, is not used in the routine detection or identification of bacteria, and so it will not be discussed further here.

Staining techniques

In order to study the shape or morphology of bacteria, they may be examined directly under a microscope, but examination of stained preparations of bacteria provides additional information.

Gram stain

A number of different staining methods may be used in microbiology, but the Gram stain is by far the most commonly used. It is quick and simple to perform (Table 3B.2), and is a fundamental test in the identification of bacteria. Developed in 1882 by Hans Christian Gram, a Danish bacteriologist, this technique has stood the test of time because Gram inadvertently discovered a stain that is able to distinguish between two important groups of bacteria, the *Gram-positive* and the *Gram-negative*. The principal difference between these two groups of bacteria lies in the structure of their cell walls. Gram-positive bacterial cell walls are composed of two layers, the inner cytoplasmic membrane and a thick outer layer of peptidoglycan-containing proteins, teichoic acids and lipoteichoic acids. Gram-negative cell walls, however, are made of three layers: (1) the cytoplasmic membrane, which is covered by (2) a thin layer of peptidoglycan, which in turn is surrounded by (3) a thick fatty layer of lipopolysaccharide. In the first stages of the staining process, crystal violet and Gram's iodine bind to peptidoglycan, resulting in a blue-black colouration. The addition of acetone or ethanol dissolves the lipid in the lipopolysaccharide of Gram-negative cell walls, thereby allowing the crystal violet–Gram's iodine mixture to leach out and the pink carbol fuchsin or safranin counterstain to enter and stain the cell wall. Acetone or ethanol, however, have a dehydrating effect on Gram-positive cells walls, fixing the blue-black crystal violet–Gram's iodine mixture in the thick layer of peptidoglycan and preventing the uptake of the pink counterstain. Hence, using the Gram stain, bacteria can be divided into Gram-positive bacteria,

Table 3B.3 Interpretation of Gram stain.

	Gram-positive bacteria	Gram-negative bacteria
Amount of peptidoglycan in cell wall	++++	+
Decolourisation with acetone or ethanol	Resisted	Easy
Final colour of Gram stain	Blue-black	Pink-red

which are stained blue-black, and Gram-negative bacteria, which look pink or red (Table 3B.3). There are also some bacteria that fail to take up the Gram stain, including the mycobacteria and mycoplasma species. It should be noted that yeasts will also take up the Gram stain, appearing blue-black, although, being fungi, they are much larger, and their cell walls have a different structure from those of Gram-positive bacteria.

The Gram stain can be applied directly to clinical samples to detect the presence of microorganisms. Examples include the examination of spun deposits of CSF in cases of possible meningitis, or specimens of synovial fluid if septic arthritis is suspected. Gram staining may also be used as a preliminary test in the identification of bacteria isolated from clinical samples.

The *Ziehl–Neelsen* (ZN) *stain* is principally used to detect mycobacteria, including *Mycobacterium tuberculosis*, the cause of tuberculosis (TB). Mycobacteria cannot be stained using the Gram stain because of the high concentration of mycolic acids that make up their waxy cell walls. ZN staining involves the application of hot carbol fuchsin, which stains bacteria pink, followed by the addition of 20% sulphuric acid, which decolourises bacteria apart from mycobacteria. This ability to retain the carbol fuchsin stain despite treatment with acid explains why mycobacteria are sometimes known colloquially as 'acid-fast bacilli'. The final stage of the ZN stain is the addition of a counterstain, either methylene blue or malachite green, to reveal bacteria other than mycobacteria. On examination under a light microscope, therefore, mycobacteria will appear pink, while other bacteria will look blue or green, depending on the counterstain employed. ZN staining of a sputum sample can lead to a rapid presumptive diagnosis of TB in a patient with suspicious clinical symptoms and signs. This is important because TB is a chronic and serious respiratory infection that is readily transmitted by the respiratory route. Early treatment of infectious cases helps to minimise the onward spread of this disease. However, *M. tuberculosis* grows slowly, taking a minimum of 2 weeks even when using rapid culture techniques, and so rapid non-cultural methods including ZN staining are used to support clinical diagnoses and allow the early institution of appropriate therapies.

Other stains may be employed for specific purposes in the laboratory. For example, Albert's stain highlights intracytoplasmic volutin granules and is used in the diagnosis of *Corynebacterium diphtheriae* (the cause of diphtheria, a life-threatening infection). Auramine is a fluorescent stain used for screening sputum samples for the presence of *Mycobacterium tuberculosis*.

The stains described in the preceding text are all examples of positive stains, where the organism that is sought takes up the stain. *Negative staining* is a different technique, where the stain is not taken up by the microorganism. Instead, the background is stained, so that the organism stands out in relief. This technique is used to aid the diagnosis of cryptococcal meningitis. This is an opportunistic fungal infection, caused by *Cryptococcus neoformans*, which occurs in immunocompromised patients including pregnant women, patients infected with human immunodeficiency virus (HIV) and solid organ transplant recipients. India ink is added to a spun deposit of CSF, staining the background black and highlighting the very thick capsules that are characteristic of this yeast.

Bacterial morphology

In addition to the Gram reaction, bacteria may also be identified by their shape and the arrangement of their cells. Gram stain is therefore used in the laboratory as one of the first steps in the identification of microorganisms cultured from clinical samples. Bacteria may be spherical (cocci), rod-like (bacilli), comma-shaped (vibrios) or spiral (spirochaetes) (see Figure 3B.1). Cocci may be seen in characteristic arrangements. When they appear in pairs, they are known as *diplococci*. The presence of Gram-negative diplococci in the Gram stain of a CSF sample would suggest the diagnosis of meningococcal meningitis caused by the bacterium *Neisseria meningitidis*. The typical appearance of staphylococci is of 'Gram-positive cocci in clusters', while streptococci and enterococci are characteristically described as 'Gram-positive cocci in chains'.

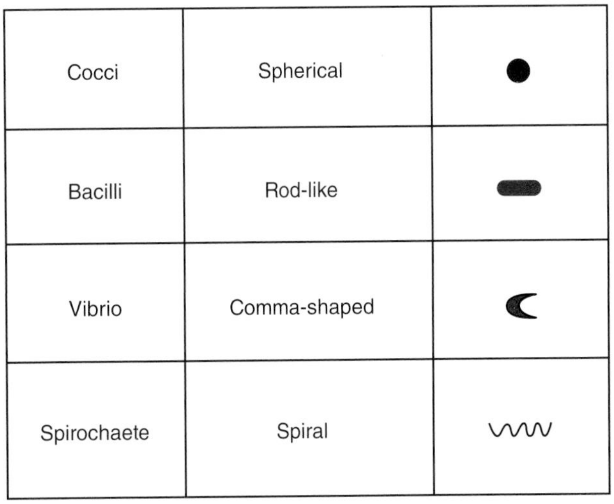

Cocci	Spherical	●
Bacilli	Rod-like	▬
Vibrio	Comma-shaped	◖
Spirochaete	Spiral	〰

Figure 3B.1 Bacterial morphology.

Culture and identification

Most medically important bacteria can be cultured in a routine diagnostic laboratory. Some have only basic nutritional requirements, while others are fastidious, and will only grow on media containing a complex cocktail of supplements. For example, *Staphylococcus aureus* can be isolated on nutrient agar, a very simple medium. The growth of *Haemophilus influenzae*, however, is enhanced by using chocolate agar, so called because of its rich brown colour. This is a very nutritious medium, made by heating blood agar to lyse the red blood cells and release additional growth factors.

There is now a wide variety of culture media available for different purposes. Culture media may be solid or liquid. Selective media contain inhibitors that prevent the growth of commensal organisms and thereby increase the detection of potential pathogens from within mixed cultures, while enrichment media generally encourage the growth of bacteria. Enrichment culture is useful for the detection of fastidious organisms, low numbers of bacteria or bacteria that have been inhibited by prior exposure to antibiotics. Indicator media, including chromogenic broths and agars, are now available. These contain specific enzyme substrates and are designed to change colour when the target organism is present. Laboratories will select appropriate combinations of media for the examination of different types of clinical specimens or the detection of specific pathogens.

The optimal *incubation requirements*, both atmospheric and temperature-related, may be used to help identify bacteria. Organisms may be 'strict aerobes', only growing in the presence of oxygen; 'strict anaerobes', which will only grow in the absence of oxygen; or 'facultative anaerobes' (also sometimes known as 'facultative aerobes'), which can tolerate both conditions. Some bacteria are known as 'microaerophilic organisms', and need to be incubated in an environment with a lower concentration of oxygen than is found in air. One example of a microaerophile is *Helicobacter pylori*, a spirochaete that is found in the stomach and duodenum and is associated with ulcer disease. Some bacteria also require the atmosphere to be enriched with additional carbon dioxide.

The majority of human pathogens will grow best at 37°C; however, some, such as *Campylobacter jejuni*, are able to tolerate higher temperatures. Others can multiply in colder conditions. For example, listeriosis, a serious systemic infection affecting pregnant women, foetuses and immunocompromised patients, is caused by *Listeria monocytogenes*, a Gram-positive rod that is able to grow on contaminated foods such as soft cheeses and patés in the refrigerator at 4°C. The growth rate is also a useful feature when identifying bacteria. Many common organisms such as staphylococci, streptococci, *Escherichia coli* and *Salmonella* require 18–24 hours (overnight) incubation, while some take longer. For example, *Pseudomonas aeruginosa* and *Bacteroides* spp. often take 2 days; *Legionella* spp. take up to 10 days; and *Actinomyces israelii* may take up to 2–4 weeks. At the far extreme, mycobacteria may take more than 6 weeks to grow using conventional solid media such as Lowenstein–Jensen agar, although more rapid liquid culture methods have now shortened this period to 2 weeks.

The macroscopic appearance of bacterial colonies growing on agar in the laboratory may also provide clues as to the identity of the organism. They may have a typical colour, size, shape or consistency. Some bacteria, including *Proteus* and *Clostridia* spp., can swarm over the surface of agar plates. Bacteria may be haemolytic if they are able to produce enzymes that lyse red blood cells. This feature may be seen when the bacteria are cultured on blood agar, and it is often enhanced by growth in an anaerobic environment. Streptococci are classified according to their haemolytic reactions. β-Haemolytic streptococci, including *Streptococcus pyogenes* (also known as β-haemolytic streptococcus Group A), an important cause of pharyngitis and cellulitis, produces a haemolysin that completely lyses red blood cells, resulting in a zone of clearing in the agar around the colonies. α-Haemolytic streptococci, including the viridans streptococci (found in the mouth) and *Streptococcus pneumoniae*, are only able partially to haemolyse red blood cells in blood agar, and this causes greening of the media. Streptococci that are unable to haemolyse blood agar are known as 'non-haemolytic streptococci'. Some bacteria produce a typical odour, although care must be taken to prevent inhalation of aerosols of the organism when examining this characteristic.

Examination of basic phenotypic characteristics will usually provide a presumptive bacterial identification. For example, Table 3B.4 outlines a simple classification scheme for bacteria using their Gram-stained appearance and atmospheric

Table 3B.4 Simple bacterial classification scheme.

		Aerobe	Facultative anaerobe	Microaerophile	Anaerobe
Gram-positive	Cocci		Staphylococcus Streptococcus Enterococcus		Peptococcus
	Bacilli		Bacillus Lactobacillus	Corynebacterium	Clostridium
Gram-negative	Cocci				
	Bacilli	Pseudomonas	Escherichia Salmonella	Haemophilus Legionella	Bacteroides Prevotella

requirements. Formal identification or speciation of bacteria, however, may require analysis of a collection of phenotypic characteristics. So, in practice, presumptive identifications are often confirmed by tests for additional features, including biochemical characteristics (such as the pattern of carbohydrate fermentation or the presence of enzymes such as urease or catalase) and the presence of antigenic determinants or special structures such as spores or flagella. Manual and automated commercial tests are available for the identification of different types of bacteria.

Bacterial typing

There are occasions when identification beyond the species level is important. This is used to help determine whether organisms are likely to be of the same strain – that is, whether they are likely to have arisen from the same original source. This is helpful for epidemiological investigations, for example, checking for possible outbreaks of infection, or to determine whether an individual patient is experiencing a relapsing infection with the same organism or a new infection with the same species of bacterium.

There are a variety of phenotypic and genotypic typing schemes available, based on different bacterial characteristics. Examples include simple tests such as the examination of the antimicrobial susceptibility pattern (antibiogram), determining different phenotypic or antigenic characteristics between bacteria from the same species (biotyping or serotyping, respectively) or examination of the proteins present in the organism (polyacrylamide gel electrophoresis, or PAGE). Other typing methods involve examination of the genetic make-up of the cell by molecular techniques. These are discussed in later sections. They include restriction enzyme analysis, restriction fragment length polymorphism (RFLP), pulsed-field gel electrophoresis, DNA hybridisation studies and genetic sequencing. The latter provides the most definitive identification, but currently largely remains a reference test.

Antimicrobial susceptibility testing

In addition to helping diagnose infections, microbiology laboratories also aim to provide guidance for their optimal management. This may include the use of antimicrobial agents, and antimicrobial susceptibility testing therefore forms a fundamental part of the work of routine laboratories. These may be tested using a number of different standardised methods, but the final report will usually classify an organism as being susceptible (or sensitive), intermediately susceptible or resistant to each antimicrobial agent tested. This classification is a clinical description suggesting the likelihood of successful treatment using the standard dose of the antimicrobial agent, taking into consideration the pharmacokinetics and pharmacodynamics of the drug. Put simply, *pharmacokinetics* may be regarded as the effect of the body on a drug, including its absorption, distribu-

tion and excretion, while *pharmacodynamics* may be thought of as the effect of a drug on the body.

Disc sensitivity testing

This is the method most commonly employed. Here, a standardised inoculum of the test organism is evenly spread across the surface of a standardised agar plate. In order to test each particular antibacterial agent, a paper disc impregnated with a specified concentration of that drug is applied to the inoculated agar plate. It is often convenient to dispense six different antibiotic-impregnated discs at one time using a dispenser. Plates prepared in this way are then incubated in the appropriate atmosphere and temperature for the test organism, usually for 18 hours, before zones of inhibition of growth surrounding the discs are measured. These are then interpreted according to agreed standards for susceptible, intermediate or resistant strains.

Minimum inhibitory concentration (MIC)

Identification of the lowest concentration of a particular antimicrobial agent that inhibits the growth of an organism *in vitro*, known as the 'minimum inhibitory concentration', can provide a more accurate description of an isolate's susceptibility to a drug. This may be important in optimising the management of deep-seated or chronic infections such as infective endocarditis. The MIC may be determined by a number of different techniques, such as agar dilution, broth macrodilution, broth microdilution and commercial tests.

In break point testing using agar dilution, a range of concentrations of the test antibiotic are incorporated into a series of agar plates. A standardised inoculum of the test organism is then spotted onto each plate. After incubation, examination of the minimum concentration that prevents the growth of the test organism can be used to determine the isolate's susceptibility to the drug tested. A similar principle is used for broth dilution testing, where a range of antibiotic concentrations are added to the liquid agar medium (broth). After incubation, the lowest concentration of the drug preventing multiplication of the organism is determined by visual inspection. Where the organism's growth has been inhibited, the broth will remain clear, while growth of the test organism will be indicated by a cloudy appearance in the broth. This type of testing can be carried out in a test tube (macrodilution technique) or in a microtitre tray (microdilution method).

These methods generally require overnight incubation. Some more rapid commercial tests are available that indirectly indicate an isolate's susceptibility pattern by detecting specific mechanisms of antimicrobial resistance. In *Haemophilus* spp., for example, rapid commercial testing can detect the presence of a β-lactamase enzyme that renders the bacterium resistant to amoxicillin. Staphylococci may be tested for the presence of an altered penicillin-binding protein, PBP2, or the gene that codes for this protein (*mecA*), which results in methicillin (meticillin) resistance.

Non-cultural diagnostic techniques

Many of the tests routinely carried out in microbiology require the presence of viable, cultivable and actively multiplying microorganisms. Sometimes, however, a retrospective diagnosis is required. The infecting organism may have been killed, for example, by prior antibiotic therapy, or it may be slow growing, difficult or even impossible to culture *in vitro*. Even for rapidly growing organisms, some of these techniques may be able to provide a more rapid and specific diagnosis than conventional methods based on bacterial isolation. In these circumstances, non-cultural diagnostic techniques – based on the detection of bacterial genes, antigens, products or the host's antibody response to the infecting organism – may be helpful. Of course, non-cultural diagnostic techniques may also have some limitations: they will not indicate whether the microbe is still alive, and they do not allow further work such as antimicrobial susceptibility testing.

Latex agglutination testing

This technique employs latex particles coated with antibodies (usually monoclonal antibodies) specific for the target organism. In the presence of the relevant antigen, antigen–antibody complexes are formed, causing visible clumping of the latex particles (see Figure 3B.2). Commercial latex agglutination tests are widely available for a variety of different target antigens, including the detection of rotavirus and adenovirus in stool samples, and for the detection of the common causes of bacterial meningitis such as *Streptococcus pneumoniae*, *Neisseria meningitidis*, Group B streptococcus and *Haemophilus influenzae* type b in CSF samples. Alternatively, latex agglutination techniques may be used as a serological test if the latex particles are coated with specific antigens, allowing the detection of particular antibodies in a patient's serum.

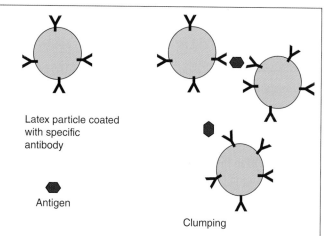

Figure 3B.2 Latex particle agglutination.

Latex particle coated with specific antibody

Antigen

Clumping

Enzyme-linked immunosorbent assay (ELISA)

These tests may be manual, automated or semi-automated, and may be used in the detection of specific antibodies or antigens in clinical samples, including serum. For example, specific antibodies can be coated onto the bottom of microtitre wells and used to bind complementary antigen if it is present in a patient's serum sample (Figure 3B.3). Non-specific unbound antigen is removed in a washing stage.

In order to detect the presence of bound antigen, a second antibody, labelled in some way and designed to attach to the bound antigen from the patient's sample, is added to the microtitre well. Any unbound labelled antibody is then removed in a second washing stage. A common method of labelling involves tagging the detecting antibody with a specific enzyme that is able to change the colour of a chromogenic substance. If the patient's serum contains the antigen being sought, at the end of the test, the microtitre well will contain a specific antibody–antigen-labelled antibody conjugate. This conjugate can then be visualised by the addition of the chromogenic substrate that will change colour. The colour change can be visualised by eye, or read and quantified using a spectrophotometer. The ELISA test is often used for serological testing, to detect the presence of a specific antibody in the patient's serum. In this case, the microtitre well of the ELISA kit is coated with a complementary antigen.

Serology

Serology, literally the scientific study of serum, is usually regarded as the diagnostic testing of serum for antibodies, although serological techniques may sometimes be applied to other clinical specimens, such as CSF samples. In microbiology, serology is used to detect the host's response to an infection. Antibodies are relatively slow to develop, and so serology will rarely provide a rapid diagnosis. However, it can be valuable in providing a retrospective diagnosis and in assessing the immune status of an individual or, in the case of serosurveys, the immunity of a population. Although it varies between different tests, serological results may generally be regarded as diagnostic when there is a fourfold or greater increase in antibody titre between acute and convalescent samples (taken 10–14 days after the acute sample), or if a specific immunoglobulin M (IgM) antibody is detected.

There are a number of different serological techniques that can be used to test for the presence of antibodies. These include agglutination tests, complement fixation tests, immunofluorescence and ELISA.

Molecular methods

A number of extremely powerful and sensitive molecular methods are available for the detection of microorganisms or microbial products, and for the typing of isolates. Although many of these tests are carried out in reference laboratories, some are already employed by routine diagnostic laboratories, and it is likely that this trend will increase over time.

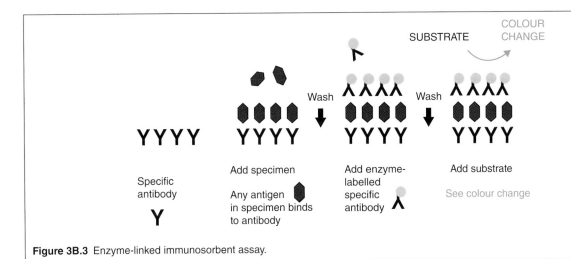

Figure 3B.3 Enzyme-linked immunosorbent assay.

Gene probes

Short segments of single-stranded DNA of known sequence, labelled with a radioactive or fluorescent tag, are known as 'gene probes'. They can be used to detect complementary segments of DNA in test samples. The test sample must first be treated to denature any DNA present so that it will be in single-stranded form. This allows the gene probe to hybridise with the DNA if it finds a complementary sequence. This method is used, for example, to identify slow-growing organisms such as mycobacteria. Once a *Mycobacterium* spp. has been isolated from a clinical specimen, it is important to know to which species it belongs as this affects the management and prognosis. For mycobacteria, some conventional identification tests can take several weeks as they depend on the growth of the organism. Gene probes are available for some of the more common species of mycobacteria such as *Mycobacterium tuberculosis* complex and *Mycobacterium avium* complex, providing a more rapid answer as compared to conventional testing.

Polymerase chain reaction (PCR)

This is a technique by which minute amounts of specific microbial nucleic acids in a test sample can be amplified *in vitro* to facilitate their detection. The process involves heating the specimen to 94°C so that the two complementary strands of the target DNA's double helix are denatured and come apart. After cooling, primers (short segments of nucleic acid sequences, specific for the microbe being sought) are added. They will bind to complementary sequences in the single-stranded DNA. Nucleotides, the building blocks for DNA, and a heat-stable DNA polymerase are then added, and the mixture is incubated at 60°C. During this stage of the cycle, new complementary strands of DNA are formed. These are then split by heating the mixture to 94°C when the cycle begins again (see Figure 3B.4).

After a series of cycles over a few hours, if there was any DNA present in the original sample, there will have been an exponential increase in its amount, providing over a million copies. These can then be detected by other molecular techniques such as gene probing or DNA sequencing. The PCR technique may be used for a variety of different applications. One example is PCR testing for *Mycobacterium tuberculosis* in CSF in order to provide a rapid diagnosis for tuberculous meningitis.

Restriction enzyme analysis

This technique is mainly used for epidemiological purposes, for comparison of isolates to determine whether they are likely to represent the same strain. Particular restriction endonucleases, enzymes that cleave DNA at specific sites, are used to cut the microbial DNA into smaller fragments. These fragments are then separated by electrophoresis on agarose gel, before being stained with ethidium bromide and examined under UV light. The resulting pattern of bands provides a 'fingerprint' that may be compared with the restriction enzyme analysis from other isolates.

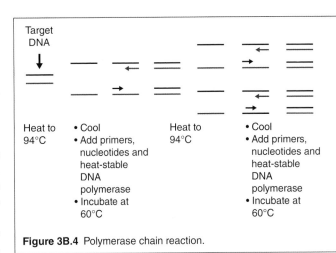

Figure 3B.4 Polymerase chain reaction.

This technique may be further refined by blotting the separated bands of DNA oligonucleotides from the agarose gel onto a nitrocellulose or nylon membrane, and then probing the DNA with specific gene probes. Known as 'RFLP analysis', this method is performed in order to detect short deletions or insertions in the DNA that change the size of the restriction fragments between different strains of the organism, but are identical in clones from the same microbe.

Pulsed-field gel electrophoresis

Similar to restriction enzyme analysis, the restriction enzymes chosen for this process cleave the DNA into relatively large fragments, unsuitable for separation by conventional gel electrophoresis. Instead, the restriction fragments are separated by pulsed-field gel electrophoresis, using an electric current with the polarity regularly reversed.

DNA sequencing

It is now possible to sequence a microorganism's nucleic acids, providing the key to its genetic make-up. Rapid methods, including automated systems, allow the order of the nucleotide bases (adenine, guanine, cytosine and thymidine) making up the microbial DNA to be determined. This powerful technique is still generally regarded as a reference or research-based tool, but it is possible that it may be more widely employed in the future.

General principles of specimen collection

Over the previous sections, common microbiological techniques for aiding the diagnosis and management of bacterial infections have been considered, but it is important to remember that these all rely on the submission of high-quality specimens to the laboratory for examination. There are a few simple tips that may help the microbiology laboratory to help the clinician. Where possible, samples should be collected before the patient has received antimicrobial therapy, since antibiotics can markedly reduce the chances of isolating a potential pathogen. If the patient is seriously unwell, such as in cases of possible bacterial meningitis, treatment should not be delayed, but a sample should be collected at the earliest possible opportunity once the patient has received empirical treatment. Contamination of clinical samples during collection should be avoided. For example, aseptic collection of a sample of pus from a dental abscess by needle aspiration will avoid potential contamination of the pus by mouth flora and provide a more accurate diagnosis. The specimens must be sent in appropriate containers. A sterile specimen pot is appropriate for many clinical samples, including urine, faeces and pus specimens. However, for the investigation of certain infections, such as amoebic dysentery (*Entamoeba histolytica*), chlamydia or gonorrhoea, samples may need to be sent under specific conditions or in particular transport media. It is always advisable to contact the laboratory in advance for advice.

Generally, specimens for microbiological examination should be transported to the laboratory as quickly as possible. If there is a delay, certain fastidious organisms may die or become inhibited or overgrown by the presence of commensal organisms. In other cases, for example, where quantification of organisms is important for the interpretation of a result (such as in the examination of urine samples), the small numbers of contaminating organisms present in the sample on initial collection may overgrow before the sample reaches the laboratory, resulting in spuriously positive results. If transport of microbiological specimens is likely to be delayed, then it is usually appropriate to store the samples in a refrigerator dedicated for this purpose. Again, if there is doubt, the laboratory should be contacted for advice.

Samples and request forms must be labelled clearly and accurately. Information should include the patient's name, date of birth and individual identifier (e.g. the NHS number or hospital identification number), the specimen type, date and time of collection, relevant clinical details, tests requested and the name and location of the requesting clinician.

Where appropriate, for example, if the patient is known or strongly suspected to be infected with a blood-borne virus, biohazard labels or flags must be attached, although care must be taken to maintain patient confidentiality. In future, the more widespread introduction of paperless computerised test requesting should help ensure that all required information is provided.

Antibacterial drugs

Antibacterial drugs can be divided into two types – *bactericidal* (the drug kills the bacterium) and *bacteriostatic* (the drug inhibits growth of the bacterial colony).

Antibacterial drugs exert their effects by the following methods:

- Interference with the production and maintenance of the bacterial cell wall
- Interference with bacterial protein synthesis
- Interference with bacterial nucleic acid production or stability
- Inhibition of bacterial metabolic processes.

This section describes the mechanisms of action of some antibacterials that dentists might prescribe. Table 3B.5 summarises the actions of some commonly used antibacterials.

Antibacterials that interfere with the bacterial cell wall

In bacteria, the cell wall is composed of peptidoglycan. In Gram-positive cells, this is a multi-layered structure, whereas in Gram-negative bacteria, it is one layer thick. Peptidoglycan does not occur in eukaryotes, and this explains the specificity of anti-cell-wall antibiotics to bacteria. Peptidoglycan is made up of chains of alternating amino-sugars, namely *N*-acetylglucosamine and *N*-acetylmuramic acid. These chains are cross-linked via side chains of *N*-acetylmuramic acid by a transpeptidase.

Table 3B.5 Actions of some commonly used antibacterials.				
Drug	Cell wall synthesis or maintenance	Protein synthesis	Nucleic acid synthesis or stability	Bacterial metabolism
Penicillins	X			
Cephalosporins	X			
Vancomycin	X			
Teicoplanin	X			
Bacitracin	X			
Tetracyclines		X		
Erythromycin		X		
Clindamycin		X		
Gentamicin		X		
Chloramphenicol		X		
Metronidazole			X	
Sulphonamides				X
Trimethoprim				X

Penicillins and cephalosporins

Penicillins and cephalosporins are β-lactam antibiotics. They are bactericidal, and interfere with the construction and maintenance of the bacterial cell wall. The main effect of β-lactams is the inhibition of cross-linking of the peptide chains. In addition to interfering with cell wall synthesis by inhibiting the enzyme that promotes cross-linkage of the peptide chains, the β-lactam antibiotics also compromise cell wall integrity by other mechanisms. There are several proteins in bacterial cells that have an affinity for penicillins and cephalosporins. These are known as penicillin-binding proteins (PBPs). The transpeptidase involved in cross-linking is a PBP; others are involved in the maintenance of cell wall shape and in septum production during division. Thus, the other effects of penicillins are the production of different shapes of bacteria and rapid lysis. The bacterial cell produces enzymes known as autolysins that can produce defects in the cell wall. Autolysins are normally suppressed; however, the β-lactams inactivate autolysin inhibitors.

Antibacterials that interfere with bacterial protein synthesis

The production of proteins depends on the action of several intracellular components, including ribosomes. Human and bacterial ribosomes differ in their structures. Mammalian ribosomes consist of 40S and 60S subunits; bacterial ribosomes are made of 30S and 50S subunits. As a result of these differences, a degree of specificity of antibiotics against bacterial ribosomes

is achieved. Protein synthesis can be divided into several steps. Some of these stages are susceptible to antibiotic action. These steps are:

- mRNA attaches to the 30S subunit of the ribosome
- tRNA brings amino acid to A site on the ribosome
- Transpeptidation of amino acid to growing peptide from P site
- Ejection of tRNA from P site
- Translocation of tRNA from A to P site with growing peptide
- Ribosome moves one codon on mRNA
- New tRNA attaches to A site

Tetracyclines

Tetracyclines interfere with the production of protein by inhibiting the binding of tRNA. Tetracyclines bind to the 30S subunit of the ribosome, and this prevents the entry of incoming acetyl tRNA to its location on the ribosome.

Erythromycin

Erythromycin exerts its action by inhibition of translocation. This is achieved by the drug binding to the 50S subunit of the bacterial ribosome.

Clindamycin

Clindamycin achieves its effect by inhibition of translocation in a method identical to that of erythromycin.

Antibacterials that interfere with bacterial nucleic acid

Bacterial DNA synthesis can be interfered with directly or indirectly via inhibition of production of essential metabolites (antimetabolic action).

Metronidazole

Metronidazole is really a prodrug. It penetrates bacterial cells, and, in susceptible anaerobes, is converted to its antibacterial form by reduction of its nitro group to a hydroxylamine moiety by the addition of four electrons. Labile intermediates produced during this reaction are the active antibacterial agents. The effects produced are:

- Inhibition of DNA replication
- Loss of helical structure of DNA
- Fragmentation of existing DNA
- Mutation of bacterial genome (at low dose)

Antimetabolic antibiotics

Some antibacterial drugs affect the production of folic acid, which is essential for nucleic acid production. Mammalian cells also require folic acid but can use the pre-formed molecule from food.

Sulphonamides and trimethoprim

These antibacterials interfere with bacterial DNA production by the following mechanisms. Sulphonamides inhibit the action of the enzyme dihydropteroate synthetase that converts *para*-amino benzoic acid (PABA) to dihydrofolic acid.

Trimethoprim interferes with dihydrofolate reductase, which metabolises dihydrofolic acid to tetrahydrofolic acid (Figure 3B.5).

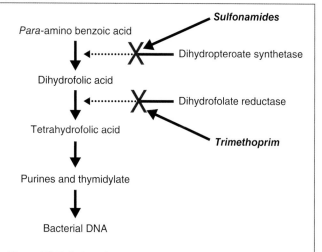

Figure 3B.5 Action of sulphonamides and trimethoprim.

Antibacterial use in dentistry

Antibacterials are used in dentistry in two ways – therapeutically and prophylactically.

Therapeutics

Therapeutically, they are used to treat infections of bacterial origin. They are not used to manage non-bacterial infections such as viral infections or non-infective inflammatory conditions such as alveolar osteitis or surgical oedema. Their main use is in the treatment of odontogenic infections; however, tetracyclines are also employed in the management of periodontal diseases. The number of antibacterials that dentists prescribe to treat odontogenic infections is small. Penicillins, metronidazole, erythromycin and clindamycin are effective in the management of over 95% of infections of dental origin.

Ideally, a sample of infected material such as pus should be taken for culture and sensitivity of the infective organism; however, therapy usually begins empirically with the prescription of a penicillin (such as amoxicillin) or metronidazole. If the prescribed medication is effective, it should be continued; if not, then the results of the sensitivity testing will inform the choice of alternative drugs.

In general practice, antibacterials will be prescribed for oral consumption. In the presence of severe life-threatening infections – for example, swelling of the floor of the mouth that causes difficulty in breathing – hospital admission and intravenous dosing of antibiotics is appropriate.

It is important to stress that antibacterials can help limit the spread of odontogenic infections. However, they do not cure the condition. At some stage in management, ideally initially, the source of the infection must be eliminated – for example, by root canal therapy or dental extraction. It should be remembered that odontogenic infections are painful, and that, in addition to the use of antibacterials, the appropriate administration of analgesics is required.

Prophylaxis

Antibacterials are used prophylactically for two reasons: first, to prevent wound infection, and second, to prevent infection at distant sites. Antibiotic prophylaxis may be considered for patients undergoing a bacteraemia-producing dental procedure in those with structural cardiac defects (see Chapter 1). Such procedures include oral surgical procedures (extractions, minor oral surgery) and some periodontal procedures such as deep scaling. The aim of prophylaxis is to prevent the patient from developing infective endocarditis.

A normal prophylactic regimen would include 3 g of Amoxil, taken orally 1 hour before the procedure. Patients allergic to penicillin would be prescribed clindamycin.

The use of antibacterials to prevent infection arising around prosthetic joints from such dental procedures as those described in the preceding text is not currently considered appropriate. There are several principles related to the use of antibacterials to prevent wound infection. First of all, the chances of wound infection must be high. Certain procedures increase the chances of wound infection. These include prolonged surgical procedures (>3 hours), implantology, transplantation and procedures in 'dirty' sites such as the gut. In general dental practice, only implantology and perhaps tooth transplantation are relevant. Therefore, most outpatient dental surgical procedures do not have an inherent risk of infection. The main cause of infection in normal outpatient dental operations is decreased patient resistance. Host resistance can be reduced as a result of local or systemic problems. Systemic problems would include severe immunodeficiency or haematological disorders. Localised effects include the end arteritis obliterans that results from therapeutic irradiation. Prophylactic antibiotics are indicated for surgical procedures (such as dental extractions) in patients with reduced resistance.

When prophylactic antibacterials are prescribed, the correct antibacterial must be chosen, and must begin at a suitable time and last for the appropriate length of time. The most suitable antibiotic is a bactericidal agent to which the patient is not allergic. A broad-spectrum penicillin such as amoxicillin is usually the drug of choice. Therapy is prophylactic, with the objective of obtaining suitable levels of drug in the blood clot of the wound. The clot becomes impenetrable to the drug 3 hours after its formation, so beginning therapy after the procedure is too late. Post-treatment therapy is of little value (a prolonged course may also increase the production of resistant organisms), so the ideal treatment is one dose before surgery.

Unwanted effects of antibacterial drugs

The unwanted effects of antibacterial drugs can be divided into global and individual. The global effect is the production of resistant organisms. The sensible use of antibiotics in dentistry as described earlier should help reduce the development of resistant organisms. The individual unwanted effects can be divided into:

- Allergy
- Minor
- Developmental
- Drug interactions

Allergy to antibacterial drugs, especially the penicillins, is common. The full range of allergic reactions may occur, including fatal anaphylaxis, the risk of which has been estimated at 1 in 100 000. It is important to establish if a patient has had an allergic reaction to a particular antibiotic as that is an absolute contraindication to the use of that drug.

Minor side effects to antibacterials include gastrointestinal upsets. Major gastrointestinal problems such as pseudomembranous colitis can occur after extended courses of clindamycin; however, such long treatments are unlikely in dentistry.

Tetracycline can produce characteristic developmental defects in teeth if taken by the patient (or pregnant female) at the time of enamel development. The defect manifests as discoloration that appears as bands corresponding to the time of drug intake. Drug interactions with antibacterials are described in Chapter 15 (titled 'Adverse drug reactions and interactions').

3C   VIRUSES AND ANTIVIRAL AGENTS RELEVANT TO DENTISTRY

Viruses relevant to dentistry

What is a virus?

The simplest (and smallest) reproducing entities known are:
- the *prions* (e.g. the causative agent of bovine spongiform encephalopathy), which appear to be composed entirely of protein.
- the *viroids* (responsible for diseases in plants), which are small single strands of naked nucleic acid.

Viruses are one level of complexity above these entities, being composed, in their simplest form, of both nucleic acid and protein. They lack any independent means of producing energy or of synthesising biomolecules. This distinguishes them from the more complex *Rickettsia* (e.g. typhus) and *Chlamydia*.

Viruses can replicate only in living cells, being parasites at the genetic level. Their nucleic acid contains information necessary for reprogramming the infected host cell to synthesise the virus macromolecules necessary for the production of viral progeny.

During replication inside the host cell, new virus proteins and nucleic acid are produced. Some of these proteins (known as 'non-structural proteins') are responsible for hijacking the host cell biosynthetic machinery and for making the new 'progeny virus nucleic acid'. Special structural proteins are also made. These assemble with the progeny nucleic acid to form virions, which are responsible for transmitting the virus nucleic acid to a fresh host cell.

Virions of different viruses vary in size (20–400 nm) and complexity. They contain only one type of nucleic acid, either RNA or DNA. The nucleic acid encodes a small number of genes – generally 3–100.

The virion nucleic acid is encased in a protein coat, the capsid, to form a 'nucleocapsid'. In the smallest virions (e.g. the parvoviruses, the rotaviruses), the nucleocapsid is naked. In many viruses, the nucleocapsid is further wrapped in a lipoprotein envelope. The function of these outer layers of the virion is to protect the nucleic acid (against inactivation by physical damage and by nucleases), and to mediate the virion's release from the infected cells and its entry into new target cells.

The proteins on the surface of the capsid in naked virions, or on the envelope, are responsible for many of the characteristics of the virus. It is via these proteins that the virus binds to and penetrates new host cells. Binding and penetration are often very specific interactions, where virus protein recognises a molecule on the surface of a host cell – for example, HIV binds to the CD4 protein, which is only present in T-cells, macrophages and some neural cells. These interactions dictate which animal species and which cell types the virus can infect. Antibodies generated by the host immune response can access surface proteins of the virus. Binding of antibodies can inhibit attachment and penetration, and thus protect against virus infection.

Capsids can have one of three basic shapes:
- *Icosahedral:* An icosahedron is a 20-faced solid. Protein molecules assemble into capsomers, and 20 capsomers assemble to enclose the nucleic acid.
- *Helical:* Protein molecules assemble into a long helical coil, forming a hollow rod around the nucleic acid.
- *Complex:* Some of the larger viruses exhibit more complex organisation.

Virus classification

Classification of viruses by the type of disease caused is very inadequate. Viruses producing very similar diseases have very different biological characteristics, and control and prevention require quite different approaches. For example, hepatitis A virus and hepatitis B virus both produce human hepatitis. Hepatitis A virus is a small, naked RNA virus that is tough and can survive outside of the cell wall enough to be transmitted by the faecal–oral route. Hepatitis B virus is an enveloped, double-stranded DNA virus that is delicate and requires intimate contact for transmission. Hence, quite different measures are obviously required to prevent the spread of the two viruses.

A more satisfactory approach is classification on the biological characteristics of the virion, the most important attribute of which is the nature of the virus genome. This classifies together similar viruses affecting humans and animals, regardless of the type of disease they cause. It is this type of classification that has pointed towards the evolution of HIV from the biologically similar viruses found in chimpanzees and other monkeys.

On this basis, viruses affecting humans are classified into viral families. Each family is split into genera and species. However, viral species are not as constant as those of higher organisms. Because they replicate so rapidly, viruses evolve very quickly, and different subtypes and strains of viruses are easily recognised. For example, the family orthomyxoviridae contains influenza A, B and C viruses. Influenza A virus is the most severe, causing repeated pandemics. A novel subtype of the virus causes each new pandemic. Following each pandemic, different strains of the pandemic subtype are isolated in the population in different parts of the world.

The major groups of animal viruses

Families of animal viruses are classified into several major groupings based on the type of nucleic acid in the virion and the mechanism of replication of the nucleic acid.

The DNA viruses

The DNA can be single stranded or double stranded. Most DNA viruses are double stranded, and include the human herpes virus family of viruses and the hepatitis B virus. For single-stranded viruses, a double strand is produced on entry into the cell, and the only common example is parvovirus B19, which is the primary cause of childhood rash.

The RNA viruses

These can be subdivided into four groups.

- *Those in which the virion RNA is a messenger.* These are the simplest, as the viral RNA can be translated into protein as soon as the nucleic acid enters the cytoplasm of the cell. The virions are not required to carry any enzymes. Examples include the enteroviruses that infect the gut and respiratory tract. Also included in the group are the flaviviruses ('flavi' = yellow), such as the yellow fever virus and the hepatitis C virus.
- *Those in which the virion RNA is negative sense.* As eukaryotic cells make mRNA only from a double-stranded DNA template, they do not have the enzymes necessary for copying DNA into RNA. If these virions are to make messages and thus proteins, they must carry an RNA polymerase in the virion to read off positive-sense mRNA from their negative-sense genomes. Examples include the influenza viruses and many other viruses that infect via the mucous membranes of the respiratory tract, including the measles and mumps viruses.
- *Double-stranded RNA virions.* These must carry the necessary enzymes for reading mRNA from a double-stranded RNA template. The only common example in humans is rotavirus, which cause, gastroenteritis, particularly in infants.
- *Those with message sense RNA that replicate via a double-stranded DNA intermediate.* These must carry a reverse transcriptase enzyme in the virion to produce double-stranded DNA from the virion RNA on entry into the cell. This double-stranded DNA then integrates into the host chromosomal DNA. Examples are the retroviruses. This group includes HIV, which causes AIDS, and the human T-cell lymphoma viruses.

Diagnosis of virus infections

A wide range of virus infections may be encountered during dental practice. Patients may present with a variety of symptoms, including oral ulceration, warts, parotitis, lymphadenopathy, respiratory infections and HIV-related disorders such as oral hairy leukoplakia and Kaposi's sarcoma.

In many cases, a virus diagnosis can be made on purely clinical grounds. However, on other occasions, the presentation may be atypical, and therefore virus diagnosis by a laboratory may be required.

Traditional techniques such as electron microscopy, virus isolation in cell culture and immunofluorescence are now rarely used. Serology is used to identify viral antibodies and viral antigens. It is most commonly used for the diagnosis of blood-borne viral infections, such as HIV and viral hepatitis. The most common serological techniques are based on the ELISA test (see discussion in preceding text). These assays are now highly automated. The PCR test (see discussion in preceding text) is a highly sensitive and specific technique for the detection of viral nucleic acid. Ideally, samples from the presumed site of infection should be tested – such as lesion swabs for vesicular lesions; nose and throat swabs for respiratory infections; and CSF for central nervous system (CNS) infections. Specific swabs for virology are required, as PCR should not be carried out on charcoal (bacteriology) swabs.

Hepatitis

Hepatitis A and E

Hepatitis A and E viruses are causes of acute self-limited hepatitis, transmitted via the faecal–oral route, and are rarely of concern in dental practice.

Hepatitis A is now rarely seen in the UK, but remains endemic in other areas of the world, particularly where socio-economic conditions are poor. It is transmitted via the faecal–oral route. Infection is often asymptomatic in children. It can be prevented by vaccination, which is recommended for travellers and other groups at increased risk of exposure.

Hepatitis E was originally thought to have a similar geographical distribution as hepatitis A. However, it is now known to be a common cause of acute hepatitis in developed countries, including the UK. Most infection in the UK is believed to be related to the consumption of undercooked pork products. Many infections are asymptomatic. Patients who are immunocompromised can fail to clear the infection, leading to chronic hepatitis.

Hepatitis B virus (HBV)

HBV can be transmitted sexually and via the parenteral route, which includes intravenous drug use and tattooing/body piercing. The virus can also be transmitted vertically, from mother to child, which is a particularly common route in endemic countries. In the healthcare setting, there is potential for transmission via needlestick injuries.

The incubation period for HBV is 2–6 months. Although some patients present with signs of acute, or even fulminant hepatitis, many acute infections are asymptomatic. Table 3C.1 lists the high-risk groups for HBV.

The majority of adults clear HBV following the acute infection, but 1–5% of immunocompetent adults go on to develop chronic infection. This occurs in over 90% of those infected perinatally. Chronic HBV infection can lead to cirrhosis, liver failure and hepatocellular cancer. Effective antiviral treatment is now available to suppress HBV replication to undetectable levels. Although infection is rarely cured, treatment results in long-term disease-free survival. Table 3C.2 lists the main serological markers used in the diagnosis of HBV infection.

HBV infection can be prevented by vaccination. HBV vaccine is a recombinant vaccine of HBsAg (hepatitis B surface

Table 3C.1 High-risk groups for hepatitis B carriage.

Patients who have received unscreened blood products

People involved with long-stay institutions

Those in occupations involving exposure to human blood (particularly surgeons)

Patients undergoing haemodialysis for end-stage renal disease

Promiscuously active individuals

Those who engage in unscrupulous tattooing/body piercing activity

Those who travel to areas with high infection rates

Those who come into contact with someone who has had a chronic hepatitis B infection

Table 3C.2 Serological markers for hepatitis B.

Marker	Description
Hepatitis B virus surface antigen (HBsAg)	Screening test. Indicates current HBV infection. Persistence in blood for over 6 months indicates chronic infection.
Antibody to hepatitis B virus surface antigen (anti-HBs)	Produced following clearance of HBV infection and following vaccination.
Antibody to hepatitis B virus core antigen (anti-HBc)	Past HBV infection. In the absence of HBsAg, indicates past (cleared) infection.

antigen). After vaccination, anti-HBs develops and confers protection. All clinical medical and dental students should be immunised against hepatitis B virus and their response checked. If a significant exposure to HBV occurs in an individual who is a vaccine non-responder, hepatitis B–specific immunoglobulin is indicated to reduce the risk of infection.

When treating dental patients, providing that the platelet counts and clotting times are normal, there is no reason why such patients should not be treated in dental practice.

Hepatitis C (HCV)

HCV is primarily transmitted via the parenteral route, and one of the commonest routes of transmission is intravenous drug use. It is less commonly transmitted sexually or vertically.

The length of incubation period for HCV is similar to that for hepatitis B. The acute infection is rarely symptomatic, but up to 80% of infected adults will develop chronic infection. Long-term chronic HCV infection is associated with cirrhosis, liver failure and hepatocellular cancer.

HCV is diagnosed by antibody testing, which may not be positive until 3 months after exposure. Further tests are needed to determine if infection is ongoing/chronic (PCR and antigen tests).

Table 3C.3 Potential causes of chronic hepatitis.

Alcohol excess

Hepatitis B or C infection

Autoimmune disease

As a complication of inflammatory bowel disease

Wilson's disease (toxic accumulation of copper in liver and brain). Inherited.

Alpha-1 antitrypsin deficiency – in adults, associated with hepatocellular cancer.

Drug-induced liver disease (e.g. from aspirin, halothane, paracetamol)

There is currently no effective vaccine against HCV. However, several direct-acting antivirals against HCV have recently been licensed, resulting in the ability to clear the virus in over 90% of cases.

Hepatitis D

Hepatitis D virus (or delta agent) is an incomplete virus. It can only replicate in the presence of HBsAg. It is transmitted via the same routes as HBV, and causes more severe hepatitis when it infects a patient with HBV infection.

Chronic hepatitis

Chronic hepatitis is defined as hepatitis persisting for longer than 6 months. The potential causes of chronic hepatitis are listed in Table 3C.3.

Blood-borne virus infections: prevention

Blood-borne viruses include HBV, HCV and HIV. Transmission of blood-borne viruses in healthcare settings can be prevented by adhering to standard infection prevention and control precautions, including measures to prevent needlestick injuries. These precautions should be applied by all staff for all patients, regardless of known infection status. Many patients remain undiagnosed or may be in the window period for infection.

The risk of transmission of infection following a needlestick injury from an infected patient is approximately 30% for HBV, 3% for HCV and 0.3% for HIV. It is important that all needlestick injuries be reported to ensure appropriate follow-up and treatment. HBV transmission can be prevented by vaccination; non-responders should receive hepatitis B virus immunoglobulin following any significant exposure. There is no post-exposure treatment for HCV, but appropriate follow-up allows early diagnosis and more effective treatment. Antiviral treatment started soon after an HIV exposure can prevent infection.

It is extremely rare for healthcare workers infected with these viruses to be a source of infection to their patients. Specific guidance is available for healthcare workers, including dentists, who are likely to be performing exposure-prone procedures (EPPs). These are defined as those invasive procedures where there is a risk that injury to the worker may result in exposure of the patient's open tissues to the blood of the worker. These include procedures where the worker's gloved hands may be in contact with sharp instruments, needle tips or sharp tissues (e.g. spicules of bone or teeth) inside a patient's open body cavity, wound or confined anatomical space where the hands or fingertips may not be completely visible at all times. Healthcare workers should be tested for HBV, hepatitis C virus and HIV prior to performing EPPs. Regulations for healthcare workers carrying out EPPs who are known to be infected with these viruses vary throughout the world, but in many cases EPP can still be performed, subject to successful treatment/suppression of viral replication and regular monitoring.

Herpes simplex virus (HSV)

Biology and epidemiology

Types 1 and 2 herpes viruses can both cause infection of the oral or genital mucosa, although the majority of HSV infections encountered in dentistry are from the type 1 virus. Geographic location, socioeconomic status and age influence the frequency of HSV type 1 (HSV-1) infection. In lower socioeconomic groups, acquisition of HSV-1 occurs in childhood. In higher socioeconomic groups, infection is often acquired later in life.

An important aspect of HSV infection is that, after primary infection of the oropharyngeal mucosa, the virus travels along the peripheral sensory nerve axons to the nerve cell body, where it lies latent. *Latency* is defined as persistence of the viral DNA in the cell but without active replication. A variety of factors can lead to the reactivation of HSV, including stress, UV light and steroid or other immunosuppressive therapy. On reactivation, HSV travels up the nerve to the epithelial surface of the skin, where it replicates.

Clinical presentation

Primary HSV infection of the oropharyngeal mucosa is usually asymptomatic. A wide range of disease manifestations can be encountered, however, including fever, sore throat, ulcerative and vesicular lesions, gingivostomatitis, localised lymphadenopathy and malaise. The incubation period ranges from 2 to 12 days, with a mean of approximately 4 days. Occasionally, severe mucous membrane disease, such as Stevens–Johnson syndrome, can occur.

Reactivation occurs intermittently throughout life. In some individuals, this results in localised vesicular lesions (cold sore). However, in most cases, reactivation is asymptomatic and contributes to viral transmission, explaining the ubiquitous nature of this virus.

Less common manifestations are herpetic whitlow, where herpetic vesicles occur on a finger due to inoculation from virus present in the oral mucosa. This is commonly seen in children who suck their thumbs, and is now less commonly seen in dentists, owing to the widespread use of gloves. HSV causes more severe symptoms in the immunosuppressed, and is also associated with rare but severe presentations such as encephalitis.

Specimen collection and laboratory diagnosis

HSV can be diagnosed clinically, where it presents as classical oral vesicles or cold sores. Where definitive diagnosis is needed, a viral lesion swab should be sent for PCR. This is an extremely sensitive test, which will also distinguish HSV-1 from HSV-2. Serology (antibody tests in blood) has no role in the diagnosis of HSV infection.

Treatment

In herpes labialis, topical administration of 5% aciclovir cream significantly reduces pain and lesion duration, but its use is limited owing to inadequate efficacy, unless used prior to the onset of lesions. Aciclovir is an effective treatment for HSV infection. For uncomplicated mucocutaneous HSV infections, it is normally given orally, and can shorten the duration of disease and reduce viral shedding. Due to poor oral bioavailability, it is required to be given five times a day. Alternatives are valaciclovir (prodrug of aciclovir) and famciclovir, which have greater bioavailability and are given orally twice daily. Aciclovir can also be given long-term at lower dosages in those with frequent recurrences to prevent symptomatic reactivation. Intravenous aciclovir is required for those with more serious HSV-related disease.

Varicella zoster virus (VZV)

Biology and epidemiology

VZV is a very contagious virus, with 80–90% of exposed individuals in a household becoming infected. Consequently, the seroprevalence in young adults is >90% in countries without a vaccination programme. The incubation period ranges from 10 to 23 days, with an average of 14 days. Transmission occurs via the respiratory route, with infection of the mucosa of the respiratory tract leading to a primary viraemia following viral replication in regional lymph nodes. A secondary viraemia occurs, delivering the virus to the skin where the characteristic vesicular rash of chickenpox occurs. Following the primary infection, manifested as chickenpox, latency is established in one or more posterior root ganglion and is life-long. Zoster (shingles) is a reactivation of VZV, with over half of cases occurring in individuals aged >50 years.

Clinical presentation

In chickenpox, vesicles develop on the skin during the first week, then dry up and finally crust. Blisters are occasionally seen on the oral mucosa during the acute phase of the disease. Zoster typically affects a single dermatome. The disease occurs

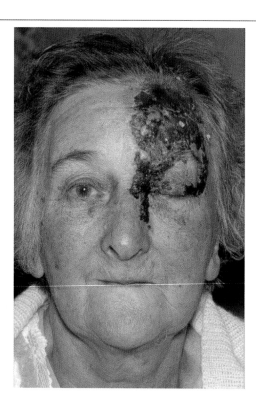

Figure 3C.1 Ophthalmic shingles – the lesions are confined to the distribution of the ophthalmic division of the trigeminal nerve.

when the virus reactivates in a single sensory ganglion, and proceeds down the associated nerve to replicate in the skin and cause the typical vesicular lesions of zoster. Ophthalmic shingles (Figure 3C.1) occurs when the ophthalmic division of the trigeminal nerve is involved. Reactivation in the geniculate ganglion of the seventh (facial) and eighth (auditory) cranial nerves is associated with facial palsy and is termed the 'Ramsay Hunt syndrome'. Zoster can be a painful disease, and post-herpetic neuralgia may occur after the rash has healed. This protracted pain may occur in 25–50% of individuals older than 50 years.

Similar to HSV, VZV is more severe and can be life-threatening in the immunosuppressed.

Sample collection and laboratory diagnosis

VZV can be diagnosed clinically where it presents as classical chickenpox or shingles. Where definitive diagnosis is needed, a viral lesion swab should be sent for PCR. Serology (antibody tests in blood) has no role in the diagnosis of VZV infection.

Treatment

Aciclovir is also effective treatment for VZV infections. However, the virus is less sensitive, and higher doses are required. As with HSV, valacyclovir and famciclovir are alternatives with greater oral bioavailability. In cases of ophthalmic zoster, antiviral therapy should be given for a minimum of 7 days, and patients with ocular symptoms or lesions on the side of the nose (Hutchinson's sign) should be referred for ophthalmological assessment.

As with HSV, intravenous treatment may be required for VZV infection in the immunosuppressed.

Prevention

VZV infection can be prevented by vaccination, and is part of routine childhood vaccination in some countries, such as the USA. It is an attenuated live vaccine. It is also recommended for healthcare workers who have not had chickenpox. A zoster (shingles) vaccine is also available. This is also a live attenuated vaccine that acts to boost immunity and prevent/reduce viral reactivation. This is part of routine vaccination in the elderly in countries such as the UK.

As the varicella vaccine is a live vaccine, it is contraindicated in pregnancy and in the immunosuppressed. As VZV infection can be severe in these groups, those without evidence of immunity who have had significant contact with chickenpox or shingles are offered varicella zoster immunoglobulin post-exposure to prevent or attenuate infection.

Cytomegalovirus (CMV)

Biology and epidemiology

CMV is a member of the Betaherpesvirinae subfamily of the Herpesviridae family. As with all herpes viruses, it remains latent in the body following primary infection. For CMV, the site of latency is white blood cells. The seroprevalence is related to socioeconomic status. In a population of high socioeconomic status, such as the UK, approximately 40% of adolescents are seropositive, with the rate increasing at 1% per year. Thus, approximately 70% of adults in this population are seropositive. Populations of low socioeconomic status have a seroprevalence of around 90%. Transmission occurs primarily through close mucosal contact with saliva.

Clinical presentation

The incubation period is between 4 and 8 weeks. Primary infection is predominantly asymptomatic. An infectious mononucleosis (glandular fever) syndrome can occur in immunocompetent young adults. Approximately 15% of cases are due to CMV, with the majority being caused by the Epstein–Barr virus. Congenital infections occur in approximately 1% of all live births, although the majority are asymptomatic; 7 percent are symptomatic at birth, with a further 10–15% developing later problems such as sensorineural hearing loss and developmental delay. Both primary and reactivated CMV are major problems following haemopoietic stem cell and solid organ transplantation. These can be severe and life threatening if untreated.

Specimen collection and laboratory diagnosis

In immunocompetent individuals, CMV is diagnosed by antibody testing in blood samples. The detection of IgM antibodies is consistent with recent primary infection. In the immunocompromised, both primary infection and reactivation can cause disease, and this is diagnosed by detecting viral DNA by PCR in blood samples. Congenital CMV is diagnosed by the detection of CMV DNA by PCR in urine.

Treatment

CMV infection is very rarely treated in immunocompetent patients. Antiviral therapy with either ganciclovir or foscarnet may be required in immunocompromised patients, although the drugs are toxic, being myelosuppressive and nephrotoxic, respectively. Oral valganciclovir, a prodrug of ganciclovir, is an option.

Epstein–Barr virus (EBV)

Biology and epidemiology

EBV is a member of the Gammaherpesvirinae subfamily of the Herpesviridae family. Latency occurs following infection of B lymphocytes, and is lifelong. The majority of EBV infection worldwide is not apparent, as asymptomatic infection occurs in young children in areas of the world where standards of hygiene are low. For example, 82% of children in Ghana, Africa, experience primary EBV infection by the age of 18 months. Approximately 90–95% of adults worldwide have serum antibodies to EBV. Infectious mononucleosis, which usually affects adolescents, occurs in countries where hygiene standards are high. Transmission occurs owing to intimate contact with oropharyngeal secretions.

Clinical presentation

The incubation period is 4–6 weeks. The most well-known clinical presentation is the infectious mononucleosis syndrome. This presents initially with malaise, headache and low fever, proceeding to tonsillitis and/or pharyngitis, cervical lymph node enlargement or tenderness and moderate-to-high fever. Splenomegaly is common, but jaundice and hepatomegaly are uncommon. A peripheral blood lymphocytosis occurs, with the detection of atypical lymphocytes. The acute symptoms resolve in 1–2 weeks, but fatigue often persists for months.

EBV is associated with the aetiology of several malignancies –particularly Burkitt's lymphoma and nasopharyngeal carcinoma in equatorial Africa and Southern China, respectively. EBV is also implicated in most cases of post-transplant lymphoproliferative disease.

Specimen collection and laboratory diagnosis

Although infectious mononucleosis can be diagnosed by a rapid monospot test on blood, this lacks sensitivity and specificity. Specific diagnosis in immunocompetent patients entails testing blood for EBV-specific antibodies.

Treatment

Antiviral therapy is not usually warranted in immunocompetent patients.

Enteroviruses

Biology and clinical presentation

Enteroviruses are RNA-containing viruses and are members of a genus of the family Picornaviridae. Over 100 enterovirus species have been isolated from humans. These include polioviruses, coxsackie A and B viruses and enteric cytopathic human orphan (ECHO) viruses. Enteroviruses identified more recently are designated with a number (e.g. enterovirus 71). Enteroviruses are small (27 nm in diameter), symmetrical particles containing single-stranded RNAs. Transmission occurs through direct contact with the nose and throat discharges and faeces of infected people. Enteroviruses cause a wide variety of diseases, including myocarditis, pericarditis, aseptic meningitis and respiratory infections. In dental practice, the two most commonly encountered enteroviral diseases are vesicular pharyngitis (herpangina) and hand, foot and mouth disease (HFMD).

Herpangina

Herpangina is an acute self-limiting disease characterised by a sudden onset of fever, sore throat and small (1–2 mm) discrete, grey, papulovesicular pharyngeal lesions on an erythematous base, which gradually progress to slightly larger ulcers. The lesions usually occur on the anterior pillars of the tonsillar fauces, soft palate, uvula and tonsils, and may be present 4–6 days after the onset of illness. Coxsackie group A viruses are usually the cause of this disease.

HFMD

HFMD is a vesicular stomatitis with skin rash. The oral lesions are more diffuse as compared to herpangina, and may occur on the buccal surface of the cheeks and gums and on the sides of the tongue. Approximately 85% of cases develop sparse vesicles on the dorsum of the fingers and on the margins of the heels. Palmar and plantar lesions appear occasionally, especially in young children. Resolution usually occurs within a week. Outbreaks usually occur in children aged <4 years, but can sometimes also occur in adults. The disease has been associated with several different enteroviruses.

Diagnosis

Diagnosis of both herpangina and HFMD is usually clinical. If laboratory diagnosis is required, then the enterovirus can be detected by PCR on a viral lesion swab.

Treatment

Only supportive care is required, and prompt recovery usually occurs.

Mumps

Biology and epidemiology

Mumps virus is an RNA-containing virus and a member of the Paramyxoviridae family. Virus particles are spherical with a lipid envelope. Transmission occurs via droplet spread and by direct contact with the saliva of an infected person. A person infected with mumps virus is infectious from 6–7 days before symptoms to 9 days after. Maximum infectivity occurs 48 hours before the onset of symptoms. The measles, mumps, rubella (MMR) vaccine was introduced in the UK in 1988. This was followed by a dramatic decline in cases of mumps. A two-dose schedule was introduced in 1996, although infection is still seen occasionally in vaccinated individuals.

Clinical presentation

The incubation period for the classic swelling of the parotid glands (parotitis) is commonly 18 days, with a range of 12–25 days. Enlargement of one parotid gland occurs in 75% of cases, followed 1–5 days later by enlargement of the contralateral gland. There is a prodrome of 1–2 days consisting of malaise, myalgia, headache and low-grade fever. Parotid swelling subsides after 4–7 days. Subclinical infection occurs in approximately 30% of individuals. The course of mumps virus infection can be very variable, and a variety of complications may occur. Orchitis, usually unilateral, occurs in 20–30% of post-pubertal males, and oophoritis in 5% of post-pubertal females. Sterility occurs only very rarely. Aseptic meningitis occurs frequently, although encephalitis is very rare. Neurological symptoms and orchitis can occur in the absence of salivary gland involvement.

Diagnosis

Laboratory diagnosis may be required for epidemiological purposes or where the clinical picture is atypical. A blood sample, collected a minimum of 4 days post-onset of illness, can be tested for the presence of mumps IgM antibody. In countries such as the UK, mumps is a notifiable condition, and the diagnosis for public health surveillance purposes involves collection of a salivary swab for antibody and PCR testing.

Treatment

Uncomplicated mumps is treated supportively using analgesics, antipyretics, rest and hydration. Currently, there is no established role for corticosteroids, antiviral chemotherapy or passive immunotherapy.

Adenovirus

Biology and epidemiology

Adenoviruses are non-enveloped DNA-containing viruses comprising several distinct serotypes that belong to the family Adenoviridae. Adenovirus infections are mostly endemic, although small outbreaks can occur in closed communities such as boarding schools, day centres and military institutions. Transmission occurs via direct contact, small-droplet aerosols and the faecal–oral route.

Clinical presentation

Clinical manifestations depend on the host and adenovirus serotype involved, and include acute respiratory infection of both the upper and lower respiratory tracts, tonsillitis, pharyngoconjunctival fever, keratoconjunctivitis and diarrhoea. Tonsillitis is a frequent manifestation in which the exudates are usually thin and follicular or net-like, but may sometimes have thick membranes. Many infections are subclinical. In severely immunocompromised children (e.g. after bone marrow transplantation), disseminated adenovirus infection can occur and may be life threatening.

Laboratory diagnosis

Viral throat or eye swabs or faeces samples can be tested by PCR.

Treatment

In immunocompetent patients, treatment is purely supportive. Infection in paediatric bone marrow transplant patients may require the early use of antiviral therapy in order to prevent or control disseminated infection.

Other respiratory infections

In addition to adenoviruses, many other viruses can cause respiratory symptoms. Examples include influenza viruses, respiratory syncytial virus (mainly causing lower respiratory infection in infants), parainfluenza viruses and rhinoviruses (the cause of many cases of the common cold). These infections are normally associated with short-lived respiratory illnesses, but can be more severe in the very young, the elderly and the immunocompromised. The primary route of transmission is via large droplet spread rather than aerosols, and therefore precautions such as using a tissue to cover the mouth when sneezing (catch it, bin it, kill it) and good hand hygiene can be effective in preventing infections. Annual influenza vaccination is available and particularly advised for risk groups, such as those with chronic conditions and the elderly. It is also important for healthcare workers.

Antiviral agents

The identification of effective antiviral agents has lagged behind that of antibiotics. Research is more difficult as many viruses cannot be easily grown in the laboratory. Viruses utilise host cell processes for much of their life cycle, and so targeting parts of the viral life cycle without adverse effects on the cell can be difficult. Antivirals tend to have a very narrow spectrum, and act specifically on a certain virus or for very closely related viruses. Viruses replicate rapidly and can evolve quickly, and antiviral resistance can be an important problem.

Despite these issues, there has been an exponential rise in licensed antivirals since the 1990s, with most of the more recently licensed antiviral agents being targeted at HIV, HBV and HCV. Many more agents are currently being developed and entering clinical trials. New antiviral compounds are being licensed every year.

Antiviral agents are currently used in dentistry for the management of oral and perioral viral infections. The condition most commonly treated is herpes labialis or 'cold-sore', which occurs on the vermilion border of the lip. Occasionally, primary herpetic stomatitis or herpes zoster infection may be treated in dental practice. Patients receiving treatment for chronic viral conditions such as HIV may be on antiviral therapy, and this can impact on dental management.

Mechanism of action of antiviral medications

Drugs such as aciclovir act to reduce viral replication by inhibition of the viral polymerase enzyme. Aciclovir is a guanosine analogue that is converted to aciclovir tri-phosphate by a combination of host and viral kinase enzymes. Once incorporated into DNA, this compound terminates the production of viral DNA, causing failure of viral replication.

Polymerase inhibition is the commonest mechanism of antiviral action, and is the mechanism of action of many antivirals active against HIV, HBV and HCV. Other licensed antivirals act to inhibit the processing of viral proteins (HIV and HCV protease inhibitors), viral integration (HIV) or viral release from infected cells (influenza).

Unwanted effects of antiviral agents

As viral replication is inherently dependent on cell processes, many antivirals have unwanted side effects. Aciclovir is a relatively safe antiviral, but can be associated with nephrotoxicity and, at high concentrations, can lead to neurotoxicity and seizures. Dose adjustment is important in those with renal failure. Particular attention should be paid to maintaining good hydration in patients on high doses of aciclovir.

Drug interactions with antiviral agents

Protease inhibitors are metabolised by cytochrome P450 enzymes. This means they have the potential to be involved in drug interactions with other medications that use this enzyme system. Important examples for dentistry include the increase in plasma concentrations of benzodiazepines that results from ritonavir therapy. Ritonavir is a drug that was previously a frequent component of HIV treatment regimes, although this is less commonly used in current treatment routines. Ritonavir can result in deep sedation when midazolam is used, and combined therapy is not advised. Similarly, the plasma concentration of local anaesthetics such as lidocaine can be higher than expected during treatment with protease inhibitors, increasing the risk of cardiotoxicity; however, this is unlikely to be a problem with the use of one or two cartridges of dental local anaesthetic in adult patients.

3D INFECTION WITH IMMUNODEFICIENCY VIRUS AND IMPLICATIONS FOR THE ORAL CAVITY: INFECTION WITH HIV

Introduction

The virus now known to cause AIDS was discovered in 1983, and is classified as a member of the lentivirus subfamily of human retroviruses. A new variant has also been isolated in patients with West African connections – HIV-II.

There are characteristic oral manifestations that are considered to be indicator diseases that occur in patients with HIV infection, and these are highlighted later in this chapter.

HIV infection begins when the individual is inoculated with the virus. Inoculation can occur either directly into the bloodstream (as during intravenous drug use from needle sharing, a needlestick injury or receipt of HIV-contaminated blood products) or by exposure of the broken skin, an open wound or mucous membranes to HIV-contaminated body fluids, such as during sexual intercourse. Inoculation may also occur by perinatal transmission from infected mother to infant.

After inoculation, the virus infects and begins to replicate in one or more susceptible cells. Circulating CD4 lymphocytes (T helper cells) and macrophages are the most commonly affected, although epithelial cells of the gastrointestinal tract, uterine cervical cells and the glial cells of the CNS may also be targets. The virus replicates sufficiently to produce detectable levels of viral copies, and the immune system responds to show host antibody production within a few weeks to months. During this period of primary HIV infection (or acute seroconversion illness), the patient often experiences a few days of clinical symptoms suggestive of a viral illness. In the majority of cases, these symptoms are probably ignored; in some cases, a glandular fever-like syndrome or some other significant symptom complex appears. This is referred to as an 'acute seroconversion illness' or 'primary HIV infection'.

Viral antigen is neutralised as the host's immune system mounts its initial antibody response to HIV. The patient usually becomes asymptomatic and remains so for a period that may range from weeks to many years. The majority of infected individuals exist in this state, and are identified by screening the serum for HIV antibody.

Epidemiology

Penile–vaginal intercourse is a low-efficiency mode of transmission, especially from women to men, but factors such as high viraemia, more advanced immunodeficiency in the infecting partner, receptive anal intercourse, sex during menses and the presence of other sexually transmitted diseases (STDs), both ulcerative and non-ulcerative, enhance the efficiency of transmission.

Globally, mother-to-child transmission during pregnancy, delivery or breastfeeding (vertical transmission) is the second major mode of spread of HIV. Mothers who themselves acquired HIV infection in the postpartum period are more efficient transmitters, presumably because of the increased viral burden associated with primary HIV infection.

The average risk of seroconversion after a needlestick injury with HIV-infected blood is approximately 0.3%. The risk of transmission after mucous membrane and cutaneous exposure to blood is estimated to be 0.09%. The risk of transmission of HIV to healthcare workers is increased when the device (such as a needlestick) causing the injury is visibly contaminated with blood, when the device has been used for insertion into a vein or artery and when the device has caused a deep injury.

Clinical presentations

HIV infection may present in any of the following ways:
- An acute viral syndrome, often resembling glandular fever.
- An asymptomatic state characterised only by laboratory evidence of HIV infection.
- A lymphadenopathy syndrome termed 'persistent generalised lymphadenopathy' (PGL), manifesting as chronic constitutional symptoms, often systemic and non-specific (weight loss, fever, night sweats).
- A chronic diarrhoea illness.
- A syndrome resulting from opportunistic infection or malignancy.
- Any combination of these.

The two main clinical manifestations of AIDS are tumours and a series of opportunistic infections. Kaposi's sarcoma (KS) is the most common original tumour described, but other tumours are now described, such as non-Hodgkin's lymphoma (NHL; usually extranodal) and squamous carcinomas of the mouth and anorectum. Most patients in North America and the UK present with *Pneumocystis carinii* (*jiroveci*) pneumonia (Figure 3D.1), followed by other opportunistic infections (Figure 3D.2).

The clinical spectrum is enlarging continuously as the survival of infected individuals is markedly improved with highly active antiretroviral therapy (HAART). There is a highly variable rate of disease progression observed in HIV-infected individuals. On the cell, CD4 is the major cellular receptor for HIV; CXCR4 and CCR5 are the identified chemokine co-receptors. Abnormalities occur in the function of all limbs of the immune system.

CD4+ T-cell dysfunction, both quantitative and qualitative, is the hallmark of HIV disease. The disease progression is closely related to virus replication. The two best laboratory parameters that have been shown to correlate with disease progression are CD4 lymphocyte count and HIV viral load.

Oral manifestations of HIV disease

Oral manifestations of HIV disease are common and include specific lesions and novel presentations of previously known opportunistic diseases (Table 3D.1). Early recognition, diagnosis and treatment of HIV-associated oral lesions may reduce morbidity. The presence of these lesions may be an early diagnostic indicator of immunodeficiency and HIV infection, may change the classification of the stage of HIV infection, and is a predictor of the progression of HIV disease.

Fungal infections

Candidiasis

Oral candidiasis is most commonly associated with *Candida albicans*, although other species, such as *C. glabrata* and *C. tropicalis*, are frequently part of the normal oral flora. Several factors predispose patients to develop candidiasis, including infancy, old age, antibiotic therapy, steroid and other immunosuppressive drugs, xerostomia, anaemia, endocrine disorders, and primary and acquired immunodeficiency. Candidiasis is a common finding in people with HIV infection. Oral candidiasis occurs most commonly with falling CD4+ T-cell count in the middle and late stages of HIV disease. Most people with HIV infection carry a single strain of *Candida* during clinically apparent candidiasis and when candidiasis is quiescent.

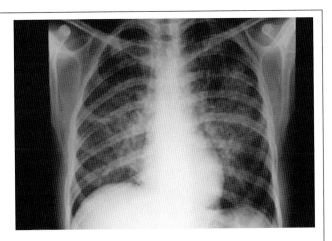

Figure 3D.1 Chest X-ray of a patient with *Pneumocystis carinii* (*jiroveci*) pneumonia.

Table 3D.1 Oral/head and neck manifestations of HIV disease.

- Fungal infections
  - Candidiasis
  - Erythematous candidiasis
  - Angular cheilitis
  - Hyperplastic candidiasis
- Histoplasmosis
- *Cryptococcus neoformans* infection
- Oral hairy leukoplakia
- Bacterial lesions (see text)
- Kaposi's sarcoma
- Oral ulceration
- Lymphoma
- Idiopathic thrombocytopaenic purpura
- Salivary gland disorders (see text)

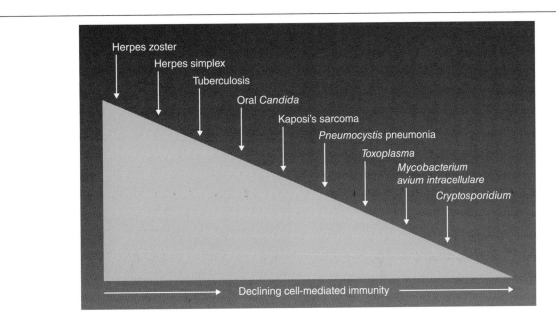

Figure 3D.2 Opportunistic infections in HIV patients as cell-mediated immunity declines.

Clinical features

The clinical appearances of oral candidiasis vary. The most common presentations include pseudomembranous and erythematous candidiasis, which are equally predictive of the development of AIDS, and angular cheilitis. These lesions may be associated with a variety of symptoms, including a burning mouth, problems eating spicy food and changes in taste. All three of these common forms may appear in one individual.

Pseudomembranous candidiasis (thrush). Characteristic creamy white, removable plaques on the oral mucosa are caused by the overgrowth of fungal hyphae mixed with desquamated epithelium and inflammatory cells. The mucosa may appear red when the plaque is removed. This type of candidiasis may involve any part of the mouth or pharynx (Figure 3D.3).

Erythematous candidiasis. Erythematous candidiasis appears as flat, red patches of varying size. It commonly occurs on the palate and the dorsal surface of the tongue. Erythematous candidiasis is frequently subtle in appearance, and may persist for several weeks if untreated.

Angular cheilitis. Angular cheilitis appears clinically as redness, ulceration and fissuring, either unilaterally or bilaterally at the corners of the mouth. It can appear alone or in conjunction with another form of candidiasis. It may be painful due to the fissuring (Figure 3D.4).

Hyperplastic candidiasis. This type of candidiasis is unusual in persons with HIV infection. The lesions appear white and hyperplastic. The white areas are due to hyperkeratosis and, unlike the plaques of pseudomembranous candidiasis, cannot be removed by scraping. These lesions may be confused with hairy leukoplakia. Diagnosis of hyperplastic candidiasis is made from the histological appearance of hyperkeratosis and the presence of hyphae (Figure 3D.5).

Differential diagnosis

Erythematous candidiasis should be differentiated from other red lesions, such as KS or erythroplakia. Histologically, oral candidiasis contains candidal hyphae in the superficial epithelium. The inflammatory responses often associated with candidal infection may be absent in immunocompromised patients. The creamy white plaques of pseudomembranous candidiasis are removable, whereas the white lesions of hairy leukoplakia are non-removable.

Diagnosis

Candida albicans is a commensal organism in the oral cavity. Candidiasis is diagnosed by its clinical appearance and by detection of organisms on smears or growth from swabs. Cultures are grown on specific media, such as Sabouraud agar. They may be positive and yet reveal very low colony counts. This probably represents a carrier state rather than active infection.

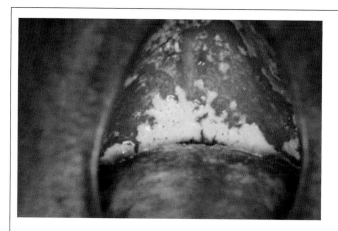

Figure 3D.3 Pseudomembranous candidiasis.

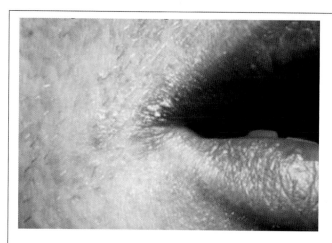

Figure 3D.4 Angular cheilitis.

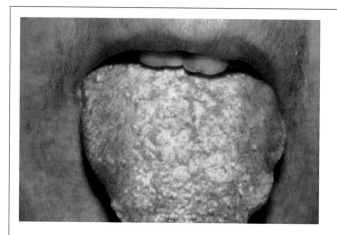

Figure 3D.5 Hyperplastic candidiasis.

Treatment

Oral candidiasis may be treated either topically or systemically. Treatment should be maintained for 7 days. Response to treatment is often good; oral lesions and symptoms may disappear in a fairly short period (ranging from 2 to 5 days), but relapses are common because of the underlying immunodeficiency.

Topical treatment

Topical treatments limit systemic absorption, but the effectiveness depends entirely on patient compliance. Topical medications require the patient to hold medications in the mouth for 20–30 min.

Clotrimazole is an effective topical treatment when dissolved in the mouth five times daily. Nystatin preparations include a suspension and an oral pastille. The Nystatin suspension has high sugar content and cannot be held in the mouth long enough to be effective. Topical creams and ointments containing nystatin, miconazole, ketoconazole or clotrimazole may be useful in treating angular cheilitis.

Systemic treatment

Several agents are effective for systemic treatment and are preferred by patients mainly because of the speed of clinical response and ease of administration. Fluconazole (Diflucan) is a triazole antifungal agent effective in treating candidiasis (50 mg tablet taken once daily for 2 weeks). Itraconazole oral suspension is also effective (200 mg daily for 2 weeks). Salivary levels of itraconazole are maintained for several hours after administration. For the rare cases of resistant candidiasis, intravenous amphotericin may have to be used.

Prognostic significance

Both erythematous and pseudomembranous oral candidiasis are associated with increased risk for the subsequent development of opportunistic infections. Several studies have shown a statistical correlation between the frequency of oral candidiasis in HIV infection and falling CD4+ T-cell counts.

Histoplasmosis

Histoplasmosis may initially present in the oral cavity. These lesions appear as ulcerations that can affect any mucosal surface. Diagnosis requires biopsy. It is rare in the UK.

Cryptococcus neoformans

Cryptococcus neoformans causing an ulcerated mass in the hard palate has been described in the literature. A biopsy of the ulcer is required for confirmatory diagnosis.

Human papillomavirus lesions

Oral warts, papillomas, skin warts and genital warts are associated with the human papillomavirus (HPV). Lesions caused by HPV are common on the skin and mucous membranes of persons with HIV disease. Anal warts have frequently been reported among homosexual men. Because the HPV types found in oral lesions in HIV-infected persons are different from the HPV types associated with anogenital warts, clinicians should probably not use the term 'condyloma acuminata' to describe oral HPV lesions.

Clinical features

HPV lesions in the oral cavity may appear as solitary or multiple nodules. They may be sessile or pedunculated, and appear as multiple, smooth-surfaced, raised masses resembling focal epithelial hyperplasia, or as multiple, small papilliferous or cauliflower-like projections.

Differential diagnosis

A biopsy is necessary for histological diagnosis.

Prognosis

There is no known association between oral HPV lesions and the more rapid progression of HIV disease, but oral warts are seen more commonly in HIV-infected persons than in the general population.

Treatment

Oral HPV lesions can be removed surgically under local anaesthesia. Carbon dioxide laser surgery can remove multiple flat warts. However, relapses occur, and several repeat procedures may be necessary.

Hairy leukoplakia and EBV

Oral hairy leukoplakia (OHL), which presents as a non-movable, corrugated or 'hairy' white lesion on the lateral margins of the tongue, occurs in all risk groups for HIV infections (Figure 3D.6). OHL occurs in about 20% of persons with asymptomatic HIV infection, and becomes more common as

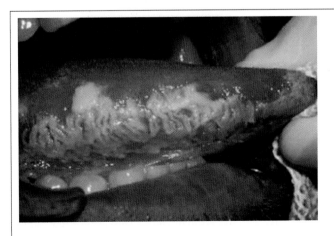

Figure 3D.6 Oral hairy leukoplakia.

the CD4+ T-cell count falls. No reports describe hairy leuko-plakia in mucosal sites other than the mouth. OHL has also occurred in non-HIV-infected people, including in recipients of bone marrow, cardiac and renal transplants.

Hairy leukoplakia and the progression of HIV disease

Diagnosis of OHL is an indication of both HIV infection and immunodeficiency. OHL correlates with a statistical risk for more rapid progression of HIV disease.

Clinical appearance and manifestations

OHL lesions vary in size and appearance, and may be unilateral or bilateral. The surface is irregular and may have prominent folds or projections, sometimes markedly resembling hairs. Occasionally, however, some areas may be smooth and flat. Lesions occur most commonly on the lateral margins of the tongue, and may spread to cover the entire dorsal surface. They may also spread downward onto the ventral surface of the tongue, where they usually appear flat. HL lesions can also occur on the buccal mucosa, generally as flat lesions. Rarely, lesions occur on the soft palate. OHL usually does not cause symptoms.

Differential diagnosis

Candida albicans may be found in association with many OHL lesions, and hyphae can be seen in specimens taken from lesions and examined using potassium hydroxide. Hyphae can be seen in stained sections. Administration of antifungal drugs may change the appearance of the lesions but does not cause them to disappear. Clinicians must distinguish them from other white lesions, such as lichen planus, idiopathic leukoplakia, white sponge naevus, dysplasia and squamous cell carcinoma.

Diagnosis

OHL can be diagnosed by incisional biopsy for definitive diagnosis. Experienced clinicians can make a presumptive diagnosis of OHL in association with HIV disease from the clinical appearance, although OHL can be confused with oral candidiasis. The typical microscopic appearance of OHL includes acanthosis, marked parakeratosis with the formation of ridges and keratin projections, areas of ballooning cells and little or no inflammation in the connective tissue.

Definitive diagnosis of OHL requires demonstration of EBV. EBV may be readily demonstrated in biopsy specimens by using a variety of techniques. Cells taken from the OHL lesion by scraping can be used for a non-invasive diagnosis using *in situ* hybridisation.

Treatment

Hairy leukoplakia usually is asymptomatic and does not require treatment. OHL is almost always a manifestation of HIV infection, and clinicians should arrange for evaluation of HIV disease and appropriate treatment for patients with OHL. OHL has disappeared in patients receiving high-dose aciclovir for herpes zoster, presumably because of the anti-EBV activity of aciclovir.

Bacterial lesions

Periodontal disease

Periodontal disease is a fairly common problem in both asymptomatic and symptomatic HIV-infected patients. It can take the form of a rapid and severe condition called 'necrotising ulcerative periodontitis'.

Differential diagnosis

The patient's history and clinical appearance make the diagnosis. It is sometimes difficult to distinguish this type of periodontal disease from non-HIV-related periodontal disease.

Different course in HIV infection

Oral flora appear to be similar to those associated with periodontal disease seen in non-HIV-infected persons. Recurrences of acute episodes are common, and response to conventional treatment may be poor. There is no known relationship yet between these conditions and the progression of HIV disease.

Mycobacterium avium intracellulare

Mycobacterium avium intracellulare that presents as palatal and gingival granulomatous masses in the oral cavity has been described. Biopsy should demonstrate the presence of acid-fast bacilli (AFB), and subsequent culture should grow *Mycobacterium avium intracellulare*.

Neoplastic lesions

Kaposi's sarcoma (KS)

KS may occur intraorally, either alone or in association with skin and disseminated lesions. Intraoral lesions have been reported at other sites, and may be the first manifestation of late-stage HIV disease (AIDS). KS occurs most commonly in men, but also has been observed in women.

Clinical features

KS can appear as a red, blue or purplish lesion. It may be flat or raised, solitary or multiple. The most common oral site is the hard palate, but lesions may occur on any part of the oral mucosa, including the gingiva, soft palate and buccal mucosa (Figure 3D.7), and in the oropharynx. Occasionally, yellowish mucosa surrounds the KS lesion. Oral KS lesions may enlarge, ulcerate and become infected. Good oral hygiene is essential to minimise these complications.

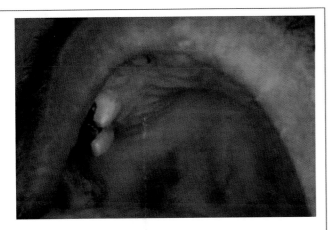

Figure 3D.7 Kaposi's sarcoma.

Differential diagnosis

KS must be distinguished from vascular lesions such as haematomas, haemangiomas, other vascular tumours, pyogenic granulomas and pigmented lesions such as oral melanotic macules. Diagnosis is made from histological examination. There are usually no bleeding problems associated with a biopsy of oral KS if due care is taken. Small, flat lesions are found in the early stages, and their histological appearance is different from the larger, nodular lesions, which are probably more advanced. Early lesions may be difficult to diagnose histologically as they resemble endothelial proliferation.

Treatment

Treatment is determined on the basis of the number, size and location of the oral KS lesions. HAART is an essential first step of KS management. If the disease burden has no visceral involvement, lesions may diminish with the response of the immune system once HAART is established. The choice of therapy depends on the effect of treatment on the adjacent mucosa, the pain associated with treatment, interference with eating and speaking, and the patient's preference. It is important to perform thorough dental prophylaxis before initiating therapy for KS lesions involving the gingiva. Response to therapy is improved if all local plaque and calculus are removed. Local application of sclerosing agents may reduce the size of oral lesions.

Local treatment is appropriate for large oral KS lesions that interfere with eating and talking. Oral KS can be treated surgically or with localised intralesional chemotherapy. Surgical removal is suitable for small, well-circumscribed lesions, such as gingival or tongue lesions. Surgical removal can be performed under local anaesthesia with a blade or with the carbon dioxide laser. Intralesional vinblastine is useful for treating small lesions, particularly on the palate or gingiva. Radiation therapy may be indicated for large, multiple lesions.

Lymphoma

Clinical features

Diffuse, undifferentiated non-Hodgkin's lymphoma (NHL) is a frequent HIV-associated malignancy. Most are of B cell origin, and EBV occurs in cells from several cases. Lymphoma can occur anywhere in the oral cavity, and there may be soft tissue involvement with or without involvement of the underlying bone. The lesion may present as a firm, painless swelling that may be ulcerated. Some oral lesions may appear as shallow ulcerations. Oral NHL may appear as solitary lesions with no evidence of disseminated disease.

Differential diagnosis

Oral NHL may be confused with major aphthous ulcers. Diagnosis of NHL must be made by histological examination of biopsy specimens.

Treatment

After diagnosis of the oral lesions, the patient must be referred for further evaluation for disseminated disease and its subsequent treatment.

Other oral lesions associated with HIV disease

Oral ulceration

Oral ulcers resembling recurrent aphthous ulcers (RAUs) in HIV-infected persons are being reported with increasing frequency. The cause of these ulcers is unknown. Proposed causes include stress and unidentified infectious agents. In HIV-infected patients, the ulcers are well circumscribed with erythematous margins.

Diagnosis

The ulcers may present a diagnostic problem. Herpetiform RAUs may resemble the lesions of coxsackie virus infection, and major RAUs may require biopsy to exclude malignancy, such as lymphoma, or opportunistic infection, such as histoplasmosis. The ulcers usually occur on non-keratinised mucosa; this characteristic differentiates them from those caused by herpes simplex.

Treatment

The RAU-type ulcers usually respond well to topical steroids in an ointment formulation. Dexamethasone elixir (0.5 mg/5 ml), used as a mouth rinse, is helpful for multiple ulcers and where topical ointments are difficult to apply. For HIV-infected persons with oral and gastrointestinal RAUs, systemic steroid therapy (prednisone 40–60 mg/day for 7–10 days) has been reported as helpful. The risks of steroid therapy, however, must be considered before administration to individuals in this population. Thalidomide (50–200 mg) has been used in Europe with some success.

Idiopathic thrombocytopaenic purpura (ITP)

Reports have described ITP in HIV-infected patients. Oral lesions may be the first manifestation of this condition.

Clinical features

Petechiae, ecchymoses and haematomas can occur anywhere on the oral mucosa. Spontaneous bleeding from the gingiva can occur, and patients may report finding blood in their mouth on waking.

Differential diagnosis

The clinician must distinguish ITP from other vascular lesions and KS. Because of potential bleeding risk, the clinician should obtain blood and platelet counts before performing other diagnostic procedures.

Salivary gland disease and xerostomia

Salivary gland disease associated with HIV infection (HIV-SGD) can present as xerostomia with or without salivary gland enlargement. Reports describe salivary gland enlargement in children and adults with HIV infection, usually involving the parotid gland. The enlarged salivary glands are soft but not fluctuant. In some cases, enlarged salivary glands may be due to lymphoepithelial cysts. The lymphocytic infiltrate is predominantly CD8 cells, unlike that in Sjögren syndrome, which is predominantly CD4 cells.

Management

Removal of the enlarged parotid glands is rarely recommended. For individuals with xerostomia, the use of salivary stimulants such as sugarless gum or sugarless sweets may provide relief. The use of salivary substitutes may also be helpful. An increase in the incidence of dental caries can occur, so fluoride rinses (which can be bought over the counter) should be used daily, and the dentist should be visited twice or thrice per year.

Diagnosis of HIV infection

HIV is now a treatable medical condition, and the majority of those living with the virus remain fit and well on treatment. Despite this, a significant number of people in the UK are unaware of their HIV infection, and remain at risk to their own health and of transmitting their virus unknowingly to others. Late diagnosis is the most important factor associated with HIV-related morbidity and mortality in the UK. Patients with specific indicator conditions should be routinely recommended to have an HIV test with informed consent.

There are two methods in routine practice for testing for HIV, involving either venepuncture and a screening assay (where blood is sent to a laboratory for testing), or a rapid point-of-care test (POCT).

The recommended first-line assay is one that simultaneously tests for HIV antibody *and* p24 antigen. These are termed 'fourth-generation assays', and they have the advantage of reducing the time between infection and testing HIV positive to 1 month, which is 1–2 weeks earlier than with sensitive third-generation (antibody-only detection) assays.

The diagnosis of HIV infection should include a good history and physical examination, followed by laboratory tests. The laboratory testing requires the sequential use of a highly sensitive screening test, followed by a highly specific confirmatory assay. The evaluation should be confidential, with appropriate counselling and informed consent of the individual. ELISA forms the basis of the common HIV infection screening system, which has a sensitivity of >99.5%.

Principles of treatment

Increased knowledge and understanding of the replicative cycle and molecular biology of HIV have made it possible to identify potential targets for antiviral treatment, as discussed in Chapter 3C (titled 'Viruses and antiviral agents relevant to dentistry').

3E   FUNGI AND ANTIFUNGAL AGENTS

Fungi

Fungi are generally larger than bacteria, and are commonly multicellular. They have a relatively thick cell wall that is rigid owing to fibrils of chitin. The chitin is embedded in a matrix of protein. Inside the cell wall is a cytoplasmic membrane that is the target of some of the antifungal agents.

Moulds or filamentous fungi grow as tubular branching filaments known as 'hyphae', and these can become interwoven to form a network or mycelium.

The yeast type of fungi are oval or spherical cells, which commonly reproduce by budding. *Candida* shows a modified form of budding. The buds elongate into filaments known as 'pseudohyphae'. These remain linked in chains and resemble the mould mycelium.

As discussed in Chapter 3D (titled 'Infection with immunodeficiency virus and implications for the oral cavity'), overgrowth of the normally commensal fungal organisms can occur in immunosuppressed patients, patients taking antibiotics, patients with poorly controlled diabetes and those using steroid inhalers. Candidal infections too were discussed in Chapter 3D.

Antifungal agents

Antifungal agents are used in dentistry in the management of oral candidiasis. They are available as lozenges, gels, ointments and oral suspensions for topical use. Systemic dosing may also be used when the infection is severe. Three groups of compounds are used. These are:

- Polyenes
- Imidazoles
- Triazoles

Amphotericin and nystatin are polyenes that are not absorbed after oral administration. They achieve their effect by interfering with the integrity of the cell wall of the organism. The antifungal agent forms a pore in the mycelial membrane, and this disrupts transmembrane transport and permeability.

The imidazoles (such as miconazole and ketoconazole) and triazoles (e.g. fluconazole and itraconazole) achieve their antifungal action by inhibiting the synthesis of ergosterol, which is the main sterol in the fungal cell membrane. This results in decreased fungal replication and also inhibits the production of candidal hyphae, which are the pathogenic forms of the organism.

Unwanted effects of antifungal medication

Antifungal drugs can cause gastrointestinal upset, and hypersensitivity reactions too can occur. Some important drug interactions can take place when patients are prescribed antifungal drugs, even during topical use. The most important interaction is with warfarin, and this is discussed in Chapter 15 (titled 'Adverse drug reactions and interactions').

FURTHER READING

Department of Health. *Health Clearance for Tuberculosis, Hepatitis B, Hepatitis C and HIV: New Healthcare Workers*. London: Department of Health; 2007. Available from: https://www.gov.uk/government/publications/new-healthcare-workers-clearance-for-hepatitis-b-and-c-tb-hiv.

Public Health England. *UK Advisory Panel for Healthcare Workers Infected with Bloodborne Viruses (UKAP)*. Available from: https://www.gov.uk/government/publications/hiv-infected-healthcare-workers-and-exposure-prone-procedures.

BHIVA – UK National Guidelines for HIV Testing; 2008.

Joint Committee on Vaccination and Immunisation. *Immunisation Against Infectious Diseases*. Chapter 18. London: Stationery Office; 2006. Available from: http://immunisation.dh.gov.uk/category/the-green-book/.

Woode Owusu M, Wellington E, Rice B, *et al. Eye of the Needle. United Kingdom Surveillance of Significant Occupational Exposures to Bloodborne Viruses in Healthcare Workers: Data to End 2013*. London: Public Health England; 2014. Available from: https://www.gov.uk/government/publications/bloodborne-viruses-eye-of-the-needle.

MULTIPLE CHOICE QUESTIONS

1. Which of the following viruses is the causative agent in cases of herpangina?
   a) Adenovirus
   b) Enterovirus
   c) Herpes simplex virus
   d) Human immunodeficiency virus
   e) Varicella zoster virus
   Answer = B

2. Which diagnostic test is indicated if laboratory confirmation of herpes labialis is required?
   a) Blood sample for HSV IgM
   b) Blood sample for HSV PCR
   c) Lesion swab for electron microscopy
   d) Lesion swab for HSV PCR
   e) Lesion swab for viral culture
   Answer = D

3. What is the risk of HBV transmission to an unvaccinated healthcare worker following a needlestick injury from an infected patient?
   a) 0.3%
   b) 3%
   c) 10%
   d) 30%
   e) 50%
   Answer = D

4. Which of the following is the commonest route of HCV transmission in the UK?
   a) Faecal–oral
   b) Intravenous drug use
   c) Respiratory
   d) Sexual transmission
   e) Vertical: mother to child
   Answer = B

5. What is the mechanism of action of acyclovir?
   a) Inhibition of the viral polymerase enzyme
   b) Inhibition of the viral protease
   c) Prevention of viral attachment to the cell
   d) Prevention of viral release from the cell
   e) Interference with cell wall synthesis
   Answer = A

6. The most common AIDS opportunistic infection in the UK is:
   a) *Pneumocystis jiroveci* (formerly '*Pneumocystis carinii*') pneumonia
   b) Cytomegalovirus retinitis
   c) Oesophageal candidiasis
   d) Squamous cell carcinoma of the tongue
   e) Kaposi's sarcoma
   Answer = A

7. The most common form of oral candidiasis in HIV-infected patients is:
   a) Hyperplastic candidiasis
   b) Angular cheilitis
   c) Pseudomembranous candidiasis
   d) Erythematous candidiasis
   e) Oral aphthous ulcerations
   Answer = C

8. The following is true regarding oral hairy leukoplakia:
   a) Only occurs in HIV infection
   b) Associated with Epstein-Barr infection
   c) Associated with oral sex
   d) Associated with poor oral hygiene
   e) Causes painful sensation
   Answer = B

9. The following are indicator diseases for HIV:
   a) Oral candidiasis
   b) Trigeminal neuralgia
   c) Obesity
   d) Insomnia
   e) Carpal tunnel syndrome
   Answer = A

10. The following is true of HIV:
    a) Transmitted by sharing a cup
    b) Late diagnosis is associated with high morbidity and mortality
    c) Treated effectively by exchange transfusion
    d) Acyclovir is an effective combination drug
    e) Only affects men who have sex with men
    Answer = B

CHAPTER 4
Immunological disease

C Stroud and H Bourne

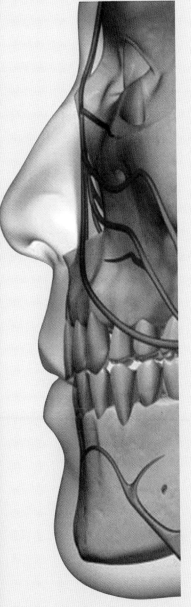

Key topics

- The normal immune response.
- Abnormalities of the immune response, including immunodeficiency, autoimmunity and allergy.

Learning objectives

- To be aware of the normal immune response, and potential disorders of the immune system and their management.
- To understand the potential impact of disorders of the immune system on oral health, and the delivery of safe dental/oral care.

Essentials of Human Disease in Dentistry, Second Edition. Mark Greenwood.
© 2018 John Wiley & Sons Ltd. Published 2018 by John Wiley & Sons Ltd.
Companion website: www.wiley.com/go/greenwood/human-disease-in-dentistry

Table 4.1 Components of innate and acquired immunity.

Innate immunity	Adaptive immunity
Phagocytic cells	T-cells
The complement system	B-cells
Barriers (see text)	

Introduction

The human immune system comprises multiple physical, chemical and cellular components to protect the individual from disease. The primary function of the immune system is to protect from infection. Disease may result, however, when parts of the immune system are absent (immunodeficiency), or when they react against inappropriate things such as drugs and food (allergy) or the body's own tissues (autoimmunity).

Traditionally, the components of the immune system have been classified as *innate* or *adaptive* (Table 4.1). The innate immune system components provide a constant level of protection. It is the first defence encountered by microorganisms. The adaptive immune system provides specific protection from the multitude of potential pathogens in the external environment. The adaptive immune system has a long-lasting immunological memory. It is so named because it adapts over the individual's lifetime to infections with an organism. While the individual components of the immune system are described separately and classified into the innate and adaptive systems, it should be clear that these individual elements work closely together to protect the body from infection, providing long-lasting immunity against microorganisms already encountered.

The first part of this chapter gives an account of the basic components of normal immune system function. The aim is to provide sufficient basic science for an understanding of the clinical problems that are addressed later in the chapter. If further details are required, the reader should consult a more detailed basic immunology text.

Overview of a normal immune response

When a microorganism enters the body through the skin or mucous membranes, the first defences encountered are those of innate immunity. These defences are constantly present and do not change following subsequent exposure to the organism. Intact skin, enzymes in tears, saliva, and acid in the stomach all provide barriers to infection.

If these barriers are breached, then the organisms will be targeted by cellular and non-cellular components of the innate immune system. Phagocytic cells are part of the innate immune system. They are able to engulf microorganisms and destroy them. Phagocytic cells include long-lived cells such as macrophages and short-lived cells such as neutrophils.

The complement system is also part of innate immunity. This system is a series of 26 proteins circulating in the bloodstream. Following activation by microorganisms, they form a cascade of proenzymes, the activation of each catalysing the activation of subsequent downstream components. The complement system protects against infection by:

- Lysing infected cells.
- Attracting phagocytic cells to the site of infection (chemotaxis).
- Coating the surface of microorganisms, so that they are more likely to be destroyed by phagocytic cells (termed 'opsonisation').

If the innate immune system fails to control the infection, then specialised cells called 'antigen-presenting cells' move from the site of infection to a specialised area (a lymph node), where an adaptive response is activated.

Within the lymph node, the cells of the adaptive immune system, the T-cells and B-cells, interact. B-cells are activated to make antibodies, and T-cells are activated to help the B-cells (also known as 'T helper cells' (Th cell) or 'CD4+ cells') or to kill infected cells (also known as 'cytotoxic T-cells' (CTLs) or 'CD8+ cells'). The adaptive response takes time to be activated, and therefore there is a delay before the immune system can initially respond. However, the adaptive immune system can modify its response on subsequent exposure to the organism, so that long-lived memory cells can respond faster and more efficiently.

What is immunodeficiency?

Immunodeficiency is the condition that occurs when one or more components of the immune system are defective or absent. This can be divided into primary causes, which patients are born with, or those secondary to events or disease processes occurring throughout life. All primary immunodeficiencies are rare. The majority of patients are diagnosed in childhood. A significant number of patients, however, do not develop symptoms until later in life, and the diagnosis is often delayed for many years. This results in significant morbidity and increased mortality. It is important to be aware of these conditions and to refer to or discuss with the local immunology department if there are any concerns. Immunodeficiency is classified in Table 4.2.

Table 4.2 Classification of immunodeficiency.

Inherited/primary immunodeficiency
- B-cells (lack of antibodies)
- T-cells
- Combined B-cells and T-cells
- Neutrophils
- The complement system

Acquired/secondary immunodeficiency
- For example, infections such as HIV, lymphoproliferative disease, malnutrition, drugs (immunosuppressives)
- Lymphomas or cancers
- Drugs that suppress the immune system
- Diseases that cause loss of immunoglobulins through the gut or renal tract

What are the consequences of immunodeficiency?

Infection

If parts of the immune system are absent, then the body is unable to defend itself from infection. Despite significant overlaps among the functions of parts of the immune system, some aspects have specific roles in the defence against certain types of microorganisms. For example, B-cells make antibodies. Antibodies cannot enter cells, and so they destroy organisms that live outside cells. If a patient is unable to make antibodies, they are unable to defend themselves effectively against microorganisms that live outside cells.

Autoimmunity and malignancy

Immunodeficient patients can also be prone to malignancies and autoimmune diseases as they have lost the regulatory and surveillance cells that keep the immune system in check.

What are the symptoms and signs of immunodeficiency?

Patients with immunodeficiency usually experience recurrent and/or serious and/or unusual infections. These infections may also be persistent and difficult to treat, such as persistent oral candidiasis. Infections may occur with unusual or rare organisms in sites where these types of infections are not usually seen. Following recurrent infections, damage in specific organs may occur – for example, bronchiectasis after repeated chest infections. Patients may also develop findings consistent with more widespread immune dysregulation such as autoimmune disease – for example, vitiligo (patches of skin depigmentation) or hypothyroidism.

Examples of specific primary immunodeficiencies seen in dental practice

Common variable immunodeficiency (CVID)

CVID is a form of antibody deficiency disorder. The cause is unknown, although it is thought to be due to multiple gene defects. Patients present with recurrent bacterial infections and may present at any age. Treatment is lifelong, with antibody replacement therapy in the form of intravenous immunoglobulin therapy given every 2–3 weeks, or subcutaneous immunoglobulin therapy administered weekly. Once on treatment, the risk of infection is reduced, but treatment with antibiotics may still be required for breakthrough infections. Patients may also have autoimmune diseases including, for example, haemolytic anaemia and granulomatous hepatitis, and are at risk of complications relating to these.

Wiskott–Aldrich syndrome (WAS)

WAS classically affects males. It is an X-linked disorder associated with eczema, low platelet counts and recurrent infections. These patients are at substantial risk of bleeding following dental treatment. In addition, antibiotic prophylaxis is required. Further management of these patients should be through liaising with the local immunology department or dental hospital.

Chronic mucocutaneous candidiasis (CMC)

CMC is a rare condition that affects both males and females. It presents with chronic candidal infection of the skin and mucous membranes. There may be an associated autoimmune endocrine deficiency. Management is through the local immunology department, and can be challenging, with the need for regular antifungal treatment at high dose and for prolonged periods.

Chronic granulomatous disease (CGD)

CGD usually presents in childhood with recurrent deep abscesses. The underlying immunological defect is the failure of the neutrophil oxidative burst, and the subsequent killing of organisms. Patients develop recurrent deep-seated abscesses that may be in unusual sites. They also develop gingivitis and tooth loss.

Deficiency of C1 esterase inhibitor (hereditary angioedema)

Defects of the control protein, C1 esterase inhibitor, may be inherited, and result in uncontrolled activation of the complement pathway. Patients develop symptoms of recurrent deep swelling with exposure to minor trauma or stress, such as during dental treatment. They can develop fatal laryngeal oedema (Figure 4.1). Urticaria does not occur in this condition.

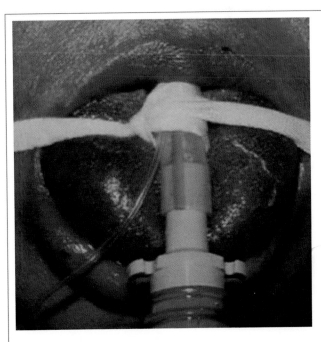

Figure 4.1 A patient with C1 esterase deficiency. The patient was intubated to protect the airway from blockage due to gross oedema.

The treatment of acute attacks is via the replacement of the enzyme or the administration of a bradykinin inhibitor. Patients may require long-term treatment with androgenic steroids and tranexamic acid. The evaluations of patients with this condition should be discussed with the local immunology department prior to dental treatment, as they may require premedication with C1 esterase inhibitor concentrate to prevent episodes of swelling.

Implications of immunodeficiency in dental practice

- Take a history:
    - Check for recurrent infections; family history (genetic).
    - Check for drugs.
- On examination:
    - Look for candidiasis, oral hairy leukoplakia, severe gingivitis, tooth loss, mouth ulceration, dry mouth, absent tonsils.
    - Skin changes (vitiligo, alopecia, telangiectasia).

Common conditions can be features of immunodeficiency

Oral candidiasis, mouth ulcers and gingivitis are common conditions that, in some patients, may suggest immunodeficiency or autoimmune conditions. The frequent causes of these conditions are listed in Table 4.3.

Table 4.3 Frequent causes of oral candida, mouth ulcers and gingivitis.

Frequent causes of oral candida
- Antibiotic therapy
- Steroid inhalers
- Dentures
- Secondary immunodeficiency (e.g. HIV, drugs)
- Connective tissue disease
- Sjögren syndrome: dry mouth
- Primary immunodeficiency (e.g. chronic mucocutaneous candidiasis)

Frequent causes of mouth ulcers
- Aphthous
- Behçet's syndrome
- Systemic lupus erythematosus (SLE)
- Cancer
- Crohn's disease

Causes of gingivitis and tooth loss
- Pregnancy
- Ciclosporin
- Scurvy
- Anticonvulsants
- Chronic granulomatous disease (primary immunodeficiency)

Allergy in dental practice

Introduction

Hypersensitivity reactions are immune-mediated antigen-specific reactions that are either inappropriate or excessive and result in harm to the host; they have been classified by Gell and Coombs (see Table 4.4). The term 'allergy' is most frequently equated with type I hypersensitivity reactions that are mediated via IgE, but is sometimes used in the context of type IV reactions. Allergic reactions, which can be severe and life threatening, can occur in dental practice, and knowledge on how to manage these conditions is therefore essential.

Incidence of allergic diseases

The incidence of allergic diseases in Western societies is increasing. More patients present with symptoms of rhinitis, conjunctivitis, food allergy, eczema and asthma. It is hypothesised that the increase in allergic disease may be due in part to the decrease in infections encountered in the Western world, and the result of immunisation regimens that have protected us from other serious infections. Our environment has also altered substantially, with changes particularly in housing that have led to increased exposure to house dust mites. The proposed hygiene hypothesis suggests that, because of the reduced exposure of the immune system to pathogens, especially at mucosal sites (gut, lungs, etc.), there is a switch of the immune system towards responses that allow the development of allergic conditions.

Allergens and irritants in dental practice

Many materials are used in dental practice that are considered to be potential allergens or irritants (see Table 4.5). Patients who feel they have a problem with these agents may present with a number of complaints, including stomatitis, mouth ulceration, soreness in the mouth from oral lichenoid lesions, burning or tingling in the mouth, cheilitis or lip swelling, oral swelling, facial eruption or more systemic features of urticaria, wheezing and even anaphylaxis.

Type I hypersensitivity (allergy)

Pathogenesis

On contact, the allergen binds to specific IgE on the surface of mast cells. This results in the degranulation of the cells and the release of pre-formed mediators, including histamine, heparin, lysosomal enzymes and proteases. A second set of chemical mediators (including leukotrienes, prostaglandins, thromboxanes, and chemotactic and activating factors) are also generated, and these are released into the local tissues about 4–8 hours later. These mediators result in a host of clinical features, described in the following text.

Table 4.4 Gell and Coombs classification of hypersensitivity reactions.

	Type I (allergy)	Type II	Type III	Type IV
Immune mediator	IgE	IgG	IgG	T-cells
Antigen	Soluble antigen	Cell surface antigens/ receptors	Soluble antigen	Soluble or cell-associated antigen
Effector mechanism	Mast cell activation and mediator release	Cytotoxic reaction	Immune complex reaction	Cell-mediated reaction
Examples of reaction	Allergic rhinitis, urticaria, asthma, systemic anaphylaxis	Transfusion reactions, acute graft rejection, autoimmune disease including Graves' disease, Goodpasture's syndrome	Cryoglobulinaemia, systemic lupus erythematosus, post-streptococcal glomerulonephritis	Contact dermatitis, chronic asthma, chronic allergic rhinitis, eczema

Table 4.5 Materials considered as potential allergens or irritants in dental practice.

Antiseptics

Metals

Impression materials

Local anaesthetics

UV radiation

Cements

Latex

Rubber dams

Acrylics

Adhesives

Mouthwashes

Other dental hygiene materials, such as chlorhexidine, formaldehyde, etc.

Table 4.6 Features of a type I hypersensitivity reaction.

Symptoms and signs	Pruritus, rhinitis, conjunctivitis, wheezing, urticaria, angioedema, vomiting, diarrhoea, abdominal cramps, dizziness, respiratory difficulties, hypotension, sense of impending doom, syncope and shock (patients may develop some or all of these features).
Onset	Rapid onset after exposure to allergen.
Recurrence	Symptoms recur after each exposure to the allergen.
Resolution	Symptoms do not occur during periods of complete allergen avoidance.

Clinical features of allergic reactions

Type I hypersensitivity (allergy) reactions usually occur within minutes of exposure to the allergen (the antigen involved in the allergic reaction). Common features of allergic reactions are urticaria (itchy wheals) and angioedema (deep mucocutaneous swelling), but breathing difficulties and cardiovascular collapse can occur. Table 4.6 highlights some of the features of allergic reactions. However, not all the symptoms and signs will be present in all patients, even when serious reactions occur. Once a patient has developed an allergy to a substance, reactions will continue to occur on re-exposure to the allergen.

Diagnosis of type I hypersensitivity reactions

The history is of great importance in diagnosing this condition. *In vitro* and *in vivo* investigations can help to make the diagnosis. Clinicians with specialist knowledge of allergy should investigate patients and interpret their test results.

Laboratory investigations

The radioallergosorbent test (RAST) was the first assay to measure specific IgE. Newer specific IgE assays have been developed that are able to use a larger number of allergens of higher quality, and non-isotopic labels are used in the detection stage. Measurement of specific IgE to various substances can be useful, but false negatives and false positives can occur. False positives are more common in patients with atopy. The finding of specific IgE to a substance to which a patient has a clinical history of allergy supports the diagnosis of allergy to that substance in the patient. Patients can have specific IgE present without any clinical features, indicating sensitisation (exposure) of the patient to that allergen.

Total IgE levels are not usually helpful in eliciting the cause of an allergic reaction, but high levels will be found in atopic patients. Atopic patients are those with a tendency to eczema, asthma or hay fever. Tryptase levels can be measured and are elevated in the patient's serum within 30–60 min of having a systemic allergic reaction. False-negative results occur. High levels should always be compared with a baseline level taken at a time of no reaction.

Skin prick tests

Skin prick tests are usually the investigation of choice, as these are cheaper, quicker and have increased sensitivity when compared with *in vitro* specific IgE testing. Skin prick testing involves the application of a small drop of allergen-containing solution onto the forearm of the patient, through which the skin is pricked with a lancet. In allergic patients, a wheal and flare reaction occurs. The wheal diameter is measured 15 min after application and compared with a positive control sample (histamine 1%) and a negative control sample (saline). The positive control should cause a wheal >3 mm, and the negative control should result in no wheal. If the allergen produces a wheal of >3 mm, this is considered to be a positive result. There are limitations to skin prick tests – including for use in patients with severe eczema; in patients dependent on antihistamines (which suppress wheal formation and therefore result in false-negative results); in young children; and in patients with dermographism (an exaggerated whealing tendency when the skin is stroked), which again results in false-positive results. In order to investigate drug allergy, intra-dermal tests may be required. In these, a small amount of diluted drug is injected into the dermis to see if this elucidates a wheal, which indicates sensitization. These can be difficult to perform and interpret, and therefore challenge testing may be required.

Challenge tests

Challenge tests can be performed if the history and test results are inconclusive. These can be difficult to standardise, and can result in patients sustaining serious reactions, including anaphylaxis. Challenges should therefore be undertaken in specialist areas with full resuscitation equipment available. Double-blind placebo-controlled challenges are required, and, if negative, they should then be confirmed by open exposure to the allergen under supervision in order to exclude the possibility of false-negative/false-positive challenges.

Causes of type I hypersensitivity reactions in dental practice

Latex allergy

Type I allergy to dental materials is uncommon; much more commonly encountered is latex allergy affecting both patients and dental surgery personnel. Anyone who routinely wears

Table 4.7 Latex-containing products.
Rubber gloves
Catheters
Intravenous tubing
Vial stoppers
Dental rubber dams
Condoms
Balloons
Adhesives
Some dental local anaesthetic cartridges

Table 4.8 Latex fruit syndrome.
Bananas
Avocado
Kiwi fruit
Potato
Chestnut
Lettuce
Pineapple
Papaya

latex-containing gloves, or is regularly exposed to natural rubber latex products (Table 4.7), may be at risk of developing latex sensitisation. The risk of this occurring appears to decline with age. Other risk factors for the development of latex allergy include spina bifida or meningomyelocele, atopy (eczema, asthma, hay fever), pre-existing hand eczema and multiple diagnostic/therapeutic interventions. A history from the patient may establish the diagnosis prior to dental treatment – for example, urticaria after contact with latex-containing gloves, reactions to condoms and wheezing after blowing up balloons. Patients may also react to multiple foods, particularly avocado, chestnut, banana and kiwi fruit. This is due to immunological cross-reactivity between conserved proteins and enzymes in latex and these foods (Table 4.8). In patients with latex allergy, contact of the skin or oral mucosa with latex-containing gloves during dental treatment can precipitate symptoms of mouth swelling (Figure 4.2) along with systemic symptoms of wheezing and urticaria, and can progress to anaphylaxis. It is therefore imperative to avoid latex-containing products when treating such patients. Latex-free products should be used where possible to avoid sensitisation of staff and patients.

Patients with latex allergy may have allergic symptoms on ingestion of these foods as a result of cross-reactivity. This list is not exhaustive.

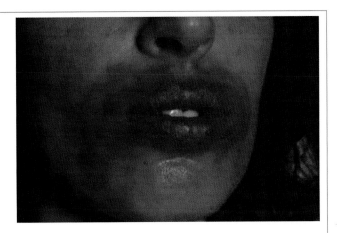

Figure 4.2 A patient allergic to latex who has undergone treatment using a rubber dam.

Table 4.9 Products containing chlorhexidine digluconate.

Mouthwash

Toothpaste

Adhesives and dressings

Ointments

Swabs for disinfection

Lubricant gels for catheterization

Other agents associated with type I hypersensitivity reactions in dental practice

Chlorhexidine

Type I hypersensitivity reactions to chlorhexidine occur, but are uncommon, given the widespread use of this chemical (Table 4.9). Minor reactions have been described, but cases of anaphylaxis rarely occur. Diagnosis is made from clinical history, specific IgE tests and skin prick tests.

Local anaesthetics

Local anaesthetics are widely used in dental practice, and allergic reactions to them are very rare. Other reactions, such as vasovagal episodes and tachycardia secondary to intravascular administration of adrenaline (contained in most dental local anaesthetic preparations), can occur. The investigation method of choice to confirm/exclude allergy to local anaesthetics is the skin prick test.

Treatment of type I hypersensitivity reactions

Allergic reactions can be subdivided into minor/limited or major systemic types.

Minor reactions

These include urticarial rashes and non-life-threatening oedema (i.e. not involving the airway). Treatment of these reactions is with oral antihistamines such as cetirizine and acrivastine rather than with the less potent, more sedating antihistamines such as chlorphenamine (chlorpheniramine). Corticosteroids are sometimes added to the treatment if the swelling is marked.

Major reactions/anaphylaxis

Anaphylactic reactions are the most serious allergic reactions. They have a rapid onset and may even lead to death. These reactions may be associated with upper airway narrowing, asthma symptoms, tachycardia, hypotension and shock. Symptoms may progress to respiratory or cardiovascular arrest. Treatment includes intramuscular adrenaline. Intramuscular/intravenous/oral antihistamine and an inhaled β-agonist may be given if there are asthmatic symptoms. Oxygen and intravenous fluids should be given when available and, if hypotensive, the patient should be placed in the supine position. Guidelines for the treatment of anaphylaxis are given in Chapter 21 (titled 'Medical emergencies'). The patient should be urgently transferred to a hospital for further management.

Other reactions

Type IV hypersensitivity reactions (contact allergy) are implicated in the pathogenesis of some other oral conditions, including stomatitis, oral erythema and cheilitis. Patch tests are widely used in the diagnosis of these reactions. Possible allergens are applied in a standardised form to a healthy area of the patient's skin. The allergens are removed 48 hours later. An eczematous reaction occurring 48–72 hours after initial application suggests that the patient is sensitised to that allergen (Figure 4.3).

Stomatitis

Oral lichenoid reactions cause patients to complain of soreness in the mouth, and can result in oral ulceration. Some patients with this condition have been found to have type IV sensitivity to mercury and other metals, including gold, cobalt, tin, silver and palladium. Patch testing may be useful in identifying this problem. Removal of amalgam adjacent to the lesions may lead to improvement even when patients are patch test negative, as these metals can also act as irritants.

Oral erythema

Redness of the mouth may also be due to type IV hypersensitivity, and implicated substances include acrylates in restorative materials and metals including palladium, gold or manganese. Interestingly, intraoral exposure to nickel before ear-piercing appears to result in a lower incidence of nickel allergy in these patients. Sensitivity to certain toothpastes can also occur in susceptible patients.

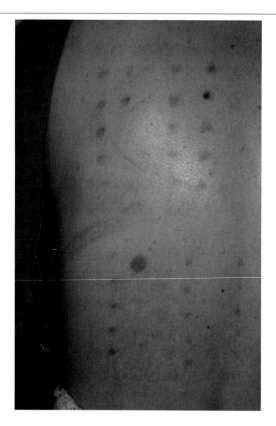

Figure 4.3 Patch testing.

Cheilitis

Cheilitis is an inflammatory eruption on the lip, and may occur due to contact allergy in some patients, but also irritancy (e.g. licking lip), atopic dermatitis and iron deficiency. Multiple substances have been described to cause cheilitis, including medicaments, toothpaste ingredients, denture cleanser components, lipstick and lip salve components, colophonium in dental floss and nickel in the mouthpiece of a musical instrument. Patch testing may be necessary to establish the cause.

Autoimmune disease

The immune system must balance the need to respond to a vast array of possible pathogens, but without reacting to its own self-molecules. If a response to self-molecules occurs, then autoimmune disease is the result. Tolerance is the mechanism by which self-reactive cells are destroyed or kept in check. Autoimmune diseases occur when there is a loss of self-tolerance mechanisms. Tolerance occurs as a multilayered mechanism in which each layer should remove the most self-reactive cells, with lower layers catching cells that slip through tolerance induction in the upper layers. These mechanisms operate both in the central lymphoid organs, where the lymphocytes are initially produced, and in the periphery, where the cells are circulating. The mechanisms involved include

Systemic autoimmune disease	Organ-specific autoimmune disease
SLE	Type 1 diabetes
Sjögren syndrome	Autoimmune thyroid disease
Behçet's syndrome	Addison's disease
Rheumatoid arthritis	Coeliac disease
Scleroderma	Pemphigus/pemphigoid

Table 4.10 Types of autoimmune disease.

deletion, inactivation of self-reactive cells and suppression. Tolerance may be broken by infections that can express molecules resembling the self-molecules, or by providing a very strong activation signal.

In order for autoimmunity to occur, an individual must express the appropriate cell surface molecules that can present a self-antigen (major histocompatibility complex, MHC). These molecules are inherited, and these types of molecules play a major role in determining susceptibility to autoimmune disease. Additional environmental factors such as drugs or infections are also required to break the layers of tolerance mechanisms.

Autoimmune disease can be classified into systemic or organ-specific varieties (see Table 4.10).

Examples of autoimmune disease seen in dental practice

Organ specific

Autoimmune thyroid disease

Hyperthyroidism is associated with symptoms of weight loss, anorexia, diarrhoea, anxiety, tremor, sweating and exophthalmos. If the patient is undiagnosed, this can be an anaesthetic risk. Carbimazole, which is used for the treatment of hyperthyroidism, can cause agranulocytosis (a marked reduction in white cells), which can lead to oropharyngeal ulceration.

Hypothyroidism is associated with weight gain, hypothermia, lethargy, dry skin, cardiac failure, ischaemic heart disease and anaemia. Analgesics and sedatives including general anaesthetics can precipitate a severe exacerbation of this condition, known as 'myxoedema coma'.

Addison's disease

Autoimmune adrenal insufficiency can present with symptoms of fatigue and depression, and it can be associated with a spectrum of other endocrine diseases. Signs of the condition include increased pigmentation of skin folds, buccal mucosa and scars. An Addisonian crisis, which can be precipitated by anaesthetics or dental treatment, will cause collapse, abdominal pain and hypotension.

Type 1 diabetes mellitus

Type 1 diabetes mellitus is associated with immunologically mediated destruction of the pancreatic islets of Langerhans, resulting in defective insulin production and hyperglycaemia. Oral complications include candidal infection, dry mouth, sialosis and glossitis. Severe periodontitis may upset glycaemic control. Patients are prone to increased superficial infections and poor wound healing. Vigorous treatment of oral and facial infections is required. Diabetes mellitus is considered more fully in Chapter 13 (titled 'Endocrinology and diabetes').

Coeliac disease

This is a common inflammatory disease of the small intestine, triggered by gluten. Gluten activates a series of immunological mechanisms that lead to small intestinal damage. Affected individuals have poor energy, failure to thrive in childhood, diarrhoea or constipation, anaemia and aphthous ulcers. Patients may also describe a blistering skin rash, called 'dermatitis herpetiformis'. The treatment is a strict gluten-free diet.

Autoimmune skin conditions

Bullous pemphigoid is seen most commonly in the elderly. The appearance is of subepidermal blisters, but the mucous membranes are usually spared. Treatment is with immunosuppression.

Pemphigus vulgaris is a rare blistering disorder associated with non-healing erosions of mucous membranes. Flaccid blisters are seen on the skin. Treatment is with high-dose steroids.

Systemic autoimmunity

Rheumatoid arthritis (RA)

RA is a common systemic autoimmune disease that is characterised by chronic inflammation of the joints, which leads to progressive joint destruction. Diagnosis is clinical. Some patients will have ulceration and neutropenia, lymphadenopathy and Sjögren syndrome (see the following text). Treatment may involve significant immunosuppression.

Scleroderma

Scleroderma is a multisystem disorder that is characterised by fibrosis of the connective tissue. Oral manifestations include periarticular involvement of the temporomandibular joint with microstomia; constriction of the oral orifice; thickened, stiffened tongue; oral telangiectasia; and widening of the periodontal membrane space without tooth mobility. If a general anaesthetic is to be considered, potential problems include dysphagia, and pulmonary, cardiac and renal disease.

SLE

SLE is a multisystem disease. There is no typical presentation, and the disease can affect multiple organ systems. Haematological complications – including thrombocytopaenia with increased bleeding tendency, low white cell counts, venous thrombosis and haemolytic anaemia – as well as hepatitis and renal disease (glomerulonephritis or nephritic syndrome) can occur. Cutaneous manifestations include mouth ulcers, photosensitive facial rash (typically butterfly distribution), alopecia and Raynaud's phenomenon (discoloration of extremities on exposure to cold). Treatment of SLE involves immunosuppressants.

Sjögren syndrome

Sjögren syndrome is the triad of dry eyes, dry mouth and associated inflammatory arthritis. In addition to the dry mouth, other dental features include increased cariogenic diet (because of impaired sense of taste), gingivitis, difficulty swallowing, candida infection, angular stomatitis and ascending parotitis. Salivary glands may be enlarged.

Vasculitis

The term 'vasculitis' refers to inflammation affecting blood vessels. The effects of this can be varied, depending on the size and location of the vessels affected. Vasculitis can be primary or secondary. Secondary causes include autoimmune conditions such as RA and SLE, drugs, infections and malignancy. Primary vasculitis may be classified based on the size and type of vessels affected, along with the presence or absence of granulomata (see Table 4.11).

Table 4.11 Classification of primary vasculitis (2012 International Chapel Hill Consensus).

Small-vessel vasculitis
- Antineutrophil cytoplasmic antibody (ANCA)–associated vasculitis
- Microscopic polyangiitis (MPA)
- Granulomatosis with polyangiitis (Wegener's granulomatosis)
- Eosinophilic granulomatosis with polyangiitis (Churg–Strauss syndrome)
- Immune complex–mediated small vessel vasculitis
- Anti-glomerular basement membrane (anti-GBM) antibody disease
- Henoch–Schönlein purpura
- Cryoglobulinaemic vasculitis
- Behçet's syndrome
- Hypocomplementaemic urticarial vasculitis (HUV)

Medium-vessel vasculitis
- Kawasaki disease
- Polyarteritis nodosa (PAN)

Large-vessel vasculitis
- Takayasu's disease
- Giant cell arteritis

Variable-vessel vasculitis
- Cogan syndrome
- Behçet's syndrome
- Single organ vasculitis
- Vasculitis associated with systemic disease
- Vasculitis associated with probable aetiology

Table 4.12 Clinical features of vasculitis.

Cutaneous	Purpuric rash, urticaria, ulceration, nodular skin lesions
Renal disease	Nephritis
Gastrointestinal	Gastrointestinal haemorrhage, colic, vomiting, pancreatitis
Pulmonary	Haemorrhage
CNS	Headache, disturbance of higher mental functions, stroke
Cardiac	Myocardial fibrosis, endocarditis, pericarditis, hypertension
Other features	Fever, weight loss, myalgia, arthralgia, conjunctivitis, uveitis, nasal crusting, sinusitis

The clinical features of vasculitis vary, depending on the conditions (see Table 4.12). Diagnosis is made using the history, along with clinical features, biopsy results and laboratory findings, including raised inflammatory markers (CRP and ESR), low complement levels and raised eosinophil count in Churg–Strauss syndrome. ANCAs may be found in Wegener's granulomatosis, microscopic polyarteritis and polyarteritis nodosa. Treatment of vasculitis includes immunosuppressant therapy. The clinical features of vasculitis are shown in Table 4.12.

Behçet's syndrome

Behçet's syndrome has significant oral manifestations, and therefore may present early to dental personnel. Patients with Behçet's suffer with the clinical triad of aphthous-type oral ulceration, genital ulcers and iritis. Ulceration can be severe, and oral symptoms may pre-date the other features. In addition, there are associated skin lesions such as erythema nodosum, folliculitis and pathergy (defined as a papule >2 mm, 24–48 hours after needle prick).

IgG4-related disease

IgG-related disease is a recently recognised disease entity. Swellings of organs or nodules of organs can occur and affect a number of organs / organ systems, including the GI tract, lymph nodes, salivary and lacrimal glands, eyes, heart, thyroid, lungs, kidneys and skin. About 60–70% of patients will have raised IgG4. Dentists would mainly encounter the disease when it affects the submandibular salivary glands (a condition previously referred to as 'Küttner's tumours'). It is a differential diagnosis for chronic obstructive sialadenitis. Around 60–90% of people with IgG4-related disease have multiple organ involvement.

Immunosuppressants

As their name suggests, this group of drugs suppresses aspects of the immune system. Most target the induction phase of the immune system, reducing lymphocyte proliferation.

Table 4.13 Immunosuppressants and their targets within the immune system.

Drug	Target within the immune system
Ciclosporin and tacrolimus	Inhibits IL-2 production and action; specific effect on T-helper cells
Corticosteroids	Inhibits cytokine gene expression
Azathioprine	Inhibits purine synthesis
Cyclophosphamide	Binds and cross-links DNA, preventing interference with DNA replication and transcription (alkylating agent)
Methotrexate	Competitive inhibitor of dihydrofolate reductase; interferes with thymidine and, therefore, DNA synthesis
Mycophenolate mofetil	Blocks synthesis of guanine
Monoclonal antibodies	Antibodies of a single specificity, available to multiple cytokine and receptor targets, and resulting in immunodeficiency and increased infection risk; examples include: • Anti-tumour necrosis factor (anti-TNF) (infliximab, etanercept, adalimumab) • Anti CD20 (rituximab) • Anti-interleukin-6 (anti IL6) (tocilizumab)

Immunosuppressants are used to treat a wide variety of autoimmune conditions, vasculitides and in the prevention of post-transplant graft rejection. Table 4.13 shows the categories of drugs that are immunosuppressants, and the aspects of the immune system they target.

Dental problems of immunosuppressed patients

All immunosuppressed patients are at increased risk of infection and malignancy as compared with untreated individuals. Oral steroids also result in poor wound healing, and there is an increased risk of peptic ulceration with aspirin and nonsteroidal anti-inflammatory drugs. In addition, some immunosuppressive drugs such as ciclosporin can have specific drug-related effects on the oral mucosa, such as gingival overgrowth.

Fungal infections

Candidiasis remains the most frequent fungal infection in these patients. Candida species are highly opportunistic, and are present in a dormant yeast phase in a significant percentage of the population. Both local and systemic factors help the yeast develop into its pathogenic (pseudohyphal) form, when it can present with a variety of clinical manifestations.

These include both acute and chronic pseudomembranous (thrush) and erythematous conditions, specific details of which can be found in most standard texts on oral medicine. Management of these infections usually involves antifungal medications and eliminating local factors, such as poor denture hygiene (see Chapter 3, titled 'Principles of infection and infection control'). However, in immunocompromised individuals, such pharmacological regimens may need to be protracted, and subsequently the infections may frequently recur. The incidence and severity of fungal infection depends on the degree of immunosuppression – the more intensive the drug regimen, the higher the risk of candidiasis. Oral candidal infections in immunosuppressed patients show a variable response to topical antifungal infections. Some are resistant to topical therapy. In these cases, systemic fluconazole is the drug of choice. However, fluconazole does inhibit the hepatic metabolism of ciclosporin, which increases the risk of ciclosporin-induced nephrotoxicity. It is important to liaise with the patient's physician if fluconazole is required in organ transplant patients.

Viral infections

The other group of oral infections that the immunocompromised are susceptible to are viral – particularly the herpes group (e.g. herpes simplex; see Figure 4.4) and the varicella zoster virus (VCV). As with *C. albicans*, a significant proportion of the population carry these viruses in a latent form, having acquired them during childhood. Later infection is the result of reactivation due to the immunocompromised host being unable to mount a sufficient immune response to the viral particles. These infections can and do occur in otherwise healthy individuals as 'cold sores' in the case of herpes simplex, and as shingles in VZV. In these instances, the infections are usually self-limiting and rarely of any long-term significance. However, in the immunocompromised individual, both infections can be more serious, and, in the case of herpes simplex, can lead to potentially life-threatening conditions such as herpes encephalitis. Obviously, in such patients, aggressive management with antiviral medication (see Chapter 3, titled

'Principles of infection and infection control') is required, and should be implemented at the earliest opportunity.

Other viral infections, such as those caused by the papilloma virus group, are also common in the immunocompromised, often presenting as papillomatous (wartlike) lesions that can occur anywhere on the skin, as well as intraorally. Other virus-related lesions that occur in immunosuppressed patients include hairy leukoplakia, which is related to the Epstein–Barr virus; this can be a feature in patients with HIV.

Immunocompromised individuals are also susceptible to a range of infections that are less likely to affect healthy persons. Careful assessment, in conjunction with the microbiology service and other clinicians involved in their care, is needed in both the diagnosis and management of these cases.

Malignancy

Immunosuppressed patients appear to be more susceptible to the development of malignant neoplasms. Malignancies that are more common in these patients include lymphomas, skin and lip cancers and Kaposi's sarcoma. It is also recognised that the various malignant neoplasms occur 20–30 years earlier in such patients than is expected in non-immunosuppressed individuals. Squamous and basal cell carcinomas appear to be a particular problem in organ transplant patients, and the dental surgeon is often the first to recognise such lesions (Chapter 11, titled 'Musculoskeletal disorders'). Any suspicious lesion should be biopsied, and the patient should be given advice on limiting exposure to sunlight and against smoking.

Ciclosporin-induced gingival overgrowth

Approximately 30% of patients taking ciclosporin experience gingival overgrowth that warrants surgical excision. If the patient is also taking nifedipine, this incidence increases to 50%. Ciclosporin-induced gingival overgrowth most frequently affects the anterior part of the mouth. The overgrowth can be extensive, affecting chewing and speech.

Risk factors for the development and expression of gingival overgrowth include the patient's underlying periodontal status, age (with young people being more susceptible), various pharmacokinetic parameters and a genetic predisposition.

Drug-induced gingival overgrowth, irrespective of the initiating drug, does impede mechanical plaque removal. The subsequent plaque-induced gingival inflammation enhances the drug-induced gingival changes. Ciclosporin-induced gingival overgrowth is characterised by a significant increase in the connective tissue component. The target cell appears to be the gingival fibroblast. The interactions among ciclosporin, gingival fibroblasts and inflammation appears to be key to the pathogenesis of this unwanted effect.

Gingival surgery (gingivectomy) remains the treatment of choice for all drug-induced gingival overgrowth. This can be completed under local anaesthesia in an outpatient setting. Recurrence of gingival overgrowth is high in all ciclosporin-treated patients, but the rate of recurrence can be reduced by

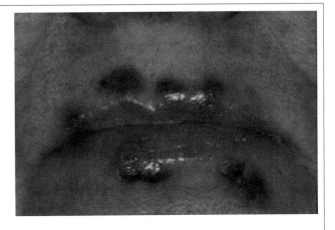

Figure 4.4 Herpetic lip infection.

treating any underlying periodontal disease. This does reduce the inflammatory component in the gingival tissues. Tacrolimus has a similar mode of action to ciclosporin; however, tacrolimus does not cause gingival overgrowth.

FURTHER READING

Additional clinical information and illustrations may be found at: www.dermnetz.org.

Online basic immunology resource: http://bitesized.immunology.org/

MULTIPLE CHOICE QUESTIONS

1. Which of the following is *not* part of the innate immune system?
   a) Tears
   b) CD8+ T-cells
   c) Neutrophils
   d) The complement system
   e) Phagocytes
   Answer = B

2. Which of the following is a true statement about the action of the complement system?
   a) Manufactures antibodies
   b) Engulfs bacteria
   c) Produces cytokines
   d) Acts as a physical defence against infection
   e) Attracts phagocytic cells to the site of infection
   Answer = E

3. Which of the following is a possible cause of a primary immunodeficiency?
   a) Lymphoma
   b) HIV
   c) Chronic mucocutaneous candidiasis
   d) Immunosuppressive drugs
   e) Protein-losing enteropathy
   Answer = C

4. Which of the following is *not* a method of testing for allergic disease?
   a) Skin prick tests
   b) Patch test
   c) Challenge tests
   d) Specific IgE tests
   e) IgG4
   Answer = E

5. Which of the following statements is true when using skin prick testing in the diagnosis of type 1 allergies?
   a) Expensive
   b) Takes a long time to perform
   c) Useful in patients with severe eczema
   d) Better sensitivity compared with specific IgE testing
   e) Can be performed in patients taking regular antihistamines
   Answer = D

6. Which of the following is *not* a risk factor for the development of latex allergy?
   a) Healthcare workers using latex gloves
   b) Hand eczema
   c) Multiple surgical procedures
   d) Spina bifida
   e) Penicillin allergy
   Answer = E

7. In anaphylaxis, the correct initial dose of adrenaline to be administered intramuscularly is:
   a) 0.5 ml 1:10 000
   b) 1 ml 1:10 000
   c) 1 ml 1:1000
   d) 0.5 ml 1:1000
   e) 1.5 ml 1:1000
   Answer = D

8. What is the mechanism of action of methotrexate?
   a) Inhibits IL-2 production and action
   b) Alkylating agent
   c) Blocks synthesis of guanine
   d) Biologic targeted monoclonal antibody
   e) Competitive inhibitor of dihydrofolate reductase
   Answer = E

9. Behçet's syndrome is *not* associated with:
   a) Oral ulceration
   b) Genital ulceration
   c) Vitamin B_{12} deficiency
   d) Iritis
   e) Pathergy
   Answer = C

10. Which of the following is defined as an organ-specific autoimmune disease?
   a) Autoimmune thyroid disease
   b) SLE
   c) Sjögren syndrome
   d) Behçet's syndrome
   e) Rheumatoid arthritis
   Answer = A

CHAPTER 5
Cardiovascular disorders

RH Jay, G Stansby, T Barakat, RA Seymour, JG Meechan, CM Robinson,
M Greenwood, S Hogg and A Balakrishnan

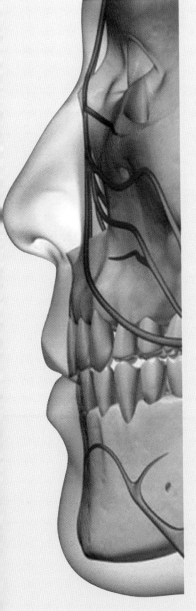

Key topics

- An overview of the major cardiovascular disorders.
- An overview of the main drugs used to treat cardiovascular disorders and their impact on the practice of dentistry.
- Current guidelines with regard to antibiotic prophylaxis in cardiac patients at increased risk from bacteraemia-producing dental procedures.

Learning objectives

- To be familiar with the common cardiovascular disorders and their relevance to dentistry.
- To be aware of the main drugs used to treat cardiovascular disorders and their potential impact on dental practice.
- To be aware of the features of cardiovascular disease and its treatment that may be encountered by dental practitioners.

Essentials of Human Disease in Dentistry, Second Edition. Mark Greenwood.
© 2018 John Wiley & Sons Ltd. Published 2018 by John Wiley & Sons Ltd.
Companion website: www.wiley.com/go/greenwood/human-disease-in-dentistry

5A INTRODUCTION TO CARDIOVASCULAR DISEASE (CVD)

The term 'cardiovascular disease' embraces those conditions affecting the heart and blood vessels. In order to understand these conditions, it is necessary to have a basic understanding of the structure and function of the heart and vascular system.

The heart and circulation

Arteries are thick-walled, high-pressure vessels that conduct blood from the heart to the tissues, while *veins* are thin-walled, low-pressure vessels returning blood to the heart. To complete a full circuit from the left ventricle, oxygenated blood must pass via the systemic arteries to a tissue capillary bed where oxygen is taken up by the tissues. Deoxygenated blood returns via the systemic veins to the right side of the heart, and thence through the pulmonary artery to the pulmonary capillaries, where it is re-oxygenated. The pulmonary veins return the blood to the left side of the heart. Figure 5A.1 represents a schematic view of the heart and blood circulation.

The heart comprises four chambers that pump the blood, with four valves to prevent retrograde flow. The left side of the heart receives oxygenated blood from the lungs, via the

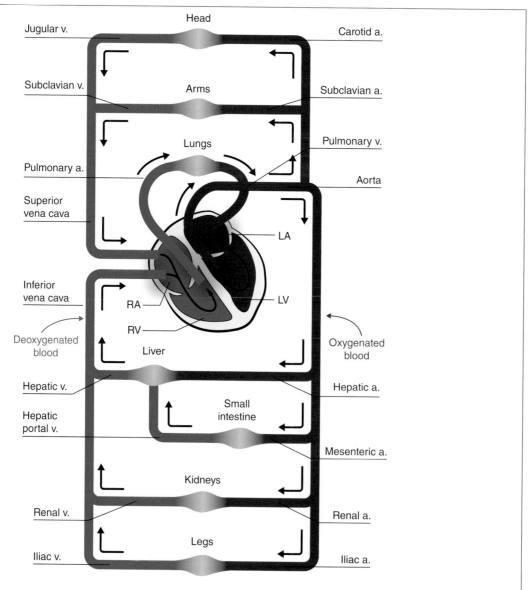

Figure 5A.1 The heart and circulation.

pulmonary veins, into the left atrium. Blood flows from here, through the mitral valve, filling the left ventricle, aided by atrial systole (contraction of the left atrium). Ventricular systole ejects blood from the left ventricle through the aortic valve into the aorta, and thence the systemic arterial circulation and capillaries. During ventricular systole, the mitral valve closes to prevent blood flowing backwards into the left atrium, and the aortic valve opens to allow forward flow from the left ventricle.

The right atrium receives deoxygenated blood from the systemic veins via the inferior and superior venae cavae. The blood passes through the tricuspid valve into the right ventricle. Right ventricular systole closes the tricuspid valve and propels the blood through the pulmonary valve into the pulmonary artery, which divides and takes the blood to both lungs.

During diastole, the heart muscle relaxes, and the mitral and tricuspid valves open to allow ventricular filling, while the aortic and pulmonary valves close to prevent retrograde flow from the aorta and pulmonary artery into the ventricles.

Electrical control

Contraction and relaxation of the cardiac muscle is coordinated by specialised electrical tissues. The sinoatrial node, situated in the right atrium, acts as the pacemaker, which stimulates atrial contraction. This occurs in a wave, with the electrical activity and consequent contraction spreading across both atria towards the atrioventricular (AV) node. The AV node detects the atrial

depolarisation and conducts it, after a short pause, via the bundle of His and the Purkinje fibres to both ventricles. These then depolarise and contract together to eject the blood. A diagram of the cardiac conduction system is given in Figure 5A.2.

Cardiac circulation

The blood supply to the myocardium is carried via the right and left coronary arteries, which branch from the aorta immediately above the aortic valve. These are 'end arteries', which means that any blockage cannot be bypassed, and will result in damage to the area of muscle supplied by the blocked artery. Venous blood passes via the coronary veins to the coronary sinus, which runs in the atrioventricular groove, and drains directly into the right atrium.

Cardiovascular pathology

CVD is the main cause of death in most Western societies. For example, in the UK, more than one in three people (38%) die of CVD, and it is also one of the main causes of premature death (death before the age of 75 years). The main forms of CVD are coronary heart disease and cerebral vascular disease.

Atherosclerosis

Atherosclerosis is the most common vascular disease, and it affects only arteries. It is important in the pathogenesis of both coronary heart disease and cerebral vascular disease.

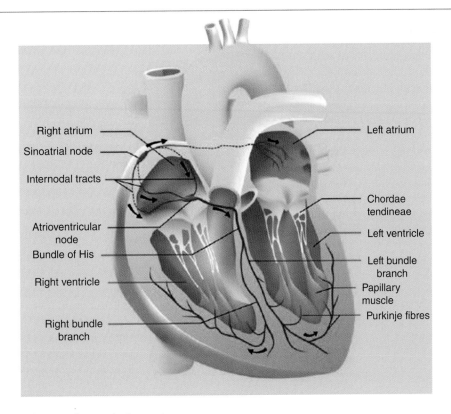

Figure 5A.2 A diagram of the cardiac conducting system.

Definitions

Atheroma is a condition that is characterised by the focal accumulation of lipid deposits in the tunica intima of arteries. The lipid deposits have a porridge-like texture and appearance, which is how the condition derives its name (*athere* is Greek for 'gruel'). Fibrosis develops in association with the lipid deposits, resulting in hardening or 'sclerosis' – hence the term 'atherosclerosis', which is used synonymously with 'atheroma'.

Risk factors

The cause of atherosclerosis is unknown; however, there are risk factors that are associated with the development of the disease (summarised in Table 5A.1).

The incidence of atherosclerosis increases with *age*. Up to the age of 55 years, the incidence in *males* is much higher than in females. In fact, significant disease is rare in women before the onset of menopause; for this reason, it has been proposed that oestrogen has a protective effect on arteries. Following menopause, the incidence of atherosclerosis in women rapidly increases, approaching the rates found in males.

Cigarette smoking increases the risk of developing the disease, and is a particularly strong risk factor in young males. *Hypertension* and *diabetes mellitus* are important systemic conditions that predispose the affected individuals to the development of atheroma. *Family history* is significant because individuals with a first-degree relative who has prematurely suffered the consequences of atherosclerosis are at increased risk of developing the disease.

Raised low-density lipoprotein (LDL) cholesterol levels in the blood is the most consistent abnormality found in patients with atherosclerosis, although the disease may also develop in those with normal levels of LDL cholesterol.

Lipid metabolism is a complex process that is influenced by both genetic and environmental factors. Some individuals have a genetic defect in an important lipid receptor, which results in persistently elevated serum levels of LDL cholesterol and the early development of coronary heart disease, usually by the fifth decade. These observations, in addition to epidemiological data and clinical evidence, led to the development of the 'diet

Table 5A.1 Risk factors for CVD.

Smoking
Hypertension
Diabetes mellitus
Hypercholesterolaemia
Family history of CVD
Sedentary lifestyle
Obesity
Age
Excess alcohol

heart hypothesis' – that high dietary fat intake leads to elevated LDL cholesterol and the development of atheroma. However, the hypothesis is controversial, and not all subscribe to this view. In contrast, elevated levels of high-density lipoprotein (HDL) correlate with reduced risk of heart disease. Other, 'weaker' risk factors include obesity, lack of exercise and low socioeconomic status.

Pathogenesis of atherosclerosis

Atherosclerosis affects medium- and large-calibre arteries and develops through three morphological stages:
- Fatty streak.
- Fibrolipid plaque.
- Complicated plaque.

The fatty streak is a subclinical lesion. The fibrolipid plaque is usually silent, but can produce clinical effects if there is significant narrowing of the arterial lumen. Progression to the complicated plaque is associated with the development of clinically significant disease. The fatty streak is an accumulation of lipid in the intima of the artery wall, just below the endothelial lining of the vessel. The lipid lies free and is also contained within macrophages, the so-called 'foamy macrophages'. Fatty streaks have been observed in all age groups, including in children.

The fibrolipid plaque is characterised by the deposition of collagen and progressive fibrosis. The lesion has a fibrous cap that bulges into the lumen of the vessel. Beneath the cap, there are pools of lipid that contain cholesterol clefts and numerous foamy macrophages. The internal elastic lamina fragments and smooth muscle cells from the tunica media migrate into the lesion, and lymphocytes also start to accumulate. In the complicated plaque, the fibrous cap becomes unstable and develops surface defects, referred to as 'ulcers' or 'intraplaque fissures'. This exposes the flowing blood to plaque contents, and, consequently, thrombosis (see the following sections) develops over the plaque (Figure 5A.3).

The thrombus may partially or completely occlude the vessel lumen. Thrombosis over a plaque will often have serious consequences, especially in narrow vessels such as the coronary arteries, and partially occlusive thrombi are a cause of embolism (see the following sections). The damaged artery may also show progressive calcification. In some cases, damage to the elastic tissue and smooth muscle of the vessel, as a consequence of inflammation, results in gradual permanent dilation of the artery, forming aneurysms (see the following sections).

Some of the molecular changes that are associated with the development of atherosclerosis have been elucidated. For example, cell adhesion molecules (ICAM-1 and E-selectin) are important in recruiting macrophages into the fatty streak and early fibrolipid plaque. Platelet-derived growth factor (PDGF) is thought to be pivotal in the progression of the lesion, as it stimulates the proliferation of smooth muscle cells and fibroblasts and increases the deposition of collagen, elastin and other matrix proteins within the lesion.

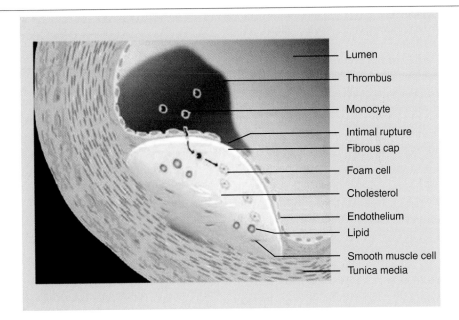

Figure 5A.3 A complicated atheromatous plaque.

Drugs used in the prevention of atherosclerosis

Various drugs are used to reduce plasma lipids. These include statins such as simvastatin, fibrates (e.g. bezafibrate), nicotinic acid, ezetimibe and bile acid sequestrants such as colestyramine.

The statins are the first-line treatment. They hinder cholesterol synthesis by inhibiting the 3-hydroxy-3-methylglutaryl-coenzyme A enzyme. Statins are of interest to dentists as they can interfere with some drugs that may be used in the management of oral diseases. Myopathy is a side effect of the statins, and the chances of this are increased if erythromycin is given to patients taking atorvastatin or simvastatin. Similarly, the antifungal agents ketoconazole and miconazole increase the risk of myopathy in individuals taking simvastatin.

Consequences of atherosclerosis

Atherosclerosis has its main effects on medium- to large-calibre arteries, and is most commonly present in areas of haemodynamic stress (e.g. at arterial bifurcations). The arteries most commonly affected are:

- Coronary arteries.
- Cerebral arteries.
- Aorta.
- Mesenteric arteries.
- Iliac and femoral arteries.

The consequences are rather distinct for each named conduit, and the clinical features are dependent on the regions that the blood vessels perfuse. In addition, the precise clinical syndrome depends on whether the atheroma causes reduction of flow to the organ or tissue, or if it completely occludes the vessel. For example, atherosclerosis of the coronary arteries will cause angina, whereas thrombosis may cause myocardial infarction (MI). Thrombosis over plaques in the vessels at the base of the brain can cause cerebral infarction (stroke).

Thrombosis over atheroma within the aorta can sometimes cause symptoms associated with systemic embolism, but the more common clinical syndrome associated with disease at this site is the *abdominal aortic aneurysm* (AAA). Thrombosis over plaques in the mesenteric vessels may produce small bowel infarction, rupture and subsequent peritonitis. Atheroma of the iliac and femoral vessels causes intermittent claudication (leg pain and weakness brought on by walking) and, when thrombosis develops, gangrene of the lower extremities.

Aneurysms

An *aneurysm* is a localised permanent abnormal dilatation of a blood vessel due to weakening of the blood vessel wall. The most common aneurysms are those that develop because of atheroma, but other conditions such as connective tissue disorders can also cause them.

Aortic atherosclerotic aneurysms form either at the arch of the aorta, the thoracic aorta or within the abdominal aorta just above the bifurcation of the iliac arteries. The last is the most frequent site for aortic aneurysm, and presents with a pulsatile abdominal mass and, sometimes, lower limb ischaemia. The biggest risk is that the aneurysm may rupture and cause a torrential and often fatal retroperitoneal bleed.

Berry aneurysm affects the circle of Willis at the base of the brain. This aneurysm is a small, saccular dilatation that develops at points of branching on the circle of Willis. They typically develop in young hypertensive individuals who have defects in the muscular wall of the arteries that comprise the circle of Willis. These defects cause areas of weakness, which predisposes to aneurysm formation. Rupture of a berry aneurysm causes subarachnoid haemorrhage.

Other aneurysms are caused by infection, and are termed *mycotic aneurysms*. Mycotic aneurysms are a consequence of localised infection of an arterial wall. One well-recognised source of infection is the embolic material produced during infective endocarditis, which can produce a mycotic aneurysm at the site of impaction (e.g. the cerebral vessels). Rupture of the latter results in cerebral haemorrhage. *Syphilitic aneurysm*, as the name suggests, is a consequence of chronic *Treponema pallidum* infection. The most common site for syphilitic aneurysm is the root of the aorta, where aortic ring dilatation and valve incompetence classically develops. Although commonly recognised in the past, it is now an exceptionally uncommon disease in Western societies.

Microaneurysms form within capillaries and typically affect cerebral and retinal capillaries. Cerebral microaneurysms are usually seen in hypertensive patients, and retinal microaneurysms in diabetics.

Dissecting aneurysm is actually a blood-filled space within the arterial wall caused by a particular pattern of rupture of the aorta rather than dilatation of the vessel *per se*. The dissecting aneurysm most commonly commences at the arch of the aorta. Initially, there is a small tear in the wall of the aorta, and the high pressures generated during cardiac systole forces blood into the defect, causing the tear to propagate. In some instances, the tear may communicate with the lumen of the aorta at some distance from the initial tear, producing a 'double-barrelled' aorta. Patients are usually elderly and hypertensive; however, dissecting aneurysms are also seen in patients with connective tissue abnormalities (e.g. Marfan's syndrome). Patients classically present with severe interscapular back pain, loss of peripheral pulses or with fatal haemopericardium and/or retroperitoneal haemorrhage.

Thrombosis, embolism, ischaemia and infarction

An understanding of these four terms is important for an understanding of CVD. The terms are inextricably linked; a thrombus once formed may undergo embolism, and both thrombosis and embolism cause ischaemia, leading to infarction.

Definitions

- A *thrombus* is a solid mass of blood constituents formed within the vascular system during life.
- An *embolus* is a mass of material floating free in the vascular system, able to become lodged within a vessel and block its lumen.
- *Ischaemia* is an inappropriate reduction in blood supply to an organ or tissue.
- *Infarction* is death of tissue due to ischaemia.

Thrombosis

There are considered to be three factors that predispose to the formation of a thrombus, known as 'Virchow's triad', first described by Rudolf Virchow, an eminent German pathologist (Table 5A.2).

Virchow postulated that changes in the surface of the vessel, the pattern of blood flow and the blood constituents are important for thrombosis to occur. However, the presence of all three factors at any one time is not an absolute requirement for thrombosis, as it may occur even if the criterion for only one of the factors is fulfilled.

Thrombosis can occur within the arterial or venous system and within the heart (cardiac thrombosis).

Arterial thrombosis

Arterial thrombosis occurs on atheromatous plaques. Smokers in particular have abnormally sticky platelets (change in the blood constituents). The atheromatous plaque protrudes into the lumen of the artery and disturbs the laminar flow of blood, setting up local turbulence (change in the pattern of blood flow). These local currents produce shear forces that can cause endothelial ulceration (changes in the wall of the vessel), which leads to platelet aggregation, activation of the coagulation cascade and deposition of fibrin. Subsequently, erythrocytes tend to get trapped in the fibrin meshwork (see Figures 5A.4, 5A.5 and 5A.6). The thrombus develops layer by layer in an incremental fashion. The first layer is composed of platelets, with a second layer of fibrin and erythrocytes, then platelets, fibrin and erythrocytes, and so on, forming a lamellated structure.

Table 5A.2 The components of thrombosis (Virchow's triad).

Changes in the constituents of the circulating blood
Changes in the flow of blood
Changes in the vessel walls

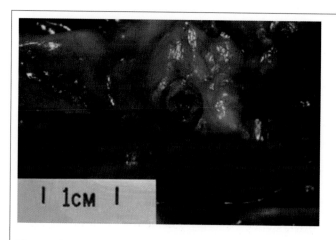

Figure 5A.4 An atheromatous coronary artery.

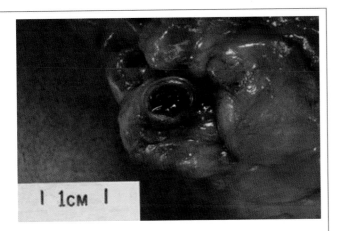

Figure 5A.5 Thrombus in a coronary artery.

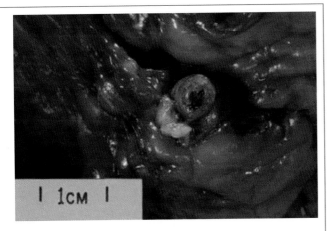

Figure 5A.6 Occluding thrombus in a coronary artery.

Table 5A.3 Risk factors for DVT.
Oestrogen replacement therapy or the oral contraceptive pill
Smoking
Immobility
History of pelvic surgery
Previous history of DVT
Pelvic tumours
Pregnancy
Surgery

painful leg, although many patients do not have typical symptoms and an ultrasound scan is required to make the diagnosis. The most clinically important consequence of DVT is pulmonary embolism. Risk factors for DVT are given in Table 5A.3.

Cardiac thrombosis

Cardiac thrombosis typically affects the chambers of the left side of the heart and occurs on the walls of the heart (mural thrombus) and the heart valves. Atrial thrombosis is caused by atrial fibrillation and mitral valve stenosis. Ventricular thrombosis occurs at the site of MI. Valvular thrombus is a feature of rheumatic fever and infective endocarditis.

It is important to appreciate that thrombosis is a dynamic process. In some instances, thrombosis is reversible, and the thrombus is effectively broken down by the fibrinolytic pathway, a process called 'lysis and resolution'. In other circumstances, there may be attempts at healing; granulation tissue grows into the thrombus, and there is organisation and fibrosis. The latter causes retraction of the thrombus, and the patency of the vessel lumen is restored. The vascular buds that comprise granulation tissue can also lead to recanalisation of an occluded vessel. Progressive fibrosis and scarring of the thrombus and vessel wall can result in a permanent stenosis (narrowing) of the vessel.

Embolism

An *embolus* is a mass of material in the vascular system that can become lodged within a vessel and block its lumen. The most common (90%) embolic material is derived from thrombi. Other causes of embolism include atheromatous debris, heart valve vegetations, tumour emboli, fat droplets, amniotic fluid, gas (caisson disease) and foreign material.

In the context of CVD, embolism caused by thrombotic debris is the most clinically significant, and can have serious consequences for the patient. It may result in sudden death.

Pulmonary embolism

Pulmonary embolism (PE) is the most common clinically recognised embolic event, and is usually derived from fragments of a DVT located in the calf or ileofemoral venous segments.

The incremental layers of the thrombus tend to accumulate on the downstream side of the atheroma, and hence the thrombus grows in the direction of the blood flow – a process called *propagation*.

Venous thrombosis

Venous thrombosis tends to initiate at valves and often develops as a consequence of venous stasis (reduction in the venous blood flow); other predisposing factors include phlebitis (inflammation of a vein) and abnormal blood coagulation factors (thrombophilia). A venous thrombus has the same basic lamellated structure as described for arterial thrombosis, but tends to have a complex pattern of layers, termed a 'coralline thrombus'. Following thrombosis, the vein may become inflamed, a condition called 'thrombophlebitis'. Venous thrombosis typically develops as a consequence of major trauma and burns, following surgery, cardiac failure, immobility and during pregnancy. The deep veins of the leg are the most common (>90%) site for venous thrombosis (deep vein thrombosis, DVT); the typical clinical sign is a swollen and

About 10% of hospital deaths are due to PE. For this reason, thromboprophylaxis with anticoagulants or anti-embolism stockings is very important in all hospital inpatients to decrease this risk. Fragments of thrombi become detached from the site of development in the vein and travel through the venous system to reach the right side of the heart. The embolus is then pumped out through the pulmonary arteries to the lungs. The size of the embolus determines the clinical effects. A large embolus may become lodged at the bifurcation of the pulmonary arteries, so called 'saddle embolus', and cause sudden death. A smaller embolus may lodge in a more peripheral branch of the pulmonary artery, resulting in a wedge-shaped infarct of lung tissue. The patient would typically complain of chest pain and breathlessness, and sometimes cough up blood (haemoptysis). Rarely, multiple tiny emboli can cause numerous small pulmonary infarctions that may be subclinical, but may lead to chronic pulmonary hypertension in some circumstances.

Systemic embolism

Systemic emboli are mainly derived from thrombi in the left side of the heart or those formed on atheromatous plaques. The clinical consequences are related to the size and number of emboli and the site where they lodge. Embolism in cerebral vessels causes cerebral infarction and a transient or permanent neurological deficit (stroke). Smaller emboli may reach the limb extremities and digits, causing areas of infarction and gangrene. Other emboli originating in the aorta may lodge in the spleen or the kidney, causing segmental infarcts, which are usually asymptomatic. Emboli lodging in the mesenteric vessels may cause death of large segments of the small intestine, with bowel perforation and peritonitis.

Ischaemia and infarction

The progression of ischaemia to infarction is determined by a number of factors: vascular anatomy, duration of occlusion, metabolic requirements of the tissue, general circulation, anaemia and the concept of reperfusion injury. If the blood supply to a tissue is predominantly from a single artery and there is little by way of a collateral blood supply, when the main artery becomes occluded, ischaemia ensues and progresses to infarction. The duration of vessel occlusion is important because transient ischaemia may not cause tissue damage. Organs with high metabolic demands (e.g. brain and heart), however, are very susceptible to damage, even from transient ischaemic events. Poor general tissue perfusion (e.g. in heart failure and anaemia) may compound the effects of localised ischaemia and lower the threshold for tissue infarction.

The degree of tissue damage as a consequence of ischaemia is only fully appreciated following reperfusion of the organ or tissue. This is considered to be due in part to the generation of reactive oxygen, causing further tissue damage,

and bystander tissue damage in the face of the ensuing inflammatory response. This phenomenon is known as 'reperfusion injury', and is one of the complications observed following treatment of ischaemia.

In MI, after 6 hours of ischaemia, there are no visible morphological changes in the myocardium. However, there are ECG changes and serological evidence of cardiac damage, which form part of the clinical information required to establish a diagnosis of MI. After 24–48 hours, the myocardium shows a zone of pallor that has a red rim (inflammation).

Microscopically, the cardiac muscle appears to be structurally intact, but the myocytes show loss of their characteristic muscle fibre striations (coagulative necrosis). After several days, the pale dead myocardium becomes soft and is at risk of rupture (haemopericardium; bleeding into the pericardial sac). If the patient survives weeks to months following an MI, the dead tissue is removed by macrophages, and there is healing by fibrosis to produce a grey scar.

Infarction in other organs (lung, kidney and spleen) shows features similar to those described for MI, and is similarly characterised by coagulative necrosis. In contrast, cerebral infarcts undergo colliquative necrosis. The brain has little by way of robust collagenous supporting tissues, and dead glial tissue and neurons undergo liquefactive degeneration (colliquative necrosis), which is essentially completely cleared by macrophages. As a consequence, a patient who survives cerebral infarction is left with a fluid-filled cystic cavity at the site of injury rather than a fibrous scar.

Clinical features of CVD

Symptoms

Chest pain is the cardinal symptom of ischaemic heart disease. In angina pectoris, the coronary arteries, narrowed by atheroma, cannot increase the blood flow to meet the increased demands of the myocardium during exercise. The patient feels a 'tight' or 'heavy' pain across the chest, which commonly radiates to the arms, neck and jaw. It is characteristically brought on by exertion, and is relieved in a few minutes by rest. A differential diagnosis for chest pain is given in Table 5A.4.

When a branch of a coronary artery becomes completely occluded by a thrombus, MI occurs. The chest pain is similar

Table 5A.4 A differential diagnosis of chest pain.

MI
Angina
Gastrooesophageal reflux disease (GORD)
Pleuritic pain
Musculoskeletal pain
Pain secondary to trauma
'Panic attack' (see Chapter 21, titled 'Medical Emergencies')

in nature, but more severe and prolonged. It may be accompanied by sweating, nausea, breathlessness and/or palpitations. It is not relieved by the antianginal drug glyceryl trinitrate (GTN).

Breathlessness, or *dyspnoea*, is a characteristic feature of heart failure. Depending on the severity, it may occur after only moderate exertion, after only minimal effort or even at rest. Back pressure from the poorly functioning left heart causes congestion of the pulmonary veins and capillaries, which can result in oedema fluid leaking into the alveoli and impairing gas transfer. Because of the changes in hydrostatic pressure with posture, breathlessness may be precipitated by lying down – *orthopnoea* – or may wake the patient from sleep – *paroxysmal nocturnal dyspnoea*.

In right heart failure, raised pressure in the systemic veins and capillaries causes leakage of oedema fluid into systemic tissues. The effects of gravity result in swelling of the ankles and legs, often worse in the evenings; this is relieved by the horizontal posture adopted while sleeping at night.

The term 'palpitations' refers to an abnormal awareness of the heartbeat. It may be a symptom of cardiac arrhythmias. A fast heartbeat may be felt as a 'fluttering', and a paused or slow heartbeat may be noted as a 'thump'. It may occur normally after exercise and can be a feature of anxiety.

Loss of consciousness due to lack of blood flow to the brain is termed 'syncope'. Low blood pressure can result in 'pre-syncope', a feeling of faintness or light-headedness without complete loss of consciousness.

Signs detectable in the clothed patient

Breathlessness may be detected by observation and measurement of the respiratory rate (see also Chapter 1, titled 'Clinical examination and history taking'). Greater than 20 breaths/min at rest is significantly abnormal. Pallor may indicate anaemia or a poor cardiac output, with associated cutaneous vasoconstriction. Under these circumstances, the peripheries may feel cold, and the capillary refill may be prolonged. This can be tested by exerting pressure on a fingertip and releasing it. The blanching of the skin produced by the pressure normally resolves in <2 sec (as the capillaries refill with blood).

The pulse may be felt in the radial artery at the wrist. Other useful sites are the brachial artery, in the antecubital fossa (on the medial side of the arm in front of the elbow) and the carotid (below the angle of the jaw). A normal pulse is regular, with a rate of 60–100 beats/min, although a resting pulse as low as 40 beats/min is found in athletic younger people. Occasional irregularities in an otherwise regular pulse usually indicate ectopic beats, and this finding is seldom of serious significance. A completely irregular pulse usually indicates atrial fibrillation. The strength or volume of the pulse can also give clues about heart disease. It may be weak or thready in states of poor cardiac output or shock. Conversely, it can be strong and 'bounding' in states of vasodilation such as thyrotoxicosis or pyrexia (due to infection). Furthermore, the strength of an individual beat is dependent on the amount of blood that has filled the heart. Thus, with an irregular pulse such as in atrial fibrillation, the beat-to-beat volume varies, with strong pulses occurring after a pause, and weak pulses ensuing when the heartbeat occurs early after the previous beat.

Blood pressure is measured using a sphygmomanometer. Automated sphygmomanometers are now widely available, which give a digital reading of the systolic and diastolic pressures. The blood pressure is taken as described in Chapter 5E (titled 'Hypertension'). It is usually measured with the patient sitting, at rest, with the arm resting approximately level with the heart.

A raised jugular venous pressure (JVP) is a sign of venous congestion in heart failure. The venous pulsation is normally visible just above the clavicle, at the root of the neck, in a patient reclining at 45°. In heart failure, the vein is distended to a higher level, and may reach the angle of the jaw or above. Chronic elevation of the venous pressure will result in detectable pitting oedema of the ankles. The swelling may be indented by gentle pressure for a few seconds, and the indentation takes a few minutes to disappear.

Peripheral cyanosis, a blue tinge due to deoxygenated blood in the peripheral circulation, may be a sign of peripheral arterial insufficiency, or may occur in states of poor cardiac output such as heart failure or shock. Central cyanosis, best detected in the lips and tongue, indicates reduced oxygenation of the arterial blood leaving the left heart, and is inevitably associated with peripheral cyanosis. Although it may occur in heart failure, it is more commonly seen in lung disease, or congenital malformations of the heart. Suspected cyanosis can be confirmed by the use of a pulse oximeter, which measures oxygen saturation by a probe on the finger or earlobe.

Clubbing of the fingers occurs in a variety of conditions, including chronic lung diseases and inflammatory bowel disease. In cardiac disease, it may indicate infective endocarditis or congenital heart malformations. Splinter haemorrhages (Figure 5A.7) in the nails are characteristic signs of endocarditis. They appear as small, dark, longitudinal marks under

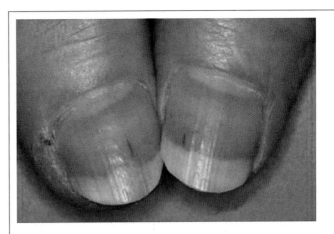

Figure 5A.7 Splinter haemorrhages in infective endocarditis (usually more than five).

the nail. A few small marks at the nail edge are common due to trauma or manual activities. In endocarditis, the splinters are greater in number (>5) and away from the edge of the nail. Other rare signs of endocarditis in the hands include Osler's nodes, which are small, painful nodules in the finger pulp, and Janeway lesions, which are red marks in the palms due to capillaritis.

A full examination of the cardiovascular system includes examination of the heart, lungs and pulses. Auscultation of the heart with a stethoscope may reveal heart murmurs, which are the sounds of turbulent blood flow, usually due to dysfunction of the heart valves. In heart failure, fine crackles or crepitations may be heard at the lung bases. Arterial bruits may be heard over narrowed arteries, and are caused by the turbulence of blood passing through the stenosed segment.

Cardiac investigations

The electrocardiogram (ECG) is recorded from skin electrodes placed over the chest and limbs (Figure 5A.8). It is the definitive test of cardiac rhythm, and can demonstrate changes of both reversible ischaemia in patients with angina and acute MI. ECG monitoring during graded exercise on a treadmill is used to diagnose angina, and to give prognostic information in ischaemic heart disease. A summary of some of the more common cardiac investigation methods is given in Table 5A.5.

The chest X-ray may show enlargement of the cardiac shadow in a variety of heart conditions, particularly heart failure. During an episode of acute left-sided heart failure, the pulmonary veins become visibly engorged, and oedema fluid in the pulmonary alveoli shows as a diffuse patchy shadowing in both lung fields.

Echocardiography provides real-time ultrasound images of the heart via a transducer moved over the chest wall. More invasive trans-oesophageal echocardiograms are used under certain circumstances. The echocardiogram shows the structure and function of the valves, the size and contractility of the chambers and can detect fluid in the pericardium.

Cardiac catheterisation involves the insertion of long catheters into the heart, usually via the femoral artery and vein in the groin, under local anaesthetics. These are used to inject X-ray contrast in coronary angiography, and to obtain measurements of intra-cardiac pressure and oxygen saturation to assess the function of the chambers and valves.

Other imaging techniques such as CT, MRI and radioisotope scanning provide additional information in certain conditions, and can provide some of the information traditionally obtained by cardiac catheterisation in a non-invasive way.

Clinical aspects of MI

MI is a medical emergency where even minutes count. It typically presents with prolonged and severe ischaemic-type chest pain, unresponsive to angina medications. Associated symptoms may include nausea and vomiting, sweating, palpitations, breathlessness and faintness. The patient should be brought by emergency ambulance directly to an emergency chest pain assessment unit or an accident and emergency department equipped to give treatment without delay. Some possible causes of chest pain are listed in Table 5A.4.

If the diagnosis is confirmed by the ECG showing elevation of the ST segment, the standard treatment is by 'percutaneous coronary intervention' – that is, coronary angiography followed by unblocking of the artery using catheter techniques, most commonly balloon angioplasty with the insertion of a stent. Since this is not available in most district hospitals, emergency ambulances are equipped to obtain and interpret the ECG, enabling immediate transport of the patient to a suitable regional cardiothoracic centre. The alternative treatment, that is, administration of thrombolytic drugs by a non-specialist, is now reserved for patients who cannot be transferred to a tertiary centre within the necessary time. MI without ST segment elevation on the ECG is usually less severe, and is initially treated in district hospitals with drugs, including antithrombotic agents and beta blockers, the diagnosis being confirmed or excluded by measurement of troponins, which are released into the blood from damaged myocardial cells.

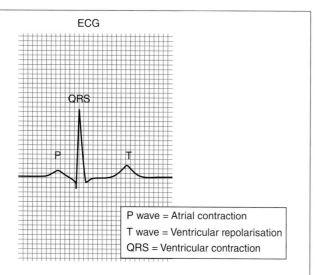

Figure 5A.8 A normal ECG waveform.

ECG

P wave = Atrial contraction
T wave = Ventricular repolarisation
QRS = Ventricular contraction

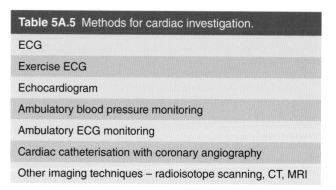

Table 5A.5 Methods for cardiac investigation.
ECG
Exercise ECG
Echocardiogram
Ambulatory blood pressure monitoring
Ambulatory ECG monitoring
Cardiac catheterisation with coronary angiography
Other imaging techniques – radioisotope scanning, CT, MRI

Other aspects of treatment of MI involve symptom relief, monitoring for and treating complications, and secondary prevention. Pain in MI is severe, and is treated with intravenous morphine or diamorphine, along with an antiemetic. The patient has continuous cardiac monitoring to detect arrhythmias or cardiac arrest. Heart failure may occur, and requires intravenous nitrates and diuretics. Echocardiography is used to assess left ventricular function, and ACE inhibitors are started if it is impaired.

All patients are treated with lipid-lowering therapy, β-blockers and antiplatelet drugs. After initial management, the patient's risk of recurrence of future complications is assessed. In particular, those with a non–ST segment elevation MI (NSTEMI) may be at imminent risk of a more severe MI, and other complications include heart failure and arrhythmias. Risk scores and further investigations are used to define the need for more invasive treatment, such as angioplasty, coronary bypass surgery or implantable defibrillators in those at significant risk of sudden death.

Following coronary interventions, most patients are treated with 'dual antiplatelet therapy', a combination of two antiplatelet drugs such as aspirin and clopidogrel, for up to a year. It is important that these not be stopped inappropriately, as there is a high risk of thrombosis with certain types of interventions, particularly drug-eluting stents.

Angina

The diagnosis of angina can often be made from the clinical history, but it is important to differentiate it from other causes of chest pain. Investigations may be required to exclude other causes and to confirm and assess the severity of angina. There are a number of 'stress tests' available to diagnose reversible ischaemia, including the exercise test, in which the ECG is monitored for ST segment changes during graded exercise on a treadmill. Other tests involve using drugs such as dobutamine or adenosine to stress the heart and bring on ischaemia, and then imaging with radioisotopes or echocardiography to detect the altered blood flow during stress.

Initial treatment of angina is with sublingual GTN, usually as a spray, to be used for rapid relief of symptoms. Several classes of drugs are used to prevent attacks, some of which may also affect prognosis. These include β-blockers, calcium channel blockers, longer-acting nitrates such as isosorbide mononitrate, and the potassium channel opener nicorandil. Preventive treatment is by risk factor control, with the routine use of lipid-lowering drugs and antiplatelet agents. In severe or resistant cases, cardiac catheterisation is undertaken and arterial stenoses relieved by either angioplasty with stenting or open coronary bypass surgery.

5B HEART FAILURE

Introduction

The term 'heart failure' refers to the inability of the heart to pump blood strongly enough to meet the body's needs. This may result in too little forward flow into the arterial circulation, resulting in low blood pressure and poor tissue perfusion. Conversely, the venous circulation becomes congested with blood, resulting in increased capillary pressure, which forces fluid from the circulation into the tissues. This increase in extravascular fluid is called *oedema*.

In physiological terms, heart failure occurs when the heart is unable to pump sufficient blood to supply the body's demands. The clinical syndrome of heart failure is characterised by a combination of breathlessness, oedema and fatigue. All of these clinical features may be caused by non-cardiac diseases, and heart failure may also be aggravated by other concomitant non-cardiac conditions.

Pathophysiology

Three clinically important considerations are:
- What is the nature of the cardiac malfunction?
- What are the body's adaptive mechanisms?
- What other conditions may be aggravating or precipitating the heart failure?

Cardiac causes of heart failure

Heart failure may result from disease of the heart muscle (myocardium), the valves or disturbances of the heart rhythm.

Heart muscle dysfunction is most commonly due to ischaemic heart disease or hypertension. The myocardium may be damaged by other causes, including drugs and alcohol, nutritional deficiencies and infections. The term 'cardiomyopathy' is used to cover a group of heart muscle disorders of uncertain cause, some of which are inherited.

Myocardial disease commonly results in left ventricular systolic dysfunction, that is, weakness of the left ventricle, which causes a reduction in the ejection fraction. Normally, >60% of the blood in the ventricle is ejected with each beat, and a reduction to 40% or below is associated with a poor prognosis. The term 'diastolic dysfunction' refers to poor relaxation of the ventricle, resulting in impaired filling. It is commonly seen in elderly and hypertensive patients, particularly if the left ventricle is hypertrophied, but is less easy to define or diagnose than systolic dysfunction. The strength of cardiac contraction is usually proportional to the degree of stretch or the filling pressure. In myocardial disease, the myocardium is less able to adapt to increased filling pressures.

Stenosis (narrowing) of a valve results in pressure overload of the chamber upstream of that valve. Thus, aortic stenosis requires an increased left ventricular pressure to eject the blood, and the ventricle becomes hypertrophied and can eventually fail. Mitral stenosis results in raised left atrial pressure, resulting in dilation of the left atrium.

Valvular regurgitation results in volume overload. For example, in aortic regurgitation, a proportion of the ejected blood returns to the left ventricle from the aorta, and has to be pumped out a second time.

Arrhythmias can precipitate heart failure in an otherwise normal heart. Severe tachycardia impairs cardiac filling during the shortened diastole, while severe bradycardia reduces the number of contractions to maintain cardiac output. The most common chronic arrhythmia is atrial fibrillation, which also impairs left ventricular filling due to the loss of atrial contraction.

Neurohormonal adaptive responses

The circulatory consequences of heart failure, for whatever causes, are:
- Reduced cardiac output.
- Increased intracardiac pressure.
- Increased back pressure in the venous circulation, resulting in increased capillary pressure and consequent leakage of fluid into the tissues (oedema).

Homeostatic mechanisms that have evolved to maintain fluid balance and blood pressure in states such as haemorrhage, dehydration or fluid overload then come into play.

Reduced cardiac output results in activation of the sympathetic nervous system and the renin–angiotensin–aldosterone system, in an attempt to maintain the blood pressure and cardiac output. Release of the catecholamines adrenaline and noradrenaline stimulates both the force and rate of contraction of the heart, and constricts the blood vessels to maintain the blood pressure. Angiotensin is also a vasoconstrictor, while aldosterone stimulates sodium retention in the kidney, and consequently water retention, increasing the circulating volume. Conversely, stimulation of stretch receptors in the atria and ventricles causes release of natriuretic peptides, which stimulate salt and water loss via the kidneys.

While many of these mechanisms may be helpful in the short term in acute heart failure, they are maladaptive in chronic heart failure. Vasoconstriction, although maintaining the blood pressure, increases the resistance against which the failing heart has to pump. Sodium and water retention aggravates oedema, and increases the circulating volume, thereby stretching the heart further. Constant stimulation of the myocardium by catecholamines results in further myocardial damage.

Exacerbating conditions

A number of non-cardiac conditions can aggravate heart failure. Indeed, clinical heart failure can occur in a normal heart if it is under sufficient external stress.

- Anaemia and hypoxia increase the cardiac workload.
- Arteriovenous shunts, including those created for haemodialysis in renal patients, necessitate increased cardiac output.
- Hyperthyroidism causes sympathetic stimulation and concomitant peripheral vasodilation, resulting in tachycardia and high-cardiac output.
- Severe renal failure impairs excretion of salt and water, resulting in fluid overload.
- Excessive intravenous fluid therapy can precipitate pulmonary oedema, even with a normal heart.

Clinical aspects of heart failure

The clinical symptoms and signs of heart failure are described in Chapter 5A. These may vary between patients. Left-sided heart failure will predominantly cause breathlessness due to pulmonary congestion, while right-sided heart failure causes systemic venous congestion, with raised venous pressure and pitting oedema. The two commonly coexist.

Clinical assessment should answer the following questions:

- Is this really heart failure?
- What is the underlying cardiac problem?
- Are there any exacerbating conditions?
- What treatment is required – initially to relieve symptoms, and ultimately to improve prognosis?

Some cases of apparent heart failure are due to other conditions. Lung disease is a common cause of breathlessness, and often coexists with ischaemic heart disease, particularly in smokers. Ankle oedema may be due to varicose veins, DVT, immobility, obesity or a decreased serum albumin concentration.

The cardiac diagnosis may be apparent clinically, but all patients should have an ECG, chest X-ray (Figure 5B.1) and an echocardiogram. The latter gives the most detailed information about the function of the cardiac chambers and valves.

Anaemia, renal failure and thyrotoxicosis may all aggravate heart failure, and full blood count, urea and electrolytes, and thyroid function tests should be performed. In ischaemic heart disease, risk factors should be assessed and treated.

Treatment of heart failure

Acute pulmonary oedema is a medical emergency requiring hospital admission. The immediate 'first aid' treatment is to sit the patient up to optimise both the haemodynamic stress on the heart and the mechanics of breathing. Oxygen should be given, and patients with ischaemic heart disease should take their GTN sublingual preparation.

In hospital, an ECG is taken to assess cardiac causes such as an acute arrhythmia or MI. Blood tests are sent, and a chest X-ray performed. Intravenous furosemide is given, which acts both as a vasodilator, reducing cardiac workload, and as a diuretic, reducing circulating volume. An intravenous nitrate infusion can be given, and morphine or diamorphine provides symptomatic relief from breathlessness. Further management depends on the underlying cause.

Chronic heart failure is assessed and treated similarly, initially with oral loop diuretics to relieve fluid overload. When the heart failure is due to left ventricular systolic dysfunction, with a low ejection fraction on the echocardiogram, a number of medications acting on the neurohormonal pathways described earlier have been shown to reduce both morbidity and mortality.

Drugs used to manage heart failure

The drugs used to treat heart failure are listed in Table 5B.1. Most of the drugs are described more fully in other parts of the chapter.

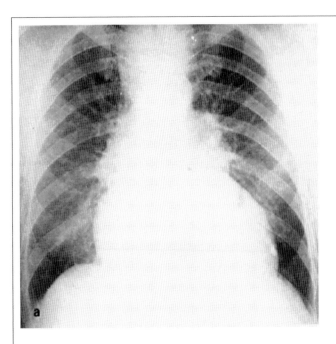

Figure 5B.1 A patient with heart failure. Pulmonary oedema is shown, with an increase in lung markings and increased heart size.

Table 5B.1 Drugs used to treat heart failure.
ACE inhibitors
Angiotensin II receptor antagonists
Loop diuretics and aldosterone antagonists
β-adrenoreceptor blockers
Vasodilators and digoxin

- ACE inhibitors reduce mortality by about 25% at all levels of severity. They have to be started at a low dose and titrated upwards with monitoring of the blood pressure, urea and electrolytes, as they can cause renal impairment and hyperkalaemia.
- Angiotensin receptor blockers act in a similar way.
- Spironolactone and eplerenone inhibit the action of aldosterone and act as potassium-sparing diuretics. They should be used with caution in patients on ACE inhibitors or angiotensin receptor blockers, which also retain potassium.
- The β-blockers carvedilol and bisoprolol reduce mortality by over 30%. β-blockade can aggravate acute heart failure, since acute adrenergic stimulation increases the contractility of the heart, and these drugs are introduced slowly once symptoms and fluid overload are controlled by diuretics.
- In some cases, where routine treatments fail to control the disease, vasodilators (such as nitrates and hydralazine) and digoxin are used for treatment.

Thus, many heart failure patients will be taking three or more medications for the heart failure itself, with additional antianginal, antithrombotic and lipid-lowering medications for their ischaemic heart disease. Care must therefore be taken with any additional prescribing. In particular, NSAIDs may cause fluid retention and acute renal failure in patients already taking diuretics and ACE inhibitors. NSAIDs are drugs that may be prescribed by dental practitioners.

Patients taking drugs for heart failure are likely to have serious cardiac problems and may be awaiting cardiac transplantation. Thus, they may only seek emergency dental treatment. Dose limitation of adrenaline in dental local anaesthetics is wise in such patients, and no more than three cartridges is recommended in an adult patient.

5C CARDIAC ARRHYTHMIAS

Pathophysiology

The normal electrical control of the heartbeat can be easily recorded using the electrocardiogram (see Chapter 5A). In normal sinus rhythm, the atrial contraction is seen as the P wave. After a short pause, the ventricles contract, producing the QRS complex. Repolarisation of the ventricles after contraction is seen as the T wave (Figure 5A.8).

The heart rate is controlled by the autonomic nervous system. Sympathetic (adrenergic) stimulation increases the heart rate and contractility, while parasympathetic (cholinergic) activity via the vagus nerve slows the heart.

Cardiac arrhythmias may be divided into tachycardias (pulse rate >100 beats/min) and bradycardias (pulse rate <60 beats/min).

Tachycardias

Sinus tachycardia, where a normal P wave occurs before each QRS complex, is a normal response to exercise, stress, fever or anaemia. A young subject may reach rates of 180 beats/min during exercise.

Supraventricular tachycardia is the term used for abnormal tachycardias originating in or above the AV node. They may arise from the atria, where a P wave will still be seen, or from the AV node itself. The ventricles are still activated normally via the His–Purkinje system.

Ventricular tachycardia arises within the ventricle. Because the electrical impulse spreads from the abnormal focus directly through the heart muscle (rather than from the fast conducting tissue), the QRS complex is wider than normal.

Atrial fibrillation is where the atrial activity becomes completely disordered, with constant electrical activity throughout the atria, and loss of coordinated atrial contraction. The AV node is randomly stimulated, and the ventricular contraction is fast and irregular (Figure 5C.1). There are no P waves.

Ventricular fibrillation is similar chaotic ventricular activity, and causes cardiac arrest.

Bradycardias

Sinus bradycardia can be normal at rest, and be caused by drugs or hypothyroidism.

Atrioventricular block (also called 'heart block') occurs when conduction of the impulse from the atria to the ventricles is impaired, as a result of disease of the AV node or bundle of His. Depending on the severity, it may simply cause a slight delay in conduction, or it may cause missed beats. In complete heart block, the ventricles receive no stimulation from above, and beat independently at a very slow rate.

Sinus node disease can cause both bradycardias and tachycardias, often alternating, due to malfunction of the sinoatrial node.

Cardiovascular reflex disorders can result in syncope due to transient bradycardias. In carotid sinus hypersensitivity, the carotid sinus baroreceptors can overreact, causing sudden, transient pauses and consequent falls or loss of consciousness. In vasovagal syncope, a variety of stimuli, including prolonged standing and emotional stress, can result in fainting, usually preceded by warning symptoms of light-headedness.

Clinical aspects of arrhythmias

Arrhythmias may be asymptomatic, or present with palpitations, heart failure or syncope. Clinical assessment at the time of the arrhythmia includes basic life support where necessary; measuring the pulse and blood pressure; and recording an ECG. However, arrhythmias are often transient and intermittent, requiring other approaches to diagnosis. Twenty-four-hour ECG recording or loop recorders attached to patients for longer periods can detect transient rhythm disturbances.

Electrophysiological studies are undertaken in special centres. Electrical catheters are introduced into the heart via the femoral vessels to stimulate and record the electrical activity in detail.

Investigation should also establish the underlying cause. This may include any form of heart disease, congenital disorders of rhythm in otherwise normal hearts, drugs and metabolic disturbances, particularly of serum potassium, magnesium or calcium.

Tachycardias are most commonly treated by drugs. Digoxin or β-blockers are commonly used to control the

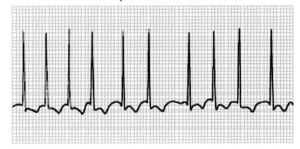

Rhythm Disturbances
Tachycardias

- Atrial fibrillation
  - The most common rhythm disturbance
  - Uncoordinated and ineffectual atrial contraction (fibrillation)
  - Results in a rapid and irregular ventricular rate
  - Reduces efficiency of the heart – heart failure

Figure 5C.1 Atrial fibrillation.

ventricular rate in atrial fibrillation, and amiodarone can sometimes revert atrial fibrillation to sinus rhythm.

In emergency situations, electrical direct current (DC) cardioversion can be used to treat not only ventricular fibrillation in a cardiac arrest, but also atrial fibrillation, as well as supraventricular and ventricular tachycardias. In the conscious patient, a short general anaesthetic or sedation is necessary before delivering the painful shock via electrodes on the chest. Elective DC cardioversion is sometimes used for chronic atrial fibrillation that causes problems despite rate-controlling drugs.

Bradycardias are usually treated with a pacemaker. This comprises a small electronic box that is buried under the skin of the chest wall and connected to one or more leads that pass through the subclavian vein into the right ventricle and atrium. The pacemaker monitors the heart's own activity, and only delivers an electric stimulus to the heart when it detects a pause. Some patients, such as those with complete heart block, are paced constantly, while the pacemaker acts as a 'safety net' in other patients with transient bradycardias, only pacing when needed.

Implantable defibrillators are increasingly being used to prevent ventricular arrhythmias and sudden cardiac deaths in high-risk patients. They are inserted in a similar way as a pacemaker, but can deliver a high-voltage defibrillating shock if a ventricular tachycardia or fibrillation is detected. Pacemakers and other implantable electrical devices have implications in the provision of dental care, and are discussed in Chapter 20 (titled 'Haematology').

Some arrhythmias can be treated by ablation of abnormal electrical tissue in the heart during electrophysiological studies, effecting a permanent cure.

Drugs used to manage cardiac arrhythmias

Drugs used to manage cardiac arrhythmias can be classified as:
- Acting on supraventricular arrhythmias (e.g. verapamil).
- Acting on supraventricular and ventricular arrhythmias (e.g. amiodarone).
- Acting on ventricular arrhythmias (e.g. lidocaine).

Alternatively, they can be categorised according to their antidysrhythmic action (Vaughan Williams classification) as:
- Class I: membrane-stabilising drugs.
- Class II: β-adrenoreceptor antagonists (β-blockers).
- Class III: agents influencing potassium channels (e.g. amiodarone).
- Class IV: calcium channel blockers.

Class I antiarrhythmics are further subdivided into Ia (e.g. procainamide, quinidine), Ib (e.g. lidocaine, mexiletine) and Ic (e.g. flecainide), depending on the kinetics of their binding to the sodium channel and their effect on the cardiac action potential. Ia drugs prolong the action potential; Ib drugs shorten it; and Ic drugs have little or no effect.

In addition to the drugs mentioned in the preceding text, cardiac glycosides are used in the management of arrhythmias.

Class I: membrane-stabilising drugs

Mechanism of action

Membrane-stabilising drugs act on the sodium channel in exactly the same way as local anaesthetics do (see Chapter 14, titled 'Pain and anxiety control'). As the binding site for these drugs is only available when the sodium channel is in the open or refractory state (see Chapter 14), accessibility to the target is governed by the rate of opening of the channel. This explains the phenomenon of frequency-dependent (use-dependent) block. The more a channel opens, the more likely the drug is to achieve its effect. Thus, antiarrhythmic drugs have a greater effect on a heart that is dysrhythmic as compared with their effect on a normal heart.

Impact on oral structures and dental management

Procainamide and quinidine may produce angioedema that may affect the lips, tongue and floor of the mouth.

Drug interactions relevant to dental practice

Local anaesthetics with marked cardiotoxicity, such as bupivacaine, should be avoided in patients taking antiarrhythmic drugs, as myocardial depression may occur. Erythromycin increases the likelihood of ventricular arrhythmias when given with quinidine. Also, antifungal agents such as itraconazole, ketoconazole and miconazole should not be prescribed to patients taking quinidine, as there is risk of ventricular arrhythmias.

Class II: β-adrenoreceptor antagonists

β-Adrenoreceptor antagonists are discussed in Chapter 5E (titled 'Hypertension').

Mechanism of action

These drugs decrease cardiac sympathetic activity by selectively blocking β_1-adrenergic receptors.

Class III: agents influencing potassium channels

The drugs that are in this class are amiodarone and the β adrenoreceptor antagonist sotalol.

Mechanism of action

By blocking potassium channels, these drugs prolong repolarisation.

Impact on oral structures and dental management

Patients taking amiodarone may complain of a metallic taste, and this drug can produce thrombocytopaenia.

Drug interactions relevant to dental practice

As with other antiarrhythmic drugs, avoidance of cardiotoxic local anaesthetics such as bupivacaine is recommended.

Erythromycin increases the risk of ventricular arrhythmias when combined with amiodarone, and should thus be avoided.

Class IV: calcium channel blockers

These drugs are discussed more fully in Chapter 5E (titled 'Hypertension').

Mechanism of action

The action of the non-dihydropyridines verapamil and diltiazem on cardiac L-type calcium channels results in slowing of the sinoatrial node pacemaker.

Cardiac glycosides

These drugs are useful in the management of arrhythmias and heart failure. The drug most commonly used is digoxin.

Mechanism of action

Cardiac glycosides inhibit the membrane-bound sodium/potassium ATPase, which results in an increase in intracellular sodium. As a consequence of this, intracellular calcium rises, producing an increase in contractility.

Impact on oral structures and dental management

Digoxin can produce a pain similar to trigeminal neuralgia in the lower part of the face.

Drug interactions relevant to dental practice

Digoxin toxicity is precipitated by hypokalaemia. As adrenaline in dental local anaesthetics can produce hypokalaemia, dose reduction (e.g. no more than two cartridges of an adrenaline-containing solution in an adult) is advised. Another drug that may cause hypokalaemia is amphotericin, and this should be avoided in patients taking digoxin. NSAIDs, erythromycin and itraconazole increase the plasma concentration of digoxin, which may lead to toxicity.

5D VALVULAR HEART DISEASE

Introduction

Malfunction of the cardiac valves is less common than ischaemic heart disease in most Western countries. However, rheumatic fever following streptococcal infections still occurs in developing countries and can cause long-term valvular heart disease.

Narrowing of a cardiac valve, restricting the forward flow, is termed *stenosis*. Leaking of the valve, resulting in backward flow, is termed *regurgitation* or *incompetence*. Valvular stenosis results in pressure overload of the upstream chamber, since higher pressures are needed to maintain cardiac output through the restricted opening. Although the flow is free and unimpeded, regurgitation results in volume overload since a proportion of the blood returns and has to be ejected a second time.

In clinical practice, mitral stenosis is seen predominantly as a late complication, occurring years after rheumatic fever. Mitral regurgitation may result from congenital valve disease or from rheumatic fever, or it may be 'functional' due to heart failure. A dilated heart results in stretching of the support of an otherwise normal valve, with resultant leaking. Aortic valve disease may be congenital, but aortic stenosis is a common degenerative finding in older people. The tricuspid valve may leak in right-sided heart failure – for instance, in patients with chronic lung disease – but disease of the right heart valves is less common than left-sided disease.

The usual clinical presentation of valvular disease is with symptoms of heart failure, or with a murmur being detected during medical examination. The various valve malfunctions can be diagnosed clinically by their physical signs, particularly the characteristics of the murmur, but the definitive investigation is the echocardiogram.

Treatment of symptoms usually involves diuretics if heart failure develops. Atrial fibrillation is a common complication of mitral valve disease in particular, and requires rate control with digoxin or β-blockers and warfarin, or one of the newer oral anticoagulants such as dabigatran, rivaroxaban or apixaban, to reduce the risk of blood clots. The risk of atrial thrombosis and embolisation is higher in atrial fibrillation due to valve disease than in other causes of atrial fibrillation, and anticoagulation is therefore particularly important.

Pathology of valvular heart disease

The two most important diseases affecting the heart valves are rheumatic fever and infective endocarditis. These two diseases are characterised by permanent damage to heart valves, which is associated with the long-term risk of developing recurrent disease and further damage to the heart. Damage to heart valves caused by rheumatic fever increases the risk of developing infective endocarditis.

Rheumatic fever

Rheumatic fever is a systemic disease that occurs 2–3 weeks after a streptococcal upper respiratory tract infection – typically, a pharyngitis caused by Lancefield group A, β-haemolytic *Streptococcus*. Rheumatic fever is uncommon in the UK. Presently, the disease most commonly affects children in Central Africa, the Middle East and India, and is associated with poor nutrition and overcrowding. The disease is characterised by inflammation at multiple sites including the heart, arteries, joints and skin.

The heart becomes generally inflamed and shows signs of endocarditis, myocarditis and pericarditis. The damaging effects of endocarditis are long-lasting, whereas the effects of myocarditis and pericarditis are transient. Endocarditis at the heart valves initially produces small irregularities on the cusps of the valve; these are called 'vegetations', and are composed of platelets and fibrin. Recurrent infections cause valvular fibrosis, fusion of valve leaflets and calcification. The mitral valve is most frequently affected, although the aortic valve may also be involved. Over time, the function of the valves deteriorates, and there is valvular stenosis and incompetence.

Inflammation of the large joints produces symptoms referred to as 'migratory' or 'flitting' polyarthritis. A skin rash develops (erythema marginatum), and subcutaneous nodules may appear. Some patients develop neurological symptoms that include chorea (involuntary movement). The disease tends to be self-limiting, but some individuals get recurrent attacks. The pathogenesis is considered to be an abnormal immunological cross-reaction; antibodies generated against the *Streptococcus* cross-react with unknown antigen moieties within the connective tissues, especially of the heart and joints. An episode of rheumatic fever increases the risk of developing infective endocarditis.

Infective endocarditis

Infective endocarditis is a disease resulting from infection of a focal area of the endocardium. It usually affects the heart valves, but infection can develop on the mural endocardium, typically at the chordae tendineae or at the site of a congenital heart defect. In the majority of cases, there is a pre-existing abnormality of the endocardium that makes it susceptible to infection. Such abnormalities include congenital heart defects, calcific aortic valve disease and damage secondary to rheumatic fever. Prosthetic heart valves (Figure 5D.1), used to replace damaged and non-functional valves, are also susceptible to developing infective endocarditis.

The infective agents are usually commensal bacteria, although infrequently fungal organisms too may cause endocarditis. These organisms reside in the oral cavity and oropharynx, gastrointestinal tract, genitourinary tract and the skin.

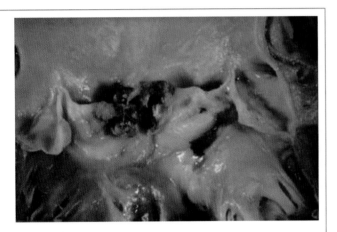

Figure 5D.1 A mechanical prosthetic heart valve.

Figure 5D.2 A vegetation on a heart valve.

Following bacteraemia, the infective agent is capable of colonising the damaged endocardium, usually resulting in a thrombotic vegetation composed of platelets and fibrin. Following colonisation, the bacteria induce further platelet aggregation and fibrin deposition and inhabit an immune-privileged niche. Although immune cells are capable of adhering to the infected endocardium, access to the organisms is hampered by the structural properties of the plaque. Bacterial growth causes enlargement of the vegetation, which develops from a small nodule to a large friable mass (Figure 5D.2).

The effects of infective endocarditis are diverse, and include both local and systemic effects. Local complications are largely a consequence of valvular destruction; the affected valve becomes incompetent, and the patient develops a heart murmur. Infected chordae tendineae are at risk of rupture, with fatal results, and local spread of infection can cause myocarditis. Systemic effects can be rather non-specific, and patients may develop an unremarkable low-grade fever with attendant weight loss and malaise. It is the development of embolic phenomena from fragments of infected vegetations that produces the stigmata of the disease. Systemic embolism produces small infarcts within the brain, spleen and kidney. Emboli typically affect the skin of the hands and feet, and the nail beds. The skin lesions may present as irregular erythematous flat macules (Janeway lesions), or as painful red raised lesions (Osler's nodes). Tiny linear subungual infarcts are termed as 'splinter haemorrhages' (Figure 5A.7), and some patients also develop finger clubbing. Small infarcts may also be observed within the mucous membranes, and retinopathy can develop following embolism to retinal vessels (Roth's spots, Figure 5D.3). The signs and symptoms of infective endocarditis are summarised in Table 5D.1.

In addition to the clinical signs and symptoms described in the preceding text, the diagnosis of infective endocarditis relies on auscultation of the heart, listening for a new heart murmur or a changing murmur, blood cultures and an echocardiogram.

Infective endocarditis is treated using a prolonged course of high-dose antibiotics. It is important that the microbiologist and cardiologist liaise at an early stage. The antibiotic will vary according to whether treatment is empirical or whether a causative organism is isolated. Surgery may occasionally become necessary if there is valvular obstruction, heart failure, repeated emboli or persistent bacteraemia. Similarly, a myocardial abscess will require drainage, and active surgical intervention will be necessary if an infected prosthetic heart valve becomes unstable.

Prophylaxis against infective endocarditis

It is important that dental practitioners be aware of the possibility of patients developing infective endocarditis after bacteraemia-producing procedures. The following cardiac conditions place individuals at increased risk.

- Previous infective endocarditis.
- Hypertrophic cardiomyopathy.
- Acquired valvular heart disease leading to stenosis or regurgitation.
- Structural congenital heart disease (sometimes including those that have been surgically treated). [Not including isolated atrial septal defect (ASD), a fully repaired ventricular septal defect (VSD) or fully repaired patent ductus arteriosus (PDA), and any device of closure that is judged to have become endothelialised].
- Valve replacements.

It is important that practitioners talk to patients about why they are at increased risk of infective endocarditis developing, and give them clear and consistent information about prevention. This should include information regarding the risks and benefits of antibiotic prophylaxis, and also an explanation as to why antibiotic prophylaxis is no longer recommended as routine (see also Chapter 1, titled 'Clinical examination and history taking'). The importance of maintaining good oral

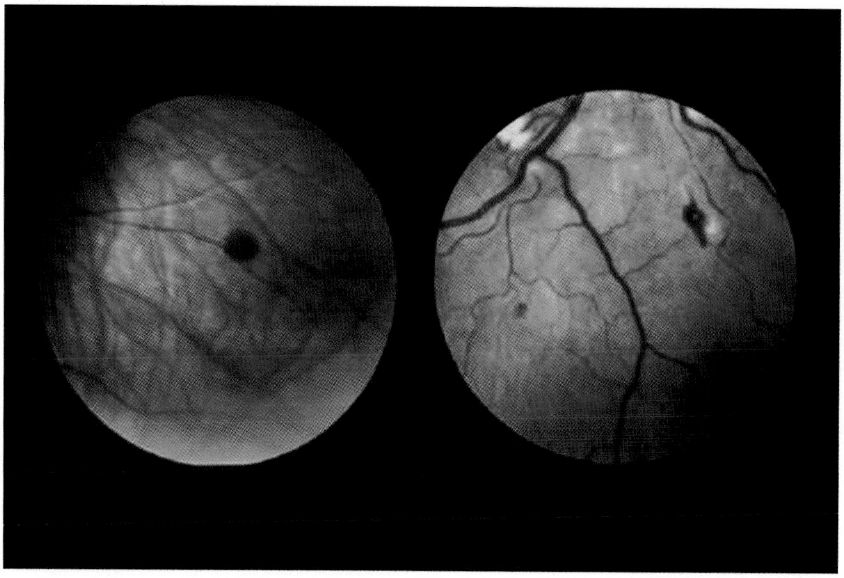

Figure 5D.3 Roth's spots.

Table 5D.1 Signs and symptoms of infective endocarditis.
Fever
Weight loss
Malaise
Night sweats
Finger clubbing
Enlarged spleen
Anaemia
Mycotic aneurysms
Heart murmur
Microscopic haematuria

health should be discussed. The risks of undergoing invasive procedures, including non-medical procedures such as body piercing and tattooing, should also be discussed where appropriate. It is important that patients (and, of course, practitioners) be aware of the symptoms that may indicate infective endocarditis, and when to seek expert advice (Table 5D.1).

Antibiotic prophylaxis against infective endocarditis is no longer routinely recommended in dentistry, but clearly high-risk cases such as those highlighted in the preceding text need special consideration (see also Table 1.2, Chapter 1). The latest guidelines from the National Institute for Health and Care Excellence (NICE) state that chlorhexidine mouthwash should not be offered as prophylaxis against infective endocarditis for patients undergoing bacteraemia-producing dental procedures.

In 2008, NICE issued guidelines stating that antibiotic prophylaxis was no longer to be used for bacteraemia-producing dental procedures. These guidelines were updated in 2016, stating that such prophylaxis may be given, but not routinely. Although the incidence of infective endocarditis has been rising in recent years, the upward trend had begun before this 2008 change in guidance.

NICE also state that any episodes of infection in people at risk of infective endocarditis must be investigated and treated promptly to reduce the risk of the patient developing infective endocarditis.

As stated in the preceding text, NICE currently state that antibiotic prophylaxis need not be given 'routinely' to patients at risk of developing infective endocarditis undergoing bacteraemia-producing dental procedures. In other words, antibiotic prophylaxis should not be given as routine, but should be seriously considered in certain risk groups (Table 1.2, Chapter 1, titled 'Clinical examination and history taking'). NICE state that 'doctors and dentists should offer the most appropriate treatment options, in consultation with the patient and/or their carer or guardian. In doing so, they should take account of the recommendations in this NICE guideline (details at the end of this chapter) and the values and preferences of patients, and apply their clinical judgement'. While clinical judgement is clearly important, high-risk patients undergoing bacteraemia-producing dental procedures would normally be offered prophylaxis. The risk categories for the development of infective endocarditis in bacteraemia-producing dental procedures are given in Chapter 1.

Traditionally, a broad-spectrum antibiotic such as 3 g of Amoxil has been used an hour before a bacteraemia-producing dental procedure as prophylaxis.

In any cases of doubt, the practitioner should consult the patient's cardiologist. The British Dental Association have also issued helpful information in this area.

5E HYPERTENSION

Raised blood pressure rarely causes symptoms in its own right, but is important because it is a major, reversible risk factor for several cardiovascular problems. It is strongly associated with stroke. Other consequences of hypertension include MI, renal failure and heart failure due to left ventricular hypertrophy (Figure 5E.1) or left ventricular dysfunction. The definition of high blood pressure is somewhat arbitrary, and is based on the threshold at which treatment has been shown to reduce complications. It is very common in the general population, increasing with age.

Pathological changes in hypertension include thickening of the blood vessel walls (arteriosclerosis), atherosclerosis and aneurysm formation. Aneurysms and arterial wall thickening may affect small arteries and arterioles, and fibrinoid necrosis of the arteriolar wall can occur in more severe cases. Hypertrophy of the left ventricle occurs due to the increased pressure load on the myocardium; pathological changes in the renal glomeruli can also be seen, and can result in permanent renal damage.

The small vessel changes can be directly visualised in life using an ophthalmoscope to observe the retinal vessels. Thickening of the arteriolar wall causes compression of the retinal venules at crossing points, the so-called 'arteriovenous nipping'. Small haemorrhages within the retina and white exudates formed from the lipids and proteins that have leaked from damaged blood vessels can also be seen.

Very severe hypertension can present as a medical emergency, with headaches, visual disturbances, changes in mental function, impaired consciousness, fits and florid retinal changes, which include swelling of the optic nerve head – the so-called 'papilloedema'. Renal function is often impaired, and diffuse intravascular coagulation can occur. This medical emergency is nowadays rare due to the effective treatment of hypertension in the population.

The higher the blood pressure, the greater the risk of complications that may arise from it. Current guidance recommends treating anyone with a blood pressure of >160/100 mmHg, aiming for a target blood pressure of 140/85 mmHg. Lower thresholds and lower target blood pressures are appropriate for high-risk groups, including those who already have symptomatic arterial disease, those with diabetes and patients with renal failure. Because the risk of complications, particularly strokes, increases sharply with age, older people should be treated at least as aggressively as the young.

Most hypertension is so-called 'primary' hypertension, with no identifiable reversible causes. Certain lifestyle habits, particularly high salt intake and alcohol excess, can aggravate hypertension. Furthermore, a small percentage of hypertensive patients do have an identifiable underlying cause, which is sometimes reversible (Table 5E.1).

Measurement of blood pressure

Blood pressure varies widely from minute to minute, depending on a wide range of factors including anxiety, exercise, posture and the state of hydration. Therefore, to confirm a diagnosis of hypertension that requires long-term treatment, at least three readings should be taken on different occasions, with the patient in a comfortable sitting position and a calm state of mind and at rest.

A standard sphygmomanometer comprises a cuff that is placed around the patient's upper arm, an inflatable air bag within the cuff to compress the brachial artery, a rubber bulb to inflate the cuff, a screw valve to allow controlled deflation and a pressure gauge that registers the cuff pressure in millimetres of mercury (mmHg).

The patient's arm should rest on a desk at approximately the level of the heart. The cuff on the upper arm should be applied closely enough that inflation of the air bag compresses

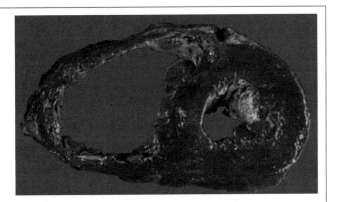

Figure 5E.1 A section through the heart showing left ventricular hypertrophy. The chamber on the right-hand side of the picture is the left ventricle, and that on the left is the right ventricle.

Table 5E.1 Causes of secondary hypertension.
Renal diseases including renal artery stenosis and polycystic kidneys
Cushing's syndrome (cortisol excess, including steroid treatment)
Conn's syndrome (aldosterone excess)
Phaeochromocytoma (catecholamine excess)
Acromegaly
Hyperparathyroidism
Coarctation of the aorta
Drugs including oral contraceptives and monoamine oxidase inhibitors

the arm, and should be high enough that the brachial artery in front of the elbow is accessible to feel and auscultate.

The cuff is inflated rapidly until the brachial or radial pulse is obliterated. The cuff is then deflated at a rate of about 2 mmHg/sec, while auscultating over the brachial artery with a stethoscope. The systolic pressure is indicated by the appearance of a knocking sound in time with the heartbeat, and the diastolic pressure by the disappearance of the sound. There are sometimes other changes in the sounds as the cuff is deflated from above the systolic pressure, described as 'Korotkoff phases' (Table 5E.2), of which only phases I and V, representing the systolic and diastolic pressures, are useful in most patients.

A wide range of automated sphygmomanometers are now available for use both in healthcare settings and by patients themselves. Some patients have consistently high clinic readings due to anxiety – the so-called 'white coat' hypertension. Automated machines that record repeated readings over 24 hours are useful in this group of patients (Figure 5E.2).

Table 5E.2 The Korotkoff phases.

Korotkoff phase	Description	Indicates
I	Sounds appear	Systolic pressure
II	Sounds disappear	Misleading 'silent gap' present in a minority of patients
III	Sounds re-appear	
IV	Sounds muffle	Previously considered to represent diastolic pressure
V	Sounds disappear	Diastolic pressure as currently defined

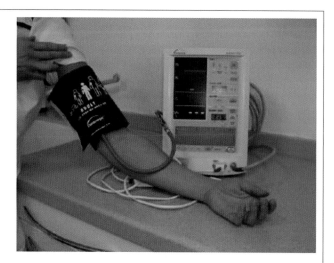

Figure 5E.2 An automated sphygmomanometer.

Drugs used to treat hypertension

The following classes of drugs are used to treat hypertension:
1 Diuretics.
2 Angiotensin-converting enzyme (ACE) inhibitors.
3 Angiotensin II receptor antagonists (ARBs).
4 Calcium channel blockers.
5 β-Adrenoreceptor antagonists (β-blockers).
6 α-Adrenoreceptor blockers.
7 Vasodilators.
8 Centrally acting drugs.

As mentioned earlier in the chapter, some of these classes of drugs have other uses, particularly in the treatment of angina and heart failure.

Diuretics and aldosterone antagonists

Diuretics are classified into:
■ Thiazides (e.g. bendroflumethiazide).
■ Loop (e.g. furosemide and bumetanide).
■ Potassium-sparing (e.g. amiloride).
■ Osmotic (e.g. mannitol).
■ Aldosterone antagonists including spironolactone and eplerenone.

Mechanism of action

All, other than osmotic diuretics, decrease reabsorption of sodium in the kidneys. This rise in excretion of sodium causes a greater loss of water, which results in a drop in plasma volume. Osmotic diuretics interfere with water reabsorption, but they are not used for the management of hypertension. Loop diuretics are used predominantly in heart failure and other causes of salt and water overload, and are not first-line antihypertensive drugs.

Impact on oral structures and dental management

A side effect of diuretic drugs is dry mouth (xerostomia). This condition can lead to an increase in dental caries and oral candidal infections.

Thiazide diuretics may produce lichenoid reactions and Stevens–Johnson syndrome.

Drug interactions relevant to dental practice

Thiazides and loop diuretics result in potassium loss, and exacerbate the hypokalaemia produced by adrenaline in dental local anaesthetic solutions. This is not a concern when low doses (one or two cartridges in an adult) of local anaesthetics are used.

Aspirin reduces the action of spironolactone and acetazolamide.

ACE inhibitors

This group of drugs includes captopril, enalapril, lisinopril, perindopril and ramipril.

Mechanism of action

The renin–angiotensin system controls the fluid volume. Renin converts angiotensinogen to angiotensin I. This latter hormone has little activity but is converted by ACE to angiotensin II, which is a potent vasoconstrictor. In addition, angiotensin II stimulates aldosterone, another important hormone involved in fluid balance. ACE inhibitors exert their antihypertensive action by inhibiting the production of angiotensin II. In addition, ACE inhibitors prevent the breakdown of bradykinin, which mediates certain allergic reactions. As bradykinin is a vasodilator, this action contributes to the antihypertensive action of ACE inhibitors. Bradykinin accumulation accounts for some of the adverse effects of this group of drugs (discussed in the following text).

Impact on oral structures and dental management

ACE inhibitors have a number of unwanted effects on perioral structures. They can produce a dry cough, dry mouth, glossitis, erythema multiforme and lichenoid reactions. Some, such as enalapril and captopril, may cause loss of taste. An important unwanted effect is angioedema. Both cough and angioedema are secondary to the accumulation of bradykinin. Importantly, this drug-induced angioedema is not responsive to hydrocortisone and adrenaline; however, it resolves normally. Captopril may cause bone marrow depression, which can result in anaemia, leukopaenia and thrombocytopaenia. A platelet count of $<50 \times 10^9$ l^{-1} is a contraindication to elective surgical procedures. A count of $<100 \times 10^9$ l^{-1} is an indication for the use of extra haemostatic measures such as suturing and the use of agents such as Surgicel®.

Drug interactions relevant to dental practice

The antihypertensive action of ACE inhibitors can be antagonised by ibuprofen. In addition, this combination may lead to hyperkalaemia and renal impairment. The absorption of tetracyclines is reduced by quinapril.

Angiotensin II receptor antagonists

These drugs include candesartan, irbesartan and losartan.

Mechanism of action

These drugs block type 1 angiotensin II receptors. This results in vasodilatation and a fall in blood pressure. These drugs therefore have many similarities of action to ACE inhibitors, but have the advantage that they do not lead to the accumulation of bradykinin, and thus have fewer unwanted effects.

Impact on oral structures and dental management

These drugs have been reported to produce taste disturbances.

Drug interactions relevant to dental practice

NSAIDs including aspirin reduce the hypotensive effects of angiotensin II antagonists and may increase renal impairment. Corticosteroids also reduce the hypotensive effects. On the other hand, anxiolytic drugs enhance hypotension in patients taking angiotensin II antagonists.

Calcium channel blockers

These can be divided into two categories:
1. Dihydropyridines (e.g. nifedipine, amlodipine, nicardipine and felodipine).
2. Non-dihydropyridines (e.g. verapamil and diltiazem).

Mechanism of action

Calcium channel blockers bind to L-type calcium channels in smooth muscles. They interfere with the entry of calcium into cells, therefore reducing contractility. They exert their effect on blood pressure by arterial vasodilatation and a negative inotropic action.

Dihydropyridines dilate coronary and peripheral vessels. Compared with non-dihydropyridines, they have a decreased effect on the myocardium. Verapamil and diltiazem reduce both the rate and force of ventricular contraction – that is, they have negative chronotropic and negative inotropic effects.

Impact on oral structures and dental management

Calcium channel blockers can cause gingival hyperplasia (Chapter 15, titled 'Adverse drug reactions and interactions'). This is exacerbated by poor oral hygiene, and often requires surgical reduction. Another side effect is taste disturbance.

Drug interactions relevant to dental practice

Calcium channel blockers increase the toxicity of lidocaine, but this is not a problem if only one or two dental cartridges are being used in adults. As with diuretics, calcium channel blockers may exacerbate the hypokalaemia induced by adrenaline in dental local anaesthetic cartridges.

Diltiazem and verapamil increase the effects of midazolam, so recovery from sedation may be prolonged in patients taking these drugs.

β-Adrenoreceptor antagonists

β-Adrenoreceptor antagonists used to treat hypertension include atenolol, labetalol, metoprolol and propranolol. Although they have been used for many years, recent evidence has shown that atenolol, the most commonly used β-blocker in the UK, is less effective than other classes of drugs. β-blockers are therefore no longer widely used as first-line treatment.

Mechanism of action

The antihypertensive action of β-adrenoreceptor blockers is complex. It does not coincide with the onset of therapy, taking a few days to occur. These drugs:

- Reduce renin release; β-adrenoreceptor agonists stimulate renin release (see the text that follows).
- Reduce cardiac output; β-adrenoreceptor action increases the rate and force of contraction of the heart.
- Reduce sympathetic activity.

Impact on oral structures and dental management

β-blockers can cause dry mouth. They may also produce intraoral lichenoid reactions. Some patients receiving β-blockers report perioral numbness.

Drug interactions relevant to dental practice

β-Adrenoreceptors may increase the toxicity of local anaesthetic agents as a result of decrease in hepatic blood flow. This is not a major concern unless large doses of local anaesthesia are administered. Although this group of drugs will counter any increase in cardiac output produced by adrenaline in local anaesthetic solutions, the unopposed α stimulation produced by the catecholamine may lead to a rise in systolic blood pressure. Again, this is unlikely unless large doses are used.

The metabolism of diazepam is reduced by β-adrenoreceptor-blocking drugs, but this is unlikely to be of any clinical significance.

Ibuprofen antagonises the antihypertensive action of β-adrenoreceptor blockers, and combined use should be avoided.

α-Adrenoreceptor blockers

Doxazosin and prazosin are selective α_1-adrenoreceptor antagonists.

Mechanism of action

Selective α_1-agonists produce vasodilatation.

Impact on oral structures and dental management

Postural hypotension is commonly seen with prazosin. Thus, care must be taken when raising the patient upright following a prolonged treatment session in the supine position. As with some other antihypertensive medications, these drugs can produce thrombocytopaenia.

Vasodilators

Some of the drugs mentioned in the preceding text such as ACE inhibitors and calcium channel blockers achieve their effect by vasodilatation; however, there are other drugs that are classed as vasodilator antihypertensives. These include hydralazine and minoxidil.

Mechanism of action

The mechanism by which these drugs achieve their effect is self-evident. They are used in combination with other agents.

Impact on oral structures and dental management

Hydralazine may produce thrombocytopaenia.

Centrally acting drugs

These drugs include clonidine and methyldopa, both of which are rarely used nowadays.

Mechanism of action

These drugs reduce blood pressure by blocking sympathetic nervous system activity. This is achieved by inhibiting adrenergic outflow from the brainstem. This results in reduced cardiac output and peripheral arterial resistance.

Impact on oral structures and dental management

Clonidine can produce pain and swelling of the salivary glands and dry mouth. Methyldopa also causes dry mouth and can lead to lichenoid eruptions and pigmented mucosal lesions. Bell's palsy and dyskinesias also occur. Methyldopa affects the liver and depresses bone marrow, and thus haemostasis can be adversely influenced.

Treatment of hypertension

Since the aim of long-term treatment is to reduce the risk of complications, it is important first to establish whether the patient has other risk factors for arterial disease, including hyperlipidaemia, diabetes and smoking, and also whether they already have any evidence of clinical atherosclerosis or other hypertensive complications. Treatment may include not only blood pressure lowering, but also smoking cessation, lipid-lowering therapy or antiplatelet drugs.

For the blood pressure itself, any adverse lifestyle factors should be identified and corrected, including obesity, alcohol excess and a high salt intake. Drug treatment may be tailored to the individual, depending on other factors. For example, diuretics may be poorly tolerated in patients with urinary problems, and β-blockers may exacerbate asthma. In a patient with both angina and hypertension, β-blockers or calcium antagonists may be doubly beneficial. ACE inhibitors protect the kidneys more effectively than other drugs in patients with diabetic nephropathy.

The British Hypertension Society has recommended the 'AB/CD' algorithm for starting or combining drugs. ACE inhibitors (A) and β-blockers (B) both have inhibitory effects on the renin–angiotensin–aldosterone system. Caucasians under 55 years of age tend to have elevated renin concentrations, and these two classes are recommended as first line. Older patients or those of the Negroid race respond less well, and calcium antagonists (C) or diuretics (D) are first line. Combination therapy is then instituted by adding a drug of the opposite group.

Recent evidence has shown that β-blockers are less effective than other drugs when used alone, and the guidance from NICE reflects this, recommending ACE inhibitors as first line in young Caucasians. Long-term monitoring is required, with blood pressure checks every few months, and other classes of antihypertensive drugs may be used according to the needs of the individual patient.

5F   ANTICOAGULANTS, DRUGS AFFECTING BLOOD CLOTTING

Anticoagulants are drugs that interfere with or block some aspect of blood coagulation. Anticoagulants can be classified as injectable, such as heparin and the newer thrombin inhibitors, and oral. Details of how these drugs interfere with the clotting cascade are given in Chapter 13 (titled 'Endocrinology and diabetes').

Heparin

Heparin is a naturally occurring substance and consists of a family of glycosaminoglycans. Fragments of heparin (referred to as 'low-molecular-weight heparins') are used increasingly in clinical practice due to the reduced risk of unwanted effects.

Pharmacodynamics

The principal mode of action of heparin is mediated via the drug's action on antithrombin III. The latter inhibits thrombin and inactivates prothrombin. In addition, antithrombin III neutralises several of the activated clotting factors, namely IXa, Xa, XIa and XIIa. Heparin activates antithrombin and accelerates its rate of action.

Pharmacological properties

Heparin is a large, highly ionised molecule that is not absorbed from the gut. It is therefore given either intravenously or subcutaneously. Heparin is metabolised in the liver, and metabolites are excreted via the kidney. After intravenous injection, heparin has an immediate onset of action. Subcutaneous heparin is effective 50–60 min after dosing. Thus, in an emergency situation, the drug is given intravenously, followed by a constant rate infusion. Low-molecular-weight heparins are only given subcutaneously. The anticoagulant effects of heparin are monitored by testing the kaolin–cephalin clotting time (KCCT), which should be increased 1.5–2.5-fold.

Low-molecular-weight heparins have now superseded intravenous unfractionated heparin for most uses. They do not need monitoring by measuring the KCCT, and are given in a dose calculated for the patient's weight, either once or twice daily.

Unwanted effects

Haemorrhage is the main unwanted effect associated with the use of heparin. Bleeding can be from any site, but commonly arises from the gastrointestinal or genitourinary tract. If haemorrhage does occur, then heparin administration is stopped, and the patient is given protamine sulphate (1 mg for every 100 units of heparin).

Approximately 25% of patients on heparin experience a mild transient thrombocytopaenia. In a few patients, however, this can be severe and paradoxically lead to a life-threatening thrombosis. Platelet counts should be carried out at regular intervals for all patients on heparin therapy. Heparin-induced thrombocytopaenia is much less common with low-molecular-weight heparins.

Commercial preparations of heparin are obtained from animal tissues and can cause allergy, especially in atopic patients. Long-term heparin therapy can cause osteoporosis, alopecia and hypoaldosteronism.

Oral anticoagulants

Warfarin is still the most widely used oral anticoagulant. Phenindione is another oral anticoagulant, but its use is restricted to those patients who develop adverse reactions to warfarin.

In many cases, warfarin is now being replaced by Direct Oral AntiCoagulants (DOAC's, previously called 'Novel Oral AntiCoagulants', or NOACs). Examples include dabigatran and Rivaroxaban. Dabigatran is an antithrombin III inhibitor and is recommended by NICE as a possible treatment to prevent thromboembolic disease in atrial fibrillation. Rivaroxaban is a direct factor X inhibitor. Both of these drugs are readily absorbed and have short half-lives in comparison to warfarin. The short half-life is advantageous in that, in the case of excess anticoagulation, the effects are relatively quickly reversed. This is particularly useful as there are currently no antidotes in widespread use, although some are being developed.

DOACs are discussed in more detail in Chapter 20 (titled 'Haematology').

Pharmacological properties

Warfarin is a coumarin-derived anticoagulant. The drug acts as an antagonist to the vitamin K–dependent clotting factors (II, VII, IX and X). Warfarin inhibits the enzymatic reduction of vitamin K to its active hydroquinone form. The latter is essential for synthesis of the aforementioned clotting factors.

Because of the varying rates of synthesis of these clotting factors, there is a delay of up to 3–4 days before a therapeutic response can be obtained following dosage. Many factors can affect warfarin's activity, including diet, small bowel disease, pyrexia, age, pregnancy, concurrent drug therapy and liver disease.

Warfarin is absorbed by the gastrointestinal tract and is extensively protein bound (98%). The plasma half-life is 35–37 hours. The drug is metabolised in the liver, and metabolites are excreted in the urine and faeces. The normal induction dose of warfarin is 10 mg, and thereafter the maintenance dose depends on the patient's international normalised ratio (INR; see the following text).

Monitoring patients on oral anticoagulants

The INR, which is based on a measurement of the prothrombin time, is the method used to measure the anticoagulant properties of warfarin. The dose is adjusted to keep the INR within the therapeutic range, which, for most indications, is 2.0–3.0 (see Table 5F.1). For certain conditions, a higher therapeutic range is needed, but there is a trade-off between effective prevention of thrombosis and the risk of haemorrhagic complications.

Unwanted effects

Warfarin is a drug with a narrow therapeutic window, and it is prone to interference from a very wide range of drug interactions. It is therefore essential to check for potential interactions before prescribing any drug in a patient on warfarin. In many cases, the drug may be used as long as the frequency of monitoring the INR is increased appropriately, in liaison with the patient's GP or anticoagulant clinic.

Haemorrhage (especially into the bowel) is the most common unwanted effect, and regular monitoring of the INR to assess the efficacy of the anticoagulant is essential for patients on anticoagulant therapy. Other haemorrhagic problems include haematuria, ecchymoses and epistaxis, and intracerebral bleeding.

Coagulation takes several days to normalise after the withdrawal of warfarin. Intravenous vitamin K will reverse the effects of warfarin within 24 hours, but, if large doses are given, then re-warfarinisation is impossible for several weeks. In an emergency situation, intravenous replacement of clotting factors with fresh frozen plasma (FFP) or other coagulation concentrates is required.

Dental management of patients on warfarin

There is a potential risk of haemorrhage in all patients on warfarin therapy. This needs to be put into perspective against the risk of life-threatening thromboembolic disorders if a patient's warfarin therapy is interrupted. Prior to any dental treatment, it is worthwhile to check the patient's INR. This can be done via the patient's GP or the local anticoagulant clinic.

If the INR is <4, then the dental treatment can be completed. Some operators would be concerned about the risk of bleeding if significant operative procedures are being carried out – for example, several extractions. In such instances, local measures such as a suture and pack is a wise precautionary treatment. Similarly, if gingival tissues are very inflamed and the patient requires root surface instrumentation, then the placing of a Coe-Pack® dressing may reassure all parties that there is little or no risk of a local haemorrhage.

If the patient's INR is >4, then they are over-anticoagulated and need to return to the clinic/GP for warfarin dose reduction. Local/national guidelines should be obtained and adhered to. The topic is comprehensively covered in the British National Formulary, where the INR for surgical management without warfarin alteration is designated the value of '4'.

An automated device for measuring the INR using a pinprick sample is shown in Figure 5F.1.

Uses of anticoagulants

Low-molecular-weight heparin is used in most clinical situations where immediate anticoagulation is required. Examples include the treatment of DVT and pulmonary embolism. Low-dose, low-molecular-weight heparin is also given prophylactically to patients who are at risk from DVT and/or pulmonary embolism. A further use of unfractionated heparin is for the maintenance of extracorporeal circuits in cardiopulmonary bypass and haemodialysis.

Warfarin is used in the prophylaxis of embolisation in rheumatic heart disease, heart valve replacement and atrial fibrillation. It is also used in the management of DVT and pulmonary embolism, where a 3–6-month course is given after initial heparin treatment.

Target INRs for patients taking warfarin are given in Table 5F.1.

Table 5F.1 Target INRs for different categories of patients on warfarin therapy.

INR	Indication
2.5	DVT, pulmonary embolism, atrial fibrillation
3.0	Patients with mechanical aortic valves
3.5	Patients with mechanical mitral valves. Patients on warfarin therapy who experience recurrent DVT or pulmonary embolism

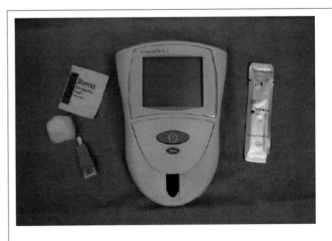

Figure 5F.1 An automated device for measuring the INR.

Antiplatelet drugs

As their name suggests, these drugs decrease platelet aggregation and may also inhibit thrombus formation in arterial circulation, where anticoagulants have little or no effect. Examples of antiplatelet drugs include aspirin, clopidogrel, prasugrel and dipyridamole. High-risk individuals are increasingly being placed on dual antiplatelets – for example, after drug-eluting coronary stenting.

Aspirin

Aspirin causes an increase in the bleeding time by reducing platelet aggregation. At all doses (75 mg and upwards), aspirin inhibits the synthesis of thromboxane A2 in the platelet by blocking cyclooxygenase. Thromboxane A2 is a prostaglandin that promotes platelet aggregation. Aspirin irreversibly acetylates the enzyme; therefore, platelets will not recover until the population exposed to the drug has been replaced (7–10 days). The effect of a single dose of aspirin on platelets (and hence the risk of haemorrhage) can last for several days.

In addition to the action on platelet cyclooxygenase, aspirin, at higher doses (>1 g/day), inhibits the synthesis of vessel wall prostacyclin. Endothelial cells synthesise prostacyclin, which causes vasodilation and inhibition of platelet aggregation. Thus, at high doses, aspirin has competing actions, blocking both the proaggregatory thromboxane A2 and the antiaggregatory prostacyclin.

Use of aspirin as an antiplatelet drug

A single dose of aspirin (150–300 mg) is given as soon as possible after an ischaemic event. Aspirin 75 mg is used for long-term maintenance or for prophylaxis in patients with established CVD. Aspirin 75 mg is also used in patients following coronary bypass surgery, in those who suffer from angina and occasionally in the treatment of atrial fibrillation.

Clopidogrel

Clopidogrel inhibits ADP-induced platelet aggregation. It is often used in combination with aspirin in the prevention of atherosclerotic events in peripheral artery disease, or following MI or stroke, as both aspirin and clopidogrel affect different aspects of platelet function. Dental extractions are usually carried out without stopping the drug, but it is important to use local haemostatic measures.

Prasugrel

Prasugrel also inhibits ADP–platelet aggregation, and is also used in combination with aspirin in the prevention of atherosclerotic events following MI or acute coronary interventions.

Dipyridamole

Dipyridamole is a phosphodiesterase inhibitor with an antithrombotic effect based on its ability to modify various aspects of platelet function such as adhesion, aggregation and survival. In addition, the drug is a potent vasodilator. The main use of dipyridamole is as an adjunct to oral anticoagulants for the prophylaxis of thromboembolism associated with prosthetic heart valves, and as an adjunct to aspirin following a stroke or transient ischaemic attack (TIA).

Fibrinolytic and antifibrinolytic drugs

Fibrinolytic drugs

Fibrinolytic drugs promote the breakdown of thrombi by activating plasminogen to form plasmin. Examples include alteplase and streptokinase, reteplase and tenecteplase. These drugs are indicated in some patients with stroke and other life-threatening thromboembolic disorders.

Alteplase

Alteplase is a tissue plasminogen activator that activates bound plasminogen. It is mainly used in the management of acute MI and pulmonary embolism. As with all fibrinolytic drugs, the main unwanted effect is haemorrhage.

Streptokinase

Streptokinase is a protein derived from β-haemolytic streptococci, which interacts with the proactivator of plasminogen to catalyse the conversion of plasminogen to plasmin. Bleeding from the site of injection is a common problem associated with streptokinase administration, and allergic reactions to the drug are common on repeat administration; hence, its use is restricted to one dose only.

Antifibrinolytic drugs

Antifibrinolytic drugs encourage the stabilisation of fibrin by inhibiting plasminogen activation. The most useful antifibrinolytic drug in dentistry is tranexamic acid, which is often used as a mouthwash in controlling persistent haemorrhage after tooth extraction. Oral tranexamic acid is used as an adjunct to factor VIII in the management of operative treatment in haemophiliacs, and also to reduce the risk of bleeding in patients with other problems with haemostasis.

5G DENTAL IMPLICATIONS OF CVD

It is clear from the preceding text that the key to the assessment of any patient with CVD is a thorough history, together with an appropriate examination. A patient who gives a history of CVD should also be questioned about the symptoms, and how well they are controlled with the medication they have been prescribed. A summary of points that are important to consider in dental patients is given in Table 5G.1.

Studies have demonstrated an association between coronary heart disease, stroke and the severity of periodontal disease. It is hypothesised that the association may be due to an underlying inflammatory response trait that places an individual at high risk for developing both periodontal disease and atherosclerosis. It is also suggested that, once established, periodontal disease provides a biological burden of endotoxin and inflammatory cytokines that serve to initiate and exacerbate atherogenesis and thromboembolic events.

Patients requiring general anaesthesia can be categorised using a system developed by the American Society of Anesthesiologists (Table 5G.2). The system is known as the 'ASA physical status classification system' and can be applied to all systems of the body.

Hypertensive patients

If possible, treatment is best carried out under local analgesia, with or without sedation. As mentioned previously, both β-blocking and non-potassium-sparing diuretics can exacerbate unwanted effects of adrenaline in local anaesthetics, and it is therefore wise to reduce the dose of adrenaline given. Similarly, patients who have had cardiac transplants may super-react to the cardiac effects of adrenaline in dental local anaesthetics, since transplanted hearts lack any sympathetic nerve supply, and therefore their receptors are upregulated to respond to circulating catecholamines. This is exacerbated by the fact that the parasympathetic nerve supply from the vagus is absent in the transplanted heart in the early post-transplant period.

The use of sedation can be valuable in patients with cardiac disease. Sedation may reduce the effects of stress, and the need for general anaesthesia may be eliminated. Dental patients undergoing intravenous sedation or general anaesthesia should continue their normal antihypertensive medication unless directed otherwise, which would be unusual.

Patients post-MI

Elective surgery under either general or local anaesthesia should be postponed for at least 3 months, and ideally 1 year in a patient who has suffered an MI. Even in emergency situations within 3 months of an MI, treatment is best carried out in consultation with the patient's physician. The incidence of further infarction after surgery in patients undergoing general anaesthesia is shown in Table 5G.3.

Other aspects of management

It is important to bear in mind that problems of direct relevance to the dentist may occur secondary to drug therapy and postoperative pain control. Drug problems that may arise include a dry mouth, which will necessitate a preventive regimen, and may require the use of artificial saliva when severe.

Table 5G.1 Important points in relation to the cardiovascular system in the history of a dental patient.

Chest pain
Angina
MI
History of coronary artery bypass graft (CABG)/valve replacement
Hypertension
Medication – particularly in relation to haemostasis
Syncope
Shortage of breath/exercise tolerance
History of rheumatic fever – may be a persisting cardiac lesion
History of infective endocarditis
Cardiac rate/rhythm
Known cardiomyopathy
Congenital disorders
Cardiac transplant
Venous or lymphatic disorders

Table 5G.2 The ASA classification.

ASA I	Healthy
ASA II	Mild systemic disease – no functional limitation
ASA III	Severe systemic disease – definite functional limitation
ASA IV	Severe disease – constant threat to life
ASA V	Moribund
ASA VI	Maintain for organ transplantation

Table 5G.3 The incidence of further MI versus time from previous infarction.

Time since infarction	Incidence of further infarction after general anaesthesia (%)
0–6 months	55
1–2 years	22
2–3 years	6
>3 years	1
No infarction	0.66

Drug-induced gingival overgrowth is well recognised, and can occur as a result of post-transplantation drugs and calcium channel blockers. The need for repeated gingival surgery is not uncommon in such patients.

The use of NSAIDs such as aspirin should be avoided in patients taking warfarin, since the anticoagulant effect is increased. Similarly, NSAIDs inhibit the hypotensive effects of antihypertensive medication, and their nephrotoxicity is increased in the presence of diuretics.

Smoking and the cardiovascular system

Smoking inhibits wound healing in the mouth and will directly affect the likelihood of success of oral surgical procedures. This particularly includes dental implantology. Smoking is a significant risk factor for oral cancer and periodontal disease.

In the context of general anaesthesia, smoking is a common cause of perioperative morbidity. In addition to its deleterious respiratory effects, the carbon monoxide that is produced by cigarettes has a negatively inotropic effect. Nicotine increases the heart rate and systemic arterial blood pressure. Carbon monoxide decreases oxygen supply and increases oxygen demand. This is particularly significant in patients who have ischaemic heart disease. These patients can get real benefit by stopping smoking 12–24 hours before surgery. It takes at least 6 weeks for there to be significant respiratory benefit from stopping smoking.

There are many factors that should be borne in mind when assessing the status of a patient with CVD who requires dental treatment. The degree of control of the disease, the complications that may arise from it and the impact of drug therapy should be remembered. A thorough history is key to safe management.

5H PERIPHERAL VASCULAR AND CARDIAC SURGICAL DISORDERS

Peripheral vascular disorders

Peripheral vascular disorders are common, particularly in elderly patients. Atherosclerotic narrowing of the peripheral arteries (peripheral arterial disease, or PAD) may result in pain on walking (claudication) or, if more severe, gangrene or ulceration leading to amputation of the leg. These are forms of chronic PAD. Ischaemia of the arm is much less common – probably because of the rich supply of collateral vessels it possesses. The peripheral arteries can be blocked acutely by embolism from the heart or acute thrombosis (acute limb ischaemia). This is a surgical emergency if the limb is to be saved. Arteries can also become abnormally wide (aneurysmal), leading to the risk of rupture, which can be life threatening when it occurs in the abdominal aorta. Important diseases of the veins include varicose veins and deep venous disorders leading to leg ulceration and DVT. Vascular surgeons are also involved in treating patients with narrowing of the internal carotid arteries.

The chronically ischaemic leg

Minor degrees of narrowing of major arteries, such as the iliac or femoral arteries, may be completely asymptomatic. As narrowing progresses, or if the vessel blocks completely, the patient may become symptomatic. For most patients with PAD, the first thing they will notice is pain in the calf muscles when they walk, called 'vascular claudication'. The pain disappears on resting for a short time but comes back in the same way when they walk again. There is no pain at rest. On examination, they may have absent pulses, but the leg usually looks normal. Using a Doppler probe, the systolic blood pressure in the leg can be measured to confirm the diagnosis, and the ankle:brachial index (ABI) can be calculated.

$$ABI = \frac{\text{Best pressure in ankle vessel (posterior tibial) or dorsalis pedis pulse}}{\text{Best pressure in arm (brachial) vessels}}$$

An ABI of <0.9 is diagnostic for the presence of PAD.

As the degree of arterial occlusion worsens, the patient may suffer increasingly shorter claudication distance before eventually getting pain at rest. Unlike the calf pain of claudication, arterial rest pain is usually felt in the foot or toes. It is typically worse at night, and the patient is woken by the pain and has to hang the foot out of bed or walk on a cold floor in order to gain some relief. The reason for this is the effect of gravity, and also that the cardiac output drops during sleep, and the warmth of the bedclothes causes vasodilation to the skin, diverting the blood from the soft tissues.

Patients who have severe arterial disease sufficient to give them rest pain are usually classified as having something called 'critical ischaemia'. Critical ischaemia can be loosely defined as ischaemia that is severe enough to threaten the loss of the limb or part of the limb. In claudication, the ABI is usually between 0.5 and 0.9. Below 0.5, the patient may start to suffer from rest pain or, if more severe, perhaps necrosis or gangrene of the toes.

Management: claudication

The presence of claudication is a marker for generalised arteriosclerosis. These patients are at a high risk of MI or stroke. Cardiovascular risk factor reduction is, therefore, the mainstay of management. Patients with claudication are around five times more likely to die of MI than they are to need an amputation of the leg.

Most patients with mild claudication are best managed conservatively, with the main advice being 'stop smoking and keep walking'. In addition, medical problems such as anaemia, hypertension, hyperlipidaemia, diabetes and heart failure should be corrected. Overweight patients should be advised to lose weight. All patients should be on an antiplatelet agent (e.g. aspirin or clopidogrel) and a statin. With such conservative treatment, most claudicants will stabilise and may even get an improvement in their walking distance as collateral vessels open up to carry blood around the blocked artery.

For more severe claudication, an angiogram (Figure 5H.1) or duplex scan can be arranged to see if there is a treatable lesion.

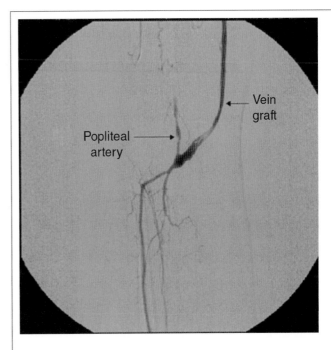

Figure 5H.1 An angiogram in a patient who has had a vein graft bypass of the lower limb.

Treatment of patients with chronic arterial disease may be carried out either by radiological intervention (balloon angioplasty) or by surgery (bypass grafting). Angioplasty is a good technique, in that it does not involve an anaesthetic and can be performed with relatively little risk to the patient. It is particularly useful for localised stenoses or short occlusions of the iliac arteries. Surgery is riskier; if it goes wrong, it can result in the loss of the leg in a small number of cases. It is used when there is either critical ischaemia or severe claudication that makes the patient's life intolerable. A variety of bypasses are possible, depending on the site(s) of blockage. The preferred choice of graft for these bypasses is usually the long saphenous vein, as the patency rate of vein grafts is higher than prosthetic grafts. In infrainguinal bypasses, the 5-year patency rate for vein grafts is 70%, as compared to 50% for prosthetic grafts.

If a suitable vein is not available, or for bypasses from the aorta or iliac arteries, artificial graft material can be used.

Management: critical ischaemia

In critical ischaemia with rest pain, ulceration or gangrene of the toes or foot, the priority is to get more blood supply into the leg before an amputation is needed. Such patients need to see a vascular surgeon as an emergency, undergo angiography or duplex scan to define the sites of blockage and have urgent revascularisation procedures by angioplasty or bypass surgery. Risk factor reduction is important in the longer term, but will not work quickly enough to save a critically ischaemic leg.

The acutely ischaemic leg

A useful way to remember the clinical signs and symptoms of an acutely ischaemic leg is the list of '6 Ps':
- Pain.
- Pallor.
- Pulselessness.
- Paraesthesias.
- Paralysis.
- Perishing cold.

Of these, 'paralysis' and 'paraesthesias' are the two that indicate severe ischaemia, threatening loss of the limb. This is because they reflect ischaemia of the two tissues most vulnerable to acute ischaemia – nerves and muscles. The two most common causes of acute ischaemia of the leg are embolism and thrombosis.

Embolism is most commonly from the heart, where a thrombus has formed because of atrial fibrillation, heart valve disease or MI. More rarely, emboli may be thrown off into the arterial circulation from aneurysms of the thoracic or abdominal aorta. Although it occurs rarely, an embolus to the peripheral arteries can come from a DVT, the so-called 'paradoxical embolus', where a DVT thrombus passes into the arterial circulation through a septal defect of the heart,

thereby getting into arterial circulation instead of causing a pulmonary embolus as it would usually do.

Thrombosis is the other main cause of acute ischaemia, and usually occurs on top of pre-existing atheroma in the peripheral arteries (such as the femoral arteries). Eventually, if an artery narrows sufficiently, it may clot off suddenly. In such cases, there may be a history of pre-existing claudication, and pulses may be absent in the opposite leg as well as in the symptomatic one.

Because of the relatively poor ability of muscle and nerve cells to cope with prolonged ischaemia, acute leg ischaemia needs to be treated as a surgical emergency, and blood flow needs to be restored within 4–6 hours if the limb is to be saved. Patients are immediately started on heparin, and, for an embolus, the patient should be taken without delay to theatre for an emergency embolectomy.

Peripheral arterial aneurysms

The word 'aneurysm' comes from the Greek word for 'widening'. Aneurysms can be found at various sites within the peripheral arterial circulation (e.g. aortic, femoral or popliteal).

Complications of aneurysms

There are a number of possible complications for any aneurysm:
- Rupture.
- Thrombosis within the aneurysm sac.
- Distal embolisation (causing acute ischaemia distally).
- Pressure on adjacent structures.
- Fistula/rupture into adjacent structures such as the vena cava.

These complications can all occur to a greater or lesser degree with arterial aneurysms at different sites.

AAAs

Aneurysms of the abdominal aorta affect the segment of aorta below the renal arteries in 90% of cases. Aneurysms that go higher than the renal arteries usually require incisions through both chest and abdomen for their repair. These are called 'thoracoabdominal' aneurysms.

Ruptured AAAs have a mortality rate of approximately 50%. The typical patient would present with collapse, shock, and abdominal and back pain. The best screening test for abdominal aneurysms is an ultrasound scan, which is cheap and provides a reliable method of sizing the aneurysm.

Infrarenal AAAs of <5.5 cm in diameter are usually managed conservatively, as the risk of rupture is low (Figure 5H.2). Aneurysms of >5.5 cm diameter will usually be recommended for surgery if the patient is fit enough. Treatment options are either open repair or endovascular repair.

Key points in assessing fitness for surgery include an assessment of cardiac, respiratory and renal problems. Patients with

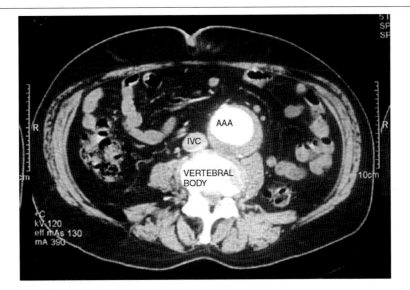

Figure 5H.2 A scan of the abdomen showing an AAA (IVC = inferior vena cava).

ruptured aneurysms should of course be taken immediately to theatre. These patients will not survive unless 'the tap is turned off'. Surgery is traditionally by 'open' operation through an abdominal incision (laparotomy). Aneurysms can sometimes be repaired using less invasive radiological techniques (this is called 'endovascular aneurysm repair').

Carotid disease

Atherosclerosis of the carotid arteries usually occurs at the point where the common carotid divides into the internal and external carotid arteries, probably because this is an area where local turbulence develops as the vessel divides. Narrowing or occlusion of the external carotid artery does not usually matter clinically because of the rich collateral arterial network within the head and neck. Stenosis or occlusion of the internal carotid artery (Figure 5H.3) is potentially much more serious, and can cause either strokes or TIAs. A TIA is defined as a neurological deficit that completely reverses within 24 hours of its onset (sometimes erroneously called a 'mini-stroke'). A stroke is a neurological deficit that persists for longer than 24 hours. *Amaurosis fugax* (means 'fleeting blindness' in Latin) is due to an embolus passing through the retinal arterial circulation, and is effectively a type of TIA.

The main investigation used to screen for carotid artery stenosis is duplex ultrasound scanning of the carotid artery. In addition, angiography may be used to confirm the severity and type of stenosis. There is good evidence that symptomatic carotid stenosis of a certain size should be treated by carotid endarterectomy in patients who are otherwise well. If these patients are treated with medical therapy only (antiplatelet drugs, lipid-lowering therapy and blood pressure control), they have a significantly increased risk of stroke as compared to patients in whom surgical endarterectomy is performed. The

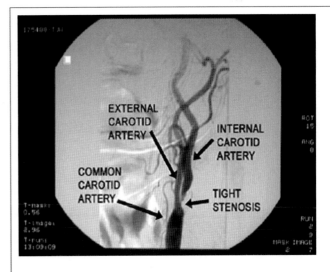

Figure 5H.3 An angiogram demonstrating carotid artery stenosis, which may lead to TIAs.

operation of carotid endarterectomy involves incision over the anterior border of the sternocleidomastoid muscle in the neck, and dissection of the common, internal and external carotid arteries. The common and internal carotid arteries are then opened using a longitudinal incision at the site of the stenosis, and the atheroma is 'cored out' and the artery closed, usually with a Dacron or bovine pericardial patch to prevent restenosis. In some patients, it may be necessary to put in a temporary plastic bypass tube (called a 'shunt') in order to maintain blood flow to the brain during this operation. The major complication of the procedure is a perioperative stroke (at the best centres, this risk is 3% or less).

Venous disease and leg ulcers

Varicose veins

Despite being so common, it is not entirely clear what causes varicose veins. They really only occur in humans, and are probably a result of mankind evolving to walk upright. When standing, the deep veins of the leg are at a much higher pressure than the superficial veins under the skin. Where the two systems join, there are valves that have the purpose of preventing the pressure within the deep system coming out into the superficial system. If these valves become incompetent, then the superficial veins dilate and appear as varicose veins (Figure 5H.4).

Varicose veins may cause problems cosmetically or may cause aching pains that are usually worse after a period of standing. If skin changes are occurring, patients may also complain of itching around the ankle, and some also find that they get swelling of the ankles. Most varicose veins in women seem to worsen after pregnancy, and occasionally abdominal or pelvic masses (including pregnancy) or malignancies can present as varicose veins due to pressure on the inferior vena cava or iliac veins. A full examination of the abdomen should therefore be part of examining a patient with varicose veins.

In patients who have had long-standing varicose veins, there may be changes of skin pigmentation (the skin is brown in colour, due to haemosiderin deposits) or lipodermatosclerosis (there is atrophy and loss of elasticity of the skin and

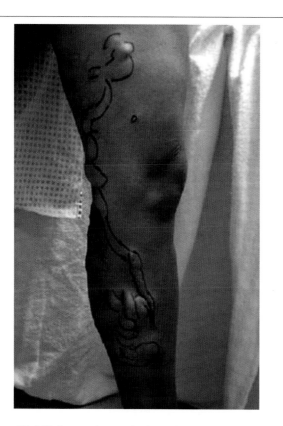

Figure 5H.4 Varicose veins, marked up prior to surgery.

subcutaneous tissues). Such venous skin changes are usually most prominent in the medial lower calf. They may also be caused by previous DVT and postphlebitic syndrome (see the following text).

DVT and pulmonary embolism

Pulmonary embolism is the most common preventable cause of death in surgical patients, usually as a result of a DVT that has formed in an immobile patient, often during surgery or immediately before or after. Its incidence is higher in sick, dehydrated, elderly patients, and particularly in those with malignancy. It is also higher in surgeries that last for long periods.

DVT

At early stages, the only sign of DVT may be an increase in warmth and dilatation of the superficial veins. As thrombosis progresses, the leg will swell. At a later stage, the leg may be extremely swollen, with impairment of skin circulation, and this may occasionally lead to venous gangrene. Many fatal pulmonary emboli arise from DVTs that were clinically insignificant in the leg. Most units now have a protocol for the diagnosis of DVT based on an integration of formalised clinical assessment, D-dimer measurements and duplex ultrasound scanning. Risk factors for DVT are given in Table 5A.3.

Most DVTs will eventually recanalise, but this will usually result in damage to the valves of the deep veins. In the long term, these patients may complain of leg swelling, venous skin changes and ultimately leg ulceration. This is sometimes called the 'postphlebitic' limb.

Pulmonary embolism

Pulmonary embolism may present in different ways. Massive pulmonary embolism will produce cardiorespiratory arrest and may initially be misdiagnosed as primary MI. A pulmonary embolism should always be suspected in a patient suffering a collapse or cardiac arrest within the first 2 weeks of a surgical procedure. Less major degrees of pulmonary embolism may produce lesser degrees of collapse, or perhaps dyspnoea or pleuritic chest pain. The treatment of DVT is anticoagulation, usually with heparin at first, followed by warfarin. Nowadays, most patients can be managed as outpatients with once-a-day injections of low-molecular-weight heparin while awaiting adequate warfarinisation. Patients with recurrent pulmonary emboli despite adequate anticoagulation should be considered for the insertion of a venacaval 'umbrella filter' via the femoral vein under X-ray control.

Prophylaxis against DVT

Patients having surgery should be considered for prophylaxis against DVT. This is particularly so if they have any risk factors. *Low risk* can be defined as surgery lasting <30 min under general anaesthesia in a person aged under 40 years with no risk factors. All others should normally have prophylaxis. The most common type of prophylaxis employed is subcutaneous low-molecular-weight heparin. It is also common practice to use thromboembolic deterrent (TED) stockings, and many units have intermittent pneumatic compression devices that work by blowing up a series of cuffs on the leg and keeping the venous pump flowing even when the patient is immobile or in theatre. Similar preventive strategies also apply to patients in bed due to non-surgical illnesses.

Leg ulceration

Ulceration can have many causes, although the most common by far is venous disease, which accounts for about 80% of ulcers.

Other causes:
- Arterial – due to major-vessel disease.
- Small-vessel disease (e.g. vasculitis, rheumatoid arthritis).
- Neuropathic (e.g. alcoholism, peripheral neuropathy, diabetes).
- Traumatic.
- Systemic disorders (e.g. pyoderma gangrenosum in ulcerative colitis).
- Neoplastic (e.g. squamous cell carcinoma).

Venous ulceration may be either superficial venous incompetence (varicose veins) or incompetence of the valves of the deep veins (e.g. postphlebitic). Venous ulceration (Figure 5H.5) will usually be found above the medial malleolous, and there will usually be the signs of pigmentation and lipodermatosclerosis.

Treatment of leg ulceration

Once the cause of the leg ulceration has been investigated, initial treatment may be directed towards underlying causative factors, such as arterial ischaemia, vasculitis, etc. The majority of leg ulcers are the result of venous disease. These are treated by dressing of the ulcer, pressure bandaging and elevation.

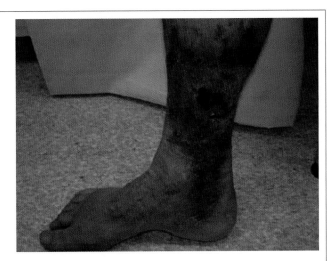

Figure 5H.5 Venous ulceration.

Elevation and pressure bandaging work by reducing the pressure in the superficial venous system.

Systemic antibiotics should be reserved for patients who have a cellulitis surrounding the ulcer. Ulcers are always affected to some degree by colonising skin organisms. Antibiotic treatment does nothing for the rate of ulcer healing, and may just breed resistant organisms. In some cases where there is a large ulcer with a clean granulating bed, it may be appropriate to consider the use of skin grafting in order to reduce the length of time required for the ulcer to heal. If there is significant superficial venous incompetence shown on duplex scan, then consideration should be given to treating this surgically to reduce recurrence of the ulcer. Unfortunately, when deep venous valve incompetence is present (usually following previous DVT), there is currently no good surgical procedure to improve deep venous function. For such patients, the mainstay of treatment is to try and get the ulcer healed using the methods discussed in the preceding text, and then to maintain healing by fitting a good-quality elastic graduated compression stocking. Patients who have their ulcers successfully treated should be encouraged to wear such stockings on a life-long basis.

Swollen legs/lymphoedema

'Swollen legs' is a common clinical problem (Table 5H.1). Most cases are due to systemic causes of peripheral oedema, such as congestive heart failure or low serum proteins. Localised causes in the leg are most often due to either venous disease such as DVT or postphlebitic syndrome (see the preceding text), or a disorder of the lymphatics – lymphoedema. This is due either to a congenital absence of the lymphatics (primary) or secondary to blockage of the lymphatics.

Primary lymphoedema can be present at birth (congenital lymphoedema), but more often it presents in the teens as lymphoedema praecox (Milroy's disease). This usually affects young females, who present with progressive swelling (non-pitting) of one or both legs. Less often, it can present

Table 5H.1 Potential causes of lower-limb oedema.

Systemic causes
- Congestive cardiac failure
- 'Right-sided heart' failure
- Hypoalbuminaemia (e.g. nephrotic syndrome)
- Fluid overload

Regional causes
- Venous obstruction (e.g. advanced pregnancy)
- Lymphatic obstruction

Local
- Sluggish venous return (e.g. poor muscle pump in a paraplegic patient)
- Acute obstruction to venous return (e.g. DVT, previous DVT)
- Cellulitis, lymphatic aplasia/obstruction

late at around the age of 30–40 years, and is then called 'lymphoedema tarda' (*tarda* = 'late' in Latin). Secondary lymphoedema can be caused by anything that damages or obstructs the lymphatics.

Causes of secondary lymphoedema

- Fibrosis (e.g. following radiotherapy).
- Infiltration (e.g. by tumour, especially lymphoma and prostate in men).
- Infection (e.g. tuberculosis, filariasis).
- Traumatic (e.g. after block dissection of lymphatics).

Treatment of lymphoedema is usually non-operative. This involves elevation and external compression stockings, and early intervention if infection develops. There are now lymphoedema nurses who use various compression devices and massage techniques that are very good at reducing the swelling in such patients. There are no curative surgical procedures available, and only the most severe cases come to surgery, which usually involves debulking procedures to improve mobility.

Cardiac surgical disorders

Cardiovascular disorders are the most common cause of death in most countries in the world. The medical management of these disorders is carried out by cardiologists. The role of cardiac surgeons is dealt with in the following section in relation to coronary artery bypass, valve disorders and congenital heart defects.

Coronary artery bypass surgery

Coronary artery bypass surgery is used when medical treatment is ineffective or insufficient.

Diagnosis

On the basis of a patient's symptoms and following a physical examination, several tests can be requested. The following tests are used to diagnose coronary artery disease and determine its extent and severity.

- ECG.
- Echocardiography. Stress testing can be done following exercise or by using drugs to speed up the heart.
- Cardiac catheterisation and coronary angiography. This involves inserting a catheter into the heart via the femoral artery in the groin. This test provides information regarding anatomy of the heart and its vessels, and can be used to perform therapeutic procedures.
- Myocardial perfusion imaging. Radionuclide tracers are used to assess myocardial blood flow.

Management

The main aim of treatment is to relieve symptoms and reduce the risk of MI. This includes measures to modify lifestyle, treat risk factors, decrease the risk of forming blood clots and the widening/bypassing of blocked/narrowed arteries.

Percutaneous coronary intervention (PCI)

The coronary arteries are accessed via a catheter inserted into the femoral artery in the groin, and then dilated with a balloon. Dilated areas can be kept open by using a stent. Drug-eluting stents have improved patency rates. For patients with single-vessel coronary artery disease, PCI offers earlier and more complete relief of angina than medical therapy, and is associated with better performance on the exercise test. The disadvantages of PCI include restenosis of treated lesions and a lesser ability to revascularise all lesions in patients with multivessel disease.

Coronary artery bypass grafting (CABG)

The procedure involves bypassing areas of narrowing/blockages with a suitable conduit (vein or artery) to achieve revascularisation. Veins for bypass grafting are usually taken from the saphenous system in the legs, while the internal mammary artery, close to the heart, can be used to provide a direct arterial supply. CABG is usually performed by opening the chest in the midline (sternotomy) or via a short left anterior thoracotomy incision. CABG can be performed with cardiopulmonary bypass ('on-pump') or without ('off-pump'). Most surgeons choose to perform CABG on-pump. There continues to be controversy and debate regarding the exact indications for CABG or PCI. In general, more severe disease may be better treated with CABG.

Education and counselling regarding diet, medication and exercise are important in the long-term management of coronary artery disease.

Valvular heart disease

Valvular heart disease principally encompasses stenosis or regurgitation, as described earlier in this chapter.

Symptoms

Patients may be asymptomatic or may have one or more of the symptoms listed in Table 5H.2. The degree of symptoms will depend on the severity of the disease.

Aetiology and individual valve lesions

Valve lesions can be congenital or acquired. The most common causes of acquired lesions are:

- Myxomatous degeneration.
- Rheumatic heart disease.
- Infective endocarditis.
- In association with connective tissue disorders (Marfan syndrome).
- Hypertension.
- Coronary artery disease.
- Atherosclerosis.
- Heart failure.

Table 5H.2 Symptoms of valvular heart disease.
Shortness of breath
Fatigue
Oedema
Dizziness
Palpitations
Fainting spells
Cyanosis
Symptoms of heart failure
Stroke due to emboli

Diagnosis

The presence of symptoms may raise suspicion, or lesions may be detected during routine physical examination. A heart murmur is usually present on auscultation, and the type of murmur can be specific for the heart valve lesion concerned. The following modalities of investigation are used:

- ECG.
- Echocardiography.
- Cardiac catheterisation.
- Magnetic resonance imaging (MRI).

Treatment

Treatment of valvular heart disease depends on the type of the lesion and the severity of symptoms. Some patients will not require treatment at all. Treatment can be broadly classified into *medical* and *interventional*.

Medical therapy

Based on the degree of symptoms and the severity of the lesions, drugs can be used to treat heart valve disease.

Interventional therapy

If medical therapy does not control symptoms, or if the condition worsens on medical treatment, intervention will be required. This includes repair or replacement of the valve. Some procedures can be performed percutaneously, but some may require open-heart surgery.

- *Balloon valvuloplasty.* A balloon catheter is inserted across the valve and inflated. Access is usually via the femoral vessels. It is used to treat mitral or pulmonary stenosis.
- *Surgical valve repair.* Valves can sometimes be repaired by open surgery on bypass. Mitral stenosis can be treated by valvotomy, and mitral valve prolapse or dilation of the mitral valve ring can also be repaired without replacing the whole valve.
- *Valve replacement.* If it is not possible to repair a valve then it can be replaced. The replacement valves can be of the following types:

- *Mechanical*: They are durable and last for several years. Patients must be anticoagulated for life, usually with warfarin.
- *Tissue or bioprosthetic valves*: They are either xenografts (porcine or bovine) or homografts (human cadaveric). Routine anticoagulation is not required, as the risk of thrombosis is low.

Cardiac transplantation

Transplantation is most commonly performed for end-stage heart muscle disease – either dilated cardiomyopathy or ischaemic heart disease – resulting in intractable heart failure. It may be used for congenital heart disease or other heart disorders that are otherwise untreatable. Patients require life-long immunosuppression and regular follow-up.

Transplantation is effective in relieving the symptoms of heart failure. Over 90% of patients report minimal limitation in activity. Heart transplantation has a high early mortality: 15–20% of recipients die within a year of the operation; 10-year survival is 50%, and 20-year survival is 15%.

Congenital heart disease

Congenital heart defects can be defined as defects in the structure and function of the heart due to abnormal heart development before birth. They are one of the most common congenital defects and can involve the walls, valves and blood vessels of the heart. They occur in about 1% of all live births. They may be asymptomatic, symptomatic or present with severe life-threatening symptoms. A proportion of babies born with congenital heart defects will need urgent treatment soon after birth. Treatment has improved significantly over the last few decades, with children born with complex defects now often growing to adulthood and leading healthy and productive lives.

Classification

Congenital heart disease can be classified according to anatomy, presentation and physiology. The presence or absence of cyanosis (bluish discoloration caused by a relative lack of oxygen) can be used to classify congenital heart disease into:

- Cyanotic heart disease.
- Acyanotic heart disease.

There are many types of congenital heart defects. They can be further classified into:

- Hole in the interior wall of the heart allowing blood from the left side of the heart to mix with blood from the right – a *septal defect*. The direction of flow depends on the pressure gradient.
- Narrowed or non-functioning valves causing obstruction or regurgitation of blood. This impairs the ability of the heart to pump efficiently.

- Complex defects that include combinations of the defects listed in the preceding points and abnormalities in the major blood vessels (aorta and its branches, and pulmonary arteries).

Some of the more common lesions are discussed in the following text.

PDA

Before birth, the aorta and pulmonary artery are normally connected by the ductus arteriosus, which is an essential part of the foetal circulation, allowing blood to bypass the circulation to the lungs. This is needed since the foetus does not use its lungs, with oxygen being provided through the mother's placenta. After birth, the ductus normally closes within a few days. In some babies, however, it remains open (patent). This opening allows blood to flow directly from the aorta into the pulmonary artery, which can put a strain on the heart and increase the blood pressure in the lung arteries. If a large PDA is not corrected, then the pressures in the pulmonary arteries may become very high and induce secondary changes, such that blood may begin to flow from the right to the left side of the heart. This situation is called 'Eisenmenger's syndrome' (there are also other causes of this). A PDA often corrects itself within several months of birth, but may require infusion of chemicals, the placement of 'plugs' via catheters, or surgical closure.

ASDs

An ASD is a hole in the septum that separates the upper (atrial) chambers of the heart. It allows blood from the left atrium (higher pressure) to flow to the right atrium (lower pressure), instead of flowing into the left ventricle (lower chamber), as it should. It can also cause pulmonary hypertension, and is another cause of Eisenmenger's syndrome (see the preceding text).

VSDs

A VSD is a hole in the septum between the ventricles (lower chambers). It allows blood to flow from the left ventricle to the right ventricle instead of flowing through the aorta, as it normally should. The heart muscle has to work harder to pump blood, and hypertrophy of the ventricular muscle results. If it is small, it may not strain the heart, but can still produce a loud heart murmur. People with unrepaired VSDs are at risk of getting endocarditis.

Coarctation of the aorta

An aortic coarctation is a narrowing, usually at the site where the ductus arteriosus was present in the proximal descending thoracic aorta. Patients may present with signs of heart failure, absent femoral pulses and very high blood pressure in the upper limbs.

Truncus arteriosus

This is a single great vessel arising from both ventricles that gives rise to the coronary, pulmonary and systemic blood vessels. It is associated with VSD.

Transposition of great vessels

In this condition, the pulmonary artery and aorta are reversed. The aorta arises from the right ventricle, and the pulmonary artery arises from the left ventricle. Other cardiac defects may also be present. Infants can only survive if they have one or more abnormal connections allowing oxygenated blood to reach the body, such as an ASD, VSD or PDA. Most babies born with this condition are very cyanotic at birth, and complex surgery is required to correct the defect.

Tetralogy of Fallot

This is a complex condition with four component lesions:
- Pulmonary stenosis.
- Right ventricular hypertrophy.
- Overriding aorta.
- VSD.

Tetralogy of Fallot typically presents with cyanosis because insufficient blood is flowing to the lungs. Some children require early surgery to place a shunt to bring more blood to the lungs. Most have open heart surgery before school age to correct the main defects.

Aetiology

Generally, the causes of congenital heart disease are unknown. Defects occur in isolation, or may be associated with other syndromes. Heredity may play a role, and various causes such as drugs, chemicals, alcohol and viral infections such as rubella during pregnancy have also been implicated.

Management

Successful treatment of congenital heart disease requires a multidisciplinary approach. Some patients require no treatment, and some do. Management of CHD can be:
- Observation with regular review.
- Cardiological with the use of drug therapy and PCI (see the following text).
- Surgery.
- Combination.

Percutaneous coronary intervention (PCI) involves simple access of a vein or artery by puncturing the skin. Several conditions are amenable to treatment via this approach, and recovery is faster as it does not involve opening the chest. Surgery is indicated if the pathology cannot be treated with PCI. Surgical procedures are used to close holes, repair/replace valves, widen arteries/openings and repair complex defects. The defects may occasionally be too complex to repair, and the child may require a heart transplant.

FURTHER READING

Available from: https://www.nice.org/guidance/cg64.

Available from: http://pathways.nice.org.uk/pathways/prophylaxis-against-infective-endocarditis.

BMJ. Available from: http://www.bmj.com/specialities/cardiovascular-medicine.

Scottish Intercollegiate Guidelines Network: Guideline 147 – management of chronic heart failure. Available from: http://www.sign.ac.uk/pdf/QRG147.pdf.

SIGN 129: Antithrombotics: Indications and management. Available from: http://www.sign.ac.uk/guidelines/fulltext/129/index.html.

MULTIPLE CHOICE QUESTIONS

1. Vascular claudication:
   a) Causes limping on walking.
   b) Is usually felt in the foot at night.
   c) Usually involves the thighs or buttocks.
   d) Is usually managed non-surgically.
   e) Is a reason to be on anticoagulants.

   Answer = D

   Explanation: Claudication does not cause limping (although it comes from the Latin word for limping); it causes muscle pain on walking. It is most often felt in the calf muscles, but can affect the thighs or buttocks, depending on the level of arterial occlusion. Vascular rest pain, not claudication, is felt in the foot or toes. Most claudicants are managed non-surgically with reduction of vascular risk factors. This includes the use of antiplatelet agents, but not usually anticoagulants.

2. Aortic aneurysms:
   a) Should be repaired as early as possible to prevent rupture.
   b) Arise most commonly in the infrarenal abdominal aorta.
   c) Are associated with hyperthyroidism.
   d) When ruptured, are associated with an overall 30–50% mortality.
   e) Are usually associated with aneurysms of the popliteal artery.

   Answer = B

   Explanation: Aneurysms should normally only be repaired if greater than 5.5 cm in size or symptomatic. If smaller, they should usually just be followed up with regular ultrasound scans, as the risk of rupture is low. They are associated with all the major risk factors for atherosclerosis in general, including hypertension but not hyperthyroidism. They most commonly affect the aorta below the renal arteries. Popliteal aneurysms are important, but are associated with only a minority of abdominal aneurysms.

3. Carotid artery stenosis due to atheroma:
   a) Is diagnosed by the presence of a bruit over the lateral aspect of the neck.
   b) Causes approximately 50% of all strokes.
   c) Can be managed with surgical endarterectomy.
   d) Can be managed with thrombolysis.
   e) Can cause a haemorrhagic stroke by producing emboli.

   Answer = C

   Explanation: A carotid bruit, although suggestive, is not diagnostic for significant internal carotid artery disease. Specific diagnosis requires imaging, most commonly by colour duplex ultrasound scanning. Narrowing at the origin of the internal carotid artery is the cause of about 15% of strokes, and if symptomatic is usually treated by the surgical procedure of carotid endarterectomy. Strokes are caused either by emboli from the stenosis or by limitation of flow due to thrombosis of the internal carotid. More recently, some cases are also being treated by percutaneous balloon angioplasty and stenting. Thrombolysis is increasingly being used for acute non-haemorrhagic (thrombotic or embolic) stroke, but it does not treat carotid stenosis.

4. The major risk factors for peripheral occlusive arterial disease include:
   a) The female sex.
   b) Premature menopause.
   c) HDL greater than 1.0 mMol/L.
   d) Diabetes insipidus.
   e) Hypertension.

   Answer = E

   Explanation: Peripheral arterial disease is associated with the same risk factors as coronary disease. The most important are smoking and diabetes mellitus (not insipidus). HDL cholesterol is protective – the higher the HDL, the lesser the risk.

5. Deep vein thrombosis:
   a) Is more common in patients undergoing lower limb surgery.
   b) Is associated with reduced D-dimer levels.
   c) Can be prevented by pre-operative warfarinisation of the patient.
   d) Always results in a swollen, painful lower limb.
   e) All patients should be screened for thrombophilia.

   Answer = A

   Explanation: There is a higher incidence of DVT in lower limb surgery due to the subsequent immobility caused, as well as the local trauma. Patients with malignancy are also at much higher risk due to their hypercoaguable state. In DVT, D-dimers are usually raised. Preventing DVT preoperatively is usually a combination of calf compression with stockings and low-molecular-weight heparinisation. A large percentage of DVTs go unrecognised, particularly when limited to the calf veins, due to lack of symptoms. The majority of pulmonary emboli are from asymptomatic DVTs. Only patients who suffer from unprovoked DVTs (i.e. in the absence of an obvious precipitant), or who present with recurrent DVTs or PEs, should be screened for thrombophilia.

6. A DVT in the popliteal vein in the leg is most likely to embolise to:
   a) The lungs.
   b) The brain.
   c) The coronary arteries.
   d) The popliteal artery.
   e) The hepatic portal vein.
   Answer = A

7. The term that describes leaking of blood from the right ventricle to the right atrium is:
   a) Mitral incompetence
   b) ASD
   c) Aortic regurgitation
   d) Tricuspid regurgitation
   e) VSD
   Answer = D

8. Which of the following is *not* a risk factor for atherosclerotic arterial disease?
   a) Cigarette smoking
   b) Female gender
   c) Diabetes mellitus
   d) Sedentary lifestyle
   e) Low HDL cholesterol
   Answer = B

9. The most common material/substance causing embolism is:
   a) Thrombus
   b) Air
   c) Fat
   d) Foreign body
   e) Misplaced medical devices
   Answer = A

10. 'Virchow's triad' refers to the components predisposing to the pathological process of:
    a) Thrombosis
    b) Embolism
    c) Ischaemia
    d) Infarction
    e) Neoplasia
    Answer = A

CHAPTER 6
Respiratory disorders

SJ Bourke and M Greenwood

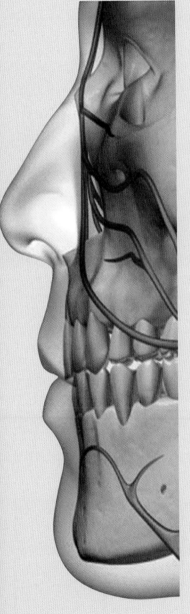

Key topics

- Major respiratory conditions encountered in dental practice.
- The impact of respiratory disorders on dentistry.

Learning objectives

- To be familiar with the main respiratory disorders likely to be encountered in dental practice – investigation and treatment.
- To understand how respiratory disorders may impact on the provision of dental care.
- To have knowledge of the common drugs used to treat respiratory disorders.

Essentials of Human Disease in Dentistry, Second Edition. Mark Greenwood.
© 2018 John Wiley & Sons Ltd. Published 2018 by John Wiley & Sons Ltd.
Companion website: www.wiley.com/go/greenwood/human-disease-in-dentistry

Introduction

The essential function of the respiratory system is to absorb oxygen from the air into the blood and to excrete carbon dioxide. Ventilation is the process of drawing air containing 21% oxygen into the lungs, and it depends on the size of each breath, the respiratory rate, the resistance of the airways and the distensibility of the lungs. Perfusion of the lungs carries deoxygenated blood to the lungs from the venous system and oxygenated blood away from the lungs to the arterial system. The processes of ventilation and perfusion bring air from the atmosphere and blood from the circulation into close contact across the alveolar capillary membrane, so that oxygen can be absorbed and carbon dioxide removed.

The respiratory centre in the brainstem controls breathing and may be affected by sedative drugs (e.g. midazolam and morphine) or brainstem disease (e.g. stroke). Respiratory diseases can affect the airways (e.g. chronic obstructive pulmonary disease (COPD) and asthma), the lung tissue (e.g. lung fibrosis and pneumonia), the pleura (e.g. pleural effusions) or the pulmonary vasculature (e.g. pulmonary embolism).

Two key features of respiratory disease are breathlessness and hypoxia. The lungs are a major interface between the person and the environment, as 8 litres of air are inhaled each minute. This air contains noxious materials. Thus, the lungs are vulnerable to infections from inhaled microbial pathogens, allergic reactions from antigens, cancer from carcinogens (e.g. tobacco smoke) and inflammation and scarring from dusts and toxins. The lungs are also vulnerable to aspiration of material from the mouth as the trachea is in direct continuity with the oropharynx. Periodontal infection can be a source of bacteria tracking down into the lungs, giving rise to pneumonia or lung abscess, and items of dental equipment or fragments of teeth can be inhaled, causing acute airway obstruction.

Clinical assessment

Respiratory disease is common and can impact on dentistry in several ways, and hence respiratory symptoms, signs and investigations are important parts of the overall medical assessment of the patient.

Symptoms

The main respiratory symptoms are breathlessness, wheezing, stridor, cough, sputum production, haemoptysis and pleuritic pain (Table 6.1). *Breathlessness* (dyspnoea) can be graded according to the patient's exercise capacity, indicated by breathlessness on climbing stairs, on walking short distances and at rest. It may be episodic, as in asthma, or persistent, as in COPD.

Many patients with severe lung disease may be more breathless when lying flat (orthopnoea), and may have difficulty in tolerating equipment that blocks their mouth during dental treatment.

Wheezing is the whistling noise produced on expiration, caused by air passing through narrowed airways. It is a

Table 6.1 Respiratory symptoms.
Breathlessness
Wheezing
Stridor
Cough
Sputum
Haemoptysis
Pleuritic pain

particular feature of asthma and COPD. *Stridor* is the noise produced on inspiration, and is a feature of obstruction of the trachea or central airways (e.g. by a tumour or an inhaled foreign body). *Cough* is a forceful expiratory blast and is a protective reflex to remove inhaled material from the lungs. It is a common symptom of many lung diseases. It may be productive of *sputum*, which is typically purulent and green in lung infections (e.g. chronic bronchitis, pneumonia, tuberculosis (TB) and bronchiectasis). *Haemoptysis* (coughing up blood) is an important symptom that always requires investigation. Patients with haemoptysis should be referred to a doctor for further assessment. Sometimes the blood may have arisen from an oropharyngeal source, but blood arising from the lower respiratory tract is a serious symptom, which may indicate diseases such as bronchial or laryngeal carcinoma, TB, severe bronchitis, pneumonia or bronchiectasis. *Pleuritic pain* is a sharp stabbing pain on breathing. It indicates irritation of the pleura by inflammation (pleurisy), infection, pulmonary embolism, tumour or an air leak from the lung (pneumothorax). It may also arise from injury to the ribs and chest wall.

Diseases of the lung can be associated with many general symptoms – such as poor appetite and weight loss from lung cancer; fever and sweating from lung infections; lethargy, malaise and peripheral oedema from hypoxia; and headaches from carbon dioxide retention. Chronic hypoxia causes a rise in pulmonary artery pressure, which may result in right ventricular failure. This is referred to as 'cor pulmonale', and it manifests as elevated jugular venous pressure and peripheral oedema.

Examination

Some signs of respiratory disease may be evident to the dental practitioner from general examination of the clothed patient. Patients with impaired lung function often have an increased respiratory rate and use accessory muscles of respiration (e.g. the sternocleidomastoids) to increase ventilation. Conversely, slow, shallow breathing may be a sign of respiratory depression during the use of sedative medication. The respiratory rate is most accurately assessed by counting it over a period of 30 sec. This is best done surreptitiously, perhaps after counting the pulse rate, as patients tend to breathe faster if they are aware that the focus is on their breathing. Wheezing or stridor may

Table 6.2 The components of Horner's syndrome.
Drooping of eyelids (ptosis)
Constriction of pupils (miosis)
Enophthalmos
Ipsilateral loss of sweating (anhidrosis)

be audible. Hoarseness of the voice may be an important clue to laryngeal disease (e.g. carcinoma), or to recurrent laryngeal nerve damage from lung cancer.

Distension of the jugular veins may indicate an elevated venous pressure from failure of the right side of the heart (cor pulmonale), or owing to obstruction of the superior vena cava from lung cancer. Enlargement of the cervical or supraclavicular lymph nodes can result from spread of disease from the chest (e.g. cancer or TB). Horner's syndrome (Table 6.2) consists of drooping of the eyelids (ptosis), constriction of the pupils (miosis), reduced prominence of the eyes (enophthalmos) and loss of sweating on one side of the face (anhidrosis). These appearances are due to damage to the sympathetic nerve supply, which may occur as a result of a tumour at the lung apex.

Pallor of the skin and mucous membranes may indicate anaemia, which can cause breathlessness. Cyanosis is a bluish discoloration of the skin and mucous membranes as a result of deoxygenated haemoglobin. It is the key sign of severe hypoxia and is best seen on the tip of the tongue. It is not usually detectable until the oxygen saturation is below 85% (normal level is 97%).

Oral candidiasis may be an adverse effect of inhaled or oral steroid therapy. Gingival overgrowth is an adverse effect of some drugs such as ciclosporin used after organ transplantation.

Tar staining of the fingers is a feature of heavy tobacco smoking, which is associated with COPD and lung cancer. Clubbing is characterised by increased curvature of the nail, with loss of angle between the nail and nail bed, such that the finger resembles a 'club' when viewed in profile (Chapter 1, titled 'Clinical examination and history taking'). It is an important sign that is associated with a number of diseases, including lung cancer, cystic fibrosis, asbestosis and fibrotic lung disease. A tremor may be due to high-dose β-agonist medication such as nebulised salbutamol. Venous dilatation, bounding pulse and flapping twitching of the hand (asterixis) are signs of severe carbon dioxide retention.

General medical history

Certain features of the patient's overall medical history are particularly important. Patients with major respiratory disease will often have had a full assessment by their general medical practitioner or hospital specialist. In complex cases, it is useful to discuss the patient's problems with their doctor, so as to coordinate and optimise medical and dental care. For example, patients receiving chemotherapy for lung cancer may be at particular risk of developing infection or bleeding after oral surgery, as a result of bone marrow suppression with reduced white cell and platelet counts.

Good dental care and hygiene are particularly important for patients receiving immunosuppressive drugs for inflammatory lung disease (e.g. the chronic granulomatous disease sarcoidosis), or after lung transplantation, as the oropharynx is a potential source of infections that can spread to the lungs.

Owing to the risks of respiratory depression, particular care is needed when considering sedation for patients with hypoxia. It is important to have a complete list of the patient's current medications and any drug allergies. Adverse effects of drug treatments may be apparent – for example, oral candidiasis from inhaled or systemic corticosteroids, gingival overgrowth from ciclosporin, or mucositis and xerostomia from anticancer chemotherapy. Potential drug interactions need to be considered – for example, macrolide antibiotics such as erythromycin and clarithromycin reduce the hepatic clearance of theophylline, and can give rise to toxic adverse effects such as vomiting or tachycardia. A small percentage of patients with asthma may develop wheezing if NSAIDs (e.g. naproxen or ibuprofen) are used for analgesia.

Aspects of the patient's environment can be important in the causation of lung disease. Tobacco smoking predisposes to lung cancer and COPD. Occupational exposure to dusts such as asbestos, coal and silica can cause lung fibrosis. Contact with pet birds can cause lung inflammation and fibrosis in the form of bird fancier's hypersensitivity pneumonitis. The lungs can be affected by systemic diseases such as rheumatoid arthritis and their treatments (e.g. methotrexate alveolitis). The lungs are particularly vulnerable to infections when the patient is immunocompromised by HIV infection or by using immunosuppressive drugs (e.g. ciclosporin or azathioprine).

Investigating respiratory disease

Some simple investigations (e.g. peak expiratory flow rate or oximetry) can be performed in the dental surgery, and are useful in assessing and monitoring the patient's respiratory status. The peak expiratory flow rate is the maximum rate of airflow during a forced expiration. It is a measure of the airway calibre, and is reduced in diseases such as asthma and COPD. Many patients own a peak flow meter and use it to monitor the activity of their asthma.

An oximeter (Figure 6.1) measures the percentage of oxygenated haemoglobin using a probe placed on a finger or ear lobe. It comprises two light-emitting diodes and a detector. Oxygenated blood appears red, whereas deoxygenated blood appears blue. Skin pigmentation or the use of nail varnish can interfere with light transmission. Oximetry is especially useful in monitoring the patient's oxygenation continuously during procedures (e.g. bronchoscopy), anaesthesia or sedation, particularly in patients with respiratory disease. Oximetry does not provide information about the patient's carbon dioxide level. In hospital practice, a sample of blood can be taken from an artery to measure oxygen and carbon dioxide levels directly.

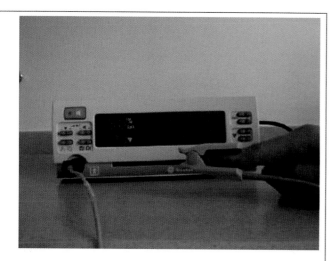

Figure 6.1 A pulse oximeter. The probe (right of picture) can be placed on a finger, and the oxygen saturation (upper figure on display as a percentage) and pulse rate (lower figure) are measured. No nail varnish is allowed.

Hospital laboratories can measure other aspects of lung function. For example, the total lung capacity is reduced in diseases that restrict the volume of the lung (e.g. fibrotic lung disease). The transfer factor measures the rate at which gas passes from the alveoli to the bloodstream, and this is reduced in diseases such as emphysema, lung fibrosis or pulmonary embolism. Clinical examination lacks sensitivity, and major disease of the lungs can be present without any detectable clinical signs. The chest X-ray, therefore, has a key role in the investigation of respiratory disease.

Computed tomography (CT) provides a much more detailed cross-sectional image, and various techniques can be used to display the lung parenchyma (e.g. lung fibrosis), mediastinal structures (e.g. lymph node enlargement in lung cancer) and vasculature (e.g. pulmonary embolism). Bronchoscopy allows direct visualisation of the main airways; biopsies may be taken for histopathological examination (e.g. lung cancer); and secretions can be aspirated for cytology and microbiology tests. Sputum microbiology is used routinely to detect microbial pathogens in diseases such as chronic bronchitis, pneumonia, bronchiectasis and TB.

Asthma

Asthma is characterised by bronchial inflammation, which results in mucosal oedema and irritability of the airways, such that they are prone to constriction of the bronchial smooth muscle. This results in symptoms such as wheezing, cough and breathlessness, and airways obstruction, which is variable and reversible with treatment. About 7% of the adult population in the UK has asthma. Asthma is multifactorial in origin, arising from a complex interaction of genetic and environmental factors.

Atopy is a constitutional tendency to produce IgE on exposure to common antigens, and atopic individuals have a high prevalence of asthma, allergic rhinitis and eczema. The prevalence of asthma is increasing, and this seems to be related to the modern urban economically developed environment. Some patients with atopic asthma develop reactions to common antigens such as house dust mite (found in carpets, soft furnishings and bedding); antigens found in pets; and antigens in the environment (e.g. grass pollens) and the workplace (e.g. isocyanates or hard wood dusts).

Attacks of asthma can be precipitated by cofactors such as respiratory tract infections, cigarette smoke, pollutants and cold air. β-Blocker drugs (e.g. atenolol) can induce bronchoconstriction, and a small percentage of asthmatics develop wheezing if given aspirin or NSAIDs (e.g. ibuprofen).

Symptoms may develop at any age, and may be episodic or persistent. Episodic asthma is a common pattern in children and young adults. The patient is often asymptomatic between attacks, but episodes of bronchoconstriction are provoked by factors such as infection or contact with an inhaled antigen. The pattern is sometimes of persistent asthma with chronic wheezing and dyspnoea. Airway remodelling in chronic severe asthma can result in permanent changes in the bronchial wall with fixed airways obstruction.

The variable nature of symptoms is a characteristic feature of asthma. Typically, there is a diurnal pattern, with symptoms and peak expiratory flow rate (PEFR) being worse early in the morning ('morning dipping'). Symptoms such as cough and wheezing often disturb sleep ('nocturnal asthma'). Symptoms may be provoked by exercise ('exercise asthma'), but many elite athletes compete at the highest level despite having asthma. Patients with asthma usually have a dramatic improvement in their symptoms and PEFR when given a bronchodilator drug or corticosteroids.

The key feature of asthma is airways obstruction, which can be measured objectively using a PEFR meter. Patients will often have a PEFR meter that they use to monitor their asthma. They may be aware of their best achievable PEFR, and they often have a self-management plan whereby they start a course of prednisolone and increase their bronchodilator medications if their PEFR falls below a set level.

Drugs used to treat asthma

In most patients, asthma can be controlled by a regular inhaled corticosteroid (to reduce airway inflammation) and an inhaled bronchodilator (to be taken as required to reverse wheezing).

Bronchodilators ('relievers')

β₂-Agonists (e.g. salbutamol, terbutaline) stimulate β-adrenoreceptors in the smooth muscles of the airways, producing muscle relaxation and bronchodilatation. They have an onset of action within 15 min, and last 4–6 hours. Adverse effects are rare, but include tremor, palpitations and muscle cramps. Patients should carry their 'reliever inhaler' with them, and it should be available when undertaking dental procedures, so that it can be used if the patient becomes wheezy. *Long-acting β*$_2$*-agonists* (e.g. salmeterol and formoterol) have a duration of action of >12 hours. *Anticholinergic bronchodilators* (e.g. ipratropium tiotropium, aclidinium, and glycopyrronium) produce bronchodilatation by blocking the bronchoconstriction effect of vagal nerve stimulation on bronchial smooth muscle. Adverse effects are rare, but some patients experience dryness of the mouth. *Theophyllines* increase cyclic adenosine monophosphate (cAMP) stimulation of β-adrenoreceptors by inhibiting the metabolism of cAMP by the enzyme phosphodiesterase. They are not available in inhaler form, and are taken as tablets. Adverse effects include nausea, headache and tachycardia. Interactions with other drugs can cause toxicity. Hepatic clearance of theophyllines is reduced by drugs such as ciprofloxacin, erythromycin and cimetidine.

Anti-inflammatory drugs ('preventers')

Inhaled corticosteroids (e.g. beclometasone, budesonide, fluticasone, mometasone and ciclesonide) are the mainstay of asthma treatment, as they control airway inflammation, which is the key underlying process in asthma. They need to be taken regularly, usually twice daily, to prevent asthma attacks. Adverse effects include oropharyngeal candidiasis and hoarseness of the voice, which can be reduced by using a spacer device and gargling the throat after inhalation. Higher-dose inhaled steroids can cause some suppression of adrenal function, increased bone turnover and skin purpura. *Leukotriene receptor antagonists* (e.g. montelukast and zafirlukast) are a new modality of anti-inflammatory therapy, given orally in tablet form. They block the effect of cysteinyl leukotrienes, which are metabolites of arachidonic acid with bronchoconstrictor and pro-inflammatory effects. *Prednisolone* (e.g. 30 mg/day for 7 days) is usually given as 'rescue treatment' for acute attacks of asthma. Patients who are prone to acute exacerbations often have their own supply of prednisolone, and are taught to start this according to a self-management plan when their PEFR falls. Adverse effects of frequent or long-term systemic steroids include osteoporosis, growth suppression, cataracts and Cushingoid features of weight gain, buffalo hump, moon face and hirsutism.

There are many different inhaler device types, such as metered-dose inhalers and breath-actuated devices. Patients need careful instruction on how to use the inhaler device that suits their needs, as poor inhaler techniques reduce the effectiveness of treatment. A spacer device improves the deposition of the drug in the lower airway and reduces the need to coordinate inspiration with actuation of the inhaler. Nebulisers may be used during acute asthma attacks to deliver high-dose bronchodilators. Oxygen or compressed air is used to nebulise the drug, which is delivered via a face mask.

When undertaking dental treatment in a patient with asthma, it is advisable to document the severity of the patient's asthma – for example, any previous hospital admissions, or severe attacks requiring admission to an intensive therapy unit.

It should be ensured that the patient's asthma is currently well controlled, with few symptoms and satisfactory PEFR. The patient should bring a bronchodilator inhaler (e.g. salbutamol or terbutaline) that can be used to relieve wheezing. Avoid using NSAIDs if the patient has previously experienced wheezing on using these medicines. Anxious patients may suffer panic attacks and episodes of anxiety-related hyperventilation during dental procedures, with overbreathing, fast pulse, sweating and anxiety. Prolonged hyperventilation can "blow off" carbon dioxide and result in dizziness, a 'pins and needles' sensation in the fingers and fainting. In contrast, an asthma attack is characterised by wheezing, respiratory distress and reduced PEFR. If the patient develops an attack of asthma, stop the procedure, sit the patient upright and administer the salbutamol or terbutaline inhaler. Failure to respond, a falling PEFR or the development of cyanosis would indicate a severe attack of asthma. In such cases, emergency medical services should be summoned, so that the patient can be treated with oxygen, nebulised bronchodilators and systemic corticosteroids.

COPD

COPD is a disease characterised by gradually worsening breathlessness due to progressive airways obstruction and comprises chronic bronchitis and emphysema. The major cause is tobacco smoking. In susceptible people, smoking causes a range of damage to the lungs that are encompassed by the term 'COPD'. *Chronic bronchitis* is the result of hypertrophy of the mucus glands, with excess secretions causing chronic cough and sputum production. Superimposed infections with bacteria such as *Streptococcus pneumoniae*, *Haemophilus influenzae* and *Moraxella catarrhalis* are common. *Airways obstruction* is the hallmark of COPD, and this is demonstrated by reduced PEFR and forced expiratory volume in 1 second (FEV_1), which is measured in hospital or general medicine practice using a spirometer.

Emphysema is the destruction of the distal bronchioles and lung tissue, and can be seen on CT scans (Figure 6.2). It is characterised by reduced gas transfer across the alveolar capillary membrane. COPD, and other lung diseases, may progress to a stage of *respiratory failure*, when the patient has hypoxia and may need long-term oxygen therapy at home. Chronic hypoxia provokes pulmonary artery vasoconstriction, as well as right heart hypertrophy and failure, which is termed 'cor pulmonale'. This is manifest as raised jugular venous pressure and peripheral oedema.

Sedentary patients may not become aware of breathlessness until there has been considerable permanent loss of lung function. Thereafter, patients with COPD usually experience gradually progressive breathlessness over the years. Those with advanced disease may have breathlessness even at rest, or on walking very short distances (e.g. 10 metres).

Exacerbations of COPD are characterised by increased breathlessness, cough and sputum. They may be precipitated by respiratory tract infections or by exposure to pollution. As lung function deteriorates, some patients develop the physiological

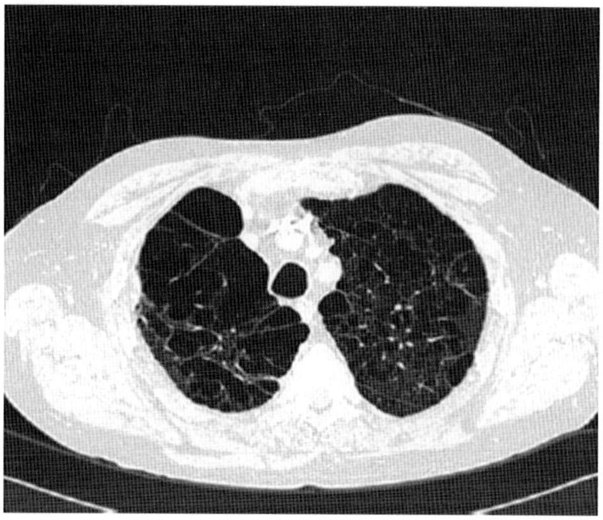

Figure 6.2 CT scan: emphysema. This 62-year-old man had smoked 30 cigarettes/day for 45 years. He developed COPD with progressive breathlessness. His CT scan shows emphysema with destruction of alveolar tissue and loss of normal lung architecture, such that the lung tissue shows areas of black cysts. He required frequent hospital admissions with exacerbations of COPD, and he developed hypoxia, requiring long-term home oxygen therapy.

response of increased ventilatory drive with a 'pink puffer' pattern, whereby they have a fast respiratory rate ('puffing') and increased use of the accessory muscles of respiration, so that they maintain their oxygen levels ('pink'). Others do not increase their ventilatory drive, and develop a 'blue bloater' pattern with hypoxia and cyanosis ('blue') and cor pulmonale with oedema ('bloated').

The most important treatment of COPD is smoking cessation. All healthcare professionals should advise patients not to smoke, and smokers should be supported in stopping smoking by using treatments such as nicotine replacement therapy. Because airways obstruction is predominantly due to structural changes in the bronchial walls and lung tissue, COPD is much less responsive to drug treatment as compared to asthma. Bronchodilator drugs (e.g. salbutamol, tiotropium and salmeterol) improve symptoms and exercise capacity. Inhaled corticosteroids reduce the frequency of exacerbations in severe COPD. Mucolytic agents (e.g. carbocisteine) may help sputum clearance by reducing its viscosity, and may reduce the frequency of exacerbations. Antibiotics (e.g. amoxicillin and tetracycline) are useful in treating infective exacerbations. Pulmonary rehabilitation is a multidisciplinary programme of care involving smoking cessation, education, exercise training, breathing control techniques and psychosocial support.

Oxygen therapy is important for hypoxic patients. Air contains about 21% oxygen. High-flow oxygen (>60%) is usually delivered via a face mask with a reservoir bag attached to an oxygen source. It is appropriate for severely hypoxic patients in an emergency – for example, after cardiorespiratory arrest or in acute asthma. Patients with COPD are usually treated with lower-dose controlled oxygen – for example, 24% or 28% masks, or a nasal cannula – at a flow rate of 2 litres/min, in order to bring their oxygen saturation to >90%. Oximetry and arterial blood gas analysis are important in initiating and monitoring oxygen therapy.

Some patients with COPD (e.g. 'blue bloaters') have chronically raised carbon dioxide levels with poor respiratory drive, such that they rely on hypoxia to maintain their drive to breathe. If they are given high concentrations of oxygen, they breathe less, resulting in increasing carbon dioxide levels, acidosis, narcosis and respiratory depression. Long-term home oxygen therapy is given to patients with severe COPD who have persistent hypoxia. This is usually provided from an oxygen concentrator machine that is installed in the patient's house. Oxygen must be delivered for at least 15 hours/day to reduce the risk of right heart failure and to improve the patient's prognosis.

Patients with COPD often have difficulty lying flat (orthopnoea), and prefer to have dental treatment sitting upright. They may also have difficulty tolerating dental equipment in their mouth if it obstructs breathing. Treatment may have to be interrupted to allow them to clear excess secretions from their airways. Particular care is needed in using sedation in patients with hypoxia and severe lung disease, and the dentist should discuss the proposed treatment with the patient's medical practitioner.

Lung cancer

Lung cancer kills about 35 000 people each year in the UK. It is a lethal disease, with only 7% of patients surviving 5 years from diagnosis. The majority of lung cancers are caused by tobacco smoking. Smoking prevention and cessation are the crucial issues in dealing with this major public health problem. About 30% of the UK population smoke, and the smoking rate is gradually falling. However, worldwide, the smoking rate is increasing, particularly in Asia.

Lung cancers are classified into two groups: small-cell carcinoma (20% of lung cancers) and non-small-cell carcinoma (80%), comprising squamous carcinoma (45%), adenocarcinoma (20%) and large-cell undifferentiated carcinoma (15%). Small-cell (oat-cell) carcinoma arises from the neuroendocrine cells of the bronchial tree. It is a highly malignant cancer that grows rapidly and metastasises early, and hence it is not suitable for surgical resection. It is treated with chemotherapy and radiotherapy. Some non-small-cell carcinomas are suitable for surgical resection if the cancer has not spread.

Patients with lung cancer may present with chest symptoms such as haemoptysis, cough, wheezing or stridor; general systemic symptoms such as weight loss and anorexia; or symptoms arising from metastases to sites such as bone, brain, liver or skin. Lung cancers sometimes secrete hormones that can cause hypercalcaemia, hyponatraemia or Cushing's syndrome (adrenocorticotrophic hormone, or ACTH). The chest X-ray is

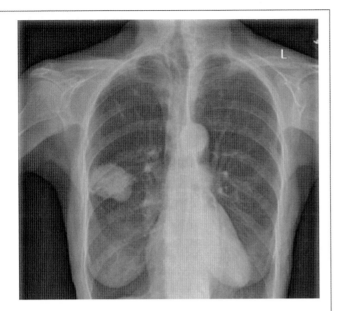

Figure 6.3 Chest X-ray: lung cancer. This 78-year-old woman presented with cough and haemoptysis. She had smoked 15 cigarettes/day for 50 years, and had clubbing of her fingers. Her chest X-ray showed a tumour in the right upper lobe, and needle biopsy showed squamous cell carcinoma. She was treated with radiotherapy.

a key investigation (Figure 6.3), and may show a variety of features such as mass lesions, lymph node enlargement, collapse or loss of lung volume from obstruction of a bronchus by carcinoma, or pleural effusion. Sputum cytology confirms malignant cells in about 40% of lung cancer cases. Bronchoscopy allows direct visualisation and biopsy of central tumours. Percutaneous needle biopsy of peripheral masses can be undertaken under radiological guidance to obtain a histopathological diagnosis.

Once a diagnosis of lung cancer has been confirmed, the next step is to determine the extent and spread of the disease. In addition to assessment of the patient's symptoms and signs, this staging process particularly involves CT scans and positron emission tomography (PET). If a non-small-cell carcinoma has been detected early, and there is no evidence of spread of the carcinoma, then surgical resection offers the best prospect of cure. The patient has to have adequate lung function and general fitness to tolerate resection of a lobe of lung. For small-cell carcinomas, and for non-small-cell carcinomas that are not suitable for surgery, chemotherapy and radiotherapy can achieve shrinkage of the tumour with improvement in symptoms and prognosis, but cure is rarely possible.

A variety of chemotherapeutic drugs are available (e.g. cisplatin or gemcitabine), but these affect all rapidly dividing cells in the body. Typical adverse effects include nausea, vomiting, hair loss, oral mucositis, loss of taste, xerostomia and bone marrow suppression, accompanied with lethargy from anaemia, a risk of infection from leukopaenia and a risk of bleeding from thrombocytopaenia.

Good dental care and oral hygiene are important in patients receiving chemotherapy. Oral surgery needs to be planned in the context of the patient's medical team. Most chemotherapy is given in cycles every 3–4 weeks, and bone marrow suppression is usually at its worst about 10–14 days after chemotherapy, and it is at this point that the risk of infection or bleeding is the highest.

Patients with lung cancer will often develop progressive cancer despite treatment, and will reach a stage when the focus is on palliative care. Mild pain may be treated by NSAIDs, paracetamol or opioids (e.g. codeine). Strong opioids (e.g. morphine or oxycodone) are used for more severe pain. Certain types of pain may be alleviated by coanalgesics such as steroids (e.g. dexamethasone) for nerve compression, and benzodiazepines, tricyclic antidepressants and antiepileptics (e.g. gabapentin or pregabalin) for neuropathic pain. Opioid analgesics tend to cause nausea and constipation, and antiemetics and laxatives may be needed. Anorexia, weight loss, fatigue and debility are common symptoms. Patients often need help with social support and with tasks of daily living.

Obstructive sleep apnoea syndrome (OSAS)

OSAS is a condition of sleep-related pharyngeal collapse in which recurrent episodes of upper airways occlusion occur during sleep, causing cessation of airflow (apnoea) in the pharynx. This provokes arousals and sleep fragmentation, resulting in daytime sleepiness. A narrow upper airway predisposes to OSAS. This is usually due to fat deposition in the neck from obesity, but other factors such as bone morphology (e.g. micrognathia), soft tissue deposition (e.g. hypothyroidism or acromegaly) or enlarged tonsils or adenoids in children may also be important. As a patient with a narrow pharyngeal airway enters deep sleep, the reduction in oropharyngeal dilator muscle tone results in collapse of the airway, with cessation of airflow (apnoea) and a fall in oxygen saturation.

The apnoea is terminated by a brief arousal from sleep and resumption of pharyngeal airflow with a burst of sympathetic nerve activity, which is accompanied by loud snoring due to vibration of the soft tissues of the oropharynx. Multiple apnoeas and arousals throughout the night disrupt sleep, resulting in daytime sleepiness, impaired concentration, road accidents and increased risk of cardiovascular disease, stroke and hypertension. The main treatment of OSAS is by delivering continuous positive airway pressure (CPAP) during sleep by using a tight-fitting nasal mask that splints the pharyngeal airway open. In some cases, mandibular advancement devices are worn over the teeth to bring the mandible forward, thereby increasing the cross-sectional area of the oropharynx. Patients with OSAS are at high risk of developing respiratory depression and carbon dioxide retention when having surgery under sedation or general anaesthesia.

Respiratory tract infections

Most upper respiratory tract infections are due to viruses (e.g. rhinovirus, coronavirus or adenovirus), and they result in clinical syndromes such as the common cold, pharyngitis, sinusitis and laryngitis. Most are self-limiting and do not require treatment. Influenza A infection, however, causes a severe illness that can result in substantial morbidity and mortality, particularly in the elderly or in patients with pre-existing lung disease. Annual influenza vaccination is therefore recommended for vulnerable patients.

Lower respiratory tract infections vary according to the circumstances of the infection, the virulence of the organism and the vulnerability of the patient. Pneumonia is an acute, severe infection of the lung parenchyma. When it is acquired in the community, the most common pathogens are *Streptococcus pneumoniae*, *Mycoplasma pneumoniae*, *Haemophilus influenzae* and viruses. Hospital-acquired pneumonia (Figure 6.4) occurs in patients who have been debilitated by other diseases or by surgery. Patients in an intensive therapy unit on mechanical ventilation via an endotracheal tube are particularly vulnerable to pneumonia. In some cases, periodontal disease may be the source of bacterial infection. The oropharynx of hospitalised patients can become colonised by Gram-negative organisms such as *Pseudomonas aeruginosa*. Poor oral hygiene and periodontal disease may promote oropharyngeal colonisation by bacteria. Aspiration of infected oropharyngeal material is more common in the presence of an endotracheal tube, as well as when the patient has a diminished cough reflex, reduced level of consciousness and general debility.

TB is an infection (caused by *Mycobacterium tuberculosis*) that may affect any part of the body, but most commonly involves the lungs. It is spread by inhaling the bacteria coughed or sneezed out by someone with infectious TB. Chronic cough, sputum, haemoptysis, fevers, sweating and weight loss are common features of TB. Cavitating consolidation in the upper lobes of the lungs is a characteristic feature of chest X-rays. Microscopy of sputum will often identify the characteristic acid- and alcohol-fast bacilli (AAFB) in patients with TB, and such patients can spread infection to others. Culture of the organism requires special media, and may take 6–8 weeks. Biopsy of the affected sites (e.g. the lung, pleura and lymph nodes) typically shows caseating granuloma.

Treatment requires a combination of isoniazid, rifampicin, pyrazinamide and ethambutol for a total of 6 months. Patients cease to be infectious after 2 weeks of treatment, and dental procedures can be safely undertaken at that stage.

Cystic fibrosis and bronchiectasis

Bronchiectasis is a chronic disease characterised by irreversible dilatation of bronchi caused by bronchial wall damage resulting from infection and inflammation. Defects in the bronchial wall can occur due to severe infections in childhood, such as whooping cough, measles or TB. Disruption of the bronchial mucosa and cilia allows bacteria to adhere to the epithelium, and the process of chronic infection, inflammation and progressive bronchial injury becomes self-perpetuating. Patients who are deficient in immunoglobulins, or who have inherited abnormalities of ciliary function (primary ciliary dyskinesia), are particularly vulnerable to developing bronchiectasis and chronic lung infection.

Cystic fibrosis is an autosomal recessive disease resulting from mutations of a gene on chromosome 7 that codes for a chloride channel in cell membranes. Loss of chloride channel function in epithelial membranes throughout the body results in a complex disease involving the respiratory, gastrointestinal, hepatobiliary and reproductive tracts. In the lungs, thick viscid secretions predispose to chronic infection with *Staphylococcus aureus*, *Pseudomonas aeruginosa* and *Burkholderia cepacia*. This results in severe progressive bronchiectasis, respiratory failure and premature death. Mucus plugging of ducts in the pancreas prevents pancreatic enzymes from reaching the intestine, with the failure to absorb fat resulting in failure to thrive and reduced nutritional status. Patients with cystic fibrosis (Figure 6.5) are treated in specialist centres with a complex regimen, including chest physiotherapy to aid sputum clearance; pancreatic enzymes and nutritional supplements to counteract malabsorption; and high-intensity oral, nebulised and intravenous antibiotics. In the later stages of the disease, respiratory failure may develop, and patients may require long-term home oxygen therapy. Lung transplantation is the main option for patients with advanced cystic fibrosis, although

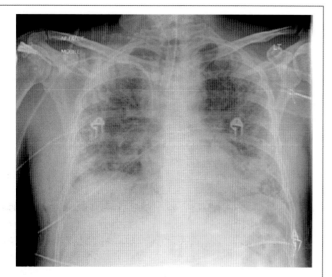

Figure 6.4 Chest X-ray: pneumonia. This 78-year-old man required emergency surgery for a ruptured abdominal aortic aneurysm. He was critically ill and required endotracheal intubation and ventilation in an intensive therapy unit. He then developed severe pneumonia. His chest X-ray shows extensive pneumonic consolidation in both lungs. Microbiology identified *Pseudomonas aeruginosa*.

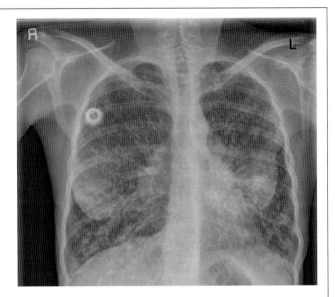

Figure 6.5 Chest X-ray: cystic fibrosis. This 20-year-old woman had developed respiratory failure due to advanced cystic fibrosis and *Pseudomonas aeruginosa* lung infection. Her chest X-ray shows severe diffuse bronchiectasis with bronchial thickening and dilatation, and areas of consolidation. An indwelling intravenous access system is in place in the right subclavian vein for administration of antibiotics. She subsequently underwent lung transplantation.

there is a shortage of donor organs. After lung transplantation, patients are maintained on long-term immunosuppressive drugs such as ciclosporin, tacrolimus, azathioprine and prednisolone to prevent rejection.

Pulmonary embolism

Most pulmonary emboli arise from thrombosis in the deep veins of the legs. Venous thrombosis tends to occur when there is a combination of venous stasis and a hypercoagulable state. Patients who are immobile on medical, surgical and obstetric wards are particularly vulnerable to thrombosis. Hypercoagulable states arise as part of the body's response to surgery, trauma and childbirth, and are also associated with malignant tumours. Recurrent thrombosis is likely where there are inherited abnormalities of the clotting system, such as factor V Leiden gene mutation, antithrombin III, and protein S or protein C deficiencies.

Pulmonary embolism typically causes acute breathlessness, pleuritic pain and haemoptysis. An acute massive pulmonary embolism can cause the patient to collapse and die, with very little opportunity for medical intervention. The diagnosis of pulmonary embolism can be confirmed by a lung perfusion scan or CT pulmonary angiogram. Heparin is given to achieve rapid anticoagulation, and then the patient is established on oral anticoagulants (such as warfarin) or direct oral anticoagulants (such as rivaroxaban, apixaban or dabigatran).

Fibrotic lung disease

Inflammation of the alveoli (pneumonitis) and scarring of the lung tissue (fibrosis) can occur in a variety of circumstances. Inhalation of asbestos or coal dust over a prolonged period in the workplace can cause pneumoconiosis with extensive lung fibrosis. Inhalation of antigens from birds or from mouldy hay can cause hypersensitivity pneumonitis in the form of bird fancier's lung or farmer's lung. Some systemic connective tissue diseases such as rheumatoid disease can also involve the lungs. Alveolitis and fibrosis can also occur as an adverse effect of drug treatment (e.g. methotrexate or amiodarone).

Sarcoidosis is a multisystem disease of unknown cause that results in granulomatous inflammation in many organs of the body, including the lungs, lymph nodes, salivary glands, skin and liver. Idiopathic pulmonary fibrosis is a severe form of progressive lung fibrosis of unknown cause, and it tends to affect patients between the ages of 60 and 70 years, often progressing to cause severe disability, respiratory failure and death. Typically, these patients have severe progressive breathlessness, clubbing and lung crackles. They may be treated with immunosuppressive drugs (such as prednisolone, azathioprine or cyclophosphamide) and anti-fibrotic drugs (such as pirfenidone or nintedanib).

Management of inhaled foreign body

The emergency management of choking is discussed in Chapter 21 (titled 'Medical emergencies'). It is important that, in dental practice, precautions be taken that protect against inhalation. In short, prevention is the key to safe management, and some methods of prevention are listed in Table 6.3. If inhalation of a foreign body is suspected, it is important that the oral cavity and the surrounding area be fully examined. If a foreign body is inhaled and passes to the lower respiratory tract (below the vocal cords), it is most likely to be found in the right main bronchus or right lung. The right main bronchus is more vertical than the left.

A finger sweep should not be performed in infants who are at risk of inhalation, as there is a risk of pushing the foreign body further back into the oropharynx. Five back blows should be given, rather than abdominal thrusts.

If a patient is suspected of having inhaled a foreign body, he or she should be referred to a hospital accident and emergency department along with a letter detailing the prior events, and

Table 6.3 Prevention of inhalation or suspicion of inhalation of foreign bodies.

Rubber dam
Mouth sponges
Instrument chains
Ensure that the foreign body has actually been inhaled!

an explanatory telephone call should be made to the department to expect the patient.

What happens in the accident and emergency department?

The history will be repeated, and the patient examined. The chest will be auscultated. Radiographs will be taken in two planes at 90° (a posteroanterior view and a lateral view of the chest). If the foreign body is suspected of being 'higher up' the respiratory tract, a lateral soft tissue cervical view may be carried out.

If the foreign body is in the lung or some other part of the respiratory tract, it must be removed. A bronchoscopy is carried out. Fine instruments with forceps at the end may retrieve the object. Rarely, open surgery may be required.

What happens if no ventilation is possible in the acute situation?

This is a rare event, as the measures detailed in Chapter 21 will usually dislodge the object. If it has fallen further in the respiratory tract, respiration will normally be possible.

In events where ventilation is not possible, however, consideration by competent personnel should be given to needle cricothyroidotomy. An outline of how this procedure is carried out is given in Table 6.4. Possible problems with cricothyroidotomy are listed in Table 6.5. One of the most important of these is the fact that cricothyroidotomy is only a holding procedure that will last for 30–45 min before a build-up of carbon dioxide occurs.

Cases of cricothyroidotomy may lead on to the need for tracheostomy. This is an elective/semi-elective procedure that is normally carried out in an operating theatre.

In summary, if inhalation of a foreign body is suspected, prompt treatment must be instituted. Any foreign body must be accounted for, and, if not, it should be considered to have been inhaled until proved otherwise. Chest radiography in these situations is mandatory. The situation of an inhaled foreign body is one that can usually be prevented.

Respiratory disorders and dentistry

When a patient gives a history of respiratory disorder, it is important that questions be asked about the effectiveness of treatment and the factors that precipitate problems. The history, in conjunction with examination of the patient, will determine the presence or otherwise of shortage of breath at rest or on exertion. A summary of the relevant points to cover in the history of a dental patient with respiratory disease is given in Table 6.6. If a patient has a productive cough, the colour of the sputum that is expectorated should be noted.

Table 6.5 Potential problems with cricothyroidotomy.

Inadequate ventilation leading to hypoxia and death – in best scenario, only good for 30–45 min.
Aspiration (blood).
Oesophageal laceration.
Haematoma.
Posterior tracheal wall perforation.
Subcutaneous and/or mediastinal perforation.
Thyroid perforation.

Table 6.6 Information that should be obtained from dental patients who have a history of respiratory problems.

Does the patient smoke?
Has there been a diagnosis of a disease (e.g. asthma, COPD, cystic fibrosis)?
Is the patient on medications (e.g. salbutamol, prednisolone)?
Is the condition stable at present?
Does the patient experience breathlessness?
Can the patient lie in a semi-recumbent position and tolerate a dental procedure?
Is there cough, sputum production or haemoptysis?
Is there a history of sinusitis?
Is there evidence of hypoxia (e.g. home oxygen treatment, cyanosis)?
Will the patient's condition affect dental treatment?
Has the patient sought medical advice for the symptoms?
Is there a need to discuss the condition with a medical practitioner?

Table 6.4 An outline of needle cricothyroidotomy.

Place the patient supine with the neck extended.
A large-bore needle is required (special kits are available).
The neck should be swabbed with antiseptic.
The cricothyroid membrane should be palpated between the cricoid cartilage and thyroid cartilage.
The trachea should be stabilised between the thumb and forefinger of one hand.
Puncture skin in the midline directly over the cricothyroid membrane. A small incision helps.
Direct needle at 45° caudally, applying negative pressure to the syringe.
Insert needle, aspirate as needle advances.
Aspiration of air signifies entry into the trachea.
Remove syringe, withdraw stylet and advance catheter – beware of puncturing the posterior wall of trachea.
High-flow oxygen is attached.

Other disorders, including sarcoidosis or ARDS (see the following text), may be guided by facts obtained earlier in the history.

Another good marker of disease severity is the necessity or otherwise for inpatient hospitalisation due to the respiratory disorder. The use (or history) of systemic steroids should be determined. The treatment that the patient may use on a permanent basis should be assessed in terms of its efficacy.

If the patient suffers from asthma, aspirin-like compounds should be prescribed with caution, as many asthmatic patients are sensitive to these analgesics.

Examination of the clothed patient

The patient's complexion may give a clue to the underlying disorder – for example, the 'pink puffer' or 'blue bloater' referred to previously. The patient may be centrally cyanosed with a bluish coloration to the tongue/lips. This is seen when there is a deoxygenated haemoglobin level of >5 g/dl. The possibility of an underlying cardiac cause for such cyanosis should be borne in mind. Signs of anaemia may be evident when the lower eyelid is gently everted but this a rather subjective sign. The presence of koilonychia or finger clubbing may also give clues about the underlying disorder. Respiratory causes of finger clubbing are discussed in Chapter 1 (titled 'Clinical examination and history taking').

Palpation of the radial pulse may reveal that it has a bounding character. Such a pulse is a sign of carbon dioxide retention in some patients with COPD. Patients who retain carbon dioxide may also have a flapping tremor of the hands when they are held outstretched, as mentioned earlier.

It may be evident that the patient is using his or her accessory muscles of respiration – a sign of significant respiratory impairment. The respiratory rate, as one of the vital signs, should be noted.

Examining the chest formally is not required, but, in many clothed patients, it is possible to make a gross assessment of the symmetry of chest movements during respiration and from the position of the trachea, which is situated centrally when palpated at the sternal notch.

Specific disorders

Asthma

Anxiety should be minimised as much as possible in asthmatic patients. Patients should have their usual bronchodilator medication (e.g. salbutamol, terbutaline) at hand, or it should be readily available in the emergency drug box. If the medication is not available, treatment should be deferred. Relative analgesia is generally preferred for anxiolysis rather than intravenous sedation.

The incidence of allergy to penicillin is increased in many asthmatic patients, and caution should be exercised in the prescription of NSAIDs. The possibility of current or past steroid use should be remembered. The incidence of oral candidiasis is increased in patients who use corticosteroid inhalers, and such patients should be encouraged to gargle with water after they have used the inhaler. Patients using β_2-agonists or antimuscarinic preparations may complain of dry mouth.

Infections

Infections of the respiratory tract may be acute or chronic, and may be of the upper or lower tract. The upper and lower respiratory tracts are separated by the vocal cords. An infection of the upper or lower respiratory tract is a contraindication to general anaesthesia, which should be deferred until resolution has occurred. An upper respiratory tract infection (URTI) will readily progress to the lower tract if this is not done. URTIs may occur as part of the common cold, as pharyngitis or tonsillitis, and as laryngotracheitis, which can cause stridor in children – that is, 'croup'.

Infections of the paranasal air sinuses can occur, and a bacterial infection may be secondary to a viral URTI. The most common bacteria implicated in acute sinusitis are *Streptococcus pneumoniae* and *Haemophilus influenzae*. Maxillary sinusitis is discussed further in Chapter 9 (titled 'Neurology and special senses').

Chronic suppurative respiratory disorders

General anaesthesia is contraindicated in active disease, as is intravenous sedation. Patients with respiratory difficulty are most comfortable in the sitting position. Those patients who are on theophylline run an increased risk of drug interactions if they are prescribed erythromycin or clindamycin.

TB

The incidence of TB is increasing. This is due to the bacillus being carried by sections of the immigrant population and immunosuppressed patients. The disease is unlikely to be transmitted in dentistry unless it is of the active pulmonary type, or if the dental staff dealing with such patients are themselves immunocompromised. If such patients require treatment, it is important that the aerosol be kept to a minimum. Ultrasonic scalers are contraindicated, and a rubber dam should be used as a precaution. General anaesthesia should be avoided if possible in the active phase, owing to possibilities of contamination of anaesthetic circuits and impaired respiratory function. Certain drugs may interfere with the drugs used in TB treatment – for example, diazepam clearance is enhanced by rifampicin. The possibility of current or previous drug abuse should also be considered.

Lung abscess

Lung abscesses secondary to inhalation during dental procedures are rare. Preventive measures should be used, including rubber dam and throat packs. If an object is suspected of being inhaled, this should never be ignored, and the procedure outlined in Chapter 21 (titled 'Medical emergencies') must be followed.

Legionnaire's disease

The stagnant water in dental units have been found to contain the *Legionella* bacterium. Studies have also demonstrated increased antibody levels in dental personnel. It is vital that measures be put in place to minimise the related risks. Such measures include flushing proprietary substances through water systems, planting devices for water purification and the effective cleansing of water lines used in dental surgeries.

Lung cancer

There is often a sensitivity to the muscle relaxants used in general anaesthesia. The cancer may lead to reductions in respiratory reserve, which is clinically significant. Metastasis of lung cancer to the jaws is unusual. A rare oral manifestation of lung cancer is pigmentation of the soft palate. Some lung cancers can produce ACTH, with concomitant effects on steroid production, as discussed earlier.

Sarcoidosis

Sarcoidosis is a multisystem granulomatous disorder that may be relevant to dentistry in terms of:
- Respiratory impairment.
- Visual impairment.
- Jaundice.
- Renal impairment.

- Steroid therapy.
- Association with Sjögren syndrome.
- Gingival enlargement.
- Cranial neuropathies.

OSAS

OSAS, as discussed earlier, is more common in obese patients. Significant implications for clinical practice include the airway during recovery from general anaesthesia and intravenous sedation. Various devices, worn orally, are marketed that claim to reduce or eliminate this problem.

Acute respiratory distress syndrome (ARDS)

Improvements in intensive care technology and medication mean that this disorder, which was almost invariably fatal some years ago, is now sometimes encountered in the medical histories of dental patients who have made a recovery. Full respiratory reserve may not be returned, however. One of the most debilitating sequelae is pulmonary fibrosis, and such patients may be taking steroids as a result.

Other causes of pulmonary fibrosis that may be encountered in dental practice include connective tissue disorders (e.g. rheumatoid arthritis), or in patients with Sjögren syndrome. Occasionally, pulmonary fibrosis occurs without any identifiable cause, and such cases are referred to as 'idiopathic'.

FURTHER READING

Asthma UK. Available from: www.asthma.org.uk.

Cystic Fibrosis Trust. Available from: www.cysticfibrosis.org.uk.

British Lung Foundation. Available from: www.blf.org.uk.

British Thoracic Society. Available from: www.brit-thoracic.org.uk.

MULTIPLE CHOICE QUESTIONS

1. If a patient with asthma becomes wheezy during an oral surgery procedure, the correct inhaler treatment would be:
   a) Budesonide
   b) Salbutamol
   c) Tiotropium
   d) Salmeterol
   e) Fluticasone
   Answer = B

   Explanation: Salbutamol is a fast-acting beta agonist bronchodilator medication that functions as a 'reliever' during an asthma attack.

2. The oxygen content of room air is:
   a) 18%
   b) 21%
   c) 24%
   d) 28%
   e) 35%
   Answer = B

Explanation: Room air usually contains 21% oxygen. High-flow oxygen (>60%) is appropriate for severely hypoxic patients in an emergency – for example, after cardiorespiratory arrest or in acute asthma. Patients with COPD are usually treated with lower-dose controlled oxygen – for example, 24% or 28% mask.

3. The key clinical feature of hypoxia is:
   a) Breathlessness
   b) Orthopnoea
   c) Wheezing
   d) Reduced peak expiratory flow rate
   e) Cyanosis
   Answer = E

Explanation: Central cyanosis is a bluish colouration of the mucous membranes of the tongue and lips, and is a cardinal sign of severe hypoxia.

4. The most common type of lung cancer is:
   a) Squamous cell carcinoma
   b) Small-cell carcinoma

c) Ductal carcinoma
d) Large-cell undifferentiated carcinoma
e) Adenocarcinoma

Answer = A

Explanation: Squamous cell carcinoma accounts for about 45% of lung cancers, with small-cell carcinoma accounting for 20%, adenocarcinoma for 20% and large-cell undifferentiated carcinoma for 15%.

5. The number of deaths in the UK each year from lung cancer is:
   a) 10 000
   b) 20 000
   c) 25 000
   d) 35 000
   e) 50 000

Answer = D

Explanation: Lung cancer kills about 35 000 people each year in the UK. It is important to ask about smoking habits, and to help and encourage patients to stop smoking.

6. OSAS is usually treated by:
   a) Bronchodilator medication
   b) Surgery
   c) Nasal steroids
   d) CPAP
   e) Oxygen during sleep

Answer = D

Explanation: OSAS is caused by occlusion of the pharynx during deep sleep. CPAP, delivered via a tight-fitting nasal mask during sleep, keeps the pharyngeal airway open, and is the main treatment.

7. A major cause of chronic lung infection in cystic fibrosis is:
   a) *Mycoplasma pneumonia*
   b) *Mycobacterium tuberculosis*
   c) *Haemophilus influenzae*
   d) Influenza A virus
   e) *Pseudomonas aeruginosa*

Answer = E

Explanation: *Pseudomonas aeruginosa* is the most common chronic lung infection in patients with cystic fibrosis, and it is often treated with long-term inhaled antibiotics such as colistin or tobramycin.

8. A typical adverse effect of an anticholinergic inhaler such as tiotropium is:
   a) Palpitations
   b) Tremor
   c) Gingival hyperplasia
   d) Dryness of the mouth
   e) Cushing's syndrome

Answer = D

Explanation: Anticholinergic bronchodilator inhalers (e.g. tiotropium, ipratropium) may cause dryness of the mouth, loss of taste, gingivitis and glossitis. Tremor and tachycardia may be the adverse effects of beta-agonist inhalers (e.g. salbutamol, terbutaline). Oral candidiasis is most common with corticosteroid inhalers.

9. Community-acquired pneumonia is most commonly caused by:
   a) *Streptococcus pneumoniae*
   b) *Staphylococcus aureus*
   c) Rhinoviruses
   d) *Pseudomonas aeruginosa*
   e) Meticillin-resistant *Staphylococcus aureus*

Answer = A

Explanation: *Streptococcus pneumoniae* is the most common cause of pneumonia when it is acquired in the community. When pneumonia occurs in patients who are ill in hospital, particularly in those on mechanical ventilation in an intensive care unit, Gram-negative organisms such as *Pseudomonas aeruginosa* are more common.

10. A typical cause of diffuse lung fibrosis is:
    a) Tobacco smoking
    b) Chronic asthma
    c) Bronchiectasis
    d) Asbestos
    e) *Pseudomonas aeruginosa* infection

Answer = D

Explanation: Asbestos is a well-recognised cause of diffuse lung fibrosis. Such patients may have a history of having worked with asbestos, which is used in pipe-lagging or as insulation material. They may have breathlessness, lung crackles on examination of the chest and clubbing of their fingers.

CHAPTER 7

Gastrointestinal disorders

M Greenwood, JG Meechan and JR Adams

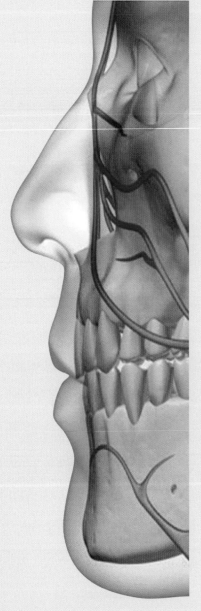

Key topics

- History and examination in relation to patients with gastrointestinal disorders.
- Dental/oral relevance of gastrointestinal disorders.

Learning objectives

- To be familiar with the major gastrointestinal disorders.
- To understand how gastrointestinal disorders may impact on dental/oral health.
- To understand how gastrointestinal disorders or their treatment may impact on dental care.

Essentials of Human Disease in Dentistry, Second Edition. Mark Greenwood.
© 2018 John Wiley & Sons Ltd. Published 2018 by John Wiley & Sons Ltd.
Companion website: www.wiley.com/go/greenwood/human-disease-in-dentistry

Introduction

Diseases of the gastrointestinal (GI) system is relevant to the dental surgeon for several reasons. The mouth may display signs of the disease itself, for example, the cobblestone mucosa, facial or labial swelling of Crohn's disease, or the osteomata of Gardner's syndrome. These are well covered elsewhere, and hence not discussed further here. The sequelae of GI disease – for example, gastric reflux producing dental erosion, iron deficiency anaemia and treatments such as corticosteroid therapy – may all impact on the management and choice of anaesthesia.

Relevant points in the history

Lethargy, dyspnoea and angina may all occur secondary to anaemia from a GI cause, but cardiorespiratory conditions should also be borne in mind. The cause of an anaemia should always be investigated. The possibility of blood loss from the GI tract should be considered. Weight loss may be the result of reduced nutritional intake secondary to anorexia, nausea or vomiting. There may be loss of protein from diseased bowel, for example, in ulcerative colitis. Cancer of the GI tract is the most significant potential cause of weight loss. The quantity and time course of the weight loss are both important. Enquiries should also be made about appetite and any changes in bowel habits.

'Heartburn' or 'indigestion' are vague terms often used by patients, and may be used to describe upper abdominal pain, gastrooesophageal regurgitation, anorexia, nausea and vomiting. Oesophageal reflux or 'heartburn' causes epigastric pain, that is, abdominal pain around the lower end of the sternum, which radiates to the back and is worse on stooping and drinking hot drinks. It can have implications for general anaesthesia (see the following text), and can be a cause of dental erosion, especially on the palatal/lingual surfaces of the teeth, as a result of the acidity of the gastric fluid. The factors promoting gastrooesophageal reflux are shown in Table 7.1.

Dysphagia, or difficulty in swallowing, is a symptom that should always be taken seriously. Plummer–Vinson syndrome is the name given to dysphagia associated with webs of tissues in the pharynx and upper oesophagus. Other components of the syndrome include glossitis, iron deficiency anaemia and koilonychia (spoon-shaped fingernails suggesting iron deficiency, but

Table 7.1 Factors promoting gastrooesophageal reflux.

Hiatus hernia
Pregnancy
Obesity
Cigarettes
Alcohol
Fatty food

also occurring in ischaemic heart disease). Some other causes of dysphagia are listed in Table 7.2.

Vomiting may be due to extraintestinal causes such as meningitis, migraine or as a result of drug therapy (e.g. morphine). In children, vomiting can be a sign of infection of various body systems. Nausea or vomiting in the morning may be seen in pregnancy, alcoholism and anxiety. Haematemesis, or vomiting of blood, may arise from bleeding oesophageal varices. The relevance of this to dentistry is mainly related to the fact that these varices may occur secondary to chronic liver disease, with its attendant implications for blood clotting and drug metabolism from hepatic impairment.

Gastric bleeding may present as haematemesis, in which case the vomit is described as resembling 'coffee grounds'. Blood altered by gastric acid appearing in the stool is described as 'melaena'; it is black and resembles tar.

A current or past history of *peptic ulcer* may be of relevance, particularly when NSAIDs are being considered. These ulcers are common, affecting around 10% of the world population. Men are affected twice as much as women. The incidence is declining in developed countries, possibly owing to dietary changes. Peptic ulcers may affect the lower oesophagus,

Table 7.2 Possible causes of dysphagia.

Oral causes
- Stomatitis
- Aphthous ulcers
- Herpetic infection
- Oral malignancy
- Xerostomia
- Tonsillitis
- Pharyngitis
- Infections involving fascial spaces of neck

Obstruction in oesophageal wall
- Oesophagitis
- Carcinoma of oesophagus
- Pharyngeal pouch
- Oesophageal web – Plummer–Vinson syndrome (iron deficiency, post-cricoid web)

External compression of oesophagus
- Enlarged neighbouring lymph nodes
- Left atrial dilatation in mitral stenosis

Disorders of neuromuscular function
- Myasthenia gravis
- Muscular dystrophy
- Stroke
- Achalasia (failure of oesophageal peristalsis and failure of relaxation of lower oesophageal sphincter)

Other
- Foreign body
- Scleroderma (see Chapter 12, titled 'Dermatology and mucosal lesions')
- Benign stricture secondary to gastrooesophageal reflux
- Globus hystericus (psychogenic)

stomach and duodenum Since the advent of effective drug therapy, the pendulum has swung away from surgery for these conditions. *Helicobacter pylori* (a microaerophilic Gram-negative bacterium) can be identified in the gastric antral mucosa in 90% of cases of duodenal ulcers, and in the body or antral mucosa in about 60% of cases of gastric ulcer. It is a common aetiological factor in peptic ulcer disease. Triple therapy regimens are used for treatment when *Helicobacter pylori* is involved – for example, a proton pump inhibitor such as omeprazole, a broad-spectrum antibiotic such as amoxicillin, and metronidazole.

The term *inflammatory bowel disease* includes ulcerative colitis, Crohn's disease (Figure 7.1) and an indeterminate type. Factors that impact on dental practice include the possibility of anaemia secondary to chronic bleeding and corticosteroid therapy in these patients. Extraintestinal manifestations of inflammatory bowel disease may occur, and are listed in Table 7.3.

Crohn's disease is a chronic inflammatory disorder characterised by granulomatous transmural inflammation. Any part of the gut can be affected, but it most commonly affects the terminal ileum and proximal colon. There may be unaffected areas, and the active areas are described as 'skip lesions'.

Ulcerative colitis is an inflammatory disorder of the colonic mucosa. It may just affect the rectum or extend to involve all or part of the colon. It is characterised by relapses and remissions.

'Irritable bowel syndrome' (IBS) is a term used to describe a group of heterogeneous abdominal symptoms for which no organic cause can be found.

A *history of GI surgery* may give clues about nutritional deficiencies that may be present – for example, iron, vitamin B_{12} or folate deficiency post-gastric surgery. Recurrent oral ulceration and glossitis may ensue.

Pancreatic disease is of relevance in a thorough history, since the consequent malabsorption of vitamin K may lead to a bleeding tendency. There is also a possibility of diabetes

Table 7.3 Extraintestinal manifestations of inflammatory bowel disease.	
Aphthous stomatitis	
Hepatic	Fatty change Amyloidosis
Gallstones	
Skin	Erythema nodosum (see the following text) Pyoderma gangrenosum (see the following text)
Arthritis	
Finger clubbing	
Eye lesions (e.g. conjunctivitis)	
Vasculitis	
Cardiovascular disease	
Bronchopulmonary disease	

mellitus or a diabetic tendency. Excessive alcohol intake can be a cause of acute pancreatitis, and a thorough social history may uncover this information. Other causes of acute pancreatitis include gallstones and some viral infections – for example, HIV and mumps. Chronic pancreatitis is of similar aetiology as acute pancreatitis. Endocrine and exocrine function both deteriorate. In both types of pancreatitis, abdominal pain is severe. *Pancreatic cancer* frequently involves the head of the pancreas, and local invasion leads to biliary obstruction, diabetes mellitus and pancreatitis. Thrombophlebitis migrans (peripheral vein thrombosis) is a common complication. Pancreatic cancer has the worst prognosis of any cancer in general terms, and treatment is usually surgical and palliative. The patient may give a history of *jaundice* or may actually be jaundiced. Jaundice is discussed later in the chapter.

Congenital disorders of relevance can occur. Familial polyposis has an incidence of 1 in 24 000, and is transmitted as autosomal dominant. People with the condition have rectal and colonic polyps. A variant is Gardner's syndrome, which also includes bony osteomata and soft tissue tumours, for example, epidermal cysts. The colonic polyps are pre-malignant, and careful follow-up of these patients is needed. Subtotal colectomy with fulguration of rectal polyps may be carried out in order to prevent malignancy.

Peutz–Jeghers syndrome is an autosomal dominant condition comprising intestinal polyps and pigmented freckles perianally extending on to the oral mucosa (Figure 7.2). The gastric and duodenal polyps have a predisposition to becoming malignant.

Some *skin disorders* may occur as part of a wider picture of GI disease. *Erythema nodosum* and *pyoderma gangrenosum* can occur in inflammatory bowel disease. The skin lesions are painful, erythematous nodular lesions on the anterior shin in

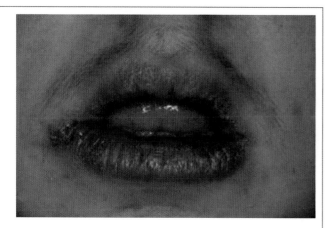

Figure 7.1 A granulomatous inflammation of the lips in a patient with Crohn's disease.

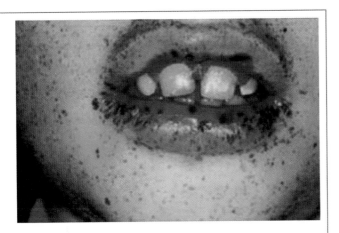

Figure 7.2 A patient with Peutz–Jeghers syndrome.

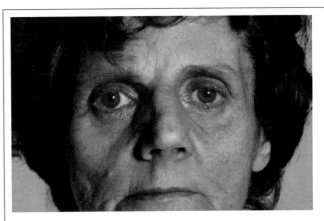

Figure 7.3 A patient with jaundice. The best place to examine for jaundice is the sclera.

erythema nodosum. Bluish-edged ulcers occur on the back, thighs and buttocks in pyoderma gangrenosum. The skin disease associated with coeliac disease is dermatitis herpetiformis, comprising an itchy papulovesicular rash mainly on the trunk and upper limbs. IgA deposits at the epithelium basement membrane zone help to establish the diagnosis. There may also be papillary tip micro-abscess formation, as well as intraoral lesions that may be erosive or vesicular, and resembling pemphigoid. Treatment is usually with dapsone. Aphthous ulcers may occur.

Coeliac disease is a permanent intolerance to gluten, leading to intestinal villous atrophy and GI malabsorption. The villous atrophy reverses when the patient is on a gluten-free diet. The disease may be complicated by anaemia and GI lymphoma.

Pseudomembranous colitis can be caused by many antibiotics, particularly clindamycin and lincomycin, and results from the proliferation of toxigenic *Clostridium difficile*. It is characterised by painful diarrhoea with mucus passage, and is treated with oral vancomycin or metronidazole.

A summary of relevant points in the history is given in Table 7.4.

Table 7.4 Relevant points in the history.

- General enquiry (e.g. lethargy, anaemia, weight loss, appetite)
- Dyspepsia, reflux
- Dysphagia
- Vomiting, haematemesis
- Change in bowel habits
- Peptic ulcer (current/past)
- Inflammatory bowel disease
- History of GI surgery
- Pancreatic disease
- Congenital disorders

Examination

Oral lesions as a manifestation of GI disease are well discussed elsewhere and are not considered further here. It is worth remembering that *cervical lymph node enlargement* is an important sign that should not be ignored. Possible causes include infection and neoplasia (primary or secondary).

Pallor can be a very subjective way of trying to assess for anaemia. The mucosa at the reflection in the inferior fornix of the eye is the best site for examination. The patient may readily become dyspnoeic secondary to anaemia, but this should be considered with an open mind because, as mentioned earlier, cardiorespiratory conditions are more likely to present in this manner.

A patient may be jaundiced for 'extrahepatic' reasons such as gallstones, cancer of the bile ducts or cancer of the head of pancreas. The sclera is a good site to examine for the yellow tint of jaundice (Figure 7.3).

Examination of the hands may reveal spoon-shaped fingernails, or 'koilonychia'. The fingers may be clubbed. GI causes of clubbing include inflammatory bowel disease (especially Crohn's), cirrhosis, malabsorption and GI lymphoma.

An enlarged lymph node in the left supraclavicular fossa (Virchow's node, Troisier's sign) can be a sign of stomach cancer. Anaemia or obstructive jaundice may complicate treatment.

Liver disease

Liver failure

Failure may occur suddenly in a liver that has been previously healthy – termed 'acute hepatic failure'. It may also occur as a result of chronic liver disease that has become decompensated – termed 'acute-on-chronic hepatic failure'. If encephalopathy occurs within 8 weeks of the symptoms of acute liver failure, the situation is described as 'fulminant hepatic failure'. The possible causes of liver failure are given in Table 7.5.

Table 7.5 Possible causes of liver failure.

Infections (e.g. viral hepatitis, yellow fever)

Drugs (e.g. paracetamol overdose, halothane)

Vascular (e.g. Budd–Chiari syndrome; see the following text)

Toxins (e.g. carbon tetrachloride)

Primary biliary cirrhosis (also termed 'primary biliary cholangitis'; see the following text)

Haemochromatosis (see the following text)

Alpha 1-antitrypsin deficiency (see the following text)

Wilson's disease (see the following text)

Malignancy

Table 7.6 Possible signs of liver disease on clinical examination that suggest a chronic problem.

Dupuytren's contracture

Palmar erythema

Finger clubbing

Leukonychia

Parotid enlargement

Jaundice

Spider naevi (Figure 7.4)

Gynaecomastia

Ascites/ankle oedema

Scratch marks (itching)

Clinical features of liver failure

The patient will be jaundiced and have a characteristic smell to the breath. The name given to this is 'foetor hepaticus'. The patient may exhibit a liver flap (see Chapter 1, titled 'Clinical examination and history taking'), and may have a constructional apraxia (inability to draw a relatively simple shape).

The clinical signs of chronic liver disease are given in Table 7.6. Such signs may include spider naevi. These comprise a central arteriole with vessels radiating from it (Figure 7.4). If compressed in the centre, the lesion can be 'emptied', and it disappears. If these are seen, acute-on-chronic liver failure should be suspected. There are several possible complications that can occur as a result of acute hepatic failure. These are wide-ranging, reflecting the nature of the liver as an organ heavily involved in storage, synthesis and haemostasis. A summary is given in Table 7.7.

Cirrhosis

The term 'cirrhosis' implies liver damage that is irreversible. Microscopically, the liver will be fibrosed with areas of nodular regeneration. The primary cause of cirrhosis is excess alcohol ingestion. Chronic infection with hepatitis B virus and hepatitis C virus are also common causes. Less common causes include primary biliary cirrhosis, chronic active hepatitis, haemochromatosis, Budd–Chiari syndrome, Wilson's disease and alpha 1-antitrypsin deficiency. These conditions are discussed further in the following text. Medications such as amiodarone and methotrexate can also cause cirrhosis. In just under one-third of cases, the cause of cirrhosis is not found – this is referred to as 'cryptogenic cirrhosis'.

Certain conditions may lead to cirrhosis becoming decompensated – that is, complications of impaired liver function arise due to some other underlying problem. Examples include infection, alcohol, imbalance of urea and electrolytes, GI bleeds or progression of the underlying disorder.

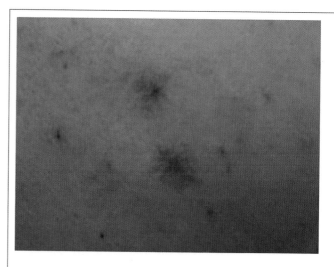

Figure 7.4 Spider naevi may be seen in chronic liver disease. They comprise a central arteriole that will empty when compressed. They occur in the distribution of the superior vena cava.

Table 7.7 Complications of acute hepatic failure.

Infection

Ascites

Bleeding

Hypoglycaemia

Cerebral oedema

Hepatorenal syndrome

Management

Nutritional supplements are required, and the diet should be low in protein if there is encephalopathy and low in salt if there is ascites. Clearly, alcohol should be avoided, but so should NSAIDs, sedatives and opiates, all drugs that can be prescribed by dental practitioners.

The overall prognosis is relatively poor, with a 5-year survival rate of approximately 50%. Interferon-α has been shown to improve liver biochemistry, and may slow the development of hepatocellular cancer in cirrhosis induced by hepatitis C virus.

Haemochromatosis

Haemochromatosis is an inherited disorder of iron metabolism in which increased iron absorption from the intestine causes deposition in multiple organs, including the liver. Other organs affected are the joints, heart, pituitary gland and pancreas. It is seen more often in middle-aged males. Females tend to present on average a decade later due to the protective effects of menstrual blood loss.

Wilson's disease

Wilson's disease is a rare inherited (autosomal recessive) disorder. It is characterised by the accumulation of copper in the liver and brain (hepatolenticular degeneration). It is treatable, and therefore all patients with cirrhosis should be checked for Wilson's disease.

Alpha 1-antitrypsin deficiency

Alpha 1-antitrypsin is a protease inhibitor that is synthesised in the liver. Such deficiency is the most common cause of genetic liver disease in children. In the adult population, it is associated with emphysema and hepatocellular cancer, as well as some forms of chronic liver disease. There is no treatment for the condition, but there are centres that use human alpha 1-antitrypsin as augmentation therapy.

Budd–Chiari syndrome

Budd–Chiari syndrome is one cause of cirrhosis. It occurs due to hepatic vein obstruction leading to acute epigastric pain or portal hypertension, ascites and jaundice. Anticoagulation therapy or surgical shunt procedures may be employed for treatment, depending on the nature of the underlying cause.

Primary biliary cirrhosis (primary biliary cholangitis) – PBC

PBC is thought to be autoimmune in origin, and 90% of patients are female, with peak presentation at 40–60 years of age. It is characterised by damage to bile ducts due to a chronic granulomatous inflammatory process that leads to cholestasis (interference with bile flow), cirrhosis and portal hypertension. Treatment is largely symptomatic and with vitamin augmentation therapy. In extreme cases, liver transplantation may be carried out.

Gilbert's syndrome

Gilbert's syndrome is an inherited metabolic disorder that is a relatively common cause of unconjugated hyperbilirubinaemia.

Onset is shortly after birth, but the condition may not be noticed for several years. Jaundice occurs if the patient becomes ill for another reason. The disorder has an excellent prognosis.

Jaundice

The term 'jaundice' refers to the yellow pigmentation seen in the skin, sclerae and mucosa, caused by a raised plasma bilirubin level. The disorder can be classified according to the type of circulating bilirubin (conjugated or unconjugated) or the site of the problem. The latter can be subdivided into pre-hepatic, hepatocellular or obstructive. The points to be considered in the history of a patient presenting with jaundice are given in Table 7.8.

Pre-hepatic jaundice

Pre-hepatic jaundice may occur as a result of excess bilirubin production. This happens in haemolysis, decreased uptake of bilirubin by the liver or decreased conjugation. If there is excess bilirubin, unconjugated bilirubin enters the blood. Being insoluble in water, it does not enter urine, resulting in unconjugated hyperbilirubinaemia.

Hepatocellular jaundice

The principal causes of hepatocellular jaundice relate to viral infections such as hepatitis A, B, C, CMV and EBV. Hepatotoxic drugs may also cause this type of jaundice. Chronic active hepatitis, cirrhosis, hepatic metastases, alpha 1-antitrypsin deficiency, Budd–Chiari syndrome and Wilson's disease are all potential causes.

Obstructive (cholestatic) jaundice

Obstructive jaundice occurs if the common bile duct is blocked, leading to excess conjugated bilirubin in the bloodstream. This is referred to as 'conjugated hyperbilirubinaemia'.

Table 7.8 Points to consider in the history of a jaundiced patient.
Colour of stool/urine
Blood transfusions
Body piercing
Intravenous drug use
Tattoos
Foreign travel
Has close contacts with people who have/or have had jaundice
Sexual activity
Medications
Alcohol consumption
Family history

As this form of bilirubin is water soluble, it is excreted in the urine, which therefore becomes dark. Less conjugated bilirubin enters the bowel, and the faeces become pale. Dark urine and pale stool is a characteristic sign of obstructive jaundice, and this question should be specifically asked of the jaundiced patient.

Causes of obstructive jaundice include gallstones and pancreatic cancer. Primary biliary cirrhosis is another cause that should be borne in mind.

Liver tumours

Metastatic deposits are the most common liver tumours. Primary tumours metastasising to the liver include tumours of the breast, GI tract and bronchus. Primary hepatic tumours occur much less frequently. They may be benign or malignant. Clinically, features are very variable, but include malaise, anorexia, weight loss, fever and pain in the right upper quadrant of the abdomen. Jaundice is a sign that tends to occur late. Tumours may rupture, leading to intraperitoneal haemorrhage. Benign hepatic tumours are usually asymptomatic.

Malignant liver tumours

Malignant liver tumours include liver metastases and hepatocellular carcinoma. Due to the anatomical structure of the liver, in carefully assessed cases, surgical resection of solitary tumours may be possible. Cholangiocarcinoma is a malignant tumour of the biliary tree. In rare cases, these cancers may be resectable.

Benign liver tumours

The most common benign liver tumours are haemangiomas. These are usually asymptomatic, and are discovered as incidental findings on imaging. Adenomas may also be seen, and can occur as a result of pregnancy or the use of contraceptive pills.

Coagulation and liver disease

Liver disease produces a complicated picture with regard to bleeding problems, owing to the multifunctional role of the liver in coagulation. Absorption of vitamin K and the synthesis of clotting factors are decreased, and abnormalities of platelet function may be seen. Malabsorption is the problem leading to decreased vitamin K uptake. Vitamin K is required for the synthesis of clotting factors II, VII, IX and X.

Prescribing in liver disease

Many drugs are metabolised by the liver. Clearly, a patient with a liver disorder will potentially have a decreased ability to metabolise such drugs. The practitioner should always bear this in mind when prescribing in these patients. When the use of a drug is necessary in a patient with severe liver disease, this should be discussed with the patient's physician. Hepatic impairment may lead to toxicity. In some cases, dose reduction is required; other drugs should be avoided completely. The antifungal drug miconazole is contraindicated if there is hepatic impairment, and fluconazole requires dose reduction. Erythromycin, metronidazole and tetracyclines should be avoided.

NSAIDs increase the risk of GI bleeding and interfere with fluid balance, and are best avoided. Paracetamol should be avoided altogether, or, after discussion with the patient's physician, the dosage should be reduced, depending on the underlying liver problem.

Nutritional disorders

Despite quality-of-life improvements in contemporary society, nutritional disorders are still seen in the developed world. Currently, the advice given in Table 7.9 is generally considered to be correct with regard to a 'good' diet.

Nutrition can be delivered by two main routes – enteral (via the gut) and parenteral (intravenous). The latter is used in patients in whom the gut route cannot be used for some reason. There have to be good reasons to use parenteral nutrition, as significant complications can arise from this. It should be used with specialist advice in hospital inpatients who would otherwise become malnourished. A period where the gut has not been functioning for at least 7 days is a prerequisite. If parenteral nutrition is the sole form of delivery of nutrients, it is designated as total parenteral nutrition (TPN). Occasionally, parenteral nutrition may be instituted when the gut is working but performing suboptimally, for example, in severe Crohn's disease.

In parenteral nutrition, the preparation is usually given through a central venous catheter, as this will last longer than delivering it into a peripheral vessel. About 2000 kilocalories/day are usually required, with 10–14 g of nitrogen. Minerals, vitamins, electrolytes and trace elements are all included. When this type of nutrition is used, it is essential that close liaison be initiated and maintained between the clinician, dietician and pharmacist.

Table 7.9 Generic advice with regard to maintaining a healthy diet.

Aim for a body mass index (BMI) of 20–25 kg/m².

Five or more portions of different fruit or vegetables (ideally with skin) should be eaten per day (one portion is represented by a piece of fresh fruit or a glass of fruit juice).

Minimise salt intake.

Restrict alcohol to the recommended limits (21 units for men, 14 units for women, per week).

Reduced intake of refined sugar.

Reduce the intake of saturated fats – food rich in omega-3 fatty acids (e.g. oily fish) is considered beneficial.

Vitamin B deficiencies

Vitamin B_{12} and folate deficiencies lead to macrocytic anaemias. If vitamin B_{12} deficiency is suspected, the Schilling test may be used to help identify the cause. This test will determine whether the low level is due to malabsorption or a lack of intrinsic factor, the latter, produced by the stomach, being necessary for vitamin B_{12} absorption. The test compares the proportion of orally administered radioactive vitamin B_{12} excreted in the urine both with and without the administration of intrinsic factor. Prior to the test, the blood is saturated with vitamin B_{12} given intramuscularly. If intrinsic factor increases the absorption, deficiency is likely to be caused by the lack of intrinsic factor. Pernicious anaemia is likely to be the cause in such cases. Possible causes of vitamin B_{12} and folate deficiency are given in Tables 7.10 and 7.11, respectively. It is usual practice to test blood for the levels of these vitamins in patients who present with recurrent oral ulceration or other mucosal lesions such as mucosal atrophy.

Beriberi is a disease caused by the deficiency of vitamin B_1 (thiamine). Lack of this vitamin can also be seen in Wernicke's encephalopathy (see Chapter 18, titled 'Care of the elderly'). This condition occurs in chronic alcoholics due to their poor diet. Hospital inpatients are prescribed multivitamins including vitamin B_1 to address any deficiency when they are admitted for whatever reason.

Pellagra is a disease caused by the lack of nicotinic acid, producing the triad of diarrhoea, dermatitis and dementia. Dietary education, electrolyte replacement and nicotinamide are the mainstay of treatment.

Table 7.10 Causes of low vitamin B_{12} levels and sources of the vitamin.

Potential causes
- Pernicious anaemia
- After gastrectomy (no intrinsic factor to allow absorption from the terminal ileum)
- Veganism or other dietary deficiency
- Crohn's disease
- Parasitic disease

Sources of vitamin B_{12}
- Best source – liver

Table 7.11 Causes of low folate levels and sources of folate.

Potential causes
- Dietary deficiency (alcoholics)
- Increased demand (pregnancy, malignancy)
- Malabsorption (e.g. coeliac disease)

Sources of folate
- Liver
- Green vegetables
- Fruit
- Synthesised by gut bacteria

Table 7.12 Possible causes of iron deficiency anaemia.

Blood loss (which may be occult)

Poor diet (unusual in adults but less so in children and babies in developing countries)

Malabsorption

Parasitic disease

Iron deficiency anaemia

Iron deficiency is seen quite commonly, particularly in menstruating women. When chronic, it leads to a microcytic and hypochromic microscopic picture. It is critical that the underlying cause of any anaemia be established (Table 7.12). Atrophic glossitis and recurrent aphthous ulceration may be seen in patients with iron deficiency anaemia. As with deficiencies of vitamin B_{12} and folate, iron deficiency anaemia too is tested for in patients who present with these conditions.

When iron supplementation is used (e.g. ferrous sulphate), such therapy should be continued until the haemoglobin level has been brought back to normal and has remained normal for at least 3 months, so that stores are replaced. The haemoglobin should rise by around 1 g/dl/week. Iron supplements lead to constipation and black stools.

Vitamin A deficiency

Vitamin A (retinol) is present in food and in the body itself as esters combined with long-chain fatty acids. It is found in liver, milk, cheese, butter, egg yolks and fish oils. Retinol is stored in the liver and transported in plasma. It is one of the fat-soluble vitamins, the others being vitamins D, E and K. Deficiency of vitamin A is the major cause of blindness in young children in the developing world, despite intensive programmes for prevention. The condition of xerophthalmia occurs in vitamin A deficiency, leading to impaired adaptation followed by night blindness. The eye becomes dry; corneal softening and ulceration eventually occur; and superimposed infection develops. Prevention is best, by using vitamin A supplementation.

Vitamin D deficiency

The body's principal source of vitamin D is that which is produced in the skin by the photoactivation of 7-dehydrocholesterol. Sunlight deficiency, rather than inadequate nutrition, is therefore more likely to produce vitamin D deficiency.

In the circulation, cholecalciferol (vitamin D) is bound to vitamin D–binding protein and transported to the liver, where it is converted to 25-hydroxycholecalciferol. After further transport to the kidney, another hydroxylation occurs to 1,25-dihydroxycholecalciferol and 24,25-dihydroxycholecalciferol, which is less metabolically active. The hydroxylating enzyme is regulated by the action of parathyroid hormone (see Chapter 12, titled 'Dermatology and mucosal lesions'), blood phosphate levels and negative feedback inhibition by 1,25-dihydroxycholecalciferol.

Deficiency of vitamin D in children results in rickets. In adults, the deficiency results in osteomalacia. Both conditions result from inadequate mineralisation of the bone matrix. In rickets, the characteristic appearance is of bow legs, and deformity at the costochondral junctions produces an appearance described as a 'rickety rosary'.

Vitamin E deficiency

Vitamin E encompasses a group of eight naturally occurring compounds. Vegetables, seed oils, cereals and nuts are the main sources of vitamin E. The vitamin is absorbed with fat and transported largely in low-density lipoproteins (LDLs). The importance of vitamin E relates to its antioxidant properties, and it also contributes to membrane stability. Vitamin E deficiency is uncommon in developed countries.

Vitamin K deficiency

Vitamin K deficiency can impact on dentistry since it is a cofactor that is essential for the production of blood clotting factors and the proteins necessary for bone formation. Deficiency of this vitamin has been discussed earlier in this chapter. Sources of the vitamin include dairy products, green leafy vegetables and soya bean oils.

Vitamin C deficiency

Scurvy is a disease that occurs because of the deficiency of vitamin C in the diet. This can be seen in developed countries in pregnancy, marked poverty or in some people with strange dietary habits. Attention to the diet is important, but ascorbic acid supplements may be prescribed. Such patients will suffer from marked gingivitis and loosening of teeth.

Dental aspects of GI system disorders

The obese patient is significant in the context of dental treatment for the following reasons: the safe provision of general anaesthesia and sedation; the possibility of iron deficiency anaemia, reflux or vomiting; and the effects of drug therapies. Useful questions to ask a patient with regard to the GI system are given in Table 7.4.

Consideration needs to be given to the choice of anaesthesia if local anaesthetics alone are not appropriate. Protocols vary between individual units, but general anaesthesia may be precluded on an outpatient basis in those above a particular BMI. This commonly used index facilitates assessment and communication between healthcare professionals. BMI is calculated as the patient's weight (in kilograms) divided by the square of the patient's height (in metres), that is:

$$BMI = Weight / (Height)^2$$

Grade 1 is a BMI of 25–30, grade 2 is 30–40, and grade 3 is >40.

Some groups of patients are at a higher risk of aspiration of stomach contents on induction of general anaesthesia. Such patients include those with a history suggestive of hiatus hernia, all non-fasted patients and pregnant patients (stomach emptying is slowed, and the cardiac sphincter more relaxed). If aspiration occurs, a pneumonitis may follow (Mendelson's syndrome).

The palatal and lingual tooth surfaces are at risk of erosion in patients who suffer from reflux of GI contents. Patients who suffer from significant gastrooesophageal reflux are usually not comfortable in the fully supine position, and this should be remembered during treatment.

Patients with pancreatic disease may have a bleeding tendency due to vitamin K malabsorption. Diabetes mellitus may complicate both pancreatitis and pancreatic cancers.

If a patient gives a history suggestive of obstructive jaundice, the main risk for the provision of safe dental treatment relates to the risk of excessive bleeding. This may occur as a result of vitamin K malabsorption. During the active phase, wherever possible, surgery should be deferred. If this is not possible, however, treatment in hospital with consideration of vitamin K supplementation is recommended.

An additional problem faced by patients with obstructive jaundice is the risk of renal failure developing after general anaesthesia – termed the 'hepatorenal syndrome'. It is thought that this syndrome occurs as a result of the toxic effect of bilirubin on the kidney. If possible, general anaesthesia should be postponed in these patients. In emergency situations, management requires the maintenance of good hydration immediately prior to administering the general anaesthetic, and the use of the osmotic diuretic mannitol.

The use of NSAIDs such as aspirin is contraindicated in individuals with peptic ulceration. Systemic corticosteroids should also be avoided in patients with peptic ulcers, as this may lead to haemorrhage or perforation, leading to abdominal pain and blood loss. Although steroids are used in the treatment of certain GI disorders, for example, inflammatory bowel disease, the duration of treatment is usually limited. It is possible to limit the duration of steroid treatment as steroid-sparing agents are usually used in the longer-term maintenance of the disease.

Ulcer-healing drugs and antacids

Ulcer-healing drugs achieve their effect by the following mechanisms:

- Inhibition of acid production.
- Increased mucus production.
- Increased bicarbonate production.
- Physical protection of mucosa.

The following groups of drugs are used:

- H_2 receptor antagonists.
- Proton pump inhibitors.
- Chelates and complexes.
- Prostaglandin analogues.
- Antacids.

H_2 receptor antagonists act as competitive inhibitors at histamine H_2 receptors to reduce gastric acid production. Examples of this group are cimetidine and ranitidine. Proton pump inhibitors block the action of the H^+/K^+-ATPase (proton pump), which catalyses the final step in gastric acid production. Examples are lansoprazole and omeprazole. These are really prodrugs, and are activated in an acidic environment. Chelates and complexes protect the gastric and duodenal mucosa by coating it. They also stimulate bicarbonate and mucus secretion, and can inhibit the action of pepsin. This group includes sucralfate and bismuth chelate.

Prostaglandins perform several actions that can protect against peptic ulceration. They stimulate mucus and bicarbonate secretion. In addition, prostaglandins inhibit the production of cAMP, which is a second messenger for histamine-induced acid secretion. The drug that is used as a prostaglandin analogue is misoprostol.

The bacterium *Helicobacter pylori*, which is involved in the aetiology of peptic ulcers, is eliminated by the so-called 'triple therapy' – that is, the use of a proton pump inhibitor, amoxicillin and either metronidazole or clarithromycin.

Unwanted effects of antiulcer drugs in the mouth and perioral structures

Ranitidine may cause staining of the tongue and, more importantly, erythema multiforme. Dry mouth can be a side effect of omeprazole and sucralfate. The latter drug may also produce a metallic taste. Antacids may cause a chalky taste. H_2 receptor antagonists can cause pain and swelling of the salivary glands.

Drug interactions

Antacids reduce the absorption of tetracyclines. Omeprazole reduces the absorption of the antifungal drugs ketoconazole and itraconazole, inhibits the metabolism of diazepam and increases the anticoagulant effect of warfarin.

Sucralfate reduces the effects of warfarin and inhibits the absorption of amphotericin, ketoconazole and tetracyclines.

FURTHER READING

Available from: www.crohnsandcolitis.org.uk/about-inflammatory-bowel-disease.

NICE Clinical Guideline 32 At Risk of Malnutrition (undernutrition) and Definition of Malnutrition (undernutrition).

MULTIPLE CHOICE QUESTIONS

1 BMI grade 1 lies in the range:
   a) 10–15
   b) 15–20
   c) 20–25
   d) 25–30
   e) 30–40
   Answer = D

2 Which of the following does *not* promote gastrooesophageal reflux?
   a) Milk
   b) Hiatus hernia
   c) Obesity
   d) Cigarettes
   e) Fatty foods
   Answer = A

3 Crohn's disease:
   a) Is confined to the terminal ileum
   b) Commonly presents with lip swelling
   c) Is characterised by transmural inflammation
   d) Is characterised by non-granulomatous inflammation
   e) Never demonstrates specific intraoral signs
   Answer = C

4 Which of the following is a proton pump inhibitor?
   a) Omeprazole
   b) Cimetidine
   c) Sucralfate
   d) Misoprostol
   e) Lisinopril
   Answer = A

5 Which of the following is a water-soluble vitamin?
   a) Vitamin A
   b) Vitamin B
   c) Vitamin D
   d) Vitamin E
   e) Vitamin K
   Answer = B

6 Beriberi is a disease caused by the deficiency of vitamin:
   a) B_1
   b) B_2
   c) B_3
   d) B_6
   e) B_{12}
   Answer = A

7 *Helicobacter pylori* is identified in the gastric antral mucosa in what percentage of cases of duodenal ulcer?
a) 15%
b) 25%
c) 70%
d) 90%
e) 100%
Answer = D

8 Which of the following is *not* normally associated with liver failure?
a) Ascites
b) Bleeding
c) Hypercoagulation
d) Cerebral oedema
e) Hepatorenal syndrome
Answer = C

9 Budd–Chiari syndrome is caused by:
a) Cirrhosis
b) Renal vein occlusion
c) Crohn's disease
d) Hepatic vein obstruction
e) Mesenteric artery infarction
Answer = D

10 Vitamin K is required for the synthesis of which of the following clotting factors?
a) Factor III
b) Factor IV
c) Factor V
d) Factor VI
e) Factor VII
Answer = E

CHAPTER 8
Renal disorders

EK Montgomery, JA Sayer, AL Brown and M Greenwood

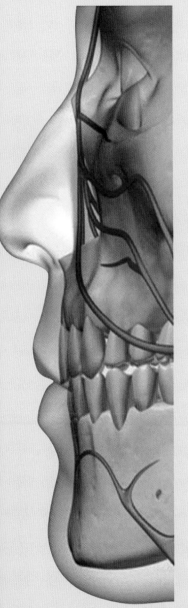

Key topics

- Normal and abnormal renal function.
- Relevance of renal disorders in dentistry.

Learning objectives

- To be familiar with the normal kidney and common renal disorders.
- To be aware of how renal disorders may impact on dental practice.
- Implications for drug prescribing in patients with renal disease.

Essentials of Human Disease in Dentistry, Second Edition. Mark Greenwood.
© 2018 John Wiley & Sons Ltd. Published 2018 by John Wiley & Sons Ltd.
Companion website: www.wiley.com/go/greenwood/human-disease-in-dentistry

Introduction

This chapter gives a simple and practical overview of normal kidney function, acute kidney injury (AKI), chronic kidney disease (CKD) and renal replacement therapy (RRT) for end-stage renal disease (ESRD). It is intended as clinically useful information for dental students and practitioners, but is not a comprehensive review of all renal diseases.

Structure of the kidneys

There are two kidneys, lying extraperitoneally on either side of the vertebral column. The kidneys are surrounded by fat in the retroperitoneal space; they move several centimetres with respiration. Each kidney consists of an outer cortex, containing the glomeruli, tubules and vessels, and the inner medulla, containing the loop of Henle and medullary collecting tubules.

The kidneys receive about 20% of total cardiac output, roughly a litre of blood per minute. Each kidney consists of approximately a million nephrons. The nephron is the functional filtering unit of the kidneys, comprising the glomerulus and the renal tubule. At the glomerulus, the afferent arteriole divides into several glomerular capillaries to form a loop of capillaries that make up the glomerular tuft. These capillary loops then recombine to form the efferent or outgoing arteriole. Each glomerulus is enclosed within an epithelial cell capsule called 'Bowman's capsule', which is continuous with the basement membrane of the glomerulus, and also with the start of the tubule. The tubule consists of the following segments – first, the proximal tubule; then, the loop of Henle; followed by the distal tubule that drains into the collecting ducts. Urine in the collecting ducts drains into the pelvis of the kidneys, and then via the ureters to the bladder.

The glomerulus

Blood circulates through the glomerular capillaries. Their specialised structure permits the production of an ultrafiltrate of plasma consisting of water containing only small solutes, which passes across the glomerular filtration barrier into the urinary space and into the tubule.

Next to the glomerulus is the juxtaglomerular apparatus (JGA), the vascular pole where the afferent arteriole arrives and the efferent arteriole leaves the glomerulus. The cells of the JGA are the source of the hormone renin, which, via the renin–angiotensin–aldosterone system, contributes to blood pressure control, salt and water homeostasis, and vascular tone.

The tubule

The ultrafiltrate of plasma is modified as it passes along the different sections of the tubule. Substances may be reabsorbed from the ultrafiltrate within the tubular lumen into the peritubular capillaries and so returned to the circulation (tubular reabsorption), or actively transported from the peritubular capillaries and secreted into the tubular lumen (tubular secretion).

The proximal tubule is where most of the ultrafiltrate is reabsorbed; about 60% of the filtered water, sodium, chloride and potassium is reabsorbed here. Glucose is normally completely reabsorbed here, unless the filtered load of glucose exceeds reabsorption capacity when the plasma glucose level is very high, resulting in glycosuria in diabetes. Phosphate and 95% of filtered amino acids are also reabsorbed in the proximal tubule.

The loop of Henle

The kidneys are able to vary the volume and concentration of urine, depending on the water intake and body fluid status. When water intake is high, water is excreted in excess of solute in a dilute urine that is hypoosmolar as compared to plasma. When water intake is low, water is retained by the kidneys, and a concentrated urine that is hyperosmolar as compared to plasma is excreted. The ability to form concentrated or dilute urine depends on the countercurrent multiplier mechanism in the loop of Henle. This depends on the different permeability properties and the different transport processes in the descending and ascending limbs of the loop. Although this mechanism is not completely understood, it is believed to depend on the development of a hyperosmotic medullary interstitium, produced by reabsorption of sodium chloride (NaCl) without water in the medullary ascending limb of the loop of Henle. This active NaCl transport out of the lumen into the interstitium results in a dilute urine and concentration of the interstitium. High urea concentrations in the interstitium also contribute to the hyperosmolarity. Because of the different permeabilities of the descending and ascending limbs of the loop of Henle, a medullary osmotic gradient is produced, which is highest at the tip of the loop in the inner medulla and papilla. As urine passes along the tubule, it equilibrates with the hyperosmolar interstitium, and water passes from the lumen to the interstitium (Figure 8.1). The collecting tubule is very impermeable to water in the absence of antidiuretic hormone (ADH). ADH is synthesised in the hypothalamus and secreted in response to hyperosmolarity or reduced circulating volume.

Measurement of renal function

Glomerular filtration rate (GFR)

Renal function is generally measured by assessing the GFR, which is described as the volume of plasma filtered by the glomerulus per unit time, and is an average of all the individual nephrons within both kidneys. The GFR varies significantly depending on age, sex, body surface area, ethnicity, physical activity and diet.

Creatinine

Serum creatinine is one of the most commonly used assessments of renal function. Creatinine is an end product of muscle breakdown. It is easy to measure using a widely available

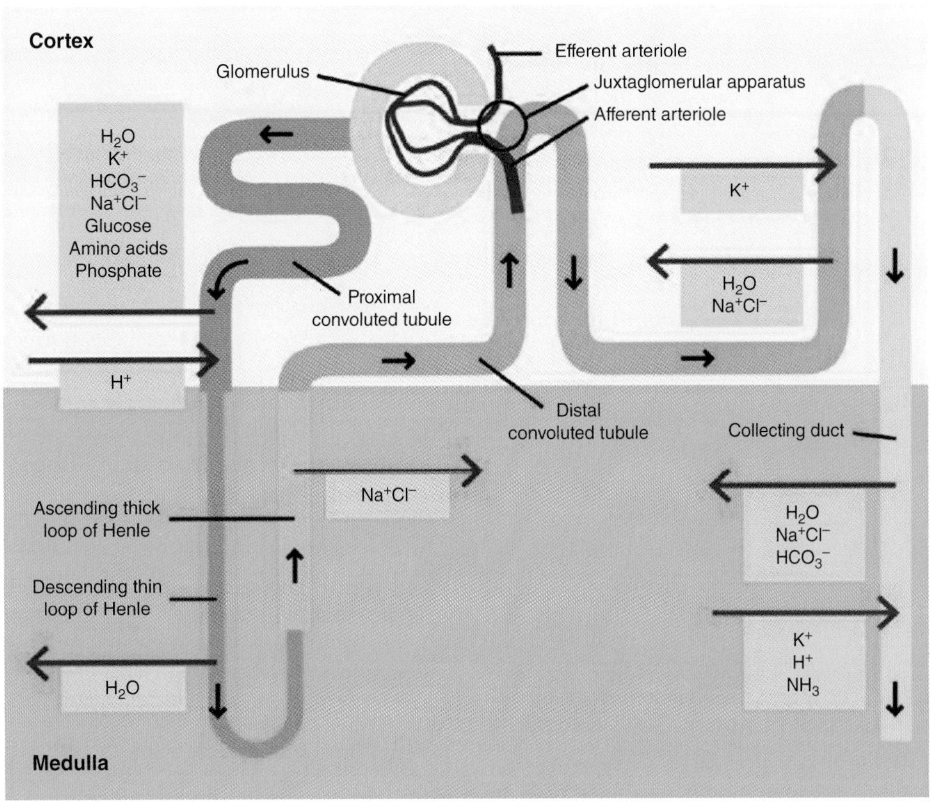

Figure 8.1 A simplified illustration of various components and their functions.

test; however, there are a large number of factors that can affect serum creatinine levels, leading to variability in results. When an individual is in a steady state with no anabolism or catabolism, serum creatinine will be produced at a steady rate proportional to muscle mass. Creatinine is small (molecular weight 113 Da) and is freely filtered at the glomerulus. It is not subsequently reabsorbed or metabolised to any significant extent, so the serum creatinine level provides a useful rough guide to GFR. However, creatinine is also secreted by the renal tubule.

Creatinine clearance (CrCl)

This is a more accurate way to measure the GFR than using serum creatinine levels alone. CrCl provides a measurement of GFR by assessing the amount of creatinine that is removed from the blood over a 24-h period. This requires the measurement of serum creatinine and a 24-h urine collection for urinary creatinine. The clearance is then calculated using the following equation:

$$CrCl = \frac{Urine\ creatinine \times volume}{Serum\ creatinine}$$

This method is not always practical, as it relies on a complete 24-h urine collection.

Formal assessment of GFR by inulin

Inulin is only cleared by filtration at the glomerulus, and hence provides a very accurate estimate of GFR. Inulin has to be infused intravenously, and so is only used in research studies.

Estimating GFR from serum creatinine measurements

As 24-h urine collections for CrCl are impractical on a regular basis, and since inulin clearance is only used as a research tool, several formulae have been developed to provide an estimated GFR (eGFR) based on serum creatinine levels and other variables. The equations are applicable to adults with stable levels of serum creatinine, and are not valid in pregnant women. The formulae are available as web tools (e.g. http://egfrcalc. renal.org/).

- *Cockcroft–Gault formula*: This is not particularly accurate when GFR > 60, and it estimates CrCl rather than GFR. Therefore, it tends to overestimate GFR (http://www. mdcalc.com/creatinine-clearance-cockcroft-gault-equation).
- *Modification of Diet in Renal Diseases (MDRD) study equation*: This involves a four-variable equation that has been validated in a large number of patients with a variety of renal diseases. It often underestimates GFR in individuals with near-normal GFR (http://egfrcalc.renal.org).

- *CKD-EPI*: This uses the same four variables as the MDRD equation; however, it analyses the variables in a different way, which enables better correction for the underestimation at higher GFR levels. It is more accurate than the MDRD equation, and is now one of the most commonly used equations in UK laboratories (https://www.qxmd.com/calculate/calculator_251/egfr-using-ckd-epi).

Control of acid–base balance

Metabolism produces hydrogen ions or protons that must be buffered to allow the body to maintain a constant pH. There are many buffer systems in the body, but the most widespread is the bicarbonate (HCO_3^-) buffer system, in which bicarbonate accepts protons and shifts to carbon dioxide (CO_2) and water, as shown in the following:

$$H^+ + HCO_3^- = H_2CO_3 = CO_2 + H_2O$$

This buffering maintains pH but cannot do so indefinitely, since the amount of buffer available within the body is limited. Eventually, the protons have to be excreted from the body, and the buffer regenerated. The kidneys regenerate bicarbonate in addition to reabsorbing filtered bicarbonate from the urine, mostly in the proximal tubule.

The kidneys achieve net excretion of protons by generating and excreting ammonium (NH_4^+) in the urine. The kidneys also excrete protons bound to other buffers – mainly phosphate, creatinine, uric acid and citrate.

Regulation of body fluid volume and composition

At the glomerulus, an ultrafiltrate of plasma is produced, consisting of water and very small solutes only. Large molecules such as proteins are normally not allowed to pass through the glomerular filtration barrier. The ultrafiltrate passes first into the Bowman's capsule and then into the proximal tubule. It is extensively modified by concentration and the active and passive ion transport as it travels down the nephron to the collecting duct.

Sodium cations (Na^+) and chloride anions (Cl^-) are the major extracellular ions and the main determinants of extracellular volume. The amount of sodium and chloride reabsorbed or excreted is key to the control of extracellular volume in the body.

Excretion (waste, drugs)

The kidneys excrete the waste products of metabolism, urea, creatinine, potassium and hydrogen ions.

The kidneys also excrete many drugs and metabolites. When kidney function is reduced, the dose of water-soluble drugs that are cleared via the kidneys must be reviewed and reduced.

Endocrine activity

The kidneys are central to calcium and phosphate metabolism. In addition to excreting and reabsorbing calcium and phosphate, the kidneys synthesise the active metabolite of vitamin D, that is, 1,25-dihydroxyvitamin D3 or calcitriol (Figure 8.2). Calcitriol acts on the gut to increase calcium and phosphate uptake, as well as on the feedback mechanism to suppress parathyroid hormone (PTH) release from the parathyroid glands and reduce osteoclast activity. The kidneys are thus essential for the maintenance of normocalcaemia and adequate bone mineralisation.

The kidneys also produce the hormone erythropoietin (EPO), which acts on the bone marrow to maintain red cell production and haemoglobin concentration.

Blood pressure control: renin–angiotensin–aldosterone system

This is one of the key regulators of salt and water balance, vasoconstriction and thus arterial blood pressure control. Renin is synthesised by the cells of the JGA in response to various stimuli. Renin cleaves angiotensin, synthesised in the liver, to angiotensin-I. This is converted by the angiotensin-converting enzyme (ACE), present in the lungs and endothelial cells, to angiotensin-II.

Angiotensin-II binds to at least two receptors, AT1 and AT2, although several additional receptors too have been identified. Most of the known effects of angiotensin-II are related to binding to the AT1 receptor, which results in vasoconstriction, aldosterone and vasopressin release, salt and water retention in the kidneys, as well as sympathetic nervous system activation. AT2 receptors are involved in antiproliferative and remodelling effects, which are thought to be important in the many cardioprotective and renoprotective effects of the renin–angiotensin blockade.

Clinical presentation of abnormal renal function

Asymptomatic patient with abnormal urinalysis or blood tests

Renal dysfunction may present as an asymptomatic finding such as nonvisible haematuria or proteinuria at routine screenings, often at a well-person clinic or check-up. Urine dipstick examination for blood and protein now forms part of the annual assessment of patients at risk of renal disease, such as those with hypertension or diabetes. Standard urine dipsticks test for urine pH, blood, protein, glucose, ketones, bilirubin and urobilinogen. Dipsticks can also be used to screen for leukocytes and nitrites, suggestive of urinary tract infection (UTI).

Proteinuria

Abnormal amounts of protein may appear in the urine as a result of damage and leakage at the glomerular filtration barrier, which overwhelm the tubular capacity for reabsorption.

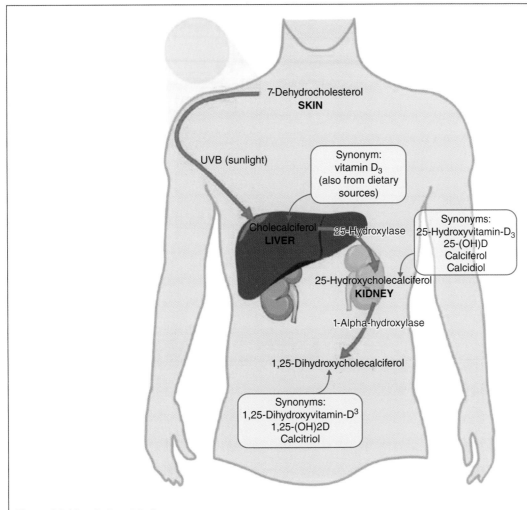

Figure 8.2 Vitamin D metabolism.

The urine normally only contains a very small amount of protein, the majority of which is Tamm–Horsfall protein (uromodulin). Proteinuria is usually quantified in the laboratory as a urinary protein creatinine ratio (uPCR) or albumin creatinine ratio (uACR), or semi-quantified in the clinic using a urinary dipstick.

Haematuria

Blood detected on urine dipstick testing may be due to blood loss from the urinary tract secondary to UTI and bladder inflammation, renal stones, interstitial kidney disease, cancer, etc. Myoglobinuria may cause a false positive urine dipstick.

Nephritic syndrome

This is a clinical presentation that may result from a variety of underlying renal pathologies causing disruption of the glomerular filtration barrier, usually due to immune-mediated inflammation and glomerulonephritis.

The nephritic syndrome comprises:

- Oliguria.
- Smoky or Coca-Cola-coloured urine due to haematuria.
- Oedema.
- Hypertension due to salt and water retention.
- Acute renal dysfunction.

Typically, there is significant haematuria and proteinuria on urine dipstick testing.

Nephrotic syndrome

Nephrotic syndrome may also be the clinical result of several underlying pathological processes, with protein leakage rather than inflammation at the glomerular filtration barrier being the major component. Nephrotic syndrome comprises:

- Significant proteinuria (uACR > 250 mg/mmol or uPCR > 350 mg/mmol).
- Hypoalbuminaemia.

- Oedema.
- Hyperlipidaemia.

Initially, renal function is usually relatively well preserved. Urine dipsticks will typically show significant proteinuria (+++).

AKI

AKI, previously known as 'acute renal failure', occurs as a result of sudden decline in GFR. This fall in GFR causes reduced elimination of nitrogenous waste products and toxins, resulting in impaired fluid and electrolyte homeostasis. It occurs over hours to days, and may be due to a wide variety of insults to the kidneys.

AKI is common, being present in 10–18% of patients admitted to the hospital. It is associated with significant morbidity, and the mortality rate ranges about 30–70%, depending on severity and the associated comorbidities. In the vast majority of cases, AKI is both preventable and treatable. Those at the highest risk of developing AKI include:

- Elderly people.
- Those with pre-existing kidney disease.
- Those with co-morbidities, including diabetes and cardiovascular disease (CVD).
- Those taking nephrotoxic medications.
- Those with hypovolaemia /dehydration.
- Those with sepsis.

There are many different definitions for AKI. The most commonly used definition is outlined in the 'risk, injury, failure, loss, end-stage renal disease (RIFLE) classification', developed by the Acute Dialysis Quality Initiative (ADQI) and later modified by the Acute Kidney Injury Network (AKIN) (Table 8.1).

AKI can also be allocated a stage from 1 to 3, increasing in severity (Table 8.2). This is based both on biochemical parameters and urine output once obstruction has been excluded.

Potential causes of AKI have classically been categorised as pre-renal, intrinsic and post-renal causes.

Pre-renal AKI

Reduced renal perfusion results in a fall of capillary filtration pressure. If there is a sustained reduction in renal perfusion over a period of time, then renal ischaemia develops, which can cause acute tubular necrosis (ATN).

Causes of pre-renal AKI include:

- Circulatory volume depletion (hypovolaemia).
- Inadequate cardiac function.
- Obstruction of blood supply to the kidneys.

Intrinsic renal AKI

This is usually due to glomerular pathology (e.g. glomerulonephritis) or tubulointerstitial disease, drugs or other nephrotoxic agents.

Table 8.1 RIFLE criteria adapted by AKIN.

Stage	Urine output	Serum creatinine	GFR
Risk	<0.5 ml/kg body weight per hour for 6 hours	1.5-fold increase	25% decrease
Injury	<0.5 ml/kg body weight per hour for 12 hours	2-fold increase	50% decrease
Failure	<0.5 ml/kg body weight per hour for 24 hours, or anuria for 12 hours	3-fold increase	75% decrease
Loss	Complete loss of kidney function for >4 weeks (need for RRT)		
ESRD	Complete loss of kidney function for >12 weeks (need for RRT)		

Table 8.2 Stages of AKI.

AKI stage	Serum creatinine	Urine output
1	Increase from baseline by 26 µmol/L, or a 1.5–2-fold increase	<0.5 ml/kg body weight per hour for 6 hours
2	Increase from baseline by 2–3 fold	<0.5 ml/kg body weight per hour for 12 hours
3	Creatinine greater than 354 µmol/L, an increase of >3-fold or the need for RRT	0.3 ml/kg body weight per hour for 24 hours, or anuria for 12 hours

Post-renal AKI

If there is obstruction to the urinary tract, the flow of urine is impeded, and the resulting back pressure results in reduced filtration and, potentially, renal ischaemia if sustained over a period of time. Obstruction may occur anywhere within the urinary tract from renal stones, as a result of an abnormality within the wall of the ureter (e.g. stricture or tumour) or from external compression from outside the ureter (compression by mass, tumour or fibrotic process). The obstruction may also occur within or below the bladder (e.g. enlarged prostate). Common causes of post-renal AKI include benign prostatic hypertrophy, renal stones and malignancy.

CKD

The National Institute for Health and Care Excellence (NICE) defines CKD as abnormalities of kidney function or structure present for more than 3 months, with implications for health.

Table 8.3 Causes of CKD.

Causes of CKD	Examples
Glomerular	Glomerulonephritis
	Diabetic nephropathy
	Lupus nephritis
Tubular/tubulointerstitial	Drug induced
	Reflux nephropathy
	Polycystic kidney disease
Vascular	Renal artery stenosis/thrombosis
	Hypertension/ischaemic nephropathy
	Vasculitis
Obstructive/urological	Renal or bladder stones
	Benign prostatic hyperplasia/prostate malignancy

The prevalence of CKD increases with age, and it is estimated that 9% of adults in the UK have CKD. There are many causes of CKD (Table 8.3). In the UK, the most common causes are hypertension, diabetes and glomerulonephritis.

Classification of CKD

CKD is classified both by rising creatinine levels or falling GFR, and by the degree of proteinuria. Stages of CKD have been recently defined by NICE (https://www.nice.org.uk/guidance/cg182/chapter/1-recommendations).

- Stage G1 denotes essentially normal renal function.
- Stage G2 is mildly reduced kidney function (GFR 60–89 ml/min/1.73 m^2). Both stages require other evidence of kidney disease (e.g. proteinuria, haematuria, structural abnormalities or genetic diagnosis of kidney disease).
- Stage G3 (eGFR 30–59 ml/min/1.73 m^2).
- Stage G4 (eGFR 15–29 ml/min/1.73 m^2).
- Stage G5 is <15 ml/min/1.73 m^2, and usually means ESRD requiring RRT.

The recent NICE classification (July 2014) also integrates the level of albuminuria with GFR, to provide risk stratification (https://www.nice.org.uk/guidance/cg182/chapter/1-recommendations). CKD management is to halt or slow the progression in renal decline as much as possible, and to treat the associated symptoms and complications. The higher the CKD stage, the more likely the patient is to progress to renal failure and develop CVD – one of the major causes of death in renal patients.

Complications of CKD

- CVD.
- Mineral and bone disorders (e.g. calcium and phosphate disorders).
- Hyperkalaemia.
- Anaemia.
- Malnutrition.

- Increased risk of other non-cardiovascular disease (e.g. infection and cancer).
- Fluid overload.
- Acidosis.

It is important to assess the rate at which a patient's renal function is declining, so that preparations can be made for RRT (dialysis or transplantation).

Management of patients with CKD

The mainstay of management for many patients is good blood pressure control, management of proteinuria, addressing cardiovascular risks, symptom control and management of CKD-associated complications.

Management of renal anaemia

Anaemia is defined as a haemoglobin level of <110 g/l. Anaemia due to renal disease may occur when the GFR falls to <60 ml/min, and it is more common in those with advanced renal disease. It is primarily due to reduced EPO production and iron deficiency. Anaemia of CKD should only be diagnosed when other causes of anaemia have been excluded.

Treatment with oral or intravenous iron is often required, along with EPO supplementation, to achieve a target haemoglobin of 100–120 g/l.

Management of mineral and bone disorders

Renal bone disease is usually due to a disorder of calcium and phosphate levels leading to the development of hyperparathyroidism. This is common particularly after CKD stage G3.

Management usually involves calcium supplementation and phosphate binders at least early in the condition. Vitamin D deficiency is also common. Reduced bone strength and increased fracture risk is common, particularly in untreated patients.

Approach to managing patients with impaired renal function

History and examination: Taking a detailed history may provide many clues to possible causes (Table 8.4). It is important to assess for a history of hypertension, diabetes or any symptoms that may be linked to autoimmune or immunological conditions such as connective tissue disorders.

Checking for a history of vascular disease such as stroke, ischaemic heart disease or peripheral vascular disease may highlight the possibility of renovascular diseases.

A urinary history should include the amount and frequency of passing urine, the presence of frothy urine (suggestive of proteinuria) or visible haematuria. A poor flow, hesitancy on initiating urination or post-micturition dribbling in a man may be suggestive of underlying prostate problems.

A detailed history of current and past medications should be taken, and specific queries made about illicit drugs and

Table 8.4 Important points to obtain in the history of patients who have renal disorder.

- History of diabetes mellitus
- Is CKD confirmed in the patient?
- Are there any related bone disorders?
- Symptoms/history of anaemia
- Questions relating to patients who are on dialysis:
  - Type
  - Frequency
  - Is there an arteriovenous fistula, graft or neck line?
- Has the patient had a renal transplant? If so:
  - When was the transplant carried out?
- Associated medications including steroids

medications bought over the counter, such as nonsteroidal anti-inflammatory drugs (NSAIDs). Details of treatment with ACE inhibitors, other antihypertensive medications and antibiotics should be sought.

A family history of renal disease is important for identifying genetic conditions such as autosomal dominant polycystic kidney disease. Lifestyle questions about smoking and alcohol consumption may also be important when looking for potential diagnoses.

General examination is performed for any signs of systemic diseases and for markers of renal impairment such as pallor due to anaemia, vasculitic rash, blood pressure, oedema, abdominal masses, palpable bladder, presence of peripheral pulses and any vascular bruits.

Investigation

Initial investigations should include full blood count, urea and electrolytes, liver function and bone chemistry, and markers of inflammation such as ESR and CRP. More detailed investigation of possible immune-mediated causes of renal failure includes autoantibody screening, including anti-neutrophil cytoplasmic antibody (ANCA), anti-glomerular basement membrane (anti-GBM) antibody, serum immunoglobulin and electrophoresis (to investigate for myeloma), and complement C3 and C4 (to look for evidence of complement activation and consumption).

Urine analysis

Dipstick urinalysis may confirm haematuria and proteinuria as a consequence of a leaking and damaged glomerular filtration barrier. Urine microscopy may reveal red cell casts, suggesting glomerular bleeding.

Imaging of the kidneys

- Ultrasound scan of the kidneys is a quick, convenient and non-invasive way of demonstrating obstruction and demonstrating renal size.
- Doppler ultrasound scanning of renal arteries and veins will demonstrate blood flow.
- Plain abdominal X-ray will show any radio-dense calcium-containing stones.
- CT IVU scan is now the preferred method of renal imaging when renal stones are suspected.
- Magnetic resonance imaging (MRI) will show details of renal anatomy and blood supply. MRI is not without some risk, as gadolinium-containing agents are sometimes used as contrast agents, and some preparations have been associated with the development of nephrogenic systemic fibrosis.
- Intra-arterial renal angiogram is the gold standard for diagnosing renal artery stenosis. Treatment of any demonstrated stenosis by angioplasty and stenting can be performed during angiography.
- Isotope renography is useful in evaluating the functioning of kidneys – particularly in looking for obstructions.

Renal biopsy

Percutaneous renal biopsy is a valuable investigation in the evaluation of kidney dysfunction. It provides a tissue diagnosis in more than 95% of cases, with a life-threatening complication rate of less than 0.1%. Renal biopsy is usually carried out under local anaesthetic, using real-time ultrasound-guided localisation to ensure the biopsy needle is correctly positioned at the renal cortex.

The kidneys and systemic disease

Diabetes mellitus

Diabetes mellitus is now the leading cause of ESRD in the USA, accounting for almost half of all cases. Microvascular lesions associated with long-duration or poorly controlled diabetes give rise to diabetic retinopathy, neuropathy and nephropathy. The underlying mechanism is believed to be by deposition of advanced glycation end products (AGEs).

In type 1 diabetes, individuals with diabetic retinopathy have a >90% chance of an associated diabetic nephropathy, so a kidney biopsy is not usually necessary to confirm the diagnosis. For type 2 diabetics, however, there is a significant incidence of other glomerular diseases, so a renal biopsy should be considered. If there are atypical features such as very short history of diabetes, very rapid progression of renal disease, marked haematuria or unusually heavy proteinuria, an alternative diagnosis should be suspected and investigated.

Microscopic vasculitis (microscopic angiitis)

Systemic vasculitis, which can affect any organ, describes a variety of clinical syndromes that are characterised by inflammation and necrosis in the wall of blood vessels. The size and type of the affected blood vessel determine the clinical presentation and disease classification. The presence of antibodies against cytoplasmic antigens (ANCA) are often identified, and can help with classification of the condition. A consideration of systemic vasculitis is given below.

- Granulomatosis with polyangiitis (GPA), previously known as 'Wegener's granulomatosis', is a necrotising vasculitis affecting small–medium-sized vessels. GPA characteristically affects the respiratory tract and the kidneys, where vasculitis of the glomerular capillaries results in a focal necrotising glomerulonephritis.
- Diagnosis of GPA depends on a combination of clinical symptoms, ANCA positivity, and biopsy evidence of small-vessel vasculitis, usually by renal or nasal biopsy.
- Untreated GPA has a mortality of almost 95% at 5 years. Treatment consists of aggressive immunosuppression with steroids, and then cyclophosphamide or rituximab. Plasma exchange is also performed for severe disease with pulmonary haemorrhage.
- Eosinophilic granulomatosis with polyangiitis (EGPA), previously known as 'Churg–Strauss syndrome', is also a necrotising vasculitis affecting small–medium-sized vessels, and is often associated with a positive ANCA test. It is classically associated with pulmonary infiltrates, asthma and eosinophilia.
- Microscopic polyarteritis (polyangiitis) is a vasculitis of small blood vessels that may affect multiple organs or be limited to one system, involving only the kidneys.
- Polyarteritis nodosa (PAN) is a vasculitis affecting medium-sized arteries, with aneurysm formation. PAN presents with hypertension and infarction in the affected organs, or bleeding from aneurysms. There is an association with hepatitis B infection. Diagnosis is by angiography, and treatment is with immunosuppression if hepatitis B has been excluded.

Anti-GBM disease

Anti-GBM disease (or 'Goodpasture's disease') is characterised by the development of autoantibodies to the glomerular basement membrane in the kidneys and the lungs. Severe glomerular inflammation with crescents may be seen on renal biopsy. There is often an AKI that progresses rapidly if not treated. Patients may also present with shortness of breath and haemoptysis suggestive of pulmonary haemorrhage.

Treatment is plasma exchange to remove the circulating anti-GBM antibodies, plus immunosuppression with steroids and cyclophosphamide to prevent further antibody formation.

Amyloid

Amyloid can be either AA amyloid, a proteolytic cleavage fragment from serum amyloid A, or AL amyloid, made up of fragments of light chains. Amyloid deposits have a very typical histological appearance, with amorphous pink deposits on light microscopy that characteristically stain apple green with Congo red when viewed under birefringent light.

Renal amyloid presents with proteinuria, usually in the nephrotic range, plus renal impairment. Diagnosis is by demonstration of amyloid deposits on biopsy, usually renal biopsy. Treatment of the underlying condition may prevent further deposition. Treatment is directed by the type of amyloid, location of deposits and suitability for treatment. Treatment usually involves chemotherapy and supportive therapy with dialysis.

IgA nephropathy and Henoch–Schönlein purpura

IgA (immunoglobulin A) nephropathy is a glomerular disease characterised by the mesangial deposition of IgA.

Henoch–Schönlein purpura consists of IgA deposition in the glomeruli, but with additional extrarenal features of a systemic vasculitis. Characteristic skin purpura is seen over extensor surfaces and buttocks, in addition to joint and gut involvement. It is most common in children, where it is usually self-limiting, although it can occur at any age. Skin biopsy of Henoch–Schönlein purpura will demonstrate IgA deposition in blood vessels.

Both conditions often present with either visible or nonvisible haematuria. IgA nephropathy is the most common type of glomerulonephritis in the UK. Management involves good blood pressure control and the use of anti-proteinuria agents (e.g. ACE inhibitors).

Sarcoid

Sarcoidosis was discussed in Chapter 6 (titled 'Respiratory disorders'). It is a disease of unknown aetiology, diagnosed when non-caseating epithelioid granulomata are demonstrated in affected organs. Typical presentation is with bilateral hilar lymphadenopathy; pulmonary infiltrates seen on chest X-ray; plus skin, eye and renal involvement.

Systemic lupus erythematosus (SLE)

SLE is an autoimmune multisystem disease, characterised by circulating autoantibodies against a number of cellular antigens. SLE is much more common in women than men, and more common in black populations than Caucasian. SLE is commonly associated with nephritis as well as problems with the heart, lungs and the nervous system.

SLE usually presents with marked systemic symptoms of rash, fatigue, malaise, muscle and joint aches, and weight loss. Pleuritic symptoms are common, as is Raynaud's phenomenon. Recurrent thrombosis may result from antiphospholipid antibodies that promote clotting (lupus anticoagulant).

The American Rheumatism Association proposed a classification of SLE, following several modifications, which requires any four or more of the criteria (Table 8.5) to make a diagnosis of SLE.

Up to half of patients with SLE will develop renal involvement (lupus nephritis). Lupus nephritis is very variable, both in presentation and histology. It may present with low-grade proteinuria, haematuria, nephrosis, slowly progressive CKD and rapidly progressive glomerulonephritis.

Table 8.5 Criteria for the classification of SLE (four or more are required for diagnosis).

Malar or butterfly facial rash
Discoid rash
Photosensitivity
Oral ulcers
Arthritis affecting two or more joints
Pleurisy or pericarditis
Renal abnormalities (persistent significant proteinuria, cellular casts)
Haematological abnormalities
Immunological disorders

Systemic sclerosis

Systemic sclerosis (SSc), or scleroderma, is an autoimmune rheumatic disease characterised by fibrotic changes affecting the skin and other organs. Scleroderma may present with localised skin changes only; as limited cutaneous systemic sclerosis; or as a systemic disorder with widespread skin involvement, pulmonary fibrosis and renal involvement. Patients often have Raynaud's phenomenon, and have typical autoantibodies, which are used to subdivide scleroderma into different categories – for example, most patients will have positive antinuclear antibodies (ANA). Anti-RNA polymerase antibodies are associated with diffuse cutaneous systemic sclerosis. Anticentromere antibody is found in limited cutaneous systemic sclerosis.

The most important renal complication of SSc is scleroderma renal crisis. This is a life-threatening complication that presents with hypertension, hypertensive encephalopathy, seizures, pulmonary oedema and AKI. Management focuses on blood pressure control with ACE inhibitors, which provide renoprotection via renin–angiotensin system blockade.

Abnormalities secondary to infections

Many renal abnormalities result from infections: infections such as septicaemia may cause AKI with acute tubular necrosis. *Escherichia coli* infection may cause haemolytic–uraemic syndrome (HUS). Chronic infection, for example, osteomyelitis or bronchiectasis, may result in amyloidosis.

HIV-related nephropathy (HIVAN)

HIV-associated nephropathy (HIVAN) has a distinctive pathological appearance with collapsing glomerulopathy, although other forms of kidney disease may also occur with HIV. Treatment with antiretroviral medication and ACE inhibitors is the mainstay of management.

Inherited renal disease

Autosomal dominant polycystic kidney disease (ADPKD)

This is the most common inherited kidney disease, with a prevalence between 1 in 400 and 1 in 1000. It is an autosomal dominant genetically determined disorder characterised by the development and enlargement of renal cysts, typically progressing to ESRD in late middle age.

Reflux nephropathy (chronic pyelonephritis)

Vesicoureteric reflux (VUR) occurs when there is a congenital abnormality of the junction between the ureter and bladder, such that urine can flow from the bladder back up the ureter into the kidneys. Such reflux of infected urine was thought to be the cause of chronic pyelonephritis or focal renal scarring, but it is now accepted that renal scarring can also occur in the absence of VUR. VUR seems to be inherited by an autosomal mechanism, such that there is an approximately 30% chance of a child inheriting VUR from an affected parent. VUR is associated with an increased risk of UTI and renal scarring, which can lead in later life to hypertension and progressive renal failure.

Renal stone disease

This is a common disorder; up to 10% of adults in the western world will suffer from a renal stone at some time. The majority of renal stones are calcium oxalate, with calcium phosphate, uric acid or cysteine stones being less common. Renal stones can cause loin pain, haematuria, UTI and obstruction. The smallest stones will pass spontaneously. Small stones may be treated by shock wave lithotripsy to disintegrate them, but larger stones may require surgical removal.

Hypertensive nephrosclerosis and atheromatous renovascular disease

Renovascular disease is a common cause of renal dysfunction in elderly patients with arterial disease. Atheromatous narrowing of the renal or intrarenal arteries can restrict blood flow to the kidneys and result in ischaemic damage. Renal artery stenosis should be suspected in association with vascular disease elsewhere (strokes, myocardial infarction, intermittent claudication).

CKD–Mineral and Bone Disorders (CKD-MBD)

The kidneys are central to the control of calcium and phosphate levels. Phosphate retention occurs in CKD because of reduced renal clearance once GFR is below 60 ml/min. Hyperphosphataemia is common once GFR is below 25–30 ml/min. At the same time, reduced vitamin D production will lead to reduced calcium absorption from the gut, leading to hypocalcaemia. This stimulus will cause increased PTH release from the parathyroid glands. PTH maintains calcium homeostasis by increasing bone remodelling to release calcium and phosphate, increasing renal reabsorption of calcium and excretion of phosphate, and increasing gut absorption of both calcium and phosphate.

If hyperphosphataemia and hypocalcaemia in CKD are not corrected, the continuing parathyroid stimulus will lead to hypertrophy of the parathyroid gland and hyperparathyroidism. Patients with CKD may have several different types of bone disease, although these are often labelled together as renal osteodystrophy or CKD-MBD. Renal bone disease may include osteomalacia, osteitis fibrosa cystica due to severe hyperparathyroidism, uraemic osteodystrophy and adynamic bone disease, which is characterised by reduced bone turnover.

In addition to bone disease, a persistent abnormality in the calcium–phosphate product is associated with the increased risk of vascular calcification, as well as calcium phosphate precipitation into joints and soft tissues such as muscles. Severe arterial calcium deposition can result in tissue ischaemia with skin necrosis, called 'calciphylaxis'. Close monitoring of bone chemistry, and strict attention to phosphate control, with dietary phosphate restriction and phosphate binders, is necessary for all patients with CKD. Similarly, monitoring and early treatment of raised parathyroid hormone levels with vitamin D supplements, while avoiding hypercalcaemia, is essential.

ESRD and RRT

When reaching ESRD, there are several therapies that can be used to replace renal function.
- Haemodialysis.
- Peritoneal dialysis.
- Renal transplantation.

Treatment with haemodialysis

Haemodialysis is usually carried out as a hospital outpatient treatment, although it is possible to learn to dialyse yourself at home. Haemodialysis requires access to the circulation, to allow the pumping of blood through the dialysis machine, and a synthetic biocompatible semipermeable membrane (dialyser), which acts as an 'artificial kidney' (Figure 8.3). This enables the removal of metabolites, toxins and excess water. By exerting a pressure difference across the semipermeable membrane, an ultrafiltrate of plasma water will be produced (ultrafiltration). As the dialysis fluid, with predetermined concentrations of small solutes such as potassium and calcium, flows to the other side of the semipermeable membrane, convective clearance down concentration gradients will also be achieved. Waste such as urea and creatinine, which are in high concentrations in the blood, will move into the dialysate, while substances at higher concentrations in the dialysate (e.g. bicarbonate) will move into the blood. Diffusion of bicarbonate

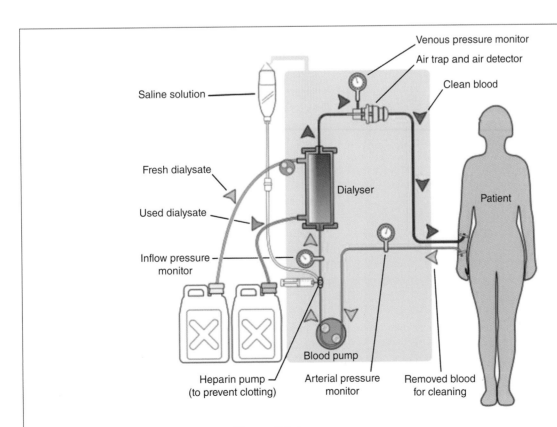

Figure 8.3 A diagram to show the process of haemodialysis.

into the blood stream will then help to correct the metabolic acidosis common in renal failure.

Circulatory access for haemodialysis will ideally give a blood flow of about 300–600 ml/min to allow efficient treatment. Such rates of blood flow allow large volumes of blood to be pumped through the dialysis circuit, resulting in efficient removal of waste products. Adequate dialysis achieves blood biochemistry parameters within internationally agreed target ranges and good blood pressure control.

Such circulatory access for haemodialysis may be obtained in an emergency by placing a central venous catheter, most commonly in the internal jugular vein, which can be tunnelled under the skin for longer-term use. Optimum access is by means of the surgical creation of an arteriovenous fistula, usually in the arm (Figure 8.4). Patients usually require anticoagulation medication, to prevent clotting of blood in the dialysis machine, and extracorporeal circulation.

Most patients with ESRD will need three haemodialysis sessions a week, each of about 4 hours duration, to give adequate waste clearance for satisfactory biochemical control, as well as adequate salt and water removal for volume and blood pressure control.

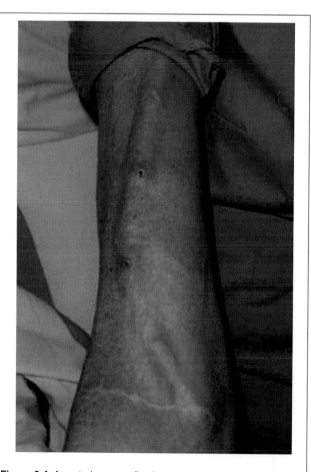

Figure 8.4 An arteriovenous fistula created to facilitate vascular access for haemodialysis.

Treatment with peritoneal dialysis

Peritoneal dialysis utilises the peritoneal membrane, which lines the peritoneal cavity, as a natural semipermeable membrane. This method of dialysis requires an intact and unscarred peritoneal membrane, so it may not be possible when there has been previous abdominal surgery leading to adhesions and scarring. Up to 2 litres of an isotonic or hypertonic solution is instilled into the abdomen via a peritoneal catheter. The fluid is left in the abdomen for a predetermined amount of time, called a 'dwell'. The metabolites and waste products then move across the membrane into the peritoneal fluid before being drained out and discarded. There are many different regimes used for peritoneal dialysis. The two main types are:

1 Continuous ambulatory peritoneal dialysis (CAPD).
2 Automated peritoneal dialysis (APD).

The peritoneal dialysis prescription must be individualised to the patient's unique requirements. It mainly focuses on two factors – the removal of fluid and the clearance of toxic metabolites.

CAPD

This usually involves 1–2 litres of dialysis fluid being run via the catheter into the peritoneal cavity. The fluid will remain in the abdominal cavity for several hours before being drained out into an empty bag by gravity. This is called an 'exchange'. Each patient will typically have between three and five exchanges per day.

APD

This works in the same way as CAPD. However, the fluid exchanges are all done at night by an automated machine.

Peritoneal dialysis is usually performed daily at home by the patient or a trained carer. It has fewer problems associated with blood pressure instability, but carries the risk of PD peritonitis, where infection is introduced into the abdominal cavity.

Renal transplantation

ESRD results in a decreased life expectancy, with a greatly increased risk of CVD in comparison with the general population. Renal transplantation offers freedom from dialysis, dietary and fluid restrictions, as well as improved survival. A further benefit is the restoration of fertility and the chance of a successful pregnancy. All CKD patients should be considered for possible renal transplantation, although not all will be medically fit, owing to other comorbid conditions.

Transplant kidneys can be from both deceased and living donors. Many patients will wait years for a suitably matched organ from a deceased donor to become available on the transplant register. However, an organ from a suitable living donor can allow timely and elective renal transplantation even before the need for dialysis. The rate of graft survival 5 years after a first adult deceased donor kidney transplant is 86%, and 92% for a living donation.

Renal transplant recipients: immunosuppressive treatment

Renal transplant recipients must take immunosuppressive drugs to prevent rejection of their transplanted kidney. Common immunosuppression regimens include the use of three agents: azathioprine or mycophenolate mofetil (MMF); ciclosporin or tacrolimus; and prednisolone. The immunosuppressive drugs mainly target the T-cell-mediated immune response, and treatment is required lifelong. If patients have experienced previous rejection, they will often be on a higher dose of medication, and hence will have a lower immune response, creating an increased risk of infection and malignancy.

Dental aspects relating to renal patients

Patients with CKD have reduced resistance to infection in addition to their renal disorder. Little modification is required in the routine dental care of renal patients, but oral hygiene is important, particularly due to the reduced resistance to infection. Standard procedures should be employed to prevent cross-infection. There is no contraindication to infiltration analgesia, but any bleeding tendencies should be excluded prior to administering a deep regional nerve block. Chronic anaemia and platelet dysfunction are associated with CKD. ESRD patients may complain of dry mouth and taste change, and may exhibit tongue coating, decreased salivary flow and poor periodontal health.

For dental procedures, most patients with renal conditions are best treated using local analgesia. Potential electrolyte disturbances, especially hyperkalaemia, could complicate general anaesthesia. Corticosteroids are often prescribed for renal patients, and it predisposes them to infection and poor wound healing.

For ease of vascular access in haemodialysis patients, an arteriovenous fistula is made (usually at the wrist). It must *not* be used by the dentist for vascular access, and the arm with the fistula should be avoided for cannulation or venepuncture.

Renal patients are often hypertensive, and this should be considered prior to any form of treatment. It is critical that good haemostasis be achieved after oral surgical procedures in terms of both possible hypertension and the bleeding tendency of these patients. Patients are best treated the day *after* haemodialysis (which is usually thrice weekly), as renal function will be optimal and the effects of the anticoagulation, usually low-molecular-weight heparin, will have worn off. It is important that consultation take place with the renal physician to ensure the timing of haemodialysis sessions and to plan any additional treatments such as blood transfusion on dialysis.

The impact of impaired renal function may not manifest itself unless the kidneys are placed under stress. Situations where this could happen are: after the administration of particular drugs, a heavy dietary protein load and pregnancy. Swallowed blood acts as a protein load and may occur, for example, from a post-extraction haemorrhage. Dietary manipulation is useful in decreasing sodium and potassium load.

Patients with renal problems may have disturbances in electrolyte levels in the blood. This can have secondary effects on the cardiovascular status of the patient. The incidence of atheroma is increased in patients with CKD, and many patients with severe nephrotic syndrome are on anticoagulation therapy.

Renal transplant recipients and many other renal patients may be on immunosuppression therapy, or may have recently received it. Therefore, any signs of oral infection should be treated immediately. It is also important to look closely for any signs of malignancy, given the increased risk in this patient group.

The impairment of drug excretion in certain groups leads to the need for care with drug prescription. Drugs such as ciclosporin and nifedipine can cause gingival overgrowth, and oral ulceration has been reported with mTOR inhibitors such as sirolimus (another type of immunosuppressant).

Prescribing in renal disease

Many drugs prescribed by dentists are excreted by the kidneys. Failure to excrete a drug or its metabolites can lead to toxicity. As a general rule, any drug that is nephrotoxic should be avoided. Other drugs may require dose reduction. Antibiotics such as erythromycin and clarithromycin will interact with immunosuppressive agents for renal transplant recipients, and should be avoided unless discussed with the renal physician. Ciclosporin and tacrolimus metabolism is altered by many drugs, leading to an increase in toxicity or risk of rejection. Resources such as *Dental Practitioners' Formulary* and *The Renal Drug Handbook* provide useful information on dose alteration for antimicrobials and many other drugs, depending on the degree of renal impairment.

NSAIDs should not be prescribed in those with more than mild renal impairment. Paracetamol would be the analgesic of choice. Agents used for dental sedation should also be used with extreme care, as a greater effect than normal may be produced.

FURTHER READING

Available from: www.renal.org/guidlines/modules/acute-kidney-injury#sthash.JMQhPi5Y.dpbs.

Formulae for estimating Glomerular Filtration Rate/Modification of Diet in Renal Diseases Study Equation. Available from: http://egfrc.calc.renal.org/.

National Institute for Health and Care Excellence – chronic kidney disease. Available from: www.nice.org.uk/guidance/cg182.

Prescribing in Renal Disease. British National Formulary. Available from: www.BNF.org.

MULTIPLE CHOICE QUESTIONS

1. Which of the following statements about kidney structure and physiology is *true*?
   a) Kidneys lie intraperitoneally on either side of the vertebral column.
   b) The kidneys receive about 80% of the total cardiac output
   c) The cells of the JGA produce the hormone 'renin'.
   d) Concentrated urine is hypo-osmolar as compared to plasma.
   e) The afferent vessel is the outgoing arteriole of the glomerulus.
   Answer = C

2. Which of the following statements about CKD is *true*?
   a) The prevalence of CKD falls with increasing age.
   b) Renal anaemia is always observed as eGR falls.
   c) Diabetes mellitus is a major cause of CKD.
   d) CKD is associated with a decreased risk of vascular disease.
   e) Most patients with CKD are symptomatic.
   Answer = C

3. In the treatment of ESRD, which of the following statements is *true*?
   a) Haemodialysis is a better treatment option than successful renal transplantation.
   b) 'Dialysis' describes the equilibration of substances across a semipermeable membrane.
   c) A fistula is always required for haemodialysis.
   d) Peritoneal dialysis cannot proceed in patients with diabetes.
   e) Haemodialysis cannot be performed in an emergency.
   Answer = B

4. Which of the following statements about AKI is *true*?
   a) AKI is uncommon among hospital admissions.
   b) AKI is diagnosed both on biochemical parameters and urine output.
   c) Renal stones may cause pre-renal AKI.
   d) Most cases of AKI are not preventable.
   e) AKI stage 1 is more severe than stage 3.
   Answer = B

5. Which of the following statements about renal impairment is *true*?
   a) Severe uraemia can cause increased bleeding risks.
   b) It is best to perform procedures on dialysis patients immediately after their dialysis session.
   c) Drug doses often need to be increased in renal impairment.
   d) NSAIDs are generally safe in renal patients.
   e) Swallowed blood from a post-extraction haemorrhage can provide a significant phosphate load.
   Answer = A

6. Which of the following statements regarding mineral and bone disorders and CKD is *false*?
   a) The kidneys can regulate serum phosphate levels even at GFR levels of <30.
   b) Dietary phosphate restriction improves hyperparathyroidism in CKD.

   c) Vascular calcification is a cardiovascular risk factor.
   d) Hyperparathyroidism may lead to increased risk of fractures.
   e) Phosphate binders may allow serum calcium levels to normalise.
   Answer = A

7. Which of the following statements about renal transplantation is *false*?
   a) Renal transplantation from a living donor may allow pre-emptive transplantation and help avoid the need for dialysis.
   b) The side effects of immunosuppression include an increased risk of skin cancer.
   c) Immunosuppressant drugs must be stopped before oral surgery.
   d) Gingival hypertrophy is a side effect of cyclosporine and tacrolimus.
   e) Tacrolimus dosage can be monitored using trough blood levels.
   Answer = C

8. Which of the following statements about dental care in patients with renal disease is *true*?
   a) Mouth infections are not more common in patients with ESRD.
   b) Reduced platelet function is seen in patients with CKD.
   c) The use of heparin in haemodialysis patients is of no concern prior to tooth extraction.
   d) Antihypertensive drugs do not contribute to gum hypertrophy/gingival overgrowth.
   e) Oral cancers are more frequent in renal transplant recipients.
   Answer = B

9. Which of the following statements about dialysis in renal disease is *true*?
   a) Peritoneal dialysis is less effective in the elderly.
   b) Peritoneal dialysis involves systemic anticoagulation.
   c) Haemodialysis is not possible in left-handed people.
   d) Peritoneal dialysis cannot be performed after major abdominal surgery.
   e) Haemodialysis cannot be performed at the patient's home.
   Answer = D

10. Which of the following statements about the causes of renal disease is *true*?
    a) Systemic sclerosis is an inherited disease.
    b) Diabetes mellitus is the commonest cause of ESRD.
    c) Renal vasculitis may be diagnosed using specialist blood tests such as ANCA.
    d) Nephrotic syndrome cannot be monitored using urine tests.
    e) HIV is not associated with kidney disease.
    Answer = B

CHAPTER 9
Neurology and special senses

M Greenwood, RI Macleod, RH Jay, JG Meechan, P Griffiths, N Ali and RJ Banks

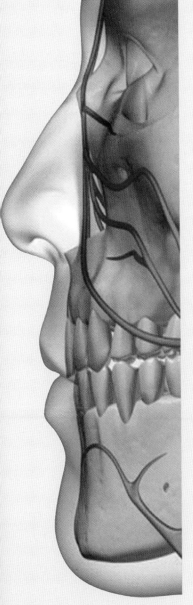

Key topics

- Major neurological disorders.
- Head injury.
- Stroke, speech and swallowing.
- ENT and ophthalmology.
- Anticonvulsant and anti-Parkinsonian drugs.

Learning objectives

- To be familiar with the major neurological disorders.
- To have an overview of the specialties of ENT and ophthalmology.
- To have knowledge of some of the drugs used to treat neurological disorders.
- To know the cranial nerves, their examination and possible dysfunction.

Essentials of Human Disease in Dentistry, Second Edition. Mark Greenwood.
© 2018 John Wiley & Sons Ltd. Published 2018 by John Wiley & Sons Ltd.
Companion website: www.wiley.com/go/greenwood/human-disease-in-dentistry

9A NEUROLOGY

Head injury

Head injuries can occur alone or accompany other trauma (e.g. to the maxillofacial region). This possibility always needs to be considered whenever such a patient presents. Knocks and bumps on the head are common, particularly in children, and fortunately most are minor in nature. Severe head injury accounts for about 50% of all trauma-related deaths, and for 15–20% of all causes of death in the 5–36-year age group.

Head injuries range from contusions, to abrasions and lacerations of the scalp; the latter can bleed profusely due to the vascularity of the tissues. It takes considerable force to fracture the skull. Fractures can involve the bones of either the base or vault. The fractures can be depressed or planar, simple or compound, the latter giving a potential portal for infection.

Significant brain injury can occur with or without damage to the overlying skull. When the skull is fractured, there will almost inevitably be an associated brain injury, although it may be less than expected, the force having been dissipated in fracturing the bone.

Signs of skull fracture

A fractured skull can occasionally result from trauma, with little in the way of specific signs apart from overlying soft tissue swelling. A history of significant head trauma, unconsciousness with the presence of a marked swelling or deep scalp laceration should certainly give rise to the suspicion of an underlying bony injury. Periorbital bruising (termed 'racoon eyes') and periauricular bruising (termed 'Battle's sign') (Figure 9A.1) are both highly suggestive of fractures to the base of the skull. The presence of blood behind the eardrum or bleeding from the ear (halo sign) (Figure 9A.2), which may indicate the presence of cerebrospinal fluid (CSF), are again indicative of underlying basal injury. In all such cases, computed tomography (CT) is indicated.

Skull fractures can be difficult to see, particularly on plain films, where they can be confused with suture lines or vessel markings. With plain films, it is essential to obtain different projections to facilitate assessment. Figure 9A.3 demonstrates the advantages of CT, with its ability to reveal any associated intracranial soft tissue damage.

The damage sustained by the brain may be focal at the site of the injury, or more diffuse. Primary damage to the brain at the site of the blow is known as the 'coup injury'; this can also affect the brain at the opposite side as it rebounds off the skull, termed the 'contrecoup injury' (Figure 9A.4). Secondary damage to the brain can arise due to cerebral oedema, ischaemia or infection, which can

Figure 9A.1 (a) Periorbital ecchymosis (racoon eyes). (b) Periauricular ecchymosis (Battle's sign). Copyright © 2005 Lippincott Williams & Wilkins. Instructor's Resource CD-ROM to accompany Smith and Mcleod's *Essentials of Nursing: Care of Adults and Children*. Reproduced with permission.

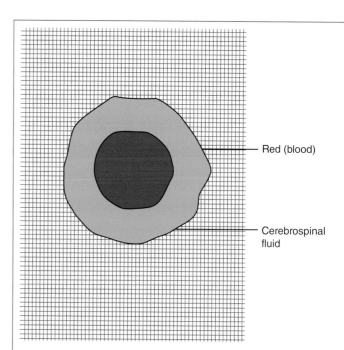

Figure 9A.2 Halo sign. Clear drainage separating from bloody drainage is suggestive of CSF. Copyright © 2005 Lippincott Williams & Wilkins. Instructor's Resource CD-ROM to accompany Smith and Mcleod's *Essentials of Nursing: Care of Adults and Children*. Reproduced with permission.

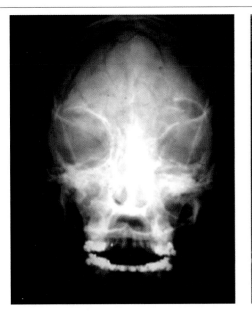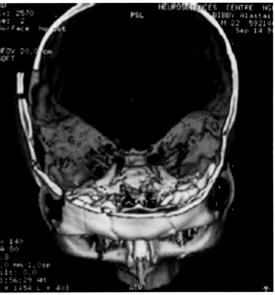

Figure 9A.3 Anteroposterior view of the skull and three-dimensionally reconstructed CT, both showing extensive skull and facial fractures.

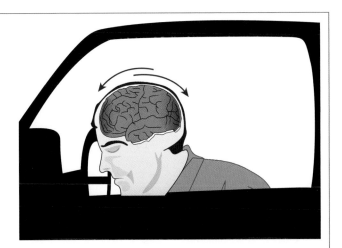

Figure 9A.4 Coup and contrecoup injuries occur at the point of contact and when the brain rebounds from the opposite direction. Copyright © 2005 Lippincott Williams & Wilkins. Instructor's Resource CD-ROM to accompany Smith and Mcleod's *Essentials of Nursing: Care of Adults and Children*. Reproduced with permission.

Table 9A.1 Glasgow Coma Scale for head injury.	
Eye opening	
Spontaneous	4
To loud voice	3
To pain	2
None	1
Verbal response	
Orientated	5
Confused/disorientated	4
Inappropriate words	3
Incomprehensible sounds	2
None	1
Best motor response	
Obeys	6
Localises	5
Withdraws (flexion)	4
Abnormal flexion posturing	3
Extension posturing	2
None	1

compound the original injury. The normal autoregulation of cerebral blood flow tends to be lost in a head injury, making the injured brain more susceptible to hypovolaemic or hypervolaemic change and hypoxia.

In general, head injuries are classified according to severity, based on the Glasgow Coma Scale (GSC; see Table 9A.1). In the UK, on average, 80% are mild (GCS 13–15); 10% are moderate (GCS 9–12); and the remainder are severe in nature (GCS 3–8). The aim of management of all head injuries is to limit the amount of brain damage.

Types of brain injury

Concussion

Concussion is one of the most common brain injuries, where the trauma is minor and the symptoms slight and short-lived. The victim may be dizzy or may lose consciousness briefly, but there is no permanent neurological damage. The person can be left feeling nauseated, have headaches, memory problems and feel tired for some time afterwards. Care needs to be taken for possible delayed intracranial bleeds.

Contusion

'Contusion' describes the condition where there is a bruise (bleeding) in the brain. Functions controlled by the damaged area will be lost or compromised. The individual may remain conscious, but severe contusions of the brainstem usually cause a coma, which can last from some hours to a lifetime.

Diffuse axonal injury

Diffuse axonal injury arises from trauma that results in the tearing of nerve structures. The result is loss of consciousness, coma and possible death. Those who survive can suffer a variety of functional impairments.

Cerebral oedema

Cerebral oedema can occur following injury. Inflammation can increase the permeability of blood vessels in the brain space and allow fluid accumulation. For this reason, anti-inflammatory drugs and intravenous mannitol are sometimes administered to moderate–severe head injury patients in an attempt to prevent cerebral oedema, which would aggravate an already existing brain injury.

Intracranial haemorrhage

Intracranial haemorrhage may result from any head trauma. Blood leaking from ruptured vessels can enter the extradural and/or subdural spaces. Accumulation of blood within the skull increases intracranial pressure and compresses the brain tissues. If the pressure forces the brainstem inferiorly through the foramen magnum, control of blood pressure, heart rate and respiration may be lost, resulting in death. Individuals who are initially lucid and begin to deteriorate neurologically are usually bleeding intracranially and require urgent investigation, usually with CT.

Extradural haemorrhage

'Extradural haemorrhage' (Figures 9A.5 and 9A.6) describes the bleeding into the space between the skull and dura mater, often from the middle meningeal artery, and can be divided into *acute* and *subacute* forms, with symptoms of the former appearing within 24–72 hours. Classically, affected individuals transiently lose consciousness at the time of injury, recover, and then, after a lucid interval, deteriorate quickly, becoming deeply comatose. They develop increased blood pressure, falling pulse rate, contralateral limb weakness and ipsilateral pupillary dilatation. The subacute variation usually presents with symptoms appearing within 2–10 days after the injury. This has a somewhat better prognosis, and symptoms include

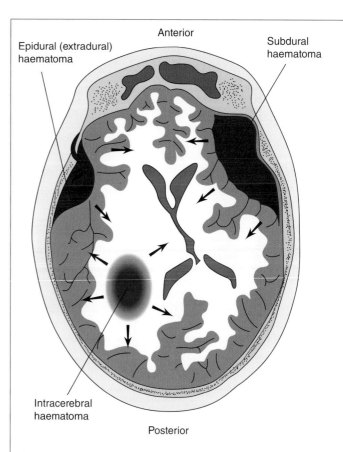

Figure 9A.5 Location of epidural, subdural and intracerebral haematomas. Copyright © 2005 Lippincott Williams & Wilkins. Instructor's Resource CD-ROM to accompany *Porth's Pathophysiology: Concepts of Altered Health States*, 7th ed. Reproduced with permission.

headache, decreasing level of consciousness and failure to show improvement.

Subdural haemorrhage

Subdural haemorrhage (Figure 9A.7) is most probably a complication of a high-velocity injury, and the patient is usually unconscious from the time of injury. Essentially, the bleeding occurs below the dura mater and spreads over the brain surface. This condition is associated with a deteriorating level of consciousness, and the underlying brain damage is more severe. As a result, the prognosis tends to be worse than for extradural haematoma.

In both extradural and subdural haemorrhage cases, the aim of surgical management is to decrease the intracerebral pressure by removing the haematoma (through burr holes or craniotomy), and to repair or seal off the damaged vessels.

Intracerebral haemorrhage

Intracerebral haemorrhage (Figure 9A.8) arises as a result of bleeding from small arteries or veins into the subcortical white

R   L

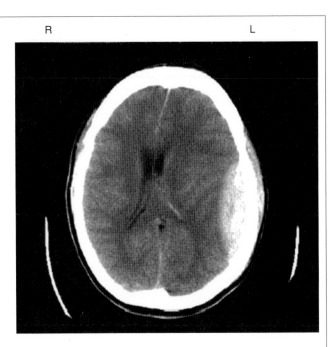

Figure 9A.6 CT image of a typical left-sided extradural haema-toma showing as a lens-shaped opacity due to the tethering of the dura mater. Note the shift of the midline to the right as a result of increased intracranial pressure.

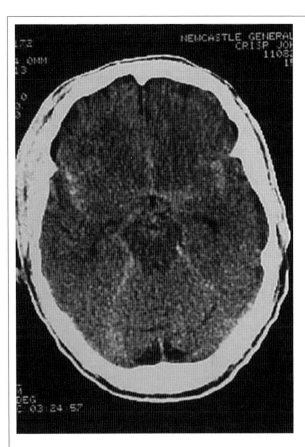

Figure 9A.8 CT of an intracerebral bleed showing diffuse spread of blood around the brain, possibly as a result of a leaking cerebral aneurysm.

R   L

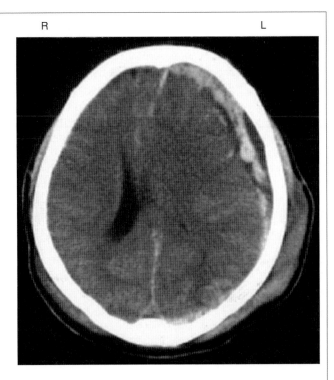

Figure 9A.7 CT showing swelling on the left side of the head from an underlying subdural haematoma, with the blood more diffusely spread around the left side of the brain. Note the pressure effects of midline shift to the right and collapse of the left ventricle.

matter, and is more common following the rupture of a vascular anomaly such as an aneurysm. Symptoms include lucid intervals followed by loss of consciousness. Focal signs tend to depend on the location of the bleed, and can include headache, hemiplegia, ipsilateral pupil dilation and progressive intracranial pressure, with potential for herniation through the foramen magnum. In these cases, management involves identifying the source of bleeding and, if possible, sealing it off. This may be achieved by a neurosurgical approach, clipping of the vessel or via a radiologically guided procedure – that is, inserting a coil into the aneurysm sac, causing the adjacent blood to coagulate and seal the vessel off.

Assessment

With any history of head injury, however minor, it is essential that the patient be fully assessed. This should include:

- GCS (see the following text).
- Vital signs.
- History of loss of consciousness.
- Pupil reflexes.
- Motor responses.

Even if normal, these should be documented as a baseline from which to monitor, as there can often be subtle or sudden changes. It is essential to look for clinical indications of expanding lesions such as:

- Localised/focal signs.
- Visual field defects.
- Eye deviations.
- Cerebral or cranial nerve signs.

In addition, there may be general signs of increased intracranial pressure, such as:

- Headache.
- Vomiting.
- Restlessness.
- Irritability.

As these signs can sometimes come on gradually within hours or even days of the incident, it is essential that friends or relatives closest to the patient be aware of the development of such signs, and be advised to return the patient to the accident and emergency department of their nearest hospital as soon as possible if the signs appear.

General signs and symptoms of brain injury

Direct injury, increasing intracranial pressure, and compression or displacement of brain tissue can all cause altered levels of awareness as well as general signs and symptoms, including:

- Altered level of consciousness.
- Altered level of orientation.
- Alterations in personality.
- Amnesia.
  - Retrograde (cannot remember events before the incident).
  - Anterograde (unaware of events after the incident).
- Cushing's reflex – increased blood pressure, slowing pulse rate.
- Vomiting (often without nausea).
- Body temperature changes.
- Changes in reactivity of pupils.
- Body posturing.

Where there is altered mental status, or the patient is unresponsive, the condition can be monitored using the GCS (Table 9A.1).

The GCS is scored between 3 (worst) and 15 (best). It is composed of three parameters: best eye response, best verbal response and best motor response.

Spinal injury

Spinal damage can accompany any other body injury, but is especially common following a high-velocity impact, such as in a fall or road traffic accident. It can range in severity from ligamentous damage, such as in a whiplash injury to the neck, to a variety of fractures of the vertebrae. The danger of such injuries is the effect on the underlying spinal cord. This can

vary from complete sectioning to partial damage, with the resultant neurological deficit being dependent on the site of the injury.

As with all neurological tissues, the spinal cord has relatively poor regenerative properties. Consequently, prevention and minimising damage are key to the prognosis. This includes careful handling of any victim in whom such an injury is suspected – such as a thorough assessment including radiological examination using plain film views or CT, and transfer to a unit specialising in the management of spinal injuries as soon as possible.

Complications

The modern management of head injuries is ideally undertaken in specialist neurosurgical units with the ability to provide the necessary intensive care with continued ventilation, management of intracranial pressure, cerebral perfusion, oxygenation and, where indicated, surgery.

These complications essentially fall into three categories – physical, cognitive and emotional – and, to some degree, depend on the site and extent of the damage.

- Physical effects include loss of motor function, coordination, paralysis, extreme tiredness, epilepsy and speech problems.
- Cognitive effects include memory loss (either for before or after the accident), reduced attention span and slower reaction times.
- Emotional effects can vary from depression, to anxiety, irrational behaviour and emotional lability, with a tendency to laugh or cry more readily than before. In some instances, the patient can develop a complete change of personality.

These effects can be extremely devastating, not only for the patient, but also for their families and friends. Some effects may ameliorate with time, but some will be permanent, as a result of the relatively poor ability of nervous tissues to repair. Affected individuals may require long periods of convalescence in specialist units, where they can receive appropriate physiotherapy, psychological support and occupational therapy to help with adaptation to disability and, where possible, learn to maintain their independence.

Brain abscess

Brain abscesses may be secondary to oral sepsis or infection elsewhere in the middle ear or paranasal sinuses. A patient with congenital heart disease is at increased risk. Such abscesses can be a complication of infective endocarditis, and this should be specifically asked about in the history of a patient suffering from a brain abscess. Brain abscess can occasionally arise from a dental source. The signs and symptoms vary, depending on the location of the abscess. CT and MRI scans are useful in localisation and diagnosis. Urgent surgical drainage is required.

Space-occupying lesions

A space-occupying lesion in the context of the brain implies the presence of a tumour, but could also be used to encompass a pathology such as a haematoma or abscess. Such lesions may affect any age group, and may lead to partial seizures, possibly developing to generalised epilepsy. Imaging is essential to determine the size and position of any suspected space-occupying lesion.

Meningitis

Meningitis is an infection of the meninges (membranes) that envelop the brain and spinal cord. The source of infection may be viral, bacterial or fungal. Fungal infections are rare, and are usually seen in immunocompromised patients. It is important to remember that bacterial meningitis can occur secondary to maxillofacial injuries involving the middle third of the face. Prompt treatment with antimicrobials (prophylactically in trauma cases) should be undertaken. The viral type of meningitis is usually mild and self-limiting. A patient with meningitis will have severe headaches, feels nauseated or has vomiting tendency, and is often drowsy. Aversion to light and a painful and stiff neck are well-known symptoms. Meningitis caused by the bacterium *Neisseria meningitidis* may produce a purpuric rash on the skin, and can progress to adrenocortical failure as a result of bleeding into the adrenal cortex.

Herpetic encephalitis is rare. When it occurs, it is essential that prompt treatment with aciclovir be instituted. A variety of infections and tumours can be seen in HIV-associated neurological disease. The neurological effects of such lesions vary, depending on the main site affected.

9B ENT

Deafness

Deafness may be of two main types – *conductive* or *sensorineural.*

Conductive deafness

This is usually due to wax in the external auditory meatus, but otitis media or otosclerosis can also cause it.

Sensorineural deafness

Potential causes of sensorineural deafness are:
- Ménière's disease.
- Acute labyrinthitis.
- Head injury.
- Paget's disease of bone (Figure 9B.1).
- Excess noise.
- Overdose of certain drugs (e.g. gentamicin).

Clinical testing

A simple test of hearing can be carried out by blocking one ear and, from behind the patient, saying a number increasingly loudly until the patient hears. Other tests can differentiate conductive from sensorineural deafness.

Rinne's test

A vibrating tuning fork should be placed on the mastoid process. When the patient can no longer hear it, the fork should be moved to a position 4 cm from the external auditory meatus. If the sound is no longer heard, bone conduction is better than air conduction (normally, the converse applies). This finding suggests possible conductive deafness.

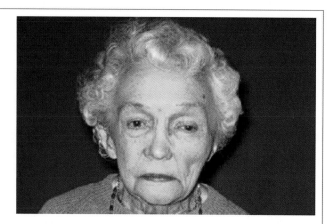

Figure 9B.1 A patient with Paget's disease of bone. The head becomes progressively enlarged.

Weber's test

A vibrating tuning fork is placed in the middle of the forehead, and the patient is asked whether the sound is located to one side or the other, or centrally. In unilateral sensorineural deafness, the sound will be heard on the 'good side'. In conductive deafness, the sound is localised to the 'bad' side.

Tinnitus

'Tinnitus' is a sound of ringing or whistling in the ears. This can occur as a result of impacted wax or Ménière's disease. The cause is sometimes never found. Clearly, any underlying cause should be removed if it can be identified.

Vertigo

Vertigo is the illusion of movement. In the majority of cases, it indicates disease of the labyrinth or its neurological connections. Ménière's disease comprises a syndrome of vertigo, deafness and tinnitus. Attacks are variable in length from minutes to hours, and can include vomiting and nystagmus. The latter is a term used to describe oscillation of the eyes on attempted fixation. It can be a physiological phenomenon, and must be maintained for a few beats to be pathological.

The treatment of Ménière's diseases is symptomatic with prochlorperazine and, sometimes, betahistine.

Dizziness

This is a very common presenting symptom to general medical practitioners. It is a less specific phenomenon than vertigo.

Infections and inflammatory disorders of the ear, nose, sinuses and tonsils

Ear infections

'Furunculosis' is the term used to denote infection of hair follicles. This is usually staphylococcal in origin. Diabetes should be considered as an underlying predisposing factor in these patients. Treatment is with heat and topical applications. If there is systemic involvement, antibiotics such as amoxicillin and flucloxacillin may be required.

Otitis externa (infection of the external ear) often occurs after excessive scratching due to an itchy skin condition such as eczema. All infected material must be removed, and topical preparations used for treatment. In otitis media (infection of the middle ear), pain in the ear may be followed by purulent discharge. The ear drum will perforate. Antibiotics are required for treatment. Continuing discharge may indicate mastoiditis (more commonly seen prior to the introduction of antibiotics). Treatment is intravenous antibiotics and myringotomy (an incision through the ear drum). In resistant cases, mastoidectomy may be required. In 'glue ear', there is an accumulation of serous or viscous material. The main predisposing factor to this is when the Eustachian tube, which normally opens during swallowing, is blocked, for example, by the adenoids. Glue ear is the most common cause of hearing loss in children. If fluid persists for longer than 6 months and there is diminished hearing, myringotomy may be required with aspiration of fluid and insertion of grommets. Removal of the adenoids is also effective.

Nasal obstruction

The most common cause of nasal obstruction is an upper respiratory tract infection (URTI). It is common for children to insert foreign bodies in the nose. In children, large adenoids or choanal atresia and post-nasal space tumours should be considered. In adults, a deviated nasal septum, either as the result of trauma or developmental in origin, can cause obstruction to the nasal passages. Polyps and chronic sinusitis are also commonly found problems. Allergic rhinitis may be seasonal or perennial – there is a significant correlation with the pollen count, and symptoms include sneezing, pruritus and rhinorrhoea. Antihistamines are the mainstay of treatment. From the maxillofacial point of view, it is important in the middle third of face fractures that CSF rhinorrhoea is actively excluded or confirmed. Fractures through the roof of the ethmoid labyrinth may result in the leak of CSF.

In cases of nasal trauma, it is important that the anterior part of the nose be examined to exclude a septal haematoma. These can cause nasal obstruction and should be immediately evacuated, as there is a risk of cartilage necrosis and nasal collapse if this is not done.

Nose bleed (epistaxis) is a common problem. Most nose bleeds come from blood vessels on the nasal septum. In older people, bleeding is more commonly arterial in origin, from a part of the nose known as 'Little's area'. Many nose bleeds are idiopathic in origin but can be associated with degenerative arterial disease and hypertension. It should always be remembered that a nose bleed, particularly in more elderly patients, may be due to a tumour in the nose or the paranasal sinuses. Patients who are anticoagulated are at increased risk of epistaxis. In terms of management, it is important that the overall physiological picture of the patient be kept in mind. Estimation of the vital signs should be carried out to exclude shock (Chapter 10, titled 'Shock'), and consideration should be given to the site of the bleeding and efforts taken to stop it appropriately. In order to reduce venous pressure, most patients with epistaxis are nursed in the sitting position. If the patients are clinically shocked, they must be placed supine. Firm and uninterrupted pressure is applied on the nostrils using the forefinger and the thumb for at least 10 min. If this does not stop the bleeding, the clot is removed from the nose, and any identified bleeding points are cauterised. If it is not possible to identify a distinct bleeding point, the nose is packed with a ribbon gauze pack soaked in bismuth iodoform paraffin paste (BIPP), or other nasal packing methods are used. In some trauma cases, an anterior pack will not be sufficient, and a posterior nasal pack needs to be placed. This can be achieved by inflating a Foley catheter after it has been passed through the nostril with the balloon lying in the post-nasal space. Once the balloon is inflated, the catheter can be pulled anteriorly to apply pressure to the bleeding area. Both nostrils will usually need to be catheterised.

Paranasal sinuses

Acute sinusitis

A secondary bacterial infection of the sinuses may occur following a viral infection. Around 10% of maxillary sinusitis infections are secondary to initial viral infections. In acute sinusitis, there may be a yellow/green nasal discharge, pain and tenderness to palpation over the affected area and raised temperature. Treatment includes analgesia, nasal inhalations and a broad-spectrum antibiotic. Swimming should be discouraged since it promotes the spread of pus within the sinuses.

Chronic sinusitis

Chronic sinusitis may present as a post-nasal drip of mucus and a bad taste in the mouth. The nose will be blocked, and there will be pain over the bridge of the nose or in the malar region. It is important to try and correct any underlying cause. Some form of drainage procedure should be instituted to prevent further problems.

Tonsillitis

Tonsillitis is a common throat condition. The appearance of a rash after 48 hours on the neck or the chest raises suspicion of scarlet fever in childhood sore throat. A rash is not seen periorally, and therefore the rash is described as having circumoral pallor. The tongue has a white coating, leaving prominent papillae – the 'strawberry' tongue. The cause is a group A *Streptococcus*. On examination, the tonsils are clearly inflamed and may have an exudate of pus. Children will often complain of abdominal pain that coexists with the tonsillitis. Older children and adults tend to complain of sore throat, fever and malaise. They may have dysphagia and palpable, painful swollen cervical lymph glands.

There is controversy regarding the use of antibiotics for the treatment of tonsillitis, as the cause will be viral in about half of the cases. If antibiotics are used, penicillin is the antibiotic of choice. Amoxicillin should not be used, as it will cause a rash in patients whose infection is due to Epstein–Barr virus (EBV). Several years ago, tonsillectomy was a commonly performed procedure in those who had recurrent tonsillitis. The number of tonsillectomies in recent years has significantly declined. Recurrent tonsillitis is, however, still an indication for tonsillectomy. In acute situations, surgical drainage is required. A peritonsillar infection, known as a 'quinsy', still often necessitates the operation of tonsillectomy. On rare occasions, tonsils can be so large as to cause cor pulmonale or obstructive sleep apnoea. If a case of tonsillitis is unchecked or untreated, a retropharyngeal abscess will develop.

Carcinoma of the pharyngeal tonsil

Cancers of the pharyngeal tonsil are most common in elderly patients. They will complain of dysphagia, odynophagia (painful swallowing) and otalgia. A particular warning sign is the case of unilateral tonsillitis. Carcinomas are usually squamous cell in origin. The precise form of treatment will depend on the histopathological nature of the tumour.

Stridor

The term 'stridor' describes noises that are produced by inspiration when the larynx or trachea has become narrowed. It may be accompanied by dysphagia. It is particularly seen in children due to the small size of their airways, but can also be seen in adults. In most adults, however, laryngeal problems tend to produce hoarseness. Due to its effects on the airway, stridor is a situation that should be treated as an emergency.

9C NEUROLOGICAL DISORDERS AND DENTAL PRACTICE

There are a number of neurological conditions that may be encountered in dental practice. It is important that a dental practitioner has broad knowledge of the main neurological conditions since they may affect the provision of dental treatment.

Relevant points in the history

The patient may give a history of 'blackouts'. It is important to be precise about what a patient means by this term as this can indicate anything from loss of consciousness to dizziness. When a history of blackouts is given, information obtained from a witness might be useful. The more that is known about the nature of such an event, the better it can be anticipated and effectively managed (or prevented). There are several cardiovascular disorders that can lead to a 'blackout'. These are also considered here.

The main points in the history are summarised in Table 9C.1.

Syncope may be vasovagal in origin (the *simple faint*), or may occur in response to certain situations such as coughing. A vasovagal attack may be precipitated by the fear of dental treatment, heat or a lack of food. It occurs due to reflex bradycardia and peripheral vasodilation. Onset is not instantaneous, and the patient will look pale, often feel sick and notice a 'closing in' of visual fields. It cannot occur when a patient is lying down, and placing the patient flat with legs raised is the treatment. Jerking of limbs may occur. In carotid sinus syncope, hypersensitivity of the carotid sinus may cause syncope to occur on turning the head. Unlike vasovagal syncope, this may happen in the supine position.

Patients may suffer from *epilepsy*. A description of the fit is useful, as this may enable early recognition. Precipitating factors should be asked about, as should questions about altered breathing, cyanosis or tongue biting during a fit. The latter is virtually a diagnostic feature of grand mal epilepsy. Medication taken and its efficacy should be assessed in terms of the degree of control achieved. Tonic–clonic or grand mal epilepsy is classically preceded by a warning or aura, which may comprise an auditory, olfactory or visual hallucination. A loss of consciousness follows, leading to convulsions and subsequent recovery. The patient may be incontinent during a fit. The 'tonic phase' gives way to a 'clonic phase', in which there is repetitive jerky movements, increased salivation and marked bruxism. After a fit of this type, a patient may sleep for up to 12 hours. If the fit continues for more than 5 min, or continues without a proper end point, 'status epilepticus' is said to be present. This is an emergency situation that requires urgent intervention with a benzodiazepine, for example, buccal midazolam or intravenous diazepam, if competent (see Chapter 21, titled 'Medical emergencies').

Absence seizures or 'petit mal' tend to occur in children who may suddenly stop speech, attention and movement. The so-called 'partial' seizures may be simple or complex. Simple seizures consist of clonic movements of a group of muscles or a limb. Complex seizures may involve hallucinations of hearing, sight or taste.

Febrile convulsions are common in infancy. They do not predict progression to later epilepsy. Keeping the child cool with fans, paracetamol and sponging with tepid water are the mainstays of treatment.

Stokes–Adams attacks describe losses of consciousness occurring as a result of cardiac arrhythmias. These may happen with the patient in any position, and may occur with no warning except for an awareness of palpitations. Recovery is usually within seconds. Other potential causes of 'blackouts' are listed in Table 9C.2.

Table 9C.1 Main points in the history of a dental patient with possible neurological disorders.

Blackouts, syncope
Epilepsy
Stroke, transient ischaemic attack
Multiple sclerosis
Facial pain
Parkinson's disease
Motor neurone disease (MND)
Cranial nerve problems (especially Bell's palsy)

Table 9C.2 Possible causes of loss of consciousness or 'blackout'.

Vasovagal syncope	Simple faint
'Situational' syncope	Cough
	Micturition
	Carotid sinus hypersensitivity
Epilepsy	
Hypoglycaemia	
Transient ischaemic attack	
Orthostatic hypotension	On standing from supine position
	Signifies inadequate vasomotor reflexes (e.g. elderly patients on tablets to lower blood pressure)
'Drop attacks'	Sudden weakness of legs usually resolved spontaneously
Stokes–Adams attacks	Transient arrhythmia
Anxiety	
Ménière's disease	Vertigo, tinnitus, hearing loss
Choking	

The patient may give a history of a stroke – that is, a *cerebrovascular accident* (CVA) or a *transient ischaemic attack* (TIA). A CVA may be haemorrhagic (subarachnoid, cerebral), thrombotic or embolic in origin. A subarachnoid haemorrhage results from rupture of a berry aneurysm of the circle of Willis, which lies at the base of the brain. Subarachnoid haemorrhages tend to affect a younger age group than the other types of CVA, and patients typically give a history of a sudden onset of excruciatingly severe headache. The prognosis is poor, but has been improved by surgical and radiological obliteration of the aneurysm. Hypertension and atherosclerosis are contributory factors to other types of CVA. Cerebral thrombosis deprives the brain of part of its blood supply, and is the most common type of stroke. Emboli leading to stroke can arise on the wall of an atrium that is fibrillating or from the wall of a heart damaged after a myocardial infarction. Typical results of a CVA are a sudden loss of consciousness and hemiplegia (on the opposite side to the cerebral lesion). There may be loss of speech or slurred speech when the CVA affects the left side of the brain. TIAs comprise a sudden onset of focal CNS signs or symptoms due to a temporary occlusion of part of the cerebral circulation. They are frequently associated with partial or complete stenosis of the carotid artery system. The symptoms resolve in <24 hours (usually much more quickly). They are the harbingers of a CVA, and the known patient will usually be taking prophylactic aspirin.

Patients with *multiple sclerosis* have a diverse condition comprising neurological signs and symptoms that are disseminated in both site and time. A viral aetiology has been postulated, but the cause is not known. Onset is variable, but optic neuritis can lead to visual disturbance or blindness, which may be a presenting feature. Weakness or paralysis of a limb can occur. Nystagmus may occur, as may ataxia (uncoordinated movements) and dysphagia. Loss of sphincter control leading to urinary incontinence may occur. The diagnosis should be considered in a young patient presenting with trigeminal neuralgia or a facial palsy. Enquiry in such cases should be directed towards other areas to check for neurological signs or symptoms elsewhere.

Facial pain

Facial pain is common and may affect up to 50% of the elderly population. A paroxysm of excruciating stabbing pain lasting only seconds in the trigeminal nerve distribution suggests *trigeminal neuralgia*, particularly in patients over 50 years of age. In the vast majority of cases, it is unilateral, most commonly affecting the mandibular and maxillary divisions. A 'trigger area' that is stimulated by washing or shaving, for example, may often be identified from the history. Talking may be enough to stimulate the pain. The diagnosis is usually simple. Carbamazepine, gabapentin or phenytoin are the mainstays of treatment. Microvascular decompression is sometimes used.

Other neurological causes of facial pain include *post-herpetic neuralgia* and *atypical facial pain*. In post-herpetic neuralgia, the patient complains of a burning pain (often in the ophthalmic division of the trigeminal nerve), which may become chronic. There is no really successful treatment; transcutaneous nerve sectioning and local anaesthetic infiltration in the painful area has been tried, as has carbamazepine. Tricyclic antidepressants have also been used.

When all other causes (including non-neurological causes of facial pain) have been excluded, some patients may still complain of facial pain – usually unilateral. The pain is described as severe, constant and not relieved by analgesics. This type of pain is more common in young females, and many are prescribed antidepressants (although not always to curative effect). 'Atypical facial pain' is the term applied to this type of facial pain.

Other disorders

Parkinson's disease results from degeneration of the pigmented cells of the substantia nigra, leading to dopamine deficiency. The incidence is equal in males and females. The disease may also result from previous head injury or cerebrovascular disease. Clinically, the patient may have tremor in the arms and hands (the latter being described as 'pill-rolling'). A so-called 'cogwheel' type of rigidity may be seen on movement. Slow movements (bradykinesia) and restlessness (akathisia) may also be noted. The patient may have an expressionless face and a stooped posture. Impaired autonomic function may lead to a postural hypotension and hypersalivation, resulting in the drooling of saliva.

Motor neurone disease (MND) comprises a group of disorders that affect motor neurones at various levels. There is no sensory loss, and this helps differentiate it from multiple sclerosis. The aetiology is unknown, but a viral agent is considered a possibility. Oral hygiene may be difficult in these patients, and dysphagia and drooling may occur.

Tumours may arise in various components of the CNS, and may be primary or metastatic, the latter being more common in the brain. Benign brain tumours are still a significant problem, as they may cause pressure effects and may not be amenable to surgery due to their location. Headaches are characteristically worse in the morning. Tumours that give rise to cerebral metastases include lung, breast, GI tract and kidney.

Impairment of vision may occur, and this may vary from mild disability to complete blindness. Diplopia or double vision may occur after a 'blowout' fracture of the orbital floor, or from injury to cranial nerves III, IV and VI. Transient visual disturbance may occur secondary to local anaesthetics that have tracked to the inferior orbital fissure.

Myasthenia gravis (MG) is an antibody-mediated autoimmune disease with a deficiency of functioning muscle acetylcholine receptors that leads to muscle weakness. The disorder more commonly affects young women. The muscle weakness is progressive and develops rapidly. Some cases are associated with Eaton–Lambert syndrome, which may occur in some patients with lung or other cancers. In Eaton–Lambert

Table 9C.3 Some possible causes of facial weakness (mostly unilateral).

Idiopathic	Bell's palsy
	Melkersson–Rosenthal syndrome
Infection	Ear infections
	TB
	Ramsay Hunt syndrome
	Glandular fever
	AIDS
Trauma	Facial lacerations/bruising in the region of the facial nerve
	Penetrating parotid injuries
	Post-parotid surgery
Neoplastic	Primary or secondary cancers
	Neuroma of facial nerve
	Acoustic neuroma
Metabolic	Diabetes mellitus
	Pregnancy
	Sarcoidosis
	Guillain–Barré syndrome
Iatrogenic	Local anaesthetic injection

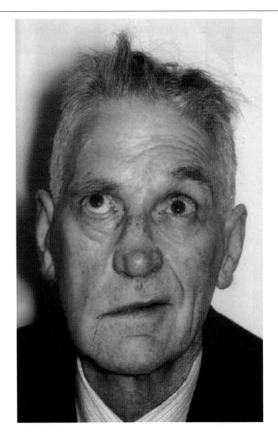

Figure 9C.1 Bell's palsy. Note the absence of wrinkles on the forehead on the affected side (patient's right). The right eye is elevated (Bell's sign).

syndrome, however, the muscles get stronger rather than weaker with activity.

A facial palsy may have a known cause or be idiopathic (Table 9C.3). If the cause is not known, the name 'Bell's palsy' (Figure 9C.1) is applied. Other causes must be excluded before this term is used. In Bell's palsy, the onset is rapid and unilateral, and there may be an ache beneath the ear. The weakness worsens over 1–2 days. If presentation is early, most clinicians give prednisolone for 5 days, the aim being to reduce neuronal oedema. An eye patch is of value to protect the cornea. The paralysis is of a lower motor neurone type, in which all the facial muscles are affected on that side. In an upper motor neurone lesion, for example, stroke, the forehead is spared, since this region is bilaterally represented in the cortex. Looking for 'forehead sparing' is thus a way of differentiating between upper and lower motor neurone causes of facial weakness.

Bilateral facial paralysis is rare. It may be seen in sarcoidosis, Guillain–Barré syndrome (idiopathic polyneuritis) or posterior cranial fossa tumours. The rare Melkersson–Rosenthal syndrome is a condition comprising tongue fissuring, unilateral facial palsy and facial swelling. The lesions are histologically similar to those of Crohn's disease.

A summary of other cranial nerve lesions is given in Table 9C.4. Nerves may be affected by a systemic cause – for example, diabetes mellitus or multiple sclerosis (MS) – or there may be a local cause. Multiple cranial nerve palsies may occur in *bulbar palsy*, which comprises palsy of the tongue, muscles of chewing/swallowing and facial muscles due to loss of function of motor nuclei in the brainstem. The onset may be acute

(e.g. in infection such as polio) or chronic (e.g. in tumours of the posterior cranial fossa).

Tics or involuntary facial movements may occasionally be seen in patients. These may be habitual (particularly in children), drug induced, or have a more organic cause. Drug-induced dyskinesias are common in the elderly on long-term phenothiazine (antipsychotic) medication, which is usually reversible on stopping the drug. Intracranial nerve compression may result in blepharospasm (contraction of both eyelids). Hemifacial muscle spasm may occur, suggesting a lesion – for example, of the cerebellopontine angle, compressing the facial nerve. Whenever a facial tic is found, consideration should be given to referral for investigation, since an underlying cause may often be treated.

In Ramsay Hunt syndrome, a profound facial paralysis is accompanied by vesicles in the pharynx on the same side, and in the external auditory meatus. It is thought that the geniculate ganglion of the facial nerve is infected with herpes zoster.

Cerebral palsy is primarily a disorder of motor function secondary to cerebral damage, most frequently associated with birth injury or hypoxia. It is the most common cause of a congenital physical handicap, the patterns of which are variable. There are three main subtypes – spastic, ataxic and athetoid. In the spastic type, the muscles are contracted, and there may be associated epilepsy. In the ataxic type, a cerebellar lesion is

Table 9C.4 Cranial nerve dysfunction and signs arising from it.

Cranial nerve		Possible problem	Sign
I	Olfactory	Trauma, tumour	Decreased ability to smell
II	Optic	Trauma, tumour, MS, stroke	Blindness, visual field defect
III	Oculomotor	Diabetes, increased intracranial pressure	Dilated pupil, ptosis
IV	Trochlear	Trauma	Diplopia
V	Trigeminal	Sensory – idiopathic, trauma, IDN/lingual damage	None, sensory deficit on testing
		Motor – bulbar palsy, acoustic neuroma	Signs in VII, IX, X, XI, XII; with acoustic neuroma also affecting VIII
VI	Abducens	MS, some strokes	Inability of eye to look laterally, eye deviated towards nose
VII	Facial	LMN – Bell's palsy	Total facial weakness
		Skull fracture	
		Parotid tumour	
		UMN – stroke, tumour	Forehead sparing – weakness
VIII	Vestibulocochlear	Excess noise; Paget's, acoustic neuroma	Deafness
IX	Glossopharyngeal	Trauma, tumour	Impaired gag reflex
X	Vagus	Trauma, brainstem lesions	Impaired gag reflex, soft palate moves to 'good' side on saying 'aah'
XI	Accessory	Polio, stroke	Weakness turning head away from affected side (sternocleidomastoid)
			Weakness shrugging shoulders (trapezius)
XII	Hypoglossal	Trauma, brainstem lesions	Tongue deviated to affected side on protrusion

IDN = inferior dental nerve; LMN = lower motor neurone; UMN = upper motor neurone.

responsible for a disturbance of balance. Writhing movements characterise the athetoid type of cerebral palsy.

In *spina bifida*, the vertebral arches fail to fuse, possibly due to a deficiency of folic acid during foetal development. The condition may lead to significant physical handicaps, such as inability to walk, epilepsy or learning difficulties. There may be an association with hydrocephalus, which often requires decompression using a shunt.

Patients with *syringomyelia* have a condition in which cavitation of the central spinal cord occurs, leading to a loss in pain and temperature sensibility. 'Syringobulbia' is the term used if the brainstem is affected – facial sensory loss may occur, as may tongue weakness.

An *acoustic neuroma* is a benign tumour occurring at the cerebellopontine angle on the vestibular part of the vestibulocochlear nerve. Cranial nerves V, VII, IX and X may also be involved, leading to tinnitus, deafness and vertigo. Facial twitching weakness or paraesthesias may occur. Other causes of facial sensory loss (innervated by the trigeminal nerve – except over the angle of the mandible, which is innervated by cervical nerves) are listed in Table 9C.5.

Table 9C.5 Potential causes of facial sensory loss.

Intracranial	
Neoplasm	Cerebral tumour
Inflammatory	MS
	Granulomatous conditions (e.g. sarcoid TB)
	Connective tissue disorders
Other	Paget's disease (nerve compression)
	Trigeminal neuropathy
	Cerebrovascular disease
Extracranial	
Neoplasm	Cancer, metastatic cancers
Inflammatory	Osteomyelitis
	Pressure from adjacent lesions
Trauma	Maxillary/mandibular fractures
Iatrogenic	Removal of mandibular third molars
	Local anaesthetic

Other neurological disorders that may be encountered include *Huntington's chorea*, which is an autosomal dominant disorder in which there is progressive dementia with marked involuntary movements. The signs do not begin to appear until middle age. *Friedreich's ataxia* is an autosomal recessive or sometimes sex-linked cord degeneration of unknown cause. Severe ataxia and deformity occurs, and there may be associated cardiac disease with arrhythmias.

General examination

The patient's gait may give an immediate clue to an underlying neurological condition – for example, the shuffling gait of Parkinsonism. A spastic gait is demonstrated by stiff limbs that are often swung around in a circular motion as the forward movement proceeds.

A patient with a neurological condition may appear confused. This may be for several reasons, and a summary of potential causes is given in Table 9C.6. Raised intracranial pressure can occur following trauma to the head – for example, in a patient with an injury associated with dental trauma. Such patients will complain of headache, and may vomit or feel restless. The classical signs of increased blood pressure and decreased pulse rate appear, and there is dilation of the pupil on the same side as the lesion. Patients with head injuries can be assessed according to the GCS, described in Chapter 9A (titled 'Neurology').

Horner's syndrome comprises four signs – a constricted pupil, ptosis (drooping of the upper eyelid), loss of sweating on the ipsilateral face and enophthalmos. It is caused by interference with the cervical sympathetic chain, for example, after a radical neck dissection, trauma to the neck or tumour.

Patients with cerebral palsy have an increased incidence of dental malocclusion and abnormal movement of the oral and facial musculature, which may cause difficulty with the dental treatment provision.

Table 9C.6 Possible causes of confusion that may be encountered in a dental patient.

Hypoxia	Ensure clear airway, care with sedatives
Epilepsy	
Infection	Significant orofacial infection, pneumonia, meningitis
Metabolic	Hypoglycaemia
Drug/alcohol withdrawal or use	
Vascular	Stroke, MI
Raised intracranial pressure	
Nutritional	Deficiency of various B vitamins

The *Sturge–Weber syndrome* describes the association between facial port-wine stains (haemangioma) and focal fits on the contralateral side. Exophthalmos and spasticity may also be evident. The fits are caused by a capillary haemangioma in the brain.

Cranial nerves

A systematic approach is needed for examining the *cranial nerves*. One approach is to consider the cranial nerves in the following groups: nerve(s) subserving the sense of smell, eyes, face, mouth, neck and ears. A summary of disorders affecting the cranial nerves and the resulting signs is given in Table 9C.4.

Any changes in the *sense of smell* may reflect a problem with the *olfactory nerve*. Colds and sinusitis may be the cause, but trauma involving the cribriform plate can also cause the nerve to have impaired function. Some operations on the nose may cause injury to the olfactory nerves.

Visual acuity may be roughly assessed by asking the patient to read a printed page. Defects of the optic nerve may also affect the field of vision. A lesion of cranial nerve III leads to complete or partial ptosis (drooping of the upper eyelid). The external ocular muscles are controlled by the actions of cranial nerves III, IV and VI. Disruption of cranial nerve III (which supplies all of the extrinsic eye muscles apart from the superior oblique and lateral rectus) causes a paralysis of internal, upward and downward movement of the eye, leading to double vision. The eye points downwards and outwards, except when looking to the affected side. A fixed dilated pupil may also be seen. Disruption of cranial nerve IV, the trochlear nerve supplying the superior oblique, prevents the eye moving downwards and medially. The double vision is worse on looking down. Disruption of cranial nerve VI (abducens supplying lateral rectus) causes an inability to abduct the eye (look to the ipsilateral side). There is deviation of the eye towards the nose and double vision.

The muscles of facial expression are innervated by cranial nerve VII (*facial nerve*). As mentioned previously, upper motor neurone lesions affecting the facial nerve (e.g. after a stroke) may be differentiated from lower motor neurone causes (e.g. Bell's palsy), since the latter causes the whole side of the face to be weakened, whereas the forehead is spared in an upper motor neurone lesion due to bilateral representation at the level of the cerebral cortex. The ipsilateral eye moves upwards on attempted closure of the eyes in Bell's palsy – this is known as 'Bell's sign' (Figure 9C.1).

In terms of *facial sensation*, the sensory division of the trigeminal (cranial nerve V) nerve subserves this over most of the face. The ophthalmic, maxillary and mandibular divisions may be compared by testing skin sensation on either side with a wisp of cotton wool. The corneal (blink) reflex is often the first clinical deficit to be seen in trigeminal nerve lesions.

The *mouth* can demonstrate signs of cranial nerve problems in the case of cranial nerves V (motor division), IX, X and XII. If the masseter muscles are palpated while asking the patient to clench the teeth, and the motor division of cranial nerve V is inactive, the masseter on that side will not contract properly. With a unilateral lesion, the mandible deviates to the weak side on opening the mouth (cranial nerve V being motor to the pterygoid muscles).

Asking the patient to say 'aah' will allow an appraisal of cranial nerves IX and X. Cranial nerve IX (glossopharyngeal) is mainly sensory for the pharynx and palate, and cranial nerve X (vagus) is mainly motor. With a unilateral lesion of the vagus, the soft palate is pulled away from the weaker side. Lesions of both nerves lead to an impaired gag reflex. Cranial nerve XII (hypoglossal) may be tested by asking the patient to protrude the tongue. The tongue deviates to the weaker side.

To test cranial nerve XI (*accessory*), patients should be asked to put their chin towards the left or right shoulder against resistance by the examiner. The sternocleidomastoid muscle (supplied by cranial nerve XI) does not function when cranial nerve XI is affected.

Cranial nerve VIII (*vestibulocochlear*) has two components – the vestibular (appreciation of position and movements of the head) and the cochlear (responsible for hearing). Lesions of the nerve may cause hearing loss, vertigo or ringing in the ears (tinnitus). Special tests are needed to check the balance and positional functions of the nerve.

Neurological disorders: management considerations in dental practice

Epileptic patients who are administered general anaesthetics should not be given methohexitone or enflurane, since these are epileptogenic. Clearly, it is important to ensure that epileptic patients have taken their normal medications on the day of their operative procedures. Intravenous sedation can be useful in the management of epileptic patients. The benzodiazepines have anticonvulsant properties, and the anxiolysis that they produce help to decrease the chances of a fit. When epileptic patients are treated with intravenous sedation, supplemental oxygen should be provided via a nasal cannula. Flumazenil, the benzodiazepine antagonist, should be avoided in epileptic patients, as the drug can itself precipitate convulsions.

Patients who have had a stroke should only be treated when their condition has been optimised wherever possible. Considerations to be factored in are that there may be a loss or impairment of reflexes, such as the swallowing or gag reflex, which has implications for the safe provision of dental treatment using local analgesia with or without intravenous sedation. The ability to protect the airway is also relevant for the provision of general anaesthesia, since the airway can be potentially jeopardised. Stroke patients may be taking anticoagulants or may be hypertensive.

Patients with Parkinson's disease may suffer from excess salivation, which can cause difficulties with visibility, leading to problems not only with the provision of dental treatment but also for the safe administration of anaesthetics. Antimuscarinic drugs will reduce the salivation and degree of tremor. Autonomic insufficiency, often seen in these patients, makes them prone to postural hypotension, and hence poor candidates for general anaesthesia.

The degree of compliance that is possible for treatment is likely to be impaired in both MS and MND patients. It is preferable to use local analgesia alone if possible. Limited mobility and/or associated psychological disorders can also lead to difficulties with treatment. These patients are best treated in the sitting position, so that any impairment of respiration is minimised. Patients with MS, particularly in early stages of the disease, may be taking corticosteroids. In patients with both MS and MND, care of the airway is particularly important, owing to the possibility of swallowing difficulties where these muscles are affected.

In MG patients, local analgesia is again preferred. Doses should be kept to a minimum. Treatment is best carried out early in the day, as muscle fatigue appears to get worse as the day progresses. The provision of intravenous sedation is not indicated in general dental practice, since respiratory impairment may be worsened. It may be acceptable to prescribe a small oral dose of a benzodiazepine if the patient is very anxious about the treatment. It is advisable to avoid general anaesthesia whenever possible, particularly since some of the agents used (e.g. the muscle relaxant suxamethonium or opioids) may have their effects potentiated in patients with MG.

Patients with cerebral palsy may not be able to tolerate treatment under local anaesthesia, and general anaesthesia may be the only modality that can facilitate it. In the athetoid type, there is an increased risk of epilepsy. The effects of cerebral palsy may be worsened by anxiety, and a suitable premedication such as diazepam can be useful.

Patients with spina bifida have an increased incidence of latex allergy. These patients are also prone to postural hypotension, and are therefore best treated when they are sitting up. Epilepsy and renal anomalies can also be associated.

9D STROKE, SPEECH AND SWALLOWING

Stroke

A *stroke* is a sudden, focal loss of neurological function due to a disturbance of blood supply to a part of the brain. Although the synonym 'cerebrovascular accident' or abbreviation 'CVA' is still sometimes used, 'stroke' is the preferred term. Strokes are a common cause of both disability and death. While the risk of strokes increases sharply with age, they can occur at any stage of life.

The term 'transient (cerebral) ischaemic attack' (TIA) refers to stroke-like symptoms that resolve spontaneously within 24 hours (usually much more rapidly); they occur due to a temporary disturbance of the cerebral perfusion. They may herald a permanent stroke, and therefore urgent preventive treatment is needed to reduce the risk of long-term disability.

Pathology of stroke

Brain tissue is dependent on its blood supply for second-to-second function, having a high metabolic rate and no metabolic reserves. This is why consciousness is lost in a few seconds after cardiac arrest, and permanent, irreversible brain damage begins after a few minutes.

The blood supply to the front of the brain comes via the internal carotid arteries, and that to the occipital lobes, cerebellum and brainstem from the vertebral arteries, which merge to form the basilar artery. The main arteries are linked at the base of the brain via the circle of Willis, so that cerebral circulation can be maintained in the event of occlusion of one of the main extracranial arteries. The intracranial vessels that lead from the circle of Willis into the brain substance are 'end arteries', with no anastomoses. Therefore, occlusion of one of these vessels results in ischaemic damage to a segment of brain.

The mechanism of damage to the brain in a stroke is by focal ischaemia, either due to occlusion of a vessel or due to haemorrhage into the brain substance. In Western Europe, only about 10% of strokes are haemorrhagic, the remainder being due to blockage of the vessel. The reverse is true in Japan, where hypertension is common, resulting in aneurysms and cerebral haemorrhage. The mechanisms of cerebral artery occlusion include atherosclerosis and thrombosis, just as in MI, but a significant proportion are due to emboli from more proximal sources. These include atheroma in the extracranial part of the internal carotid artery, or even the common carotid or aorta, and also emboli from the heart, most commonly in atrial fibrillation.

Risk factors and prevention

The major risk factors for stroke are similar to those for other arterial diseases (Table 9D.1). Age is important in both sexes, and hypertension is more important than in MI. Smoking, hyperlipidaemia, diabetes and coagulation disorders also contribute, with prothrombotic conditions increasing the risk of thrombosis or embolism, and anticoagulation or bleeding disorders increasing the risk of haemorrhage. Atrial fibrillation is the major risk factor for cardiogenic emboli, but these can also occur with ventricular aneurysms in ischaemic heart disease, or with infective endocarditis, resulting in septic emboli from vegetations.

Primary prevention (in patients without clinical evidence of cerebrovascular disease) is by effective treatment of the risk factors. In the case of atrial fibrillation, anticoagulation with warfarin is used. The non–vitamin K oral anticoagulants (DOACs) dabigatran, rivaroxaban and apixaban are now trialled and licensed for this indication, and do not require coagulation monitoring. Further developments in this field are imminent within the lifetime of this book. In most other situations, antiplatelet treatment with aspirin is used in those at high risk.

Secondary prevention is important in those who have suffered a TIA or a non-disabling stroke, and it is important to distinguish a haemorrhage from an infarct by CT or MRI scanning. For the small percentage due to haemorrhage, treatment of hypertension is of paramount importance, and antithrombotic therapy should be avoided. For occlusive strokes and TIAs, risk factors must be effectively treated, including hypertension, and antiplatelet treatment given, most commonly with clopidogrel.

Surgical endarterectomy or stenting of the carotid artery can also greatly reduce the risk of stroke in patients with a recent TIA and a carotid stenosis of more than about 70%. Since the risk of stroke is highest immediately after a TIA, rapid-access clinics are set up to ensure that patients can have imaging of both the brain and the cerebral circulation, start appropriate medical treatment and, where appropriate, be scheduled for surgery within 2 weeks. The ABCD^2 score (Table 9D.2) can estimate the risk of a stroke following TIA, and this is used to guide urgency of referral – those with a score of 4 or above should have specialist assessment within 24 hours, and may need admission.

Table 9D.1 Risk factors for stroke.

Age
Hypertension
Smoking
Hyperlipidaemia
Diabetes mellitus
Coagulation disorders (increased risk of either thrombosis or haemorrhage)
Atrial fibrillation
Septic emboli from endocarditis

Table 9D.2 The ABCD² score of risk of stroke following TIA.

Risk factor	Points
Age 60 or over	1
Clinical features of TIA	
• Unilateral weakness with or without speech impairment	2
• Speech impairment alone	1
Duration of TIA	
• 60 min or longer	2
• 10–59 min	1
Diabetes	1

Table 9D.4 The ROSIER score assessment of stroke.

Feature	Score
Loss of consciousness or syncope	−1
Seizure activity	−1
New, acute onset of:	
• Asymmetric facial weakness	+1
• Asymmetric arm weakness	+1
• Asymmetric leg weakness	+1
• Speech disturbance	+1
• Visual field defect	+1

Table 9D.3 Types of stroke.

Total anterior circulation stroke (TACS)
Partial anterior circulation stroke (PACS)
Lacunar stroke (LACS)
Posterior circulation stroke (POCS)

Clinical features of stroke or TIA

Stroke results in sudden focal loss of brain function, and the nature of this clearly depends on the part of the brain that is affected. Stroke is not a cause of loss of consciousness, except in very severe cases involving most of the brain. Four broad types of stroke are recognised, reflecting the site and extent of damage (Table 9D.3).

- *Total anterior circulation stroke* (TACS). Occlusion of the middle cerebral artery affecting the majority of the anterior part of one cerebral hemisphere. It causes contralateral impairments affecting movement (hemiparesis), sensation (hemianaesthesia), vision (homonymous hemianopia affecting the same half of the visual field in both eyes) and higher-cerebral-function disturbance – for example, loss of speech, neglect of affected side and difficulty performing tasks (dyspraxia).
- *Partial anterior circulation stroke* (PACS). As in the preceding point, but less severe, and without higher-cerebral-function involvement.
- *Lacunar stroke* (LACS). Small stroke with limited deficit – for example, weakness of one arm or one side of the face. LACS are usually in the white matter beneath the cerebral cortex, and due to disease of the small vessels within the brain substance.
- *Posterior circulation stroke* (POCS). Stroke affecting structures supplied by the vertebrobasilar system, including the cerebellum, brainstem cranial nerve nuclei, occipital lobe and long motor/sensory tracts. Effects include cranial nerve palsies, incoordination of movement due to cerebellar ataxia, visual field loss from occipital lobe damage and hemiparesis due to involvement of the nerve pathways from the cortex passing through the brainstem.

Management of acute stroke

An acute stroke is a medical emergency where even minutes count, since it can be treated with intravenous thrombolysis where indicated, but the treatment has to be given as early as possible – within 4.5 hours of onset as a maximum. The 'recognition of stroke in the emergency room' (ROSIER) score (Table 9D.4) is designed to aid rapid assessment of stroke in the emergency room, and to minimise delays in treatment. A score of over 0 indicates a probable stroke.

An urgent CT scan is needed to exclude a haemorrhagic stroke before thrombolysis can be given. At present, many patients present too late for this treatment (see Chapter 21, titled 'Medical emergencies'). Hence, attempts are being made to alert the public to the importance of early presentation, and to streamline emergency ambulance services and reorganise hospital services to improve thrombolysis rates.

On arrival, the patient needs a neurological examination, including assessment of swallowing, and cardiovascular examination, including auscultation for heart murmurs or bruits over the neck vessels that might indicate a source for emboli. Initial investigations include a cerebral CT scan, ECG, chest X-ray, plasma glucose and lipids, and routine haematology and biochemistry profiles. The CT scan will show a haemorrhage as a radiodense mass, and may sometimes reveal an alternative diagnosis such as a brain tumour, but the changes of an infarct as seen on a scan take time to develop.

Once a haemorrhage has been excluded, aspirin treatment is started. Heparin is avoided, since this can increase the risk of secondary haemorrhage into the infarcted area. Careful monitoring and correction of oxygen saturation, blood pressure, temperature and blood glucose are thought to minimise the area of brain damage in the partially ischaemic boundary zone surrounding the infarct.

Further treatment involves prevention of complications such as DVT, pneumonia or pressure sores, alongside rehabilitation and secondary prevention. Patients are treated aggressively for hypertension and hyperlipidaemia, and started on antiplatelet therapy. Smoking cessation and diabetes control are also important. Those with less disabling strokes are investigated by duplex carotid ultrasound with a view to carotid endarterectomy.

Stroke rehabilitation

Rehabilitation is the restoration of patients to their maximal physical, psychological and social functions. It is undertaken by a multidisciplinary team, initially in hospital, but continued in the community.

- Physiotherapists concentrate on exercises aimed at restoring lost function.
- Occupational therapists help with learning new ways of coping with loss of function, including provision of aids and appliances, and adaptations.
- Speech therapists assess and treat swallowing disorders as well as speech problems.
- Social workers provide help at home for tasks the patient can no longer perform, or arrange for long-term residential or nursing home care.
- Others team members include clinical psychologists, orthotists, continence advisors, nurses and doctors.

Dental aspects of stroke

Stroke patients may require special help on account of their disability. They may use aids and appliances such as wheelchairs or walking aids. Also, communicating with patients who have speech problems can take time and effort. Those with severe disability are likely to attend with a carer who can help them, speak for them and ensure that any advice from the dentist is put into action.

Certain specific aspects of dental care may cause problems:
- Patients may need help with oral hygiene, fitting of dentures, etc.
- The gag reflex and mechanisms protecting the airway may be impaired, requiring care during procedures.
- Patients may be on several drugs that either affect the delivery of dental care (e.g. anticoagulants), or have direct oral side effects (e.g. antihypertensive drugs).
- They may be more sensitive to adverse effects from sedatives or opioid analgesics.
- Care is needed with adrenaline-containing anaesthetics in patients on antihypertensive medication.

Speech

Dysarthria is difficulty in articulating speech, due to structural/functional problems with the mouth or tongue. *Dysphasia* is loss of cerebral cognitive language skills due to damage to the speech-controlling areas of the cerebral cortex. *Dysphonia* is failure of the voice, usually indicating a problem with the larynx or its nerve supply.

Strokes can cause all three problems, but dysphasia is particularly common in major strokes of the dominant (usually left) hemisphere, and therefore occurs in strokes paralysing the right side of the body. Broca's area of the cerebral cortex lies in front of the lateral sulcus (Sylvian fissure), and is involved in speech production. Wernicke's area lies behind and below the lateral sulcus, and governs language comprehension. In strokes, expressive dysphasia or Broca's dysphasia is often more severe than receptive, or Wernicke's dysphasia, so patients can understand more than they can express.

Dysarthria may occur in strokes that affect the movement of the tongue or palate, or in cerebellar strokes affecting the coordination of these movements. Dysarthria can occur in other neurological conditions, such as MND (which often presents with a bulbar palsy, paralysing the orofacial muscles), cerebellar degeneration, Parkinson's disease and multiple sclerosis. It has a wide range of other causes, including dry mouth, ill-fitting dentures and alcohol intoxication.

Patients with speech problems following a stroke require thorough assessment by a speech and language therapist (SALT). Language can sometimes be regained with time, practice and exercises. In other cases, language aids are needed, for example, picture charts for a dysphasic patient to request food, drink, the toilet, etc., by pointing, or a keyboard-based writing system for a patient with severe dysarthria due to bulbar palsy.

Swallowing

Dysphagia is the term for difficulty swallowing, not to be confused with 'dysphasia' (see the preceding text).

Elements of swallowing

The oral stage comprises mastication, formation of a food bolus and manoeuvring the bolus to the pharynx. During the pharyngeal stage, the pharynx and larynx elevate, and the soft palate and glottis close, thus preventing food or drink from entering the nose or trachea. The contraction of the pharyngeal muscles moves the bolus into the oesophagus. This sequence of events is automatic, but under voluntary control. The oesophageal stage is involuntary, in that the peristaltic propulsion of the bolus towards the cardiac sphincter occurs by automatic reflexes set off by the entry of the food into the upper oesophagus.

Swallowing disorders

Strokes may affect the oral and pharyngeal phases of swallowing, resulting in danger of aspiration of food or drink into the lungs, causing pneumonia. Other neurological diseases such as MND and MS may do the same.

Mechanical obstruction of the oesophagus may occur due to oesophageal cancer, or due to benign stricture formation from recurrent gastrooesophageal acid reflux, causing the formation of a fibrotic scar. The oesophagus may also be compressed by adjacent structures such as cancers affecting the lung or mediastinal lymph nodes.

Oesophageal motility disorders include incoordinate peristalsis due to old age, 'corkscrew oesophagus' (which results in a characteristic appearance on barium swallow), and achalasia, a condition of unknown cause in which damage to the neuronal plexus causes impaired relaxation of the cardiac sphincter with atonic dilatation of the oesophagus above.

Assessment and treatment of swallowing problems

The history usually gives a clue to the cause. Patients with a mechanical obstruction to the oesophagus complain of difficulty swallowing solids, while liquids pass more easily. Large pieces of food such as meat can cause a complete obstruction and, if they are not successfully regurgitated, can present acutely with total inability to swallow. Patients with neurological disorders may already have a known diagnosis, and they usually describe coughing or choking after swallowing, and have more trouble with liquids than solids.

In suspected mechanical obstruction, a barium swallow X-ray or upper gastrointestinal endoscopy are the tests of choice. For suspected malignancy, an endoscopic biopsy is necessary to confirm the diagnosis, and CT scanning can assess the extent of disease. Oesophageal incoordination can be confirmed by a barium swallow or oesophageal manometry. Oropharyngeal dysfunction should first be assessed clinically by a speech and language therapist, who may then perform an X-ray study of the swallowing reflex by video-fluoroscopy while the patient swallows radio-opaque foods of differing consistency.

Treatment depends upon the cause. A benign oesophageal stricture can be dilated and treated with proton pump inhibitors to reduce gastric acid production. A malignant stricture may be cured by oesophagectomy, or treated palliatively by radiotherapy or dilatation with the placement of a stent. Neurological swallowing problems affecting the oral and pharyngeal phases may be managed by training the patient to eat carefully in an upright position, and to 'double swallow' food. The texture of the food can be modified – solids can be pureed, and liquids can be thickened with cellulose-based thickeners to reduce the risk of aspiration into the lungs.

Long-term tube feeding into the stomach is undertaken in some cases. Nasogastric tubes are usually only used for temporary feeding, and a permanent percutaneous endoscopic gastrostomy (PEG) tube is inserted when long-term feeding is required. The procedure is undertaken under sedation and local anaesthesia, using an endoscope to place a guidewire from the abdominal wall into the stomach, and out through the mouth. The guidewire is then used to pull a flanged tube into place that allows direct feeding into the stomach. The track of the tube heals to prevent leakage into the peritoneal cavity, and the tube can be changed periodically without recourse to repeat endoscopy.

9E OPHTHALMOLOGY

Measurement of vision

There is no single measurement that will accurately encompass all aspects of the visual system. Visual acuity, or resolving power of the eye, should be measured in any case with suspected eye involvement, including midfacial fractures, and can assume great medicolegal significance in this setting.

In clinical situations, visual acuity is usually measured with the Snellen chart, which consists of a series of letters ranging from the largest at the top of the chart to the smallest at the bottom (Figure 9E.1). The largest letter at the top of the chart would normally be readable at 60 metres. Visual acuity is recorded as a fraction. The numerator refers to the distance at which the chart is viewed during testing, and the denominator denotes the normal reading distance for the lowest line that can be read (usually given in small digits near the respective lines). For example, a visual acuity of '6/60' means that, at 6 metres, the patient could only read a letter that should be readable at 60 metres. A visual acuity of '6/6' corresponds to normal vision, although many young patients can do better than this and score 6/5. The patient should have one eye covered, and, if glasses are used for distance vision, these should be worn. Testing is usually performed at 6 metres.

In emergency situations, when no distance vision chart is available, it is acceptable to measure near vision using a newspaper to indicate whether small print or only large headlines can be read.

If the vision is too poor to read any letters, check whether the patient can count the fingers of your hand at 1 metre or 0.5 metre; whether he or she can perceive a hand moved in front of the eye; or, finally, whether he or she can perceive a pen torch shone into the eye, ensuring the other eye is covered completely.

Common causes of visual loss

Age-related macular degeneration

The macula is the area in the centre of the retina that is rich in cones and responsible for colour detection, as well as fine, detailed vision. At the centre of the macula is the fovea, a small yellowish depression where there is no nerve fibre layer and the photoreceptors are most densely and regularly arrayed. Anything that prevents the macula from functioning results in loss of central vision, causing, in particular, difficulty in reading and recognising faces.

Age-related macular degeneration (AMD) is the most common cause of registration as severely visually impaired. With the ageing of the general population, particularly in the so-called developed world, the prevalence of AMD is rising.

The end result of macular degeneration is an island of missing vision in the centre of the visual field. Peripheral vision

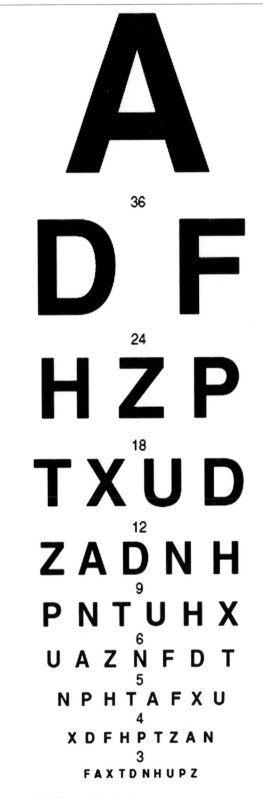

Figure 9E.1 The Snellen chart.

remains intact, however, so that most patients with macular degeneration maintain independent living.

Until recently, there was no treatment available for macular degeneration. It is possible now, however, to modify the natural history of the so-called 'wet type' of macular degeneration by injecting inhibitors of vascular endothelial growth factor into the vitreous cavity. This can result in the regression of subretinal new vessels with preservation of vision. It remains to be seen what effect this will have on the epidemiology of visual impairment from macular degeneration.

Cataract

A *cataract* is an opacity of the human crystalline lens that degrades the image falling on the retina. The most important risk factor is age, but diabetes, smoking and exposure to UV light may also play a part.

Once vision is degraded to the point where reading is no longer possible, or vision has dropped below the legal requirements for driving, cataract surgery is the only treatment option.

Cataract extraction with intraocular lens insertion is the most common operation performed in National Health Service hospitals. Recent advances in surgery have transformed both the visual outcome and speed of rehabilitation. The aim of cataract surgery is to remove the lens contents while leaving the capsular bag in place, as this is best place to insert a new intraocular lens implant (Figure 9E.2). This is usually achieved by *phacoemulsification*, a surgical procedure in which a probe vibrating at ultrasonic frequencies is used to break the lens nucleus into fragments and then emulsify and aspirate them. The surgery is performed through a small, self-sealing wound.

Open-angle glaucoma

Open-angle glaucoma is the most common neuropathy affecting the optic nerve. It results from the apoptosis of ganglion cell axons leaving the eye through the optic nerve. Because the

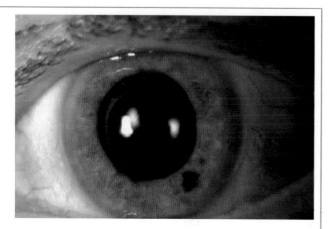

Figure 9E.2 Postoperative cataract extraction showing an intraocular lens implant in the capsular bag.

axons that are lost are not replaced by glial tissue, the size of the redundant space in the optic nerve head, called the 'cup', increases. This results in a change in the appearance of the optic nerve, termed 'cupping', which is visible on ophthalmoscopic examination. The loss of ganglion cell axons eventually results in loss of the visual field.

The most important risk factor for open-angle glaucoma is raised intraocular pressure. Aqueous humour is produced by the ciliary epithelium by a combination of active secretion and ultrafiltration. Aqueous humour exits the eye through the porous tissue of the trabecular meshwork in the angle of the eye. The balance between inflow and outflow maintains an intraocular pressure of about 16 mmHg on average. If the outflow resistance of the trabecular meshwork increases, the intraocular pressure will rise. Over time, by mechanisms that are not fully understood, raised intraocular pressure results in progressive damage to the optic nerve.

Although there are other risk factors operating, the only treatments for glaucoma that are proven to be effective work by lowering intraocular pressure. This can be achieved by using topical eye drops that either reduce inflow by reducing ciliary body secretion of aqueous humour, or increase outflow through the trabecular meshwork.

Diabetic retinopathy

Diabetic retinopathy, in common with many of the other complications of diabetes, is a microangiopathy. It causes visual loss by two main mechanisms: diabetic maculopathy and proliferative retinopathy.

In the case of diabetic maculopathy, progressive microvascular changes and retinal ischaemia result in outpouchings called 'microaneurysms', which develop from the venous side of capillaries. These microaneurysms can leak fluid, protein and phospholipids into the surrounding retina.

Proliferative diabetic retinopathy is potentially more serious and can result in total blindness. Increasing retinal ischaemia results in the release of diffusible vasoproliferative factors that cause new vessel growth, typically on the optic disc and on the vascular arcades. These new vessels can bleed into the vitreous gel, resulting in a catastrophic loss of vision, and the associated contractile glial cells may form a fibrosing membrane that results in detachment of the neurosensory retina. The prognosis in proliferative diabetic retinopathy has been transformed by argon laser photocoagulation to the retina outside the vascular arcades, which promotes regression of new vessels.

Interacting with the visually impaired patient

Most visually impaired people will still have some vision. It is therefore important to make written material accessible by using a larger font of at least size 14, having plenty of contrast and avoiding patterned backgrounds or glossy paper.

The acute red eye

Inflammation in any organ leads to an increase in blood flow and dilation of blood vessels. The eye is unique in that its covering tissues are transparent, so these dilated blood vessels are visible directly to the clinician. A red eye is the most common presentation of a wide range of ocular pathologies. It is the time course of the onset, the location of the vascular engorgement and the associated symptoms that help discern the cause. The two most important symptoms in this regard are *pain* and *visual loss*.

The presence of either or both of these two cardinal symptoms – pain and loss of vision – is alarming, and means that serious pathology needs to be excluded. Conversely, a red eye without pain or loss of vision, even if the redness is dramatic, is very rarely of concern. As with all generalisations in medicine, however, exceptions to this rule do exist.

Although there are many causes for an acute red eye, six are discussed in the following, of which the first three are common but not sight-threatening, and the second three are rarer but can threaten sight.

Conjunctivitis (very common, no pain, no loss of vision)

The translucent mucous membrane that covers the white of the eyeball and the inside of the eyelids is termed the 'conjunctiva'. It is commonly the site of viral and bacterial infections. Symptoms include puffy eyelids, watering, stickiness and grittiness. Often, both eyes are affected. The white of the eye shows diffuse redness. Both viral and bacterial conjunctivitis are self-limiting conditions and do not usually require treatment. Antibiotic drops or ointment are still often prescribed. Viral conjunctivitis can persist for several weeks, and is often highly contagious. Advice on avoiding close contact and not sharing towels should be given. A health worker with conjunctivitis should avoid patient contact until full resolution.

Subconjunctival haemorrhage (very common, no pain, no loss of vision)

This is the most dramatic presentation of the acute red eye, but also the least concerning. Subconjunctival haemorrhage occurs spontaneously and very commonly, and makes part or all of the white of the eye go a bright, dense red colour. Pain is absent, but patients often complain of grittiness. Resolution occurs over a week or two, and reassurance is all that is required.

Episcleritis (common, mild pain, no loss of vision)

Inflammation of the covering layer of the eye beneath the conjunctiva is called 'episcleritis'. This common condition is identified by the pattern of redness on the eye. It usually affects a single sector of the white of the eye, leaving the rest of the eye unaffected. Mild discomfort is the norm; more severe degrees of pain suggest a more serious condition. Treatment is with NSAIDs or steroid drops, and recurrence is common.

Corneal ulceration (severe pain, possible loss of vision)

The cornea is the curved, colourless, window overlying the iris and pupil, and its purpose is to refract incoming light. The optical requirements of the cornea demand that it be essentially free from blood vessels, which would scatter light and degrade the image. This avascularity of the cornea means that infection within it is not handled well by the immune system, as blood-borne components of the body's defence system cannot readily gain access. Corneal infection can rapidly lead to corneal thinning and perforation of the eye, which may result in blindness. Even if the infection is cleared, scarring often results, which, in the central part of the cornea, can seriously impair sight. Infection of the cornea is therefore an important cause of acute red eye.

Viral infection is commonly by herpes simplex, and is essentially the ocular counterpart of a cold sore on the lips. Bacterial infection can be due to a wide range of Gram-positive and Gram-negative organisms, and is often secondary to contact lens use. For both types, symptoms include an intensely red eye, with watering and photophobia (aversion to light). Lesions affecting the central cornea will cause reduced vision; more peripheral corneal ulcers may not. Close inspection of the cornea reveals a white spot for bacterial cases; viral ulcers may not be visible initially. The addition of a drop of fluorescein, a commonly used vital dye, shows an area of corneal epithelial loss, which glows green under blue illumination. Urgent ophthalmic referral is required. Treatment is with topical antiviral or antibiotic agents.

Acute uveitis (uncommon, pain, loss of vision)

The uvea is the middle layer of the three concentric layers that make up the eye, and comprises the choroid, ciliary body and iris. The anterior part of the uvea is most commonly affected, and acute uveitis is also sometimes called 'iritis'. Many cases are idiopathic, although some are part of a systemic inflammatory disorder such as seronegative arthritis or sarcoidosis.

Most cases of uveitis present with an acute red eye, with photophobia, pain and mild–moderate loss of vision. Intensive topical steroid drops, with dilating drops to widen the pupil, are the mainstay of treatment.

Acute glaucoma (very uncommon, severe pain, marked loss of vision)

The dynamics of aqueous humour production and drainage have been outlined in the preceding section on open-angle glaucoma. Whereas open-angle glaucoma is a silent and insidious destroyer of vision, acute angle closure causes the intraocular pressure to rapidly rise to very high levels, resulting in severe pain and acute visual loss. In acute (or angle closure) glaucoma, there is a sudden increase in the resistance to aqueous outflow when the pupil is in mid-dilation, as the peripheral iris becomes apposed to the trabecular meshwork. Left untreated, such high levels of intraocular pressure will bring irreversible damage to the optic nerve or cause interruption to the retinal blood flow, resulting in permanent loss of sight.

Acute glaucoma mainly affects the elderly, and is more common in long-sighted people. Symptoms include a severely painful red eye, along with headache, nausea and vomiting. An incorrect diagnosis of intracranial pathology such as a subarachnoid haemorrhage is occasionally made. The vision is usually profoundly reduced, and the pupil is invariably unreactive to light and enlarged, as compared to the unaffected eye. Acute glaucoma is one of the few ophthalmic emergencies, and patients should be seen urgently by an ophthalmologist to commence pressure-lowering treatment.

Conditions of common interest

Giant cell arteritis

Giant cell arteritis (GCA) is the most common systemic vasculitis. It is almost never found below the age of 50, and its incidence rises sharply with age. It primarily affects the extracranial branches of the carotid arteries but can cause more widespread problems. GCA can present to many different specialties, each of which is familiar with a slightly different spectrum of a disease that has a common underlying pathology.

GCA is of interest to the ophthalmologist because it is a cause of preventable blindness, and to the dentist because it can be a cause of facial and lingual pain. Inflammation and occlusion of the posterior ciliary arteries can result in optic nerve infarction or anterior ischaemic optic neuropathy (AION) with loss of sight of the affected eye. Untreated, about 50% of patients with arteritic AION in one eye will go on to lose sight in the other eye. Arteritic AION typically presents with sudden and complete loss of vision in one eye. The affected optic nerve is swollen and becomes pale as nerve fibres die off. Prior to the onset of visual loss in one eye, patients may have a variety of symptoms, including malaise, weight loss, shoulder ache and stiffness, and headaches. The headaches are usually maximal in the temporal regions, and are associated with superficial tenderness.

About 40% of patients with GCA experience jaw claudication, which refers to an ache in the muscles of mastication brought on by sustained chewing. Other oral presentations include toothache, lingual pain or even tongue infarction. Diagnosis is difficult, and no one symptom, sign or test is completely diagnostic. Most patients with GCA have raised inflammatory markers. The ESR is usually markedly elevated, often >100 mm/hour. CRP is usually also raised, and diagnostic accuracy is improved by combining these two tests.

The definitive confirmation comes from temporal artery biopsy, which shows granulomatous inflammation with giant cells, disruption of the internal elastic lamina and luminal occlusion or narrowing. As a result of skip lesions, not all biopsies are positive, so it may be necessary to treat in the absence of a confirmatory biopsy. GCA is treated with high doses of systemic steroids.

Sjögren syndrome

Sjögren syndrome is an autoimmune condition in which exocrine glands such as the lacrimal and salivary glands are attacked and destroyed. Although pulmonary, renal and brain involvement can occur, the principal sites of involvement are the eyes and the mouth. It is commonly associated with rheumatoid arthritis, and it affects women more commonly than men.

For normal functioning, the cornea and conjunctiva must always be kept moist. The tear film is complex; there is a layer of glycoproteins attached to the corneal and conjunctival epithelium – an aqueous layer secreted by the lacrimal gland, and a lipid monolayer on the surface secreted by meibomian glands at the lid margin. The aqueous component of tears is produced by the lacrimal gland, which is a tubuloacinar gland with histological and antigenic similarities to the salivary glands. It is therefore not surprising that dry eyes and dry mouth often coexist with a connective tissue disorder such as rheumatoid arthritis.

The deficient tear film can result in poor corneal wetting, with dry spots developing between blinks. Vital dyes such as fluorescein will often show an interpalpebral pattern of staining. Aqueous tear deficiency is managed by the use of topical tear substitutes such as hypromellose or polyvinyl alcohol, and sometimes by inserting silicone plugs into the lacrimal puncta to prevent normal tear drainage.

Behçet's disease

Behçet's disease is a complex multisystem inflammatory disease of unknown aetiology. The principal features are oral ulceration, genital ulceration and ocular inflammatory disease. The ocular involvement consists of retinal venous vasculitis or inflammation of the iris with transudation of protein and cells into the normally clear aqueous. Patients usually complain of blurred vision and floaters, although there may also be a painful red eye if the iris is involved.

Behçet's disease can be difficult to control, and, even with immunosuppression, devastating visual loss can occur.

Ophthalmic complications of dental anaesthesia

Fortunately, ophthalmic complications of dental anaesthesia are very rare indeed, and are usually transient. Given the frequency with which dental anaesthesia is performed, some of the reported complications are probably coincidental. Complications include double vision due to lateral rectus palsy, transient loss of vision in the ipsilateral eye, Horner's syndrome and ptosis.

Mechanisms include: diffusion from the pterygomaxillary fossa into the orbit through bony defects or through lymphatic and venous networks; inadvertent injection into the orbit through the inferior orbital fissure; inadvertent intra-arterial injection into the superior alveolar artery; and trauma to arteriolar walls stimulating the sympathetic nervous plexus on the surface.

Transmission of infections through the ocular surface

It should be remembered that the ocular surface is a potential portal for the transmission of systemic infections such as Creutzfeldt–Jakob disease (CJD), HIV, HBV and HCV. There have been cases of CJD and rabies being transmitted by infected corneal grafts from hosts, who were not known to be affected at the time of harvesting.

All dental surgeons are likely to operate on patients who, unknown to them, harbour potentially transmissible viruses. Therefore, sensible precautions should be applied in all cases.

In situations where bone is being drilled, it has been shown that microscopic fragments can penetrate the cornea. There is no doubt that potentially contaminated aerosols can make contact with the eye. Although the risk of viral transmission from dental procedures is difficult to determine, the wearing of adequate eye protection during dental procedures is recommended.

Facial trauma and the eye

Facial trauma is frequently associated with eye injuries. The risk of ocular damage is greatest for comminuted zygomatic fractures followed by orbital floor fractures. As a result, all patients with midfacial fractures should have their visual acuity documented. Full details of traumatic injuries to the face are given in standard maxillofacial textbooks.

9F   ANTICONVULSANT AND ANTI-PARKINSONIAN DRUGS

Anticonvulsant drugs

Anticonvulsant medications are used to treat epilepsy and neuralgias. Dentists may prescribe these drugs in the management of trigeminal neuralgia, and may encounter patients receiving such therapy in practice. Some of these medications have unwanted effects in the mouth, and they impact on dental care. In addition, the medical emergency of status epilepticus is a condition that dentists may have to manage. Thus, an anticonvulsant should be available in the emergency drug box (see Chapter 21, titled 'Medical emergencies').

Drug classification

The following are the main drugs used as anticonvulsants:
- Phenytoin.
- Sodium valproate.
- Carbamazepine and oxcarbazepine.
- Ethosuximide.
- Gabapentin and pregabalin.
- Lamotrigine.
- Benzodiazepines.
- Barbiturates.

Unfortunately, no single drug controls all types of seizures, and different patients need different medications. Concurrent therapy is often required to establish good management. Other drugs with anticonvulsant activity (such as levetiracetam and topiramate) are used as 'add-on' drugs to improve control.

Oral administration is the normal route for prophylaxis; however, during the medical emergency of status epilepticus (see Chapter 21, titled 'Medical emergencies'), intravenous administration of midazolam or diazepam is required if the topical route of midazolam administration fails.

Mechanism of action

Anticonvulsant drugs achieve their effect by one or more of the following mechanisms:
- Reduction of membrane excitability by ion channel blockade (sodium or calcium channels).
- Increase of inhibitory neurotransmitter (γ-aminobutyric acid (GABA)) activity.
- Decrease of excitatory neurotransmitter (glutamate) activity.

Table 9F.1 summarises the ion channels and neurotransmitters influenced by the various anticonvulsant drugs.

Unwanted effects of anticonvulsant medication

Anticonvulsant drugs produce several unwanted effects in the mouth and perioral structures, and can impact on the management of dental patients. Among the unwanted effects of phenytoin in the orofacial region are:
- Gingival overgrowth.
- Root shortening.
- Root resorption.
- Hypercementosis.
- Salivary gland hypertrophy.
- Cervical lymphadenopathy.
- Cleft lip and palate.

Similarly, carbamazepine causes:
- Xerostomia.
- Glossitis.
- Oral ulceration.
- Cervical lymphadenopathy.
- Cleft lip and palate.

Many of the anticonvulsants produce haematological effects that can affect patient management. Phenytoin and carbamazepine

Table 9F.1 The ion channels and neurotransmitters influenced by various anticonvulsant drugs.

Drug	Sodium channel	Calcium channel	GABA	Glutamate
Phenytoin	X	X		
Sodium valproate	X	X	X	
Carbamazepine	X	X		
Ethosuximide		X		
Gabapentin			X	
Pregabalin			X	
Lamotrigine				X
Vigabatrin			X	
Benzodiazepines			X	
Barbiturates			X	

cause anaemia and agranulocytosis. In addition, these drugs and sodium valproate can produce thrombocytopaenia. If carbamazepine is prescribed to treat trigeminal neuralgia, then full blood counts should be taken on a regular basis (every 3 months), and gross changes, such as a drop in the white cell count to <3000, indicate a change in therapy.

Drug interactions are not uncommon with anticonvulsants, especially carbamazepine and phenytoin. A glance at Appendix 1 of the British National Formulary will demonstrate the many interactions that can occur with carbamazepine. Anyone prescribing this medication should carefully elicit a history of concurrent drug therapy from the proposed recipient. Examples of drugs that increase the action of carbamazepine are alcohol, allopurinol, clarithromycin, omeprazole and verapamil. The effect of the anticonvulsant is reduced by cisplatin and fluoxetine. Carbamazepine and phenytoin reduce the anticoagulant effect of warfarin and decrease the action of corticosteroids, doxycycline and oral contraceptives.

Anti-Parkinsonian drugs

Drugs used to treat Parkinsonism aim to counter the disruption in balance between reduced dopamine and increased acetylcholine.

Drug classification

The drugs are divided into two groups:
- Dopaminergic.
- Antimuscarinic.

Some dopaminergic drugs are:
- Levodopa.
- Bromocriptine.
- Cabergoline
- Lisuride.
- Pergolide.
- Pramipexole.
- Ropinirole.
- Amantadine.
- Benserazide.
- Carbidopa.
- Selegiline.
- Entacapone.
- Tolcapone.

Some antimuscarinic drugs are:
- Benzatropine.
- Orphenadrine.
- Procyclidine.
- Trihexyphenidyl.

Mechanism of action

Dopamine itself is not used, as it cannot cross the blood–brain barrier. Dopaminergic drugs do not all achieve their effects in the same way, but all lead to increases in effective dopamine levels. They can act as:
- Dopamine precursors (e.g. levodopa).
- Direct dopamine receptor agonists (e.g. bromocriptine).
- Stimulators of dopamine release (e.g. amantadine).
- Dopa-decarboxylase inhibitors (e.g. benserazide).
- Monoamine oxidase inhibitors (e.g. selegiline).
- Catechol-*O*-methyltransferase (COMT) inhibitors (e.g. entacapone).

Figure 9F.1 demonstrates the site of action of dopaminergic drugs.

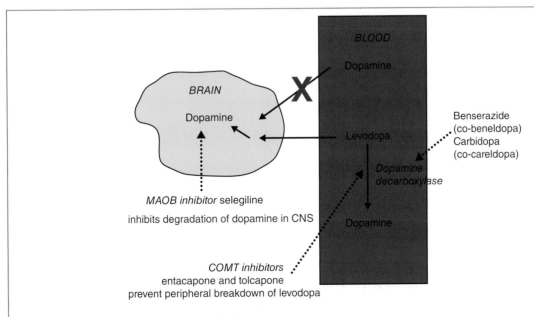

Figure 9F.1 The site of action of dopaminergic drugs.

Unwanted effects

The major unwanted effect of antimuscarinic drugs is dry mouth. Dopaminergic medications can also produce xerostomia, as well as taste disturbance, stomatitis, oral ulceration, headache and dyskinesias.

Some dopaminergic drugs interact with medication that dentists may prescribe. Levodopa is antagonised by benzodiazepines; erythromycin increases bromocriptine toxicity; and selegiline increases the CNS toxicity of opioids. As catechol-*O*-methyltransferase is the enzyme involved in the initial metabolism of exogenous adrenaline, it is probably wise to limit the amount of adrenaline-containing local anaesthetic cartridges administered to patients on this drug, although no evidence of any serious interaction is available.

FURTHER READING

BMJ. Available from: http://www.bmj.com/specialties/neurology.

Epilepsy Action. Available from: http://www.epilepsy.org.uk/.

SIGN Guideline 119: Management of patients with stroke: identification and management of dysphagia. Available from: http://www.sign.ac.uk/guidelines/fulltext/119/section2.html.

MULTIPLE CHOICE QUESTIONS

1. Which of the following is unlikely to be caused by stroke?
   a) Loss of one side of the visual field in both eyes.
   b) Unilateral arm weakness.
   c) Loss of consciousness.
   d) Word-finding difficulties.
   e) Unilateral facial drooping.
   Answer = C

2. The term for difficulty in using or understanding words is:
   a) Dysphrasia.
   b) Dysarthria.
   c) Dysphagia.
   d) Dysphonia.
   e) Dysphasia.
   Answer = E

3. Food sticking in the throat is most likely to be caused by:
   a) Stroke.
   b) MND.
   c) Oesophageal stenosis.
   d) Multiple sclerosis.
   e) Cerebellar degeneration.
   Answer = C

4. Which of the following is *not* a treatment for swallowing difficulties caused by a stroke?
   a) Oesophageal dilation with stenting.
   b) Thickened fluids.
   c) Nasogastric feeding.
   d) PEG feeding.
   e) Soft diet.
   Answer = A

5. Which of the following is *not* part of the emergency management of an acute occlusive stroke?
   a) Urgent CT scanning.
   b) Carotid artery stenting.
   c) Swallowing assessment.
   d) Intravenous thrombolysis.
   e) Oral aspirin.
   Answer = B

6. Which of the following assessment scales is used to estimate the risk of a stroke following a TIA?
   a) ABCD^2.
   b) ROSIER.
   c) CURB65.
   d) CHADSVASC.
   e) FAST.
   Answer = A

7. Which of the following is *not* appropriate for secondary prevention of stroke after a TIA?
   a) Oral antiplatelet treatment.
   b) Carotid endarterectomy.
   c) Warfarin for patients in atrial fibrillation.
   d) Tranexamic acid for patients with haemorrhagic strokes.
   e) Lipid-lowering therapy.
   Answer = D

8. 'Battle's sign' is demonstrated by the clinical appearance of:
   a) Periorbital ecchymosis.
   b) Periauricular ecchymosis.
   c) Perizygomatic ecchymosis.
   d) Peritonsillar ecchymosis.
   e) Perimandibular ecchymosis.
   Answer = B

9. A typical appearance of extradural haemorrhage on a CT scan is of:
   a) A biconvex-shaped opacity.
   b) A biconcave-shaped opacity.
   c) Ventricle opacity.
   d) Circumferential opacity.
   e) Extracranial opacity.
   Answer = A

10. Which of the following is *not* likely to be a cause of sensorineural deafness?
    a) Acute labyrinthitis.
    b) Head injury.
    c) Paget's disease of bone.
    d) Overdose of certain drugs (e.g. gentamicin).
    e) Impacted wax in the external auditory meatus.
    Answer = E

CHAPTER 10
Shock

S Clark

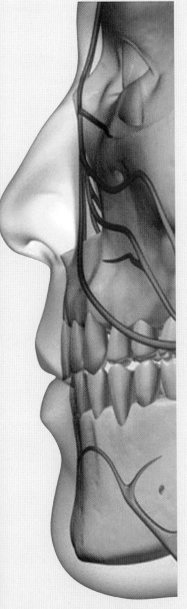

Key topics

- Definition of *shock*.
- Types of shocks and their pathophysiology.

Learning objectives

- To be able to define *shock*.
- To understand the principles of management of shocked patients.

Essentials of Human Disease in Dentistry, Second Edition. Mark Greenwood.
© 2018 John Wiley & Sons Ltd. Published 2018 by John Wiley & Sons Ltd.
Companion website: www.wiley.com/go/greenwood/human-disease-in-dentistry

Introduction

Shock is the acute alteration of the circulation in which inadequate perfusion leads to cellular damage, dysfunction and failure of major organ systems. It is a clinical term, and is a generalised failure of the circulation. It does not imply the cause of shock.

Since the effects are seen within the cardiovascular system, the causes of shock and the cardiovascular system can be compared to a central heating system (Figure 10.1).

- True hypovolaemic shock – lack or loss of fluid in the system.
- Apparent hypovolaemic shock – failure of the pipes in the system.
- Obstructive shock – failure of the fluid to return to the pump.
- Cardiogenic shock – pump failure.
- Failures that lead to cellular hypoxia/organ failure – malfunctioning radiators.

Pathophysiology

Shock involves inadequate cardiac output to meet tissue or organ demands, either because of pump or peripheral circulatory failure.

$$\text{Cardiac output} = \text{heart rate} \times \text{stroke volume}$$

A decrease in blood volume in the cardiovascular system can result in reduced venous return to the heart. This activates baroreflexes, which increase the heart rate and cause peripheral arteriolar constriction. This sympathetic stimulation is enhanced by the rising levels of the hormones adrenaline, aldosterone, noradrenaline and angiotensin II. The increased heart rate improves cardiac output. Therefore, the first sign of shock is often an increase in heart rate. The increased peripheral resistance helps maintain arterial blood pressure. This may result in systolic blood pressure being normal when there has been significant loss of blood volume, and cellular perfusion may be inadequate. A normal blood pressure does not equate with an absence of shock.

The peripheral vasoconstriction in hypovolaemic shock is most marked in the skin and splanchnic circulation in an attempt to redistribute and preserve blood flow to maintain perfusion to vital organs. This gives rise to the cold, pale, clammy skin and weak thready rapid pulse seen in hypovolaemic shock.

Sympathetic venoconstriction increases the blood flow back to the heart and the stroke volume.

As a result of impaired oxygen delivery, anaerobic metabolism will occur. This leads to elevated blood lactate and decreased pH. This metabolic acidosis is detected by chemoreceptors, stimulating the respiratory centre. The respiratory rate increases in an attempt to blow off CO_2 and compensate for this acidosis. An increase in respiratory rate is a marker of established shock and impending deterioration.

The anaerobic metabolism resulting from suboptimal oxygen delivery is poorer at energy production than aerobic metabolism. The vital cell functions dependent on this energy production become impaired and deteriorate with enzyme malfunction and disrupted ion exchange across the cell. This causes cell death and, ultimately, organ failure.

Cardiac physiology may be considered as *preload, myocardial contractility* and *afterload*.

Preload is the volume of venous return to the heart, and is dependent on the blood volume and pressure gradient of the venous system. The greater the pressure and pressure gradient, the greater the venous return to the heart.

The venous return determines cardiac muscle fibre length and its contractile properties –*myocardial contractility*. This follows Starling's law. Therefore, too little venous blood in the chambers of the heart results in an inefficient, low cardiac output. Overfilling of the chambers overstretches the muscle, resulting in impaired contractility, and cardiac output falls. There is an optimal stroke volume in maximum cardiac output that appropriate rapid fluid resuscitation in shock aims to achieve. Medical treatment, such as inotropes to modify contractility and vascular resistance, may be considered to treat shock after establishing the optimal fluid volume.

Afterload is the pressure that the heart must generate to eject blood from the heart. If afterload increases, the stroke volume and, subsequently, cardiac output decreases.

In all causes of shock, the physiological response of the patient depends on previous medical conditions, age, medication and the speed and adequacy of resuscitation and interventions. These affect the body's normal compensation mechanisms. In adults, deterioration may be gradual. In children and infants, compensatory mechanisms may be abruptly overwhelmed with sudden and dramatic deterioration.

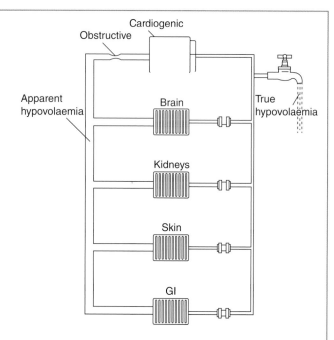

Figure 10.1 Causes of shock and the cardiovascular system (comparative diagram).

Shock is an acute failure of circulation. Gradual circulatory failure allows autoregulation to preserve fluid delivery as well to activate as more long-term compensatory mechanisms – for example, thirst.

Aetiology of shock

Identifying the underlying cause is important in treating shock (Table 10.1).

Hypovolemic shock

This is the commonest cause of shock in trauma situations, where fluid loss leads to reduced venous return and low cardiac output. It may arise from:

1. Haemorrhage.
2. Loss of gastrointestinal fluid, such as in vomiting and diarrhoea.
3. Burns with direct loss of fluid from the burn surface and tissue fluid sequestration.
4. Renal loss of water and electrolytes, as seen in diabetic ketosis.

The effects of blood loss on various organs and the cardiovascular signs can be seen in Table 10.2.

Cardiogenic shock

Cardiac output falls with cardiogenic shock owing to abnormalities of the heart. This may be commonly seen in acute myocardial infarction. Other cardiac impairment or malfunction may be seen acutely in cardiac contusion, arrhythmia or valve rupture. Any pre-existing cardiac disease will compound this shock and the response of the heart to other types of shock.

Obstructive shock

Obstructive shock describes falling cardiac output that is caused by mechanical obstructions to the circulation. This can be the restriction of venous return to the right atrium, as in tension pneumothorax (increasing intra-thoracic pressure reduces the pressure gradient of venous return); obstruction of the pulmonary system, as in pulmonary embolism; or restriction in cardiac filling, as in cardiac tamponade. These obstructions impair the stroke volume and, subsequently, cardiac output.

Apparent hypovolemia

These causes all relate to a redistribution of blood/plasma in the vascular system. Sepsis and septic shock arises from organisms, toxins or inflammatory mediators causing peripheral vasodilation. This apparent redistribution of blood causes an increase in heart rate to maintain cardiac output, and accounts for the warm, well-perfused extremities. Subsequently, while an increase in temperature may be a hint to a diagnosis of septic shock, an index of suspicion, in combination with blood lactate or arterial blood gas analysis, may be required. This may also give an indication of the severity of the impaired cell metabolism. In the early stages of septic shock, high cardiac output may occur. This may progress to low cardiac output

Table 10.1 Classification of shock.

Type of shock	Causes			
True hypovolemia	Blood loss	Plasma loss	Saline loss	Dehydration
Apparent hypovolemia	Sepsis	Neurogenic	Anaphylaxis	Adrenal insufficiency
Obstructive shock	Pulmonary embolism	Cardiac tamponade	Tension pneumothorax	
Cardiogenic shock	Myocardial infarction	Myocardial contusion	Cardiac failure	Cardiac arrhythmia

Table 10.2 Classification of blood loss.

	Class I	Class II	Class III	Class IV
Blood loss (ml)	Up to 750	750–1500	1500–2000	>2000
Blood loss (% blood volume)	Up to 15%	15–30%	30–40%	>40%
Pulse rate (beats/min)	<100	100–120	120–140	>140
Blood pressure (mm Hg)	Normal	Normal	Decreased	Decreased
Pulse pressure (mm Hg)	Normal or increased	Decreased	Decreased	Decreased
Respiratory rate	14–20	20–30	30–40	>35
Urine output (ml/hour)	>30	20–30	5–15	Negligible
CNS/mental status	Slightly anxious	Mildly anxious	Anxious, confused	Confused, lethargic

Table 10.3 Clinical features of sepsis.

Early	Late
Restlessness and slight confusion	Decreased conscious level
Tachypnoea	Tachypnoea
Tachycardia	Tachycardia
High cardiac output	Low cardiac output
Systolic BP normal or slightly decreased	Systolic BP <80 mmHg
Oliguria	Oliguria
Metabolic acidosis, elevated blood lactate	Metabolic acidosis, elevated blood lactate
Warm, dry, suffused extremities	Cold extremities

without intervention as the responses or interventions are overcome and sepsis becomes overwhelming (Table 10.3).

Neurogenic shock arises from the loss of sympathetic control increasing the size of the vascular bed. This increased capacity of the veins to hold blood reduces venous return and cardiac output. This is seen briefly in a vasovagal attack or faint. A true neurogenic shock is an impaired sympathetic outflow, as seen in spinal transection or brainstem injury.

Anaphylaxis is a massive immune-mediated response where inflammatory mediators cause rapid vasodilation and a fall in vascular resistance and venous return.

Adrenal insufficiency/endocrine shock involves acute adrenal failure when a sudden lack of cortisol results in reduced vascular resistance and venous return.

Clinical features

In true hypovolaemia, the cause may be obvious. There is a reduction in blood flow to the organs. The severity of the hypovolaemia can then be assessed and measured by the changes seen in each organ (Table 10.2). Cold, clammy extremities are seen, owing to a capillary refill time of greater than 2 seconds. The lack of blood volume results in flat, collapsed veins.

Traumatic causes of hypovolaemia involve significant loss of blood volume in one of five places: thorax, abdomen, pelvis, within the lower limbs or exsanguination from any other site. Assessment and treatment of these areas after the A and B steps of resuscitation (the 'ABC' process is discussed later in text) could prevent the progression of shock, as well as clinical deterioration.

In cardiogenic shock, the circulating blood volume remains the same, but the sympathetic response still occurs, maintaining cardiac output. A failing pump dams back fluid in the venous system. This may be detected by an elevated jugular venous pressure (JVP) and engorged neck veins, or signs of pulmonary oedema. An electrocardiogram (ECG) may show compromised functions seen in infarction or ischaemia. Both of these are common causes of cardiogenic shock. Valve rupture or contusions may be caused by trauma. Unusual heart sounds, supplemented by echocardiography may be required to diagnose valve abnormalities.

In obstructive shock, blood is again dammed back in the venous system, and engorged, dilated neck veins may again be present. Penetrating trauma may be the cause in tension pneumothorax or cardiac tamponade, although both these and pulmonary embolism can occur without trauma. All these three are immediate life-threatening conditions. Tension pneumothorax can be identified by auscultation with no breath sounds, and hyper-resonance on percussion on the affected side. A deviated trachea can occasionally be seen. Cardiac tamponade is identified with muffled heart sounds. A focused assessment sonography in trauma (FAST) may clinch the diagnosis. A pulmonary embolus may be suspected by decreased air entry, D-dimer blood tests, ECG changes and, ultimately, perfusion or CT scans.

Apparent hypovolaemia may be identified by a dynamic, high-cardiac-output circulation with pyrexia in early sepsis. Late sepsis may resemble hypovolaemic shock (Table 10.3). Neurogenic shock, anaphylaxis and adrenal insufficiency may only become apparent through examination, index of suspicion and patient history.

Principles of management

The airway, breathing, and circulation (ABC) steps of resuscitation take precedence. The concerns are maximising oxygen delivery and improving cardiac output. Therefore, oxygen administration and fluid infusion are the first steps in the treatment of shock. While such treatment is instigated, a full patient assessment is undertaken, and attempts can be made to achieve a definitive diagnosis. The ABC process involves the following steps:

1. Examine the <u>A</u>irways to ensure there are no obstructions to oxygen delivery. Oxygen should be given in a non-rebreathing mask at 15 litres per minute.
2. Examine the neck and chest to ensure air entry is not obstructed, and check <u>B</u>reathing to ensure gas exchange is not impaired. Listen to heart sounds.
3. Good intravenous access with short and wide cannula is needed. The <u>C</u>irculation is assessed to optimise blood delivery to vital organs and restore perfusion. In adults, fluid administration is with warmed crystalloids at a rate of 10 ml/kg if normotensive, and 20 ml/kg if hypotensive. If class 3 or 4 hypovolaemic shock is present, give blood early. If a patient is exsanguinating through a visible wound, apply firm pressure. Surgery may be required to prevent further blood loss – that is, 'switching off the tap' in Figure 10.1.

An ECG will detect arrhythmias, ischaemia or infarction, and help identify the cardiogenic components of shock.

Checking the capillary refill time (longer than 2 seconds being a sign of reduced perfusion), temperature, and character of pulse may all give further clues before progressing to patient history (trauma/administration of drugs, known adrenal disease).

If septic shock is suspected, give the appropriate antibiotics promptly.

Inotropic support (e.g. noradrenaline) may be needed to improve cardiac output, particularly in late septic shock.

The response to treatment is important, since shock is a dynamic event. The assessment and reassessment of the patient for improvement or deterioration is essential.

Monitoring

The basic parameters such as pulse, BP, respiratory rate and temperature are all measured. ECG leads and a pulse oximetry sensor are attached. Pulse oximetry may be unreliable in a patient who is peripherally shut down.

Central venous pressure monitoring is an accurate guide to the administration of fluid volume replacement and venous return to the right atrium. This optimises output, making use of the principles of Starling's law.

Monitoring of the clinical response to any intervention and restoration of fluid volume can be seen in the improvement in organ function. An accurate assessment of organ response is with urinary catheterisation and the measurement of hourly renal output. Urine output should be 0.5 ml/kg/hour. Urea and electrolytes, arterial blood gases and lactate levels all allow the impact and progress of treatment or shock to be assessed.

While fluid resuscitation refills the system, efforts must be made to prevent continued loss. This may involve surgery.

Refractory shock

It is necessary to reassess the underlying causes in case of shock that fails to respond to intravenous fluids. There may be more than one cause for shock; the possible causes include:

1. Underestimation of the degree of hypovolaemia.
2. Failure to arrest haemorrhage.
3. Presence of underlying obstructive causes (e.g. cardiac tamponade or tension pneumothorax that has since developed).
4. Underlying sepsis.
5. Secondary cardiovascular effects of pump failure.

There may be a full response to resuscitation – for example, in sepsis, where support of the cardiovascular system with the appropriate intravenous antibiotics resolves the cause.

There may be a transient response – for example, in hypovolaemic shock, where blood loss is replaced but ongoing, and operative treatment may be required to stop the loss.

There may be no response to treatment, requiring urgent operative resuscitation, or the quick consideration of another cause of shock.

SUMMARY

A working knowledge of the causes and possible effects of shock is important for the practice of dentistry in its widest sense. Prompt recognition and treatment is critical.

REFERENCES

American College of Surgeons Committee on Trauma. *Advanced Trauma Life Support (ATLS)*, 9th edition; 2012.

Royal College of Surgeons of England. *Care of the Critically Ill Surgical Patient*, 3rd edition; 2010.

MULTIPLE CHOICE QUESTIONS

1. Which of the following is the best definition of the term 'shock'?
   a) Shock is the alteration of the circulation in which inadequate perfusion leads to cellular damage, dysfunction and failure of major organ systems.
   b) Shock is the acute alteration of the circulation in which reduced perfusion leads to cellular damage, dysfunction and failure of major organ systems.
   c) Shock is the alteration of the circulation in which inadequate perfusion leads to cellular damage and failure of major organ systems.
   d) Shock is the acute alteration of the circulation in which inadequate perfusion leads to cellular damage, dysfunction and failure of major organ systems.
   e) Shock is the acute alteration of the circulation in which inadequate cardiac output leads to cellular damage, dysfunction and failure of major organ systems.

   Answer = D

2. Which of the following does not impair venous return to the heart?
   a) Reduced blood volume.
   b) Increased intrathoracic pressure.
   c) Venoconstriction.
   d) Spinal transection.
   e) Lack of cortisol.

   Answer = C

3. In what types of shock would engorged neck veins be an anticipated clinical sign?
   a) Cardiogenic and apparent hypovolaemic.
   b) True hypovolaemic and cardiogenic.
   c) Obstructive and apparent hypovolaemic.
   d) Cardiogenic and obstructive.
   e) True and apparent hypovolaemic.

   Answer = D

4. In class 3 true hypovolaemic shock, which of the following is seen?
   a) Blood loss of 25%.
   b) Increased pulse pressure.
   c) Urine output of 15 ml/hour.
   d) Respiratory rate of 25 breaths/minute.
   e) Lethargic mental status.

   Answer = C

5. Which of the following is not a sign of reduced tissue perfusion?
   a) Increased respiratory rate.
   b) Reduced urine output.
   c) Cool peripheries.
   d) Restlessness and anxiety.
   e) Capillary refill time of >2 seconds.

   Answer = E

6. Which of these is not an accurate guide to the treatment of hypovolaemic shock?
   a) Temperature.
   b) Central venous pressure.
   c) Urine output.
   d) Pulse.
   e) Respiratory rate.

   Answer = A

7. Which of these is not an immediate life-threatening cause of shock?
   a) Blood loss of 1.5 litres.
   b) Cardiac tamponade.
   c) Anaphylaxis.
   d) Tension pneumothorax.
   e) Myocardial infarction.

   Answer = A

8. Which of the following parameters are compatible with class 2 hypovolaemic shock?
   a) Normal BP, increased pulse pressure, pulse 125.
   b) Normal BP, decreased pulse pressure, pulse 120.
   c) Normal BP, normal pulse pressure, pulse 120.
   d) Normal BP, increased pulse pressure, pulse 120.
   e) Normal BP, decreased pulse pressure, pulse 125.

   Answer = B

9. What does Starling's law refer to?
   a) Heart rate.
   b) Myocardial arrhythmias.
   c) Myocardial contractility.
   d) Myocardial contusion.
   e) Blood pressure.

   Answer = C

10. Which of the following pre-existing patient factors influences the response to shock?
    a) Pacemaker.
    b) Beta blocker medication.
    c) Patient at the extremes of age.
    d) Steroid insufficiency.
    e) All of the above.

    Answer = E

CHAPTER 11
Musculoskeletal disorders

F Birrell, M Greenwood and RH Jay

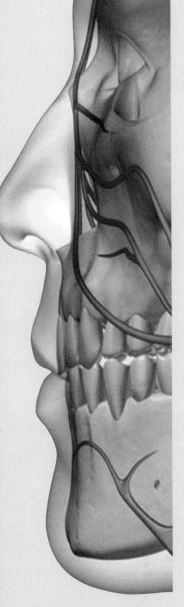

Key topics

- Major musculoskeletal disorders, and arthritis in particular.
- Impact of musculoskeletal disorders on dentistry.

Learning objectives

- To be familiar with the more common musculoskeletal disorders that dentists may encounter.
- To understand how musculoskeletal disorders may impact on the provision of dental care.

Essentials of Human Disease in Dentistry, Second Edition. Mark Greenwood.
© 2018 John Wiley & Sons Ltd. Published 2018 by John Wiley & Sons Ltd.
Companion website: www.wiley.com/go/greenwood/human-disease-in-dentistry

Introduction

There are many ways in which disorders of the musculoskeletal system can impact on dental management. For example, cervical spine involvement may lead to poor neck extension, disorders of bones may impact on surgical management and muscular disorders can cause difficulties with the safe provision of intravenous sedation or general anaesthesia.

Musculoskeletal problems are diagnosed by recognising the pattern of disease (Table 11.1). Duration divides acute arthritis (<6 weeks duration) and chronic arthritis (≥6 weeks). Inflammation is found in varying degrees in all types of arthritis, but osteoarthritis typically has mild or short-lived inflammation, as compared to the prolonged and/or severe inflammation of a true inflammatory arthritis, such as rheumatoid arthritis. The presence of deformity strongly suggests chronicity, but the type of deformity is often diagnostic (e.g. ulnar deviation of the hands in rheumatoid arthritis).

If one joint is involved (monoarthritis), then infection, crystal arthritis or seronegative arthritis are the likely causes. Involvement of two to four joints (oligoarthritis) is most commonly caused by seronegative arthritis. Polyarthritis involves five or more joints.

The impact of the disease on the patient's activities of daily living are very important. Functional limitation is a significant consideration in determining treatment.

Classifying musculoskeletal problems

The key distinction is the presence of inflammation. All the disorders shown in Table 11.2 have prominent inflammatory elements. They are known collectively as 'seronegative arthritides'.

In contrast, the presence of inflammation in a second group of disorders is mild, or absent and mechanically driven. These disorders include osteoarthritis, back and neck pain, and sports injuries. Finally, there are connective tissue disorders, where the defect is immunological, but the main manifestations are distant from the joint. Such disorders include Sjögren syndrome, systemic lupus erythematosus (SLE), scleroderma and myositis.

Table 11.1 Key features for the diagnosis of joint disease.

Features	Findings
• Timing	Acute versus chronic
• Inflammation	Yes/no
• Deformity	Yes/no (mild/moderate/severe)
• Pattern	Mono/oligo/polyarthritis
• Impact	
• Impairment	For example, bent knee
• Activity restriction	Cannot walk
• Participation	Cannot go to the pub

Table 11.2 Seronegative arthritides and disorders with prominent inflammatory components.

Rheumatoid arthritis
Psoriatic arthritis*
Enteropathic*
Ankylosing spondylitis*
Reactive arthritis*
Juvenile idiopathic arthritis
Crystal arthritis (gout, pseudogout)

*These are collectively known as 'seronegative arthritides', remembered with the mnemonic 'PEAR'.

Osteoarthritis

Osteoarthritis is a mechanically driven, but biochemically mediated, disease of synovial joints. It is a group of allied diseases where there is an imbalance between cartilage synthesis and degradation. It is characterised by pain, tenderness, decreased range of movement and variable inflammation. There are changes to the cartilage and classical radiographic changes, as will be described.

In clinical practice, the presence of pain plus typical changes on radiographs is generally accepted for diagnosis.

Clinical features

Signs of generalised osteoarthritis are often found in those with one painful joint. The typical pattern is involvement of the hands, knees and hips, although foot disease may often be unrecognised.

Symptoms

Patients complain of localised pain that, in the case of the hip, is increased on weight bearing. Advanced disease causes non-weight-bearing/nocturnal pain (probably due to raised intraosseous pressure). There may be short-lived or absent early-morning joint stiffness, or no symptoms.

Signs

In the hand, outgrowths known as 'nodes' may be seen on the fingers. Distal interphalangeal (DIP) nodes (towards the end of the finger) are termed as 'Heberden's nodes', whereas proximal interphalangeal (PIP) nodes are termed as 'Bouchard's nodes' (Figure 11.1). There is generalised muscle wasting.

The radiographic signs of osteoarthritis are summarised in Table 11.3. A radiograph of a knee joint showing the changes of osteoarthritis is shown in Figure 11.2.

Risk factors for osteoarthritis

In primary osteoarthritis, there is incomplete understanding of the aetiology. The incidence and prevalence increase with age, and it is usually more common in women. Osteoarthritis is

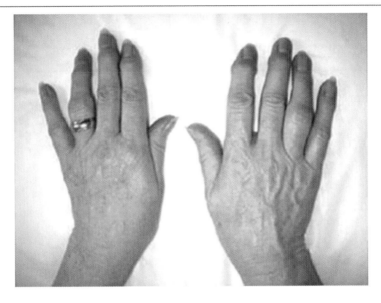

Figure 11.1 Osteoarthritis in the hands.

Table 11.3 Radiographic signs of osteoarthritis.
Joint space narrowing
Osteophytes
Sclerosis
Subchondral bone cysts

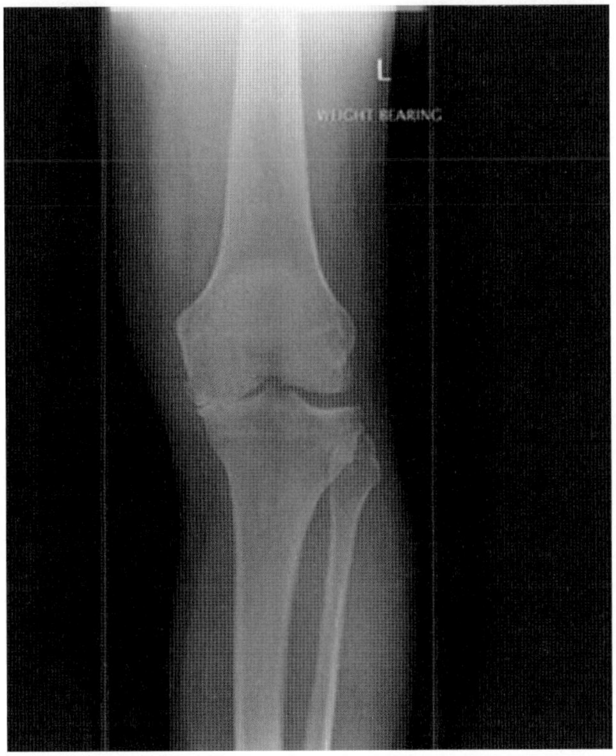

more common in occupations and populations where the load on joints is greater, for example, in the obese and runners (knee). There are recognised genetic associations for some subgroups.

Secondary osteoarthritis occurs earlier with more predictable severity in damaged joints – for example, after a cruciate ligament injury of the knee.

Demographic changes

The incidence of osteoarthritis is increasing; this is mainly due to the ageing population. There is estimated to be at least a 40% increase in the numbers needing total hip replacements (THRs) in the future.

Management

The management of osteoarthritis can be divided into pharmacological and non-pharmacological methods.

The pharmacological route relies on analgesics, particularly NSAIDs, starting with topical and progressing to oral if needed. Recent evidence shows that paracetamol has all of the toxicities of an NSAID, but does not have a clinically important benefit in osteoarthritis, so there is no longer a routine recommendation that paracetamol be the first oral agent. Indeed, many rheumatologists would never use it, especially in combination with other more effective NSAIDs such as ibuprofen or naproxen. Injections of steroids may also be used, but hyaluronan is not recommended.

Non-pharmacological methods include exercises to develop musculature – for example, in the lower limb, exercises to develop the quadriceps muscle, weight loss and the provision of aids. Education and support are also valuable.

Surgical treatment is discussed later in the text. It is reserved for recalcitrant cases.

Figure 11.2 Radiographic changes of osteoarthritis (see Table 11.3).

Rheumatoid arthritis

Rheumatoid arthritis is an autoimmune systemic inflammatory illness, characterised by symmetrical joint inflammation and variable extra-articular features. It may be defined according to the criteria shown in Table 11.4, derived from the American College of Rheumatology.

In clinical practice, the presence of symmetrical joint swelling with prolonged early morning stiffness (≥30 min), lasting for 6 weeks or longer, is generally accepted.

Clinical features

The typical pattern is of involvement of the peripheral joints, including the upper and lower limbs, but sparing the DIP joints.

Symptoms

There will be pain in or around the joint, sometimes with myalgia (muscle pain), which may be increased in the morning or with rest (gelling). The early morning stiffness of ≥30 min may be severe or prolonged. Patients may have dry eyes, dry mouth or other extra-articular symptoms.

It is important to recognise that rheumatoid arthritis is a multisystem disorder that may involve diverse systems. A summary is given in Table 11.5.

Signs

On examination, there is a 'boggy swelling' of affected joints that may be hot, tender and sometimes red. Typical deformities seen are the swan-neck/boutonnière deformity of the fingers (so-called due to their shape), or a Z-thumb. Classically, there is ulnar deviation at the metacarpophalangeal (wrist) joints (Figure 11.3).

Periarticular signs of rheumatoid arthritis include rheumatoid nodules (rubbery swellings, typically over elbows or other extensor surfaces, although they can be found anywhere). Bursitis/tenosynovitis may also be seen.

Extra-articular signs are seen in Sjögren syndrome. Osteoporosis may be seen.

Table 11.4 American College of Rheumatology criteria used to define typical rheumatoid arthritis.

Symmetrical arthritis
Hand joints
At least three areas
Morning stiffness
Rheumatoid nodules
Serum rheumatoid factor
Radiographic changes

Table 11.5 The multisystem nature of rheumatoid arthritis.

Cardiovascular
- Myocarditis
- Pericarditis
- Valve inflammation

Respiratory
- Pulmonary nodules/fibrosis

Renal
- Amyloidosis

Liver
- Hepatic impairment

Skin
- Palmar erythema
- Subcutaneous 'rheumatoid' nodules

General
- Malaise
- Anaemia of chronic disease
- Thrombocytopaenia

Radiographic signs of rheumatoid arthritis

The radiographic signs of rheumatoid arthritis are summarised in Table 11.6, and shown in Figure 11.4.

Burden of rheumatoid arthritis

Rheumatoid arthritis affects around 1% of the population, and is twice as common in women as compared to men. There is an increasing incidence and prevalence after age 50.

Management of rheumatoid arthritis

Education with regard to the nature of the disease is important. Various splints and devices can be used for joint protection. Analgesics, including NSAIDs, are used. There have been many developments in recent years of disease-modifying anti-rheumatic drugs (DMARDs). DMARDs aim to reduce symptoms and prevent joint damage. They require very close monitoring to check for side effects, which can be significant. They are slow in their action.

Recent advances in rheumatoid arthritis treatment are summarised in Table 11.7.

Reactive arthritis

Reactive arthritis is an autoimmune inflammatory condition, triggered by an infection characterised by (usually self-limiting) inflammation of one or more joints. It is a clinical diagnosis based on the development of a typical mono- or oligoarthritis,

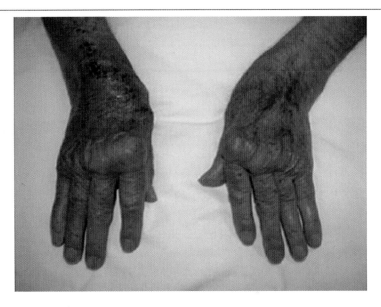

Figure 11.3 Clinical features of rheumatoid arthritis – ulnar deviation of the hands.

Table 11.6 Radiographic signs of rheumatoid arthritis.
Early
• Periarticular osteoporosis
• Periarticular erosions (action of synovitis on the 'bare area' of bone)
Late
• Joint space narrowing
• Subluxation/dislocation
• Ankylosis

developing 10–14 days after being triggered by a gastrointestinal or genitourinary infection.

Clinical features

Monoarthritis or oligoarthritis of large joints occur most commonly the knee. Therefore, septic arthritis may need to be excluded by joint aspiration. A triggering infection, for example, by *Campylobacter* or *Salmonella*, can be identified in up to 50% of cases, and should be actively sought to aid effective treatment.

Reiter's syndrome may be found. This is an association of reactive arthritis with conjunctivitis and urethritis. Reiter's syndrome may be associated with a rash of the hands and feet, histologically indistinguishable from psoriasis. Keratoderma blennorrhagica is the name given to the rash on the hands and feet.

Viral infections, especially parvovirus B19 and Coxsackie viruses, can cause reactive polyarthritis with a rheumatoid arthritis-like pattern, but which is self-limiting.

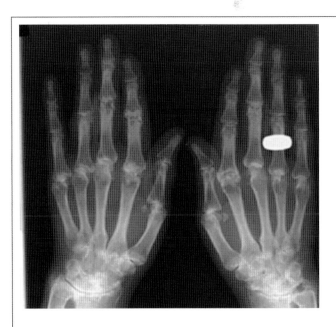

Figure 11.4 Radiographic features of rheumatoid arthritis (see Table 11.6).

Signs and symptoms

The signs are consistent with the pattern of involvement. Symptoms include pain and morning stiffness in the affected joint(s). Symptoms may be improved by exercise or NSAIDs.

Radiographic signs of reactive arthritis

There are usually no radiographic changes. If radiographic changes are seen, then a reconsideration of the diagnosis should take place.

Table 11.7 Recent advances in rheumatoid arthritis treatment.

- Parenteral methotrexate
- Combination therapy: 'triple therapy' (methotrexate/sulfasalazine/hydroxychloroquine methotrexate/leflunomide)
- Anti-TNF agents ('biological therapy')
- Infliximab (humanised anti-TNF mouse monoclonal antibody)
- Adalimumab (fully human anti-TNF monoclonal antibody)*
- Certolizumab (PEGylated monoclonal)
- Golimumab (fully human anti-TNF monoclonal antibody)
- NICE guidance requires that two DMARDs (including methotrexate) be used prior to anti-TNF therapy
- Anti-CD20 monoclonal (rituximab)
- Anti-IL-6 (tocilizumab)
- Anti-CTLA4 Ig (abatacept)

Commonly used

- Hydroxychloroquine
- Sulfasalazine
- Leflunomide
- Myocrisin®
- Oral steroids (not usually regarded as DMARDs, but does slow erosions, probably with greater morbidity)

Less commonly used

- Minocycline
- Ciclosporin
- Azathioprine
- Penicillamine

*Caution, due to infection risk – especially dissemination/tuberculosis, autoimmune disease such as SLE and potential for increased primary or recurrent malignancy. DMARD = disease-modifying antirheumatic drug; TNF = tumour necrosis factor.

Management of reactive arthritis

Reactive arthritis is usually self-limiting. NSAIDs are usually beneficial, and DMARD therapy may occasionally be needed. There is a 50% recurrence rate.

Other joint disorders

Juvenile chronic arthritis may lead to an increased incidence of caries and periodontal disease, owing to difficulties in maintaining good oral hygiene. In addition, if the temporomandibular joint (TMJ) is involved, facial growth may be disturbed.

As mentioned earlier, one of the early signs of the development of rheumatoid arthritis may be stiffness of the fingers, particularly in the early morning ('early morning stiffness'), which usually decreases during the day. In more advanced disease, the direction of the fingers appears to drift away from the thumb – 'ulnar deviation'. The onset is often slow, but it can be acute with malaise, fever and joint pain. There is anaemia that is normocytic and normochromic – the so-called 'anaemia of chronic disease'. Treatment in the early stages is usually with NSAIDs. Second-line treatment includes a variety of agents such as gold and the chemotherapy agent methotrexate (this may lead to folic acid deficiency, with the potential for secondary oral problems). Corticosteroids have been used for treatment, as have antimalarial medications. The mainstay of physical treatment involves occupational therapy, and includes household device modification – for example, modified toothbrush handles and modified kitchen appliances. The recommendation of electric toothbrushes to aid oral hygiene in these and other patients with musculoskeletal disorders should be considered. Felty's syndrome consists of rheumatoid arthritis, splenomegaly leading to leukopaenia, anaemia and lymphadenopathy.

The skin disorder psoriasis may have an associated arthritis that usually resembles a less severe version of rheumatoid arthritis. The arthritis may be deforming, and is termed 'arthritis mutilans'. Blood tests are normal; oral lesions are rare. Occasionally, treatment might be with methotrexate.

Gout may be of a primary or secondary type. In primary gout, raised serum levels of uric acid lead to deposition of urates especially in joints, leading to arthritis. In secondary gout, certain drug treatments may precipitate the condition. An alcoholic binge can instigate gout in those predisposed to it. Gouty tophi may occur where masses of urate crystals become deposited in joints or extra-articular sites – for example, the subcutaneous nodules of the helix of the ear. The classic joint affected by gout is that of the great toe. Gout may lead to renal failure. The treatment in an acute attack is usually indomethacin, but longer-term maintenance requires allopurinol, which decreases uric acid production.

Disorders mainly involving soft tissues

Ankylosing spondylitis is a chronic inflammatory disease affecting the spine, mainly seen in young males. Over 90% of cases are HLA B27 positive – the disease is partly genetically determined. There is ossification of ligaments and tendons, and the onset is insidious. The patient often complains of low back pain. A quarter of the patients may develop eye lesions. Patients may also have aortic valvular disease or cardiac conduction defects. As intervertebral ossification develops, the radiograph takes on a so-called 'bamboo spine' appearance. The spinal curvature results in the patient developing a stooped 'question mark'–shaped posture. Treatment is with anti-inflammatory medications. There are implications for general anaesthesia, and these are discussed later in the text.

Marfan syndrome is an autosomal dominant condition that comprises skeletal, ocular and cardiovascular malformations.

The patients are conspicuously tall and have lax ligaments. They are predisposed to lung cysts, leading to the risk of pneumothorax. Ocular lens dislocation can occur. Aortic dissection is possible, leading to aortic and mitral incompetence. The palatal vault is high, and there is an increased incidence of TMJ dysfunction.

In Ehlers–Danlos syndromes, the patient's principal complaints are of lax joints and easy bruising (due to deficient platelet function). The skin is elastic, and there is a predisposition to mitral valve prolapse. This disorder of collagen formation may be autosomal dominant, but some types are recessive.

Muscular disorders may be of relevance in dental treatment. Duchenne muscular dystrophy is a sex-linked disorder comprising widespread muscle weakness. This tends not to affect the head and neck, but may be relevant in terms of ease of access to treatment or the provision of general anaesthesia/sedation (owing to the effects on respiratory muscles). The affected muscles appear to be enlarged, known as 'pseudohypertrophy'. Cardiomyopathy and respiratory impairment may occur.

Acquired myopathies include polymyositis and dermatomyositis (the latter if there is an associated skin disorder). These are rare and immunologically mediated inflammatory myopathies comprising pain and muscle weakness. There are often circulating autoantibodies present. The female incidence is twice that of males. Speech and swallowing may be difficult. The characteristic rash may occur in up to one-third of polymyositis cases, which consists of a butterfly-shaped violet rash across the bridge of the nose and cheeks. There may be associated Raynaud's disease (a vasospastic disorder resulting in the excessive reaction of extremities to cold) or other connective tissue disorders – for example, Sjögren syndrome. Treatment often involves corticosteroids.

Cranial (giant cell) arteritis and polymyalgia rheumatica (PMR) are disorders of blood vessels that cause muscle pain due to ischaemia. Inflammation and luminal obliteration of medium-sized arteries occur. Giant cells may be found histologically. The affected area may be cranial/temporal, or more widespread in the case of PMR. In cranial arteritis, the eye can be involved, leading to blindness. In this form of arteritis, there is a unilateral throbbing headache usually affecting middle-aged or older females. A biopsy of the temporal artery confirms the diagnosis. To prevent blindness, early administration of prednisolone is mandatory if the disorder is suspected.

Ischaemic pain may be felt in the muscles of mastication, and this must be differentiated from TMJ pain. Unlike TMJ pain, it tends to have a later onset (middle aged or older), and there is no diurnal variation. The pain is more severe, and there is increased ESR. In trigeminal neuralgia, the pain may be associated with mastication, but the ESR is normal, and it may thus be differentiated from cranial arteritis. In cases of PMR, a similar age and sex distribution are seen as compared to cranial arteritis.

Management of fractures and joint replacements

A *fracture* may be defined as the breaking of a part, especially a bone. Various types of fractures are recognised. A fracture may be *simple* or *comminuted*. The latter suggests that the bone is in several pieces. A *greenstick fracture* refers to a fracture that is an incomplete break, where one side of a bone is broken but the other is merely bent. Greenstick fractures are commonly seen in children. Fractures may also be *closed*, meaning that the soft tissue coverings remain intact, or may be *open* or *compound*, when the soft tissue covering is also disrupted.

The principle of fracture treatment is that the fracture should be repositioned to its original anatomical state (termed 'reduction'), and then secured by 'fixation'. It is essential to obtain direct access to the fracture site in most cases; as a result, the procedure is known as 'open reduction and internal fixation' (ORIF). Various methods of fixation can be used, ranging from wires to screws to plates, usually made of titanium. Once the fracture has been reduced and fixed, the soft tissue envelope is carefully repaired.

Occasionally, fractures can be treated conservatively if function is adequate and the fractured bony components are well aligned and stable. One example could be a fractured mandibular condyle that is minimally displaced with a normal dental occlusion. Such cases are usually treated without operative intervention. This would be described as 'conservative management'.

It may be possible in some cases to treat a fracture in a closed manner by manipulation. This is often unsatisfactory, however, since the bone fragments may not be stable after they have been manipulated. Such management would be described as a 'closed reduction'.

Joint replacements

Joint replacements are indicated when the natural joint is so affected by disease that both function and pain experienced by the patient are unacceptable. The most commonly replaced joint is that of the femoral head where it articulates with the pelvis – a 'hip replacement'. This is usually described as a total hip replacement (THR), as both the femoral head and the acetabulum are replaced.

Patients who are assessed for THR have several factors that need to be considered. Effects on daily living are clearly important, and will vary to some extent with the lifestyle of the individual. Most surgeons are keen to delay THR for as long as possible since, if the procedure is carried out at a very young age, a further procedure will inevitably be required, although the mechanical components have a lifespan of several years.

Joint replacements may be carried out in patients with osteoarthritis or rheumatoid arthritis. The former is more common, since rheumatoid arthritis is a multisystem disorder. However, joint replacements are also performed in patients with rheumatoid arthritis, and these may on occasion be carried out in some of the smaller joints. Occasionally, a procedure known as *arthrodesis* is opted for, which involves the surgical induction of joint ossification between two bones. In arthrodesis, the surgeon will place the limb or digit in a conformation that is the most useful – a position of function.

In patients who have had joint replacements, antibiotic prophylaxis is not indicated when they are about to undergo a dental procedure that may cause a bacteraemia.

Metabolic bone disease and calcium

Physiology of calcium metabolism

Calcium is required for a wide range of bodily functions, including the electrical stabilisation of nerve and muscle membranes, and the formation of hydroxyapatite, the main mineral component of bone. It is absorbed from the gastrointestinal tract, stimulated by vitamin D, and is carried in the blood. Approximately half of plasma calcium is bound to albumin, where it is inactive, and half is ionised or 'free' calcium, which is metabolically active.

A normal adult ingests about 1 g of elemental calcium daily, of which 20% is absorbed, and 80% passes into the faeces. Of the extracellular free calcium pool, about 0.5 g per day is exchanged with bone calcium. The renal glomeruli filter 10 g of calcium per day, of which 9.8 g is reabsorbed by the tubules. The remaining 0.2 g is lost in the urine, balancing dietary absorption in the steady adult state. These various calcium fluxes are under hormonal control by vitamin D and parathyroid hormone (PTH).

Vitamin D is a fat-soluble vitamin derived from cholesterol, and structurally related to steroid hormones. It occurs in two forms, ergocalciferol (vitamin D_2) and cholecalciferol (vitamin D_3), which have equivalent metabolic pathways and actions. Cholecalciferol is synthesised in the skin through the action of sunlight, and both forms are absorbed from dietary sources (vitamin D_2 from plants and vitamin D_3 from animals). Vitamin D undergoes two hydroxylation steps to reach its active form. The liver converts it to 25-hydroxyvitamin D, and the kidney creates the active form of 1,25-dihydroxyvitamin D, which is also known as *calcitriol*. The liver also inactivates vitamin D by hydroxylation at the 24 position, creating 24,25-dihydroxyvitamin D. The active form stimulates bone formation and the gastrointestinal absorption of calcium.

PTH is a peptide hormone secreted from the four pea-sized parathyroid glands embedded in the thyroid gland in the neck. Its function is to maintain a stable level of ionised calcium in the plasma. The parathyroid cells themselves monitor the plasma level, increasing PTH secretion in response to falls in plasma calcium, and suppressing secretion if calcium rises. PTH raises the plasma calcium by three main mechanisms: it causes bone resorption, stimulates vitamin D hydroxylation by the kidneys (which increases gastrointestinal calcium absorption) and promotes renal calcium retention and phosphate loss (Figure 11.5).

Calcitonin, a peptide hormone that is secreted by the interstitial cells of the thyroid gland, and which antagonises some actions of PTH, has some therapeutic uses in metabolic bone disease and hypercalcaemia. In normal human physiology, however, it is essentially inactive.

The principal bone cells are the *osteoblasts*, which lay down both the protein matrix of bone and the hydroxyapatite mineral content, and the *osteoclasts*, which resorb bone. In normal bone remodelling and repair, a local cycle of activity occurs on the surface of the bone. Osteoclastic resorption of the mineral and bone matrix is followed by the osteoblastic deposition of a new matrix, which then becomes mineralised, and the bone then enters a quiescent phase, with osteocytes covering the surface.

Investigations of bone disease

When metabolic bone disease is suspected clinically, there are two groups of tests that are commonly used: *biochemical tests* give information about bone metabolism, hormones and cellular activity; and *imaging tests* are used to detect abnormal bone structure, and to locate areas of abnormal function.

Biochemical tests

The 'bone biochemistry profile' is a set of blood tests that reflect calcium/bone metabolism. It includes the following:
- Total serum calcium.
- Serum albumin is measured to allow the correction of calcium for abnormal protein levels. Albumin often falls in systemic illness and gives a falsely low calcium, that is, a low total calcium when the metabolically active ionised calcium is normal. Measurement of ionised calcium can be performed in clinical laboratories, but is not a routine test.
- Phosphate levels are often not useful, as they can fluctuate widely depending on diet. Phosphate levels rise in renal failure, due to impaired phosphate excretion, and falls in hyperparathyroidism, since PTH stimulates phosphate excretion and calcium retention by the renal tubules.
- Alkaline phosphatase (ALP) is a plasma enzyme derived from osteoblasts. Levels rise in conditions with increased bone turnover – for example, fracture healing, vitamin D deficiency, bone metastases and Paget's disease. Levels are higher in children due to normal bone growth. ALP is also released from the liver and bile ducts, and is part of the routine 'liver function tests'. In cases of doubt about the origin of a raised ALP, isoenzymes can be separated to distinguish hepatobiliary and bone isoforms.

Plasma PTH and 25-hydroxyvitamin D can also be measured, and several other blood and urine markers of bone turnover and osteoblastic/osteoclastic activity are available for specialist use.

Imaging tests

The simplest form of bone imaging is the plain radiograph, which gives good information about the abnormalities of bone structure.

Bone scintigraphy is a radioisotope scan using a radiolabel that is taken up and deposited by osteoblasts. The whole

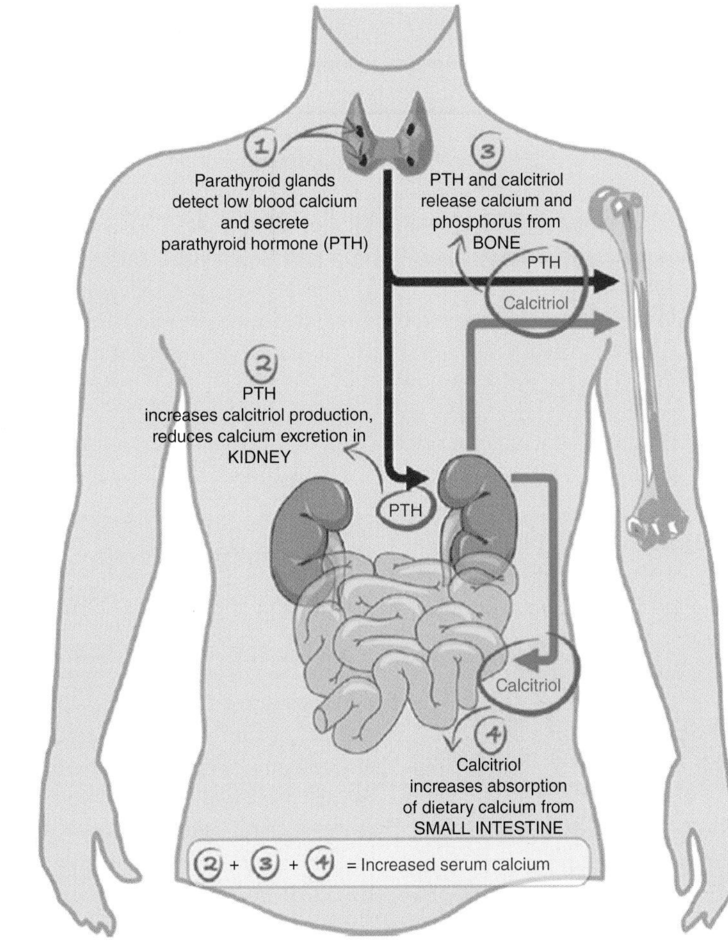

Figure 11.5 Calcium metabolism.

skeleton is then imaged using a gamma camera. 'Hotspots' indicate increased turnover – for example, fractures, metastases and Paget's disease. It is useful for locating the site of a bone abnormality, but other evidence is required to distinguish the various causes. The most common use is in screening for bone metastases in cancer. Multiple myeloma can affect the bones without causing hotspots, and an X-ray skeletal survey is used in this condition.

Dual-energy X-ray absorptiometry (DEXA) scanning is used to assess osteoporosis. It gives a highly reproducible measure of the amount of bone mineral per area of the image, and can be used to monitor the effects of treatment, as well as in diagnosis.

Other imaging techniques include CT and MRI scanning, and are used in special situations.

Drugs used in bone disease

Calcium and vitamin D supplements are available in a variety of doses and formulations. They are commonly used in the malnourished elderly, and as an adjunct to other treatments for osteoporosis. The UK pharmaceutical spelling of vitamin D_3 is now 'colecalciferol'. Active forms of vitamin D are used, particularly in renal disease, where renal 1-hydroxylation is impaired. Calcitriol is 1,25-dihydroxyvitamin D, and alfacalcidol is 1-hydroxyvitamin D. The main side effect of vitamin D preparations is hypercalcaemia, and monitoring is essential in patients on pharmacological doses or active metabolites.

Bisphosphonates (formerly called 'diphosphonates') are used in a variety of conditions to inhibit osteoclastic bone resorption. They all contain two phosphate groups attached to a carbon atom, and are incorporated into hydroxyapatite in place of calcium phosphate. When ingested by osteoclasts, they cause apoptosis, thus inhibiting bone resorption.

Both oral and intravenous preparations are available, and the drugs, although effective orally, have poor gastrointestinal bioavailability. Absorption is impaired by the presence of calcium in the intestine, and they should therefore be taken on an empty stomach, separated from food and calcium preparations. The most common side effect of oral treatment is oesophagitis, caused by direct mucosal contact with the tablet, which should therefore be swallowed with a large glass of water.

Alendronate and *risedronate* are bisphosphonates that are commonly used as once-weekly preparations in osteoporosis. *Zoledronate* is used intravenously for bone metastases, Paget's disease and hypercalcaemia of malignancy, as well as for osteoporosis. Several other bisphosphonates (all ending in '-dronate') are available.

Dental patients who are taking bisphosphonates need special care when undergoing dental extractions. The altered bone metabolism seen with high-dose therapy can lead to osteonecrosis, which is a significant clinical problem. The risk is less with the commonly used low-dose weekly oral therapy for osteoporosis, but cases have been reported, usually following several years of treatment. In terms of management, the risk of osteonecrosis is minimised in much the same way as the risk of osteoradionecrosis, but extractions should be avoided where possible and ideally carried out before the bisphosphonate therapy is started.

Established osteonecrosis is rarely treated surgically as trimming/removal of bone usually induces necrosis of further bone on an advancing front. Use of topical chlorhexidine gel to keep the necrotic bone clean has been reported. Osteonecrosis is discussed in Chapter 15 (titled 'Adverse drug reactions and interactions').

Strontium ranelate is now rarely used in osteoporosis, since it increases the risk of thrombosis and ischaemic heart disease.

Denosumab is an antibody against RANKL, a cytokine that stimulates osteoclasts. Its use is increasing, and it is given by subcutaneous injection every 6 months for osteoporosis. It is also used for bone metastases. It is a potent osteoclast inhibitor that can cause hypocalcaemia, so vitamin D and calcium nutrition must be adequate before treatments starts. It can also result in osteonecrosis of the jaw.

Parathyroid disorders

Hypoparathyroidism

Failure of PTH secretion may occur due to autoimmune destruction of the glands, but the most common cause is surgical removal – for example, in total thyroidectomy for thyroid cancer. The glands may be unintentionally removed or damaged in any thyroid operation, and observation for this complication is part of routine postoperative care.

The symptoms are those of hypocalcaemia, which leads to neuromuscular excitability. Paraesthesias, numbness and tingling occur in the extremities and around the mouth. Muscle cramps occur, and the arms may adopt the characteristic posture described as 'main d'accoucheur' (obstetrician's hand), in which the wrist is flexed, and fingers flexed at the metacarpophalangeal joints, bringing the fingertips and thumb together at a point. If this is not present spontaneously, it may be induced by the application of a sphygmomanometer cuff – called 'Trousseau's sign'. Percussion with the fingertip over the facial nerve may elicit contraction of the facial muscles – called 'Chvostek's sign'.

Severe hypocalcaemia with these features is a medical emergency, and requires intravenous calcium infusions to prevent complications such as convulsions or laryngospasm, which obstructs the airway. The diagnosis is confirmed by finding hypocalcaemia with a low PTH level. Long-term treatment of hypoparathyroidism is not by means of PTH replacement, but rather by giving active metabolites of vitamin D such as calcitriol or alfacalcidol. Doses are adjusted to maintain a normal total and ionised calcium level.

Several rare, genetic disorders of PTH metabolism may be associated with disordered dentition. These include MEDAC syndrome, with multiple autoimmune endocrine deficiencies and candidiasis, and pseudohypoparathyroidism, in which end-organ resistance to the action of PTH is associated with mental retardation, short stature and abnormal bone and tooth development.

Hyperparathyroidism

The most common cause of an elevated level of PTH, above the laboratory 'normal range', is the appropriate response of the parathyroid glands to calcium levels. This 'secondary hyperparathyroidism' may be seen in the nutritional deficiency of calcium or vitamin D, or in gastrointestinal malabsorption. It is also seen in renal failure as a result of the failure in the activation of vitamin D to the 1,25-hydroxy form by the kidneys, and due to the fall in plasma calcium that occurs when a high phosphate concentration causes precipitation of calcium and phosphate in tissues. In secondary hyperparathyroidism, although the PTH level is raised, the plasma calcium is normal or low.

'Primary hyperparathyroidism' refers to autonomous overproduction of PTH, resulting in hypercalcaemia. The most common cause is a benign adenoma of one of the four parathyroid glands, with hyperplasia of all four glands occurring in a minority of cases.

The clinical features are those of hypercalcaemia, and the phrase 'stones, bones, abdominal groans and psychic moans' is a useful mnemonic for this. There is an increased risk of kidney stones, which can cause infections or severe colicky pains radiating from the loins to the groin area. Hypercalcaemia also impairs the kidney's ability to concentrate the urine, which can result in an increased volume of dilute urine. Bone pain can be diffuse and nonspecific, and its cause can be unrecognised until the diagnosis of hyperparathyroidism is made biochemically. The gastrointestinal effects of hypercalcaemia include peptic ulceration, pancreatitis and constipation. Hypercalcaemia can cause mental apathy, confusion and depression.

Hyperparathyroidism is not the only cause of hypercalcaemia. It also commonly occurs in malignant disease, either due to the production of PTH-related peptide (PTHRP) or from the effects of bone metastases. Another rare cause of hypercalcaemia is increased calcium or vitamin D intake from supplements or from calcium-containing antacids and milk in patients with acid-related indigestion – the so-called 'milk–alkali syndrome'.

Investigation of primary hyperparathyroidism is initially by finding high plasma calcium with inappropriately high PTH. If the PTH is suppressed, then other causes of hypercalcaemia need to be sought. These include malignant disease and excessive vitamin D or calcium intake. The parathyroid glands can be imaged by a variety of methods, including isotope scanning, ultrasound and MRI.

Severe hypercalcaemia can result in dehydration and renal failure. It is a medical emergency that requires intravenous rehydration and intravenous bisphosphonate therapy while the underlying cause is being investigated.

The treatment of primary hyperparathyroidism is by surgical excision of the offending gland or glands. Where surgery is not possible and the patient is symptomatic, the PTH and calcium levels can be controlled by cinacalcet, a drug that mimics the effect of calcium on the parathyroid cells.

Important bone conditions

Osteomalacia and rickets

Vitamin D deficiency may be caused by poor sunlight exposure, poor dietary intake or intestinal malabsorption of fat and fat-soluble vitamins. Activation of vitamin D is impaired in renal failure. Major deficiencies are rare in developed countries, but subclinical deficiencies are common in frail, institutionalised older people with poor nutrition.

In childhood, deficiency of vitamin D or calcium results in rickets, with abnormal bone growth, soft bones and characteristic skeletal deformities. These include enlarged epiphyses, visible at the costochondral junctions as a row of swellings called the 'rickety rosary'. Ends of the long bones of the limbs are also enlarged and visible on X-rays. Softening of the bones causes bowing, particularly of the tibia and fibula, and the pull of the diaphragm on the lower ribs can cause a horizontal groove along the lower border of the thorax, called 'Harrison's sulcus'.

In adults, the same deficiency is called 'osteomalacia'. The bones are fully formed, so deformities do not occur in the same way as in children, and the symptoms are often vague and nonspecific. Diffuse bone or muscle pain and tenderness can occur, and weakness of the proximal muscles may give a waddling gait. Occasionally, tingling and tetany can occur due to severe hypocalcaemia. Demineralisation of the bones occurs due to secondary hyperparathyroidism. *Looser's zones* are focal areas of demineralisation around nutrient arteries visible on X-rays, and pathological fractures may occur in severely weakened bones.

The biochemical changes of osteomalacia and rickets are inconsistent, but characteristically include low levels of calcium and phosphate, and raised alkaline phosphatase. The 25-hydroxyvitamin D level will be low, and the PTH level should be raised. The secondary hyperparathyroidism may succeed in maintaining a normal plasma calcium.

Treatment of both osteomalacia and rickets is by supplementing calcium and vitamin D. In simple dietary deficiency, oral supplementation is effective. In malabsorption, the underlying gastrointestinal cause should be investigated and treated, and higher doses may be needed. In renal disease, the active metabolites alfacalcidol or calcitriol are required.

Osteoporosis

Osteoporosis is a generalised skeletal disorder in which the risk of fracture is increased due to loss of bone mineral and matrix, and deterioration in the microarchitectural structure of bone. It is asymptomatic until a fracture occurs, the most common sites being the vertebrae, distal radius and neck of femur. Pain due to vertebral crush fractures often goes unrecognised, and the diagnosis can be missed. Osteoporosis is considered to be a major risk factor for periodontal disease.

The key investigation is the measurement of bone mineral density by DEXA scanning. The World Health Organisation has defined *osteoporosis* as a bone density of >2.5 standard deviations below the population mean for young adults. Bone density declines with age, and deteriorates more rapidly in women after menopause. Therefore, asymptomatic osteoporosis is very common in the older population.

Risk factors for the development of osteoporosis include age, female gender, early menopause and family history. It is aggravated by dietary calcium and vitamin D deficiency at levels too mild to cause full-blown osteomalacia. Several medical conditions can aggravate osteoporosis, including malabsorption, chronic liver disease and chronic kidney disease. Corticosteroid treatment is a major cause of osteoporosis. All patients on long-term steroid treatment should have their bone density monitored, and preventive treatment given to those at high risk.

The most common treatments for osteoporosis are low doses of alendronate or risedronate, given orally once a week. Other bisphosphonate preparations are sometimes used, both oral and intravenous. In addition to bisphosphonates, calcium and vitamin D supplements are given to those with reduced dietary intake. Denosumab (see the preceding text) is a relatively new treatment whose use is increasing.

Bone metastases

Bones are a common site to which malignant diseases of other organs can metastasise. The most common sources of secondary spread to bone are carcinomas of the bronchus, breast and prostate. However, a wide range of other tumours too can cause bone metastases, and primary bone tumours can also occur, although they are uncommon. Myeloma, a malignant proliferation of plasma cells in the bone marrow, can also cause lesions in the bone.

Most tumours within the bone may stimulate osteoclastic bone resorption – the so-called 'lytic' metastases, seen on radiographs as holes in the bone. Some tumours, particularly prostate cancer, stimulate osteoblastic bone formation, resulting in 'sclerotic' metastases, which appear on radiographs as areas of increased bone mineralisation.

Bone metastases may be asymptomatic, or may present as bone pain; a sudden, spontaneous fracture; or with pressure on adjacent structures such as the spinal cord or nerve roots in vertebral metastases. Radioisotope bone scanning helps to detect the site of metastases, and then imaging by plain X-ray, or sometimes CT or MRI scanning, shows the extent of the tumour and any potential complications.

Radiotherapy is a useful palliative measure for bone pain or to prevent the progression of a metastasis likely to cause a fracture or compression. Sometimes, the surgical fixation of a bone or decompression of the spinal cord is required. Bisphosphonates, usually given intravenously in high doses, are effective at preventing the progression of bone deposits in a variety of solid tumours and in myeloma, and these drugs are being used increasingly in the treatment of malignancy. Denosumab has similar actions, but has not yet been investigated so extensively.

Paget's disease of bone

Sir James Paget also described a form of localised cancer affecting the nipple, not to be confused with the bone disease of the same name. Paget's disease of bone is a condition of uncertain cause, in which the organised maintenance of bone structure by a regulated cycle of osteoclasts and osteoblasts is disrupted. Bone resorption and formation become disorganised, resulting in a characteristic 'moth-eaten' appearance on a radiograph. The bone cortex can become thickened, and deformity can occur.

The disease is characteristically focal in nature, and may slowly spread along a limb bone from one end to the other (Figure 11.6). Just as with bone metastases, it is often asymptomatic, but may present with pain, fractures or compression of adjacent structures. The last of these is particularly true when it affects the skull, which becomes thickened, resulting in a characteristic head shape. Expansion of the bone at the base of the skull can cause compression of the hindbrain and spinal cord at the foramen magnum, in addition to cranial nerve compression, most commonly affecting the auditory nerve and causing deafness.

Treatment is with bisphosphonates to inhibit the excessive, disorganised bone resorption. Surgery is sometimes needed for fractures or for compression of the spinal cord or nerves.

In Paget's disease, there may be hypercementosis of the teeth. This leads to potential difficulties in dental extractions, and therefore many teeth may need to be removed surgically rather than by conventional extraction.

Other bone disorders

Osteopetrosis is a condition in which the bone density is increased but the bone is nevertheless structurally weak. The patient may suffer fractures or bone pain, but is often asymptomatic. Decreased marrow activity may lead to anaemia. Some patients who are taking corticosteroids may be prone to osteomyelitis or fracture. Dental extractions should be as atraumatic as possible; flaps should be avoided if possible, and antibiotics prescribed until healing is complete.

Osteogenesis imperfecta is a rare autosomal dominant condition consisting of a defect in collagen formation; it may be

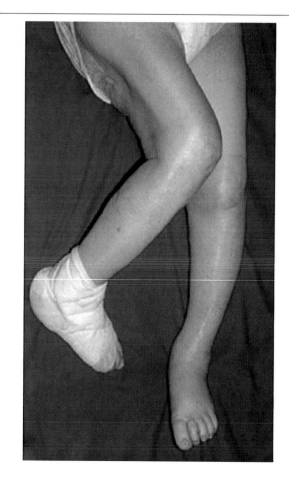

Figure 11.6 A patient with Paget's disease of bone, showing the characteristic 'sabre tibia'.

associated with dentinogenesis imperfecta. The patient may give a history of multiple fractures secondary to relatively minor trauma. There may be associated deafness, and the patients tend to have weak tendons and bruise easily. Heart valve problems may occur, and, as a result, patients are potentially at risk from infective endocarditis. It is rare to fracture the jaw as a result of dental treatment. Classically, the patients have blue sclera.

Fibrous dysplasia is a condition that may affect a single bone (monostotic) or multiple bones (polyostotic). It consists of an area of bone replaced by fibrous tissue, leading to local swelling. In the polyostotic disorder, there may be associated skin pigmentation (café au lait patches). Rarely, there may be mucosal pigmentation. The disease is usually self-limiting, although, in the craniofacial region, it may interfere with occlusion and vision.

Cleidocranial dysplasia occurs as a result of a defect in membrane bone formation, inherited as autosomal dominant. It mainly involves the skull and clavicles. The head is large and brachycephalic, with a persistent frontal suture. The clavicles are absent or stunted, conferring the ability to approximate the shoulders anteriorly. There is a persistent deciduous dentition, often unerupted permanent teeth, dentigerous cysts and supernumeraries.

In cases of polyostotic fibrous dysplasia associated with pigmentation and precocious puberty in females, the name 'Albright's syndrome' is applied. Radiographically, the bone has a ground-glass appearance. Serum calcium and phosphate levels are normal. Surgical treatment consists of 'debulking' lesions.

Dental treatment in patients with musculoskeletal disorders

There are many musculoskeletal conditions that can impact on dental management. The key to safe management is a thorough history underpinned by a working knowledge of common musculoskeletal disorders. A summary of the conditions that may present in a history is given in Table 11.8.

Table 11.8 Points in the history that may be of relevance in musculoskeletal disease.

Bone disorders

- Osteoporosis
- Rickets and osteomalacia
- Fibrous dysplasia
- Paget's disease of bone
- Osteopetrosis
- Cleidocranial dysostosis
- Osteogenesis imperfect
- Achondroplasia

Joint disorders

- Osteoarthritis
- Rheumatoid arthritis
- Psoriatic arthritis
- Gout
- Mouth opening
- Neck extension

Muscular disorders

- Duchenne muscular dystrophy
- Polymyositis
- Dermatomyositis
- Cranial arteritis
- Polymyalgia rheumatic

Other disorders

- Ankylosing spondylitis
- Marfan syndrome
- Ehlers–Danlos syndromes
- Reiter's syndrome

Patients with a history of radiotherapy to the head and neck are at risk of osteoradionecrosis (ORN). This is considered further in Chapter 15 (titled 'Adverse drug reactions and interactions').

Patients with osteoporosis may have impaired respiratory function due to vertebral collapse leading to secondary thoracic deformity. In fibrous dysplasia patients, there is an increased risk of hyperthyroidism or diabetic tendency. In patients with Paget's disease of bone, there is the possibility of cardiac failure and chest deformities. Patients with osteogenesis imperfecta may have secondary chest deformities that can be severe enough to compromise respiratory function. This has clear implications for the provision of general anaesthesia and intravenous sedation. Patients with osteopetrosis may be anaemic or taking corticosteroid therapy, and both of these will have a bearing on management.

Patients with syndromes

Patients with Marfan syndrome may have lung cysts that predispose to spontaneous pneumothorax. This syndrome is an autosomal dominant connective tissue disease. Minor signs include a high arched palate. Curvature of the spine in an anteroposterior direction (kyphosis) or lateral direction (scoliosis) may lead to thoracic deformities and respiratory impairment. Patients with Ehlers–Danlos syndromes are predisposed to mitral valve prolapse and cardiac conduction defects. Patients with ankylosing spondylitis may have decreased mouth opening, making dental treatment problematic and making intubation difficult for general anaesthesia. The characteristic spinal deformity seen in ankylosing spondylitis may lead to thoracic deformity with consequent effects on respiratory function. These patients can also have associated aortic valve problems.

Patients with joint disorders

It is important to remember that patients with osteoarthritis and rheumatoid arthritis may have impairment of cervical spine mobility. This can pose problems in positioning the patient appropriately, both to allow dental treatment and to facilitate the provision of general anaesthesia (where the neck needs to be extended). Patients with rheumatoid arthritis may wear a cervical collar. Corticosteroid treatment may be used in both types of arthritis. Usually, however, these will be administered locally to the affected joint(s). It should be remembered that rheumatoid arthritis is a multisystem disorder. The TMJ is often asymptomatic in patients with rheumatoid arthritis, but there may be impaired function leading to limitation in mouth opening. Patients with gout are at an increased risk of hypertension, ischaemic heart disease, diabetes mellitus and renal disease.

As mention earlier, it is not considered necessary to prescribe prophylactic antibiotics for bacteraemia-producing procedures in patients who have undergone joint replacement surgery.

Other disorders

The possibility of cardiomyopathy and respiratory disease should be taken into account when treating muscular dystrophy patients. Such patients are also sensitive to the muscle relaxant suxamethonium, and are predisposed to developing malignant hyperthermia if a general anaesthetic is administered.

SUMMARY

There are many musculoskeletal conditions that can impact on dental management. The key to safe management involves obtaining a thorough history. Conceptually, musculoskeletal disorders are best defined as bone disorders, joint disorders and muscular disorders. Some musculoskeletal disorders are associated with disease in other body systems.

Musculoskeletal conditions cover a wide spectrum of disease. The dental practitioner should be wary about their potential implications for dental treatment.

REFERENCES

BMJ. Available from: http://www.bmj.com/specialties/rheumatology.

SIGN 142: management of osteoporosis and prevention of fragility fractures. http://www.sign.ac.uk/guidelines/fulltext/142/index.html.

MULTIPLE CHOICE QUESTIONS

1. Bisphosphonates work by:
   a) Stimulating osteoblasts.
   b) Inhibiting osteoclasts.
   c) Inhibiting osteoblasts.
   d) Stimulating osteoclasts.
   e) Stimulating both osteoclasts and osteoblasts.
   Answer = B

2. Which of the following does not cause osteonecrosis of the jaw?
   a) Oral bisphosphonates.
   b) Subcutaneous denosumab.
   c) Intravenous bisphosphonates.
   d) Phosphorus poisoning.
   e) Oestrogen replacement therapy.
   Answer = E

3. Features of hypocalcaemia include:
   a) Skin pigmentation.
   b) Bone pains.
   c) Tetany.
   d) Dehydration.
   e) Diarrhoea.
   Answer = C

4. Which of the following statements about vitamin D is false?
   a) It is derived from cholesterol.
   b) It is activated by hydroxylation in the kidney.
   c) It inhibits parathyroid hormone release.
   d) Deficiency in adults results in osteomalacia.
   e) It is made through the action of sunlight.
   Answer = C

5. Primary hyperparathyroidism:
   a) Is a normal response to the deficiency of vitamin D.
   b) Is a cause of hypercalcaemia.
   c) Is often caused by renal failure.
   d) Is most commonly caused by parathyroid cancer.
   e) Is usually congenital, associated with defective dentition.
   Answer = B

6. Which of the following is *not* a risk factor for osteoporosis?
   a) Age.
   b) Female gender.
   c) Male gender.
   d) Family history.
   e) Early menopause.
   Answer = C

7. Rheumatoid arthritis:
   a) Is one of the autoimmune disorders.
   b) Is confined to the joints.
   c) Has no cutaneous manifestations.
   d) Has the same aetiology as osteoarthritis, but affects different joints.
   e) Has no potential cardiac manifestations.
   Answer = A

8. Ulnar deviation of the hands is characteristically seen in:
   a) Paget's disease of bone.
   b) Osteoarthritis.
   c) Psoriatic arthritis.
   d) Rheumatoid arthritis.
   e) Ankylosing spondylitis.
   Answer = D

9. 'Sabre tibia' is seen in:
   a) Osteoarthritis.
   b) Lower limb osteotomy.
   c) Rheumatoid arthritis.
   d) Ankylosing spondylitis.
   e) Paget's disease of bone.
   Answer = E

10. Which of the following is *not* normally seen in radiographs of joints affected by osteoarthritis?
    a) Joint space widening.
    b) Joint space narrowing.
    c) Osteophytes.
    d) Sclerosis.
    e) Subchondral bone cysts.
    Answer = A

CHAPTER 12

Dermatology and mucosal lesions

K Staines

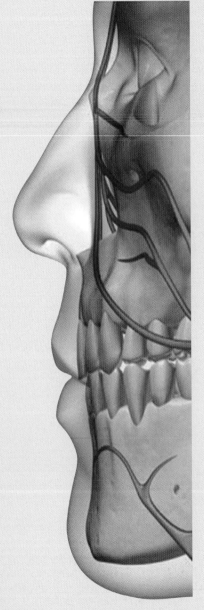

Key topics

- Major dermatological disorders
- Dermatological disorders and their oral manifestations

Learning objectives

- To be familiar with some of the more common dermatological disorders.
- To have knowledge of those dermatological disorders with oral/perioral manifestations.

Essentials of Human Disease in Dentistry, Second Edition. Mark Greenwood.
© 2018 John Wiley & Sons Ltd. Published 2018 by John Wiley & Sons Ltd.
Companion website: www.wiley.com/go/greenwood/human-disease-in-dentistry

Introduction

A patient may present to a general dental practitioner with skin lesions noted as an incidental finding. In other circumstances, patients may present with oral lesions potentially related to existing skin lesions. It is therefore appropriate that a dental practitioner have a working knowledge of common dermatological diseases, with a special focus on conditions with oral manifestations. Understanding the process of assessment of skin lesions and developing a working knowledge of systemic diseases with dermatological and oral manifestations are hence important from a dental surgeon's perspective.

Assessment of a patient presenting with skin lesions

The assessment of a patient presenting with lesions involving the skin is not dissimilar to the process undertaken for a patient presenting with oral mucosal disease.

The *history of presenting complaint* should include:

- Site.
- Spread.
- Duration.
- Fluctuation in size.
- Persistence.
- Exacerbating and relieving factors.
- Any associated symptoms, such as pain or pruritus.
- Overall impact of the skin complaint on the patient's quality of life.

The medical history should include a complete systems review, with particular focus additionally on:

- Any past history of dermatological symptoms, investigations and treatment received, including the clinical setting in which this occurred.
- A history of atopy (hypersensitivity to multiple triggers).

The drug history should include a detailed account of any medications that the patient is taking, including use of over-the-counter medications and herbal remedies. Details of any topical or systemic medication taken currently or in the past by the patient for the skin complaint should be elicited and recorded. Also, details about any allergies to drugs or contact allergens should be elicited, and their nature recorded.

The family history should include the relevant family history of skin disorders.

The social history should include details of factors such as occupation and travel. It is important to record how the skin complaint may be having an impact on the patient's occupation and social life.

Examination of the patient's skin relies mainly on inspection and palpation of the lesions. Good lighting is important. It is vital that consent be sought from the patient, and the underlying rationale for such an examination be explained and understood by the patient. It is often impractical and, indeed, possibly inappropriate to expect the patient to expose skin, which may be perceived as unusual in a dental clinic. Hence, examination is often confined to skin areas that are exposed or can be exposed with minimal effort, such as by rolling up the sleeves. In a specialist setting, provided adequate privacy and clinical justification is present, further examination of unexposed skin areas may be indicated and appropriate. The need for a chaperone is important.

Key points to focus on during examination includes determining the sites that are involved and ascertaining whether the disease is localised/generalised and symmetrical/asymmetrical in terms of distribution. Examples of clinical signs to look out for include:

- Rashes.
- Blisters.
- Alterations of pigmentation.

Nail changes

'Nail dystrophy' is the collective term used to describe pathological changes consequent to nail disease.

Nails should be examined with appropriate lighting and, if possible, with magnification. To avoid any changes in blood flow, it is important to ensure that the digits are not pressed against any surface. A range of conditions, including trauma, infection, inflammation and tumours, may result in nail changes and signs. Lichen planus (LP), for example, may involve the nails, resulting in signs ranging from longitudinal ridging to onycholysis (distal separation of nail from the nail bed).

Finger clubbing

Finger clubbing results from an increased curvature of the nail plate, in both transverse and longitudinal dimensions. The angle between the nail plate and nail bed is increased to greater than 180°. An increase in the overall dimensions of the fingertip is generally evident. Potential causes of finger clubbing are discussed in Chapter 1 (titled 'Clinical examination and history taking').

Diseases of the skin

Eczema and dermatitis

'Dermatitis' is a broad term describing inflammation of the skin. In lay terms, both 'dermatitis' and 'eczema' are often used synonymously. The patient may complain of itchy, uncomfortable, reddened skin. Clinical examination may reveal erythematous areas of skin with a degree of swelling and scaling. Fissuring and thickening may also be observed. Due to the pruritus that may accompany these changes, patients often scratch the affected areas and cause secondary changes such as excoriation.

Atopic dermatitis (eczema)

'Atopy' describes the condition of excessive hypersensitivity to multiple triggers commonly encountered within the environment, such as pollen, dust mite and perfumes. Atopic individuals may develop, often early in childhood, a chronic inflammatory skin condition, aptly termed 'atopic eczema'. The condition tends to wax and wane, while in some patients it may pursue a chronic course. In a minority of patients, the condition may persist into adult life.

The regions involved tend to be localised around the thinnest skin areas in contact with the allergen, such the periorbital skin or wrists.

Urticaria

The underlying pathophysiology is the subepithelial release of inflammatory mediators such as histamine, resulting in tissue swelling and formation of wheals, accompanied by intense pruritus. Urticaria may be triggered by various factors, including certain medications, infections, autoimmune processes and foods. In a significant number of cases, no underlying cause is identified. Urticaria can be classified as either acute or chronic.

Contact dermatitis

The underlying pathophysiology is a T-cell-mediated hypersensitivity reaction to one or more allergens such as nickel or epoxy resin. A careful history is critical, including detailed accounts of work or hobbies where allergens may be encountered. Epidermal skin patch testing may help identify one or more allergens.

Disorders of keratinization

Psoriasis

Psoriasis is a complex immune-mediated disease. There is a genetic predisposition, as well as other risk factors such as smoking, obesity, alcohol and vitamin D deficiency. Clinical presentation typically will include well-defined erythematous plaques with scaling (Figure 12.1). Nail involvement may also be a feature. Psoriasis is mainly a skin disease; however, various

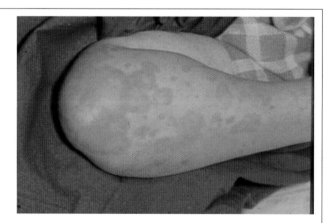

Figure 12.1 Psoriasis.

malignancies, as well as autoimmune and cardiovascular diseases, are reported to occur more frequently in this group of patients. The underlying mechanisms remain elusive. Additionally, these patients have increased risk of developing other associated disorders such as psoriatic arthritis.

Infections and skin manifestations

Superficial bacterial skin infections

Folliculitis

Folliculitis is an infection of one or more hair follicles, resulting in localised discomfort aggravated by movement of the hair within the follicle. Itching is an additional prominent symptom. The usual infecting organism is *Staphylococcus aureus*. Infection is initially localised, with pustules forming within the individual hair follicles. With persistence of infection, the adjacent skin may become involved, with erythema and crusting becoming evident. Folliculitis may follow a chronic course.

Impetigo

Impetigo is another skin infection that has *Staphylococcus aureus* (and/or *Streptococcus pyogenes*) as the causative agent(s). This is a highly transmissible skin infection that may arise *de novo* or complicate pre-existing skin disease such as eczema.

Deep bacterial skin infections

Cellulitis

Cellulitis is an infection of the skin and subcutaneous tissues, usually caused either by *Streptococcus pyogenes* or *Staphylococcus aureus*; however, other bacteria including anaerobic and gram-negative bacteria may be implicated. Rarely, fungal infections in immunocompromised patients may result in cellulitis. The presence of a predisposing skin condition such as eczema or a venous leg ulcer that impacts on the skin barrier may increase the risk of cellulitis. Systemic immunosuppression, diabetes mellitus, poor circulation and lymphoedema may also predispose towards the development of cellulitis.

Clinical signs are pain, erythema and localised oedema. The legs are most frequently involved, but cellulitis can occur anywhere on the body. Spread of infection into the bloodstream may result in septicaemia, while local spread may result in abscess formation, or necrotising fasciitis. Facial cellulitis, especially in children, may result in meningeal spread, causing meningitis.

Erysipelas

Erysipelas is a superficial form of cellulitis typically caused by Streptococci; however, other bacteria such as *Staphylococcus aureus* may be involved It often presents as an erythematous facial rash.

Bacterial exanthemata

Lyme disease

Lyme disease is caused by *Borrelia burgdorferi*. Transmission occurs through tick bites; however, only a minority of patients will be aware of the bite, which simply manifests as a red flat lesion (macule) or raised lesion (papule) on the skin. Then the patient, over the course of days or weeks, characteristically develops multiple systemic symptoms such as fatigue, lymphadenopathy and skin lesions.

Syphilis

Syphilis is a sexually transmitted infection (STI) caused by the bacterium *Treponema pallidum*. It is characterised by periods of active disease and latent periods, with the patient remaining infective throughout the course.

Transmission may occur through sexual activity involving infected ulcers in the genital and anal areas, the lips or mouth. Microtrauma and transmission through infected blood during sexual activity is also possible. Other less common routes of transmission include through the placenta to an unborn baby, and by way of blood transfusions, although screening of blood products prevents this.

- *Primary syphilis*: In the first stage of syphilis, a papule develops at the site of infection, which is most commonly the genital area – however, it may also be the lips or oral mucosa. The papule will rapidly form into a painless non-healing ulcer (syphilitic chancre), only to heal after several weeks. Regional lymphadenopathy will accompany the chancre.
- *Secondary syphilis*: Secondary syphilis develops 6–8 weeks following resolution of the chancre. A widespread skin rash is typically present. Oral lesions such as snail track ulceration and white patches may also develop.
- *Tertiary syphilis*: The hallmark lesion of tertiary syphilis is the gumma, which is a non-caseating granulomatous ulcerative lesion that may extend to involve underlying structures such as the bone. Skin is the most common site; however, gummata may develop on internal organs such as the liver (visceral gumma). The oral site most frequently involved is the palate. Tertiary syphilis has been historically associated with leukoplakia, which more commonly involves the tongue (syphilitic leukoplakia).

Gonorrhoea

Gonorrhoea is caused by the bacterium *Neisseria gonorrhoeae*, transmitted predominantly by means of sexual contact resulting in infection of the mucous membranes. Manifestations differ in males and female patients. Male patients may complain of a burning pain on urination, and testicular pain. Female patients tend to experience symptoms during more advanced stages of the disease, such vulvar discomfort, pus-like or bloody vaginal discharge and painful urination. Signs and symptoms may, however, be absent, despite the patient remaining infective. A rash may be present in some patients, typically presenting as small papules that turn into pustules involving the limbs, palms, soles and trunk, but sparing the face, scalp and mouth. Patients may complain of pharyngitis and oral lesions. The latter are rare, but, if present, typically present as oral ulceration with surrounding erythema and a grey pseudomembrane involving one or more mucosal surfaces.

Fungal infections (mycoses)

Fungal infections of the skin are generally mild in immunocompetent patients. In immunosuppressed patients, fungal disease can cause significant and potentially life-threatening infections. Superficial fungal infections affect the skin (outer layers), nails and hair. Examples include candidal infections and dermatophytic infections (tinea).

Tinea

This is caused by fungal organisms confined to non-living parts of the body, and hence only affect the nails and the keratinised components of hair and skin, resulting in localised inflammation partly secondary to the local immune host immune response.

Transmission is usually through direct contact with humans or infected animals (such as cats or dogs).

Localised predisposing factors include heat, humidity and macerated skin. Systemic predisposing factors include conditions such as diabetes mellitus.

Tinea pedis (athlete's foot) is probably the most well-known type of tinea infection. This infection is transmitted in environments such as swimming pools. The resultant signs are those of localised erythema and scale formation, typically involving the sole of the foot and the toe web area.

Candidal infections

Skin infections caused by *Candida* organisms are usually associated with systemic predisposing factors. Local factors include pre-existing skin diseases such as chronic eczema or psoriasis, and a warm humid climate, particularly with occlusion of the skin – for example, prolonged contact of a wet nappy in children may result in a localised candida skin infection. Examples of systemic predisposing conditions include diabetes mellitus, iron deficiency, malnutrition and immunodeficiency.

Examples of candida skin infections include:
- Intertrigo – involving the skin folds, for example, at the junction of the breast and chest in females.
- Angular cheilitis – involving the dermal portion of the corners of the mouth.
- Vulvovaginal candidiasis – vaginal and vulvar symptoms caused by yeasts, most often *Candida albicans*.
- Balanitis – involving the penile area in men.

Examples of candidal infections of the nails include:
- Onychomycosis – an infection of the nail plate.
- Chronic paronychia – a nail-fold infection.

Chronic mucocutaneous candidiasis

This term describes a range of syndromes involving immuno-logical/endocrine/congenital disorders with resultant candida infections. These infections are typically recurrent or persistent, involving multiple sites of the mucosae, skin and nail tissues. Presentation is usually in infancy or childhood. The oral mucosa may be one of the sites involved.

Oral lesions secondary to fungal infections

Oral candidiasis can result in various oral clinical conditions, some of which are listed here:

- Acute pseudomembranous candidiasis – removable white patches involving localised or diffuse areas of the oral mucosa.
- Chronic hyperplastic candidiasis – non-removable white patches involving the commissures.
- Chronic erythematous candidiasis – develops in denture-bearing areas (denture stomatitis).
- Candidal-associated lesions – such as median rhomboid glossitis, manifest with an area of rhomboid-shaped depapillation on the dorsum of the tongue.

Viral infections of the skin

Shingles

Varicella zoster virus–induced inflammation of cranial nerve and peripheral ganglia results in limited areas of involvement, confined to the dermatomal distribution of the involved nerve. Sensory nerves are most commonly involved; however, motor nerves may be involved too. One example is the involvement of the facial nerve resulting in facial paralysis in Ramsay Hunt syndrome. Trigeminal nerve involvement is most commonly that of the ophthalmic division.

The prodrome results in symptoms consistent with itching, altered sensation and pain, which is typically followed, often days later, by the development of a rash within the area involved.

The skin lesions are initially macular erythemas with vesiculation, ulceration and crust formation, unilaterally distributed within the sensory nerve dermatome, with surrounding erythema of the adjacent skin. The involved area may exhibit altered sensation, accompanied typically by severe burning pain.

Immunocompromised patients may present with bilateral or even widespread involvement beyond the confines of the affected dermatome.

Transmission risk resolves only when the lesions completely crust over.

Herpetic whitlow

Herpetic whitlow is caused by the herpes simplex virus (HSV) types I or II, typically involving the distal area of one or more fingers.

Primary infection can occur secondary to inoculation. Dental surgeons may acquire herpetic whitlow through the saliva of infected patients especially if infection control is poor – for example non-wearing of gloves.

The main symptoms are reported as pain and swelling of the affected area, and examination reveals localised erythema, blistering and painful swelling involving the distal aspect of the finger involved. A transmission risk is present and relevant for dental surgeons.

Herpes labialis 'cold sore'

Following primary infection, HSV may remain latent within the trigeminal ganglion. Reactivation may result in the development of herpes labialis, often on a recurrent basis. Precipitating factors include factors such as exposure to sunlight, and stressful or adverse events.

Clinical examination reveals a group of vesicles along the vermillion border that then ulcerate, followed by crusting.

The lesions will resolve generally over 7–10 days in immunocompetent patients, but may persist longer in immunocompromised patients.

Oral lesions secondary to viral infections

Viral ulceration may be a single episode (e.g. primary herpetic gingivostomatitis) or recurrent (e.g. recurrent intraoral herpes ulceration, or RIOHU). Oral ulceration may be secondary to a range of causes in HIV.

Epstein–Barr virus (EBV) causes oral hairy leukoplakia (OHL), which clinically appears as white patches on the lateral aspect of the tongue.

Dermatological manifestations of systemic disease

Deficiency states

Anaemia

The signs and symptoms of iron deficiency depend on the rapidity of development of the anaemia and its severity. Iron deficiency is the most common cause of anaemia. Patients may report symptoms such as fatigue and shortness of breath. Clinical examinations may yield the following signs:

- Nail changes – vertical ridging, brittleness and spoon-like shape (koilonychia).
- Angular cheilitis – erythematous lesions at the corners of the mouth.
- Atrophic glossitis – smooth, often painful tongue.
- Hair – increased loss and thinning.
- Skin – pallor.

Vitamin C deficiency (Scurvy)

Scurvy is a condition caused by prolonged deficiency of vitamin C (ascorbic acid), which is required for the formation of collagen, which in turn is a building block of connective tissue structures, including blood vessels. Vitamin C is also integral to the functioning of the immune system and for other physiological activities.

Scurvy may be seen in alcoholics, in those who have inadequate nutrition secondary to anorexia or bulimia, and in those with inflammatory bowel disease.

Pellagra

Pellagra, a disease caused by the deficiency of niacin (vitamin B_3), is characterised by the '3Ds': diarrhoea, dermatitis and dementia. Pellagra may develop as a primary process due to dietary deficiency. Also, when there is sufficient niacin (or tryptophan) in the diet, pellagra can develop as a secondary process, owing to ineffective absorption in conditions of chronic alcoholism, liver cirrhosis or inflammatory bowel disease.

Dermatological clinical features include skin lesions initially resembling symmetrical areas of sunburn, which thereafter assume a brownish discolouration. Areas affected include the hands, lower legs, face, neck and lips.

Dermatological manifestations of GI disease

The oral manifestations of Crohn's disease, which affects the gastrointestinal tract, are indistinguishable from those of orofacial granulomatosis (OFG), which occurs in the absence of Crohn's disease. The clinical manifestations of OFG are therefore characterised by chronic or recurrent swelling of the orofacial tissues, resulting in oral manifestations similar to those of oral Crohn's disease. Oral ulceration may also be present in about half of all patients, with aphthous-like ulcers being the more common ulcer type. Histopathologically, on biopsy, non-caseating granulomata are identifiable as in oral Crohn's disease; however, there is no evidence of gastrointestinal involvement in OFG.

Dermatological manifestations of endocrine disease

Hyperthyroidism

Hyperthyroidism results from excess circulating thyroid hormone causing increases in the body's metabolic rate. Skin manifestations include facial flushing, warm moist hands and hair thinning. Nail changes include nail distortion, which may additionally be complicated by a process known as onycholysis, where the nails lift off from the nail bed. Myxoedema secondary to an excess of glycosaminoglycans within the dermis results in red nodules developing within the shins (pretibial myxoedema). A goitre may be present (enlarged thyroid gland), which can be evident on inspection and/or palpation of the head and neck.

Hypothyroidism

Hypothyroidism results from abnormally reduced levels of circulating thyroid hormone, which in turn causes a reduction in the body's metabolic rate. Clinical manifestations may include dry skin, thinning of hair, nail changes and psychological disturbances, including depression. A goitre (enlarged thyroid gland) may be present, which can be evident on inspection and/or palpation of the head and neck.

Diabetes mellitus

Diabetes mellitus may result in skin problems secondary to the associated increased risk of infections such as impetigo. Diabetic dermopathy may develop in the presence of poor diabetic control, and result in harmless skin lesions that resolve with improvement in the patient's glycaemic status. A significant complication of diabetes is the risk of developing leg ulcers. The nerve and vascular complications of diabetes may result in peripheral neuropathy with reduced sensation, increasing the risk that any injury (including defective footwear) may go unnoticed, resulting in skin blisters. These blisters may develop into ulcers, and infection may then supervene, with the risk of cellulitis and gangrene as potential complications.

Cushing's syndrome

Cushing's syndrome is caused by systemic exposure to high levels of cortisol derived from exogenous or endogenous sources. The most characteristic feature is the development of a round puffy face (moon face), and also a buffalo hump – both consequences of the differential depositing of fats. Further effects include osteoporosis, fatigue, muscle weakness, hypertension, poor glycaemic control and psychological/ psychiatric manifestations.

Other potential dermal manifestations include the development of fragile skin, bruising and purpura consequent to capillary leakage, striae involving abdomen and buttocks, and excess hair growth (hirsutism).

Actinic disorders of the skin

Actinic keratoses

The clinical appearance of these lesions is typically that of well-defined, scaly, multisite lesions associated with increased thickening of the skin (hyperkeratosis and acanthosis). The lesions may exhibit changes in pigmentation – typically brown or reddish changes in coloration. There are several clinical variants of actinic keratosis – such as actinic cheilitis (involving the vermillion border of the lip), which is particularly relevant.

Prevention involves sun care advice; however, existing lesions can be treated with local excision or topical treatments options such as cytotoxic preparations (e.g. 5-fluorouracil).

Actinic cheilitis

Risk factors for actinic cheilitis include outdoor activity, fair skin and site (lower lip in particular). The clinical findings typically include dryness of the lower lip with scaling, potential colour changes, pigmentation change, atrophy and development of white patches or plaques. Actinic cheilitis is considered

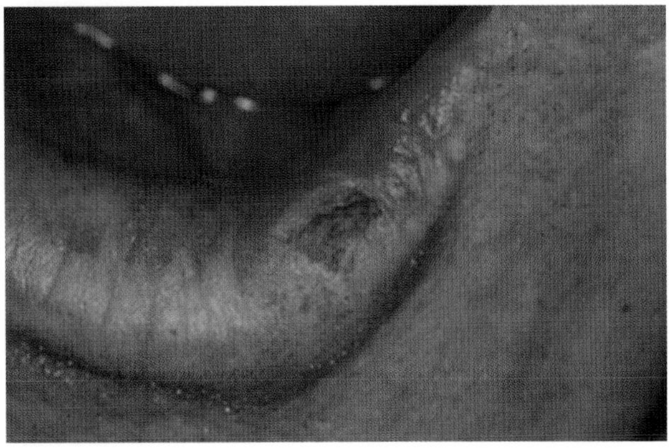

Figure 12.2 Squamous cell carcinoma of the lower lip.

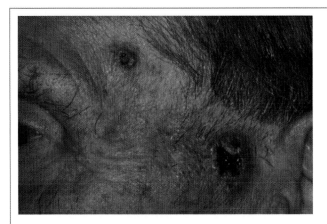

Figure 12.3 Basal cell carcinoma.

to increase the risk of malignant transformation more than two-fold. Additionally, since the risk of metastasis from a lip squamous cell carcinoma is much higher than from a skin lesion, the importance of prevention, diagnosis and treatment is even more significant.

Squamous cell carcinoma of the skin (SCC)

Squamous cell carcinoma is a malignant tumour of skin keratinocytes. Typically, lesions develop on sun-exposed skin, with approximately half of the lesions occurring in the head–neck region, and around one-quarter presenting on the upper extremities. Other associated factors may be chronic irritation and immunosuppression. Patients with fairer skin types are at a higher risk than those with pigmented skin types.

Clinical presentation is typically that of a (rapidly) enlarging painless ulcer with a margin exhibiting features of induration. The lesion may also have an area of underlying nodular swelling complicated by bleeding, crusting or an exudate. Histopathological diagnosis consequent to a tissue biopsy is required to confirm the diagnosis (Figure 12.2). Metastatic spread may occur via local draining lymph nodes.

Basal cell carcinoma (BCC)

Basal cell carcinoma is a carcinoma of the basal layer of the epidermis. It typically affects older, fair-skinned patients who have experienced actinic damage, with the facial skin often involved. Up to one-third of patients may experience multiple lesions. BCC is the most common skin cancer, approximately four times as common as squamous cell carcinoma of the skin. It most commonly affects fair-skinned individuals, and its incidence is related to sun exposure. Lesions most commonly affect the face, and may be multiple. Clinical presentation is that of a white nodule, which, if left untreated, results in the development of an ulcer with rolled margins (Figure 12.3).

As the lesions typically do not metastasise, treatment is by cryotherapy; curettage is done for small lesions, while surgery or local radiotherapy is considered for larger lesions. The lesions may recur; however, such recurrences are amenable to retreatment. Metastasis is extremely rare, and hence treatment with excision, curettage, cryotherapy or radiotherapy is often curative, with a good prognosis.

Referral of patients with suspected skin malignancy

Patients should be referred through a defined suspected cancer pathway referral (2 week rule referral) if clinical findings raises the suspicion of skin malignancy.

Keratoacanthoma

Keratoacanthoma is a benign tumour of the epidermis that is thought to arise from hair follicles. It may mimic a squamous cell carcinoma clinically, and share some features histopathologically. The facial skin is a common site. The disease manifests with the development of a symmetrical nodule with a keratin-containing central core, reaching a couple of centimetres in size, or larger in certain instances. While the lesion may resolve without any treatment and leave behind some scarring, surgical excision results in an improved aesthetic appearance.

Disorders of skin and oral pigmentation

Physiological pigmentation in the skin and oral mucosa depends on:

- Number of melanocytes (specialised pigment-producing cells present in the basal cell layer of the skin and mucous membranes).
- Amount of melanin produced by melanocytes.

External or internal causes that result in an increase or decrease in either of these parameters may result in changes of pigmentation in the skin and oral cavity. Deposits of external agents such as mercury may also cause a localised increase in pigmentation. Pigmented skin lesions are typically bluish-black or brown in colour.

External causes of pigmentation of skin

Pigmentation may occur secondary to the deposition of external agents, such as in the case of tattoos. Heavy metal deposition in skin secondary to heavy metal poisoning may result in skin pigmentation, although this is extremely rare. Actinic (sun) damage can result in changes in skin pigmentation.

Internal causes of pigmentation of skin and oral mucosa

Generalised/multiple areas of pigmentation

- *Racial pigmentation*: Pigmentation of the oral mucosa may be perfectly normal in darker-skinned individuals. There is, however, a huge range among individuals of the same race in terms of both distribution and intensity of pigmentation. This is related to melanocyte activity, as there is no difference in melanocyte numbers between dark- and fair-skinned populations.
- *Addison's disease*: Melanocyte activity is influenced by the adrenocorticotropic hormone (ACTH). ACTH levels may be increased in Addison's disease secondary to low serum cortisol levels, resulting in stimulation via hormonal hypothalamic–pituitary–adrenal feedback (HPA axis). Increased melanocyte activity may manifest as increased pigmentation of the skin and oral mucosa.
- *ACTH-producing tumours*: Some tumours, such as bronchogenic carcinoma, may produce ACTH, which can influence melanocyte activity and manifest as increased pigmentation of the skin and oral mucosa.
- *Physiologic pigmentation of pregnancy (melasma)*: This is physiologically normal, with increased pigmentation of the skin and nipples. Pigmentation may occasionally develop intraorally.
- *Peutz–Jeghers syndrome*: This is a genetically inherited syndrome that results in perioral pigmentation, which clinically looks like multiple freckles. Lip and intraoral pigmentation may be possible. The pigmentation may fade after puberty. Clinical diagnosis is important as there is a genetic risk of bowel cancer. Therefore, screening is recommended for the patient and family members.
- *Post-inflammatory melanin incontinence*: This is inflammation caused by mucosal diseases such as oral LP (OLP) or periodontal disease. It causes melanocytes to leak pigment, resulting in localised pigmentation.
- *Drug-induced pigmentation*: Some drugs such as antimalarial drugs can also cause increased pigment production and deposition, resulting in pigmentation.

Localised pigmented skin lesions secondary to melanin accumulation in the skin cells (no melanocytic proliferation)

Freckles

Freckles are typically evident on the face, most commonly in fair-skinned people, and are evident as small, brownish, non-raised pigmented lesions.

Melanocytic pigmented lesions of the skin

Solar lentigo

This is a flat pigmented skin lesion that develops secondary to ultraviolet damage proliferation of melanocytes and accumulation of melanin within the skin cells in a localised fashion. These lesions tend to arise in patients over 40–50 years of age.

Naevi

In lay terms, the most common naevus is known as a 'mole', which in medical terminology, however, is more appropriately termed a 'melanocytic naevus'. Naevi can be found on any skin surface.

Naevi are composed of groups of melanocytes forming clusters. Some naevi are acquired during life, while others are present at birth (congenital). The majority of acquired naevi can be classified into three types: junctional, compound and intradermal.

Moles are readily diagnosed on a clinical basis; however, it is important to consider more serious diagnoses such as melanoma (see the following text).

Melanoma

Melanoma is a malignancy of the melanocytes that are present in the skin and mucosae. In the UK, although it is the third most common type of skin cancer, it results in more deaths than all the other skin cancers aggregated. It can spread via lymphatics initially, and thereafter haematogenously, most commonly to the brain, liver and lung.

Melanoma most commonly arises from exposure to the ultraviolet light present in sunlight, or through the use of sunbeds. However it can also arise in non-sun-exposed areas such as the oral cavity (Figure 12.4) or nasal mucosae.

Manifestations of melanoma include either a new black or brown lesion that has developed on the skin, or indeed a

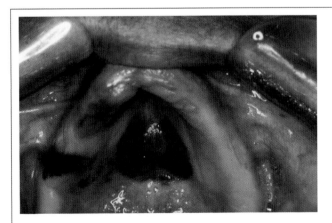

Figure 12.4 An intra-oral melanotic lesion. On biopsy, this proved to be a malignant melanoma.

pre-existing pigmented lesion such as a mole. The following changes in an existing mole should prompt urgent referral for expert assessment.

- Bleeding.
- Crusting.
- Asymmetry.
- Change to edges of lesion.
- Colour variation.
- Diameter >6 mm.

Rarely, melanomas can arise in the oral mucosa. The most common sites of oral involvement is the palate and the maxillary gingivae. Oral involvement can also occur secondary to metastatic spread. Malignant melanomas are generally clinically silent and may be mistaken for a benign pigmented lesion. Hence, with localised pigmented lesions where a definable clinical diagnosis is not possible on clinical grounds, a biopsy is required to confirm the diagnosis and exclude other differential diagnoses.

Amelanotic melanomas do not present with increased pigmentation, and instead appear as white or red lesions. They may rarely present within the oral cavity.

Pigmentation of the oral mucosa

External and internal causes of diffuse oral mucosal pigmentation are common to those outlined in the preceding text, causing diffuse skin pigmentation. Isolated/localised areas of pigmentation within the oral mucosa pose a challenge to the dental practitioner, as they cannot readily be distinguished on clinical grounds from a mucosal melanoma.

The most common pigmented lesion is an amalgam tattoo, caused by deposits of amalgam. The availability of clinically documented evidence that the pigmented lesion has been unchanged in the same area for several years and/or radiographic evidence of amalgam fragments obviates the need for histopathological confirmation. In other cases where clinical doubt exists, a biopsy may be required to confirm the diagnosis and exclude other differential diagnoses.

An oral melanotic macule is an idiopathic pigmented lesion caused by melanin deposition. It is also known as an 'ephelis'. It is considered the equivalent of a skin freckle, and has no risk of malignant transformation.

Naevi (benign melanocytic hyperplasias) are relatively uncommon within the oral cavity. Melanoma of the oral cavity accounts for less than 1% of all melanomas, and less than 2% of all malignancies of the head and neck.

Clinical management of intra-oral pigmentation

The clinical approach should be directed towards determining the potential cause and excluding potential systemic and drug induced causes. Pigmentation may be a manifestation of serious systemic disease such as Addison's disease, tumours producing ACTH and Peutz–Jeghers syndrome.

It is important to be aware that, despite the rarity of malignant melanomas within the oral cavity, these do occur. As the initial appearances are clinically similar to any other cause of localised pigmentation, any idiopathic area of pigmentation merits careful assessment, including biopsy and histopathological examination.

Autoimmune dermatological disease

LP

LP is a T-lymphocyte-driven chronic autoimmune disease that predominantly involves the stratified squamous epithelium of the oral mucosa, skin and genitalia. Current thinking is that LP has a multifactorial aetiology.

Dermatological manifestations of LP

Papular, purplish, pruritic skin lesions typically present on the flexor aspect of the forearms and shins (Figure 12.5). Scalp lesions may be present, which may result in localised hair loss. Genital involvement may be a presenting or accompanying feature with lesions, including reticular keratosis and erythema and/or ulceration. Complications of genital involvement include pain and discomfort and, in the longer term, scarring and stricture formation. Oral and genital involvement may be present concomitantly in oral vulvovaginal syndrome. Oesophageal involvement is rare, but has been described and can result in stricture formation.

Oral manifestations of LP

OLP may occur as an isolated oral disease, or in combination with skin LP and/or other mucosal diseases (such as vulvovaginal LP).

Commonly implicated aetiological factors in OLP are drugs (drug-induced OLP) or mercury (amalgam-associated OLP). Associations between hepatitis C virus infection (HCV) and autoimmune diseases such as autoimmune thyroiditis have been postulated. In clinical practice, it is often not possible to identify any potential cause or trigger.

OLP has a prevalence of around 1–2% in the UK, and is more common in middle-aged females. Clinical symptoms associated with OLP may range from being totally asymptomatic to marked soreness and pain.

Intraoral OLP lesions typically have a reticular (web-like) pattern of keratosis, involving one or more mucosal surfaces (Figure 12.6). Other patterns, such as annular (ring-like) or plaque-like keratosis, may be present. Such lesions may be associated with areas of atrophic thinning, mucosal erosion, ulceration and bullous lesions. A desquamative gingivitis (full-thickness gingivitis involving the attached gingivae with desquamation evident or demonstrable with the slight application of direct pressure) is often additionally evident, albeit not invariably. While clinical

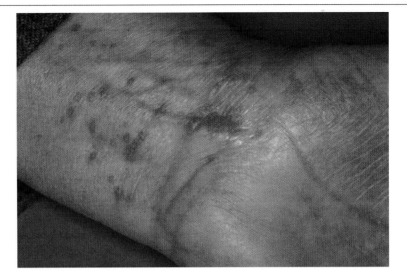

Figure 12.5 The forearm rash of a patient with LP.

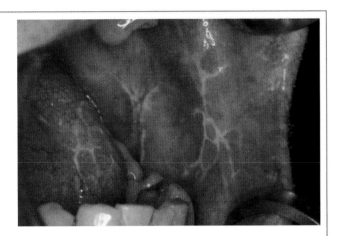

Figure 12.6 A classical intra-oral appearance of LP.

'Desquamative gingivitis' is a descriptive term identifying the presence of desquamation *and /or* erythema *and /or* erosion on the buccal aspect of attached gingivae. Desquamative gingivitis is typically associated with OLP, oral MMP and oral pemphigus vulgaris.

findings are often characteristic, histopathological confirmation of the diagnosis is often sought in specialist practice.

The World Health Organisation considers OLP as one of the potentially malignant oral conditions owing to the increased risk of malignant transformation as compared to non-affected individuals with heathy oral mucosa.

Pemphigoid

Mucous membrane pemphigoid (MMP)

MMP is an autoimmune disease whose underlying pathophysiology involves antibodies directed at antigen(s) in the epithelial basement membrane, resulting in a split and blister formation at this level. The lesions may or may not involve the skin, but they invariably tend to affect mucous membranes such as the oral, ocular and genital mucosae.

Presentation varies, depending on the severity of disease activity and extent of involvement. At one end of the spectrum, the sole manifestation may be desquamative gingivitis, while, on the other end, there may be extensive eye, oral, pharyngeal and genital involvement, with ulceration, blistering and scarring.

Skin lesions may present as itchy erythematous papules and blisters. Genital lesions may result in erosions, and, at a later stage, be complicated by scarring.

Eye involvement may present with non-specific symptoms of ocular irritation or burning. Conjunctival inflammation may be an isolated sign in one or both eyes in the early stages, while, with advanced ocular disease, the resultant complications of scarring may be evident. Long-term complications include corneal scarring and potential blindness.

Involvement of the nasal mucosa may result in ulceration with secondary crusting and/or epistaxis. Pharyngeal involvement may result in stricture formation, with consequent symptoms of odynophagia (pain on swallowing), dysphagia or even shortness of breath, depending on the level at which such narrowing develops.

Intraoral findings may include the following:

- Mucosal erosion and frank ulceration, including the hard and soft palates.
- Blister formation – may be seen intact or burst.
- Desquamative gingivitis.
- Scarring of oral mucosa.

Clinical findings require laboratory-based confirmation of the diagnosis. A tissue sample (skin or mucosal tissue) is typically sent for histopathological examination, and another sample is sent for direct immunofluorescence (DIF) analysis. Identification of IgG, IgA and C3, with linear deposits of IgG or IgA and C3 at the basement membrane zone (BMZ), would substantiate the clinical diagnosis. There are blood-based investigations that can confirm the presence of antibodies directed at the BMZ, such as indirect immunofluorescence (IF) for IgG, IgA and C3.

> *Indirect IF* as an investigation is carried out by taking a clotted blood sample, from which serum is separated. The serum (possibly containing antibodies directed against basement membrane components in case of MMP) is incubated with a substrate such as monkey oesophagus. The antibodies will then bind to the target antigen. The rest of the serum is washed away, leaving the bound antibodies, which can then be targeted with an antihuman antibody with a fluorescent marker. The resultant histopathological pattern is thereafter interpreted.

Mild cases of MMP, confined to the oral mucosa, can be managed with topical steroids such as Betnesol (betamethasone phosphate) mouthwash. In case of more severe inflammation, systemic therapy may be required. If there is extra-oral involvement, such as eye inflammation, then the treatment needs are dictated by such involvement. The management of patients with extra-oral involvement requires multidisciplinary care with medical disciplines such as ophthalmology and dermatology.

Bullous pemphigoid

The clinical presentation often involves skin lesions on sites such as the thighs and flexor aspects of the forearms. Such lesions may be pruritic eczematous or erythematous papules, coupled with large blisters. The frequency of oral mucosal involvement is low, especially compared to MMP, and hence these patients are more likely to present to physicians.

Erythema multiforme (EM), Stevens–Johnson syndrome and toxic epidermal necrolysis

EM is an acute, immunologically mediated disease in response to various antigens, with herpes simplex infection being reported as its most common trigger – termed 'Herpes-associated EM' (HAEM). About 90% of minor EM cases are caused by HSV, either following a clinically evident infection or secondary to asymptomatic shedding of the virus. Other microbial triggers are organisms such as *Mycoplasma pneumoniae*. Drugs – ranging from NSAIDs, penicillin to carbamazepine – have been reported to cause EM. Foods with additives such as benzoic acid have also been reported to trigger EM. Young adults are predominately affected, although presentation may occur at any age.

The presentation ranges from limited disease, possibly involving the oral mucous membrane, to severely widespread disease, involving multiple mucous membranes such as eyes, genitals, pharynx, mouth and skin. Oral involvement generally is with widespread ulceration and blistering. A desquamative gingivitis may be present.

Skin lesions classically have a target appearance, with the upper and lower extremities being frequent sites of involvement (Figure 12.7). Eye involvement is particularly dangerous, as it can lead to blindness.

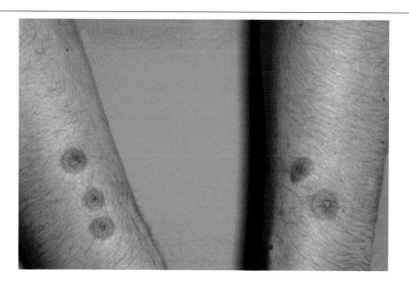

Figure 12.7 The target lesions of EM.

Traditionally, EM has been classified as *minor* or *major*, and a *chronic/recurrent* variant is also well described.

EM minor tends to involve one mucous membrane site and skin. This is the most likely form to be encountered by dental surgeons, with mucous membranes of the oral mucosa and lips being involved.

Major EM involves two mucous membrane sites and skin (involvement of less than 10% of the skin surface area). The severity of the disease is greater than that observed in minor EM.

Patients with a diagnosis of chronic/recurrent EM experience recurrences that are frequent.

Diagnosis is mainly based on clinical findings. Biopsy of a lesion may reveal certain histopathological findings. However, these are not specific enough to formulate a diagnosis. Identification of the trigger is an important part of the diagnostic process – for example, identification of a cold sore or initiation of drug therapy prior to the episode. Specialist care is recommended in all but the mildest cases. Supportive care with hydration, pain relief and antiseptic mouthwashes, provided on an outpatient basis, should be sufficient in milder cases; however, inpatient care is required in more severe cases.

Antivirals may be initiated in cases of HAEM, and antimicrobial therapy if EM is secondary to *Mycoplasma* pneumonia. In cases where EM has developed secondary to a drug, cessation of the culprit drug would be indicated. Systemic corticosteroid use is still widespread. However, there is some disagreement about its utility and safety in the literature. Topical steroid therapy for oral lesions – for example, Betnesol mouthwash – may be helpful and safe for treatment of oral lesions secondary to EM.

Stevens–Johnson syndrome and toxic epidermal necrolysis

These conditions tend to be caused secondary to a drug-induced hypersensitivity reaction. Carbamazepine is an example of such a drug. Both are now considered to be separate conditions to EM; however, they do share certain clinical features. They are significantly more severe in terms of involvement and severity, with patients being acutely unwell and hence unlikely to present initially to their dental surgeon.

The hallmark of these conditions is the severity and associated morbidity of the acute drug reaction, with oral, genital and ocular mucosal involvement in nearly all patients. Hospitalisation is required on an inpatient basis, and there is a potential need for admission to a high-dependency unit. The hallmark target lesions may be present; however, skin lesions are often atypical, large and macular, with blister formation. Differentiation between the two relies on estimation of the extent of body surface area involvement – with a less than 10% involvement indicating Stevens–Johnson syndrome, and a 30–100% involvement indicating a diagnosis of toxic epidermal necrolysis. These conditions have the potential to be fatal, with fatality rates in the literature ranging from around 5% for Stevens–Johnson syndrome to around 30% for toxic epidermal necrolysis.

Pemphigus

This group of disorders includes pemphigus vulgaris, pemphigus vegetans, pemphigus foliaceus, paraneoplastic pemphigus and other variants. Antibodies are directed against desmosomal antigens such as Desmoglein (DSG) 1 and DSG 3, and also to several non-desmoglein antigens.

Pemphigus vulgaris

Pemphigus vulgaris is the variant most likely to be encountered by dentists; however, all other variants have the potential to present with oral manifestations. Oral mucosal lesions tend to precede skin lesions. Other mucosal sites that may be involved include conjunctiva, larynx, nasal mucosa and vagina.

Presentation varies, depending on the severity of disease activity and the extent of epithelial involvement. At one end of the spectrum, the sole manifestation may be a desquamative gingivitis, while there may be extensive eye, oral, pharyngeal and genital involvement on the other end, with ulceration and blistering. Skin lesions may be observed, such as itchy erythematous papules, erosions and easily ruptured blisters.

Intraoral findings may include mucosal erosion, frank ulceration and oral blister formation –thereafter, the blisters burst easily, leaving an area of frank ulceration. A desquamative gingivitis is often evident, and simple pressure may result in the formation of a blister – the so-called 'Nikolsky's sign'.

The clinical findings require laboratory-based confirmation of the diagnosis through histopathological assessment, while a second specimen should be sent as a fresh sample for DIF analysis for IgG or IgA.

A tissue sample (skin or mucosal tissue) is typically sent for histopathological examination, while another sample is sent for DIF analysis. Identification of IgG, IgA and C3 with an intercellular epithelial distribution will confirm the clinical diagnosis.

There are blood-based investigations that can confirm the presence of antibodies directed against intercellular epithelial structures such as indirect IF for IgG, or IgA, C3 or ELISA for antibodies directed against intercellular epithelial antigens such as Desmoglein 1 and 3. Mild cases can be managed with topical steroids, such as a clobetasol/Orabase combination therapy. More often, more severe inflammation is present that requires systemic therapy. Management of pemphigus vulgaris in patients with extra-oral involvement requires multidisciplinary care with dermatology and other specialities. Admission for hospital inpatient treatment may be necessary for the treatment of pemphigus.

Dermatitis herpetiformis

Dermatitis herpetiformis manifests as a chronic skin condition with papules and vesicular eruptions on the elbows and scalp. The disease is associated with known or latent coeliac disease. The oral mucosa is rarely involved.

Lupus erythematosus (LE)

LE is an autoimmune systemic disease, broadly classified into systemic and discoid LE.

Systemic lupus erythematosus (SLE)

SLE is a multi-organ disease with connective tissue involvement and vasculitis. Antibodies such as antinuclear antibodies and anti-double-stranded DNA are associated with this disease. The postulated mechanism involves interaction of environmental factors, such as infections, in genetically predisposed individuals. Despite SLE having a wide range of presentations, cutaneous lesions are the most common.

Discoid lupus erythematosus (DLE)

Skin lesions often present in the head and neck. The oral lesions of SLE and DLE clinically resemble OLP.

Behçet's syndrome (BS)

BS is a chronic multi-system disorder, classically described as a triad of oral and genital ulceration and uveitis (eye inflammation). Oral ulceration tends to be severe, recalcitrant and aphthous-like, with a mixture of minor, herpetiform and major-type ulcers. BS is more common in Eastern Mediterranean and East Asian countries, and has HLA and MHC associations.

The differential diagnosis would include other syndromes that cause oral and mucocutaneous ulceration together with eye inflammation, such as SLE.

Graft versus host disease (GVHD)

GVHD is an acute or chronic reaction that may occur following allogenic transplantation (most frequently following bone marrow transplantation). GVHD results when immunologically competent cells in the graft react immunologically to antigens on the recipient cells. Both acute and chronic GVHD have oral manifestations.

Indeed, chronic GVHD may cause lesions similar to OLP at both clinical and histopathological levels.

Drug-induced causes of oral/ dermatological lesions

Nicorandil (a potassium channel activator), a drug often prescribed for patients with acute coronary syndrome, has the potential to cause oral and/or skin ulceration. Oral ulcers are painful, with one or more large occurrences, mostly involving the tongue or the inner aspect of the cheeks. Dose reduction may be sufficient; however, some cases will only respond to complete cessation of the medication.

Lichenoid lesions

Several drugs, such as oxybutynin, have been reported to cause lichenoid skin lesions. Oral lichenoid reactions can occur in isolation or accompany skin lesions. Differentiation from idiopathic OLP can be challenging, since resolution, especially of oral lesions, can be delayed and partial following selective withdrawal of the culpable drug.

Fixed drug eruption

Solitary fixed drug eruptions may involve the skin and, rarely, the oral mucous membrane, with bullous formation and ulceration. The lesions may be associated with other mucocutaneous lesions. Drugs ranging from tetracyclines to oxybutynin have been implicated.

Drug-induced bullous disease

Pemphigus vulgaris may be induced by drugs with a sulphydryl group in their chemical structure, such as captopril, the angiotensin-converting enzyme inhibitor. Presentation with bullous disease, involving the skin and oral mucosa with a relevant drug history, should raise clinical suspicion and be included in the differential diagnosis. MMP may also be drug induced, and have similar clinical considerations in terms of diagnosis.

FURTHER READING

BMJ. Available from: http://www.bmj.com/specialities/dermatology.

Colven RM. Dermatology. *Medical Clinics of North America* 2015; **99**(6): xvii –xviii.

Crispian Scully. *Oral and Maxillofacial Medicine: The Basis of Diagnosis and Treatment*, 3rd edn. Edinburgh: Churchill Livingstone; 2013 (ISBN 9780702049484).

Richard B Weller, Hamish JA Hunter, Margaret W Mann. *Clinical Dermatology*, 5th edn. Chichester: John Wiley & Sons Inc; 2015 (ISBN: 1118850971).

MULTIPLE CHOICE QUESTIONS

1. Pigmentation of the oral mucosa is most likely to be a feature of:
   a) Hypothyroidism.
   b) Addison's disease.
   c) Psoriasis.
   d) Syphilis.
   e) Gonorrhoea.
   Answer = B

2. Skin blisters are likely to be caused by:
   a) Iron deficiency anaemia.
   b) Pemphigus vulgaris.
   c) Cushing's disease.
   d) Peutz–Jeghers syndrome.
   e) OLP.
   Answer = B

3. Regarding the varicella zoster virus (HHV-3), which one of the following statements is most likely to be correct?
   a) May cause shingles.
   b) May cause herpes labialis.
   c) May cause recurrent EM minor.
   d) May cause pemphigus vulgaris.
   e) May cause oral hairy leukoplakia.
   Answer = A

4. Regarding herpes simplex virus (HHV-1)–induced herpes labialis (cold sore), which one of the following statements is most likely to be correct?
   a) Is considered to be a potential predisposing factor for the development of lip squamous cell carcinoma.
   b) May be precipitated by stress.
   c) Is considered to be a manifestation of vitamin D deficiency.
   d) Is considered to be a predisposing factor for the development of squamous cell carcinoma.
   e) Is considered to be a risk factor for the development of actinic cheilitis.
   Answer = B

5. Pellagra is likely to be associated with:
   a) Vitamin D deficiency.
   b) Vitamin B_{12} deficiency.
   c) Zinc deficiency.
   d) Vitamin B_3 deficiency.
   e) Is not usually associated with any deficiency state.
   Answer = D

6. Oral and conjunctival inflammation are more likely to be a recognised complication of:
   a) MMP.
   b) Psoriasis.
   c) Primary syphilis.
   d) LP.
   e) Hyperthyroidism.
   Answer = A

7. Which one of the following diagnoses is most likely to be associated with a relatively poorer prognosis?
   a) Basal cell carcinoma.
   b) Malignant melanoma.
   c) Squamous cell carcinoma.
   d) Lentigo maligna.
   e) Discoid lupus erythematosus.
   Answer = B

8. Which one of the following statements most appropriately describes the salient clinical features of Behçet's syndrome?
   a) Aphthous-like ulceration of the oral and genital mucosa.
   b) Snail-track-like ulceration of the oral and genital mucosa.
   c) Snail-track-like ulceration of the oral and pharyngeal mucosa.
   d) Aphthous-like ulceration of the oral mucosa and conjunctivae.
   e) Granulomatous ulceration of the oral and genital mucosa.
   Answer = A

9. LP is most likely to involve which of the following sites?
   a) Sclera.
   b) Conjunctivae.
   c) Oesophagus.
   d) Nasal mucosa.
   e) Genital mucosa.
   Answer = E

10. Regarding basal cell carcinoma, which one of the following statements is most likely to be correct?
    a) Regional lymph node metastasis is present in approximately one-third of patients at diagnosis.
    b) Regional lymph node metastasis is present in approximately half of patients at diagnosis.
    c) Is a premalignant/potentially malignant condition.
    d) Is recognised as a common complication of vitamin D deficiency.
    e) Regional lymph node metastasis is rarely present at diagnosis.
    Answer = E

CHAPTER 13
Endocrinology and diabetes

RH Jay, M Greenwood and JG Meechan

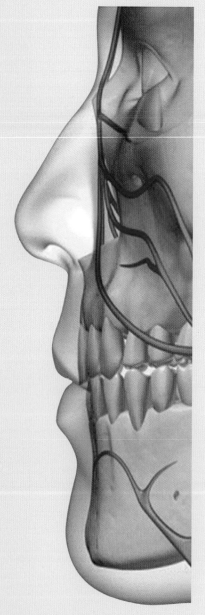

Key topics

- Major endocrine gland disorders.
- Pregnancy.
- Dental aspects of endocrine disorders, and implications for patient management.

Learning objectives

- To be familiar with the more common endocrine disorders.
- To understand the effects of endocrine disorders on patient management in dentistry.

Essentials of Human Disease in Dentistry, Second Edition. Mark Greenwood.
© 2018 John Wiley & Sons Ltd. Published 2018 by John Wiley & Sons Ltd.
Companion website: www.wiley.com/go/greenwood/human-disease-in-dentistry

Introduction

Endocrinology is the branch of medicine that deals with the endocrine system and its disorders, including hormones and the glands from which they are secreted. *Hormones* are molecules secreted directly into the bloodstream from one organ, with regulatory actions at distant sites. Some, such as insulin, act via cell surface receptors, while others, including thyroxine (T_4) or steroid hormones, bind to intracellular receptors.

Endocrinology covers a wide spectrum of diseases, some very uncommon. The most common endocrine condition is diabetes mellitus, which is dealt with separately in this chapter. Certain specialist areas, such as disorders of fertility and reproduction, will not be covered in this chapter, which will instead focus on the more common endocrine syndromes, or those of specific importance to the practice of dentistry.

Several endocrine glands secrete steroid hormones, and there is potential confusion in the way the term 'steroids' is used.

- The technically correct use includes all hormones that have a basic molecular structure based on four rings, derived from cholesterol. This covers the sex steroids (such as testosterone and oestrogens), adrenal steroids (including cortisol and aldosterone), and also the active form of vitamin D.
- In clinical medical terminology (and in this chapter), the term 'steroids' is often used to mean anti-inflammatory and immunosuppressive drugs that act via the cortisol receptor, such as prednisolone or dexamethasone.
- In lay terminology, the term is often understood to mean the artificial androgens misused by athletes to stimulate muscle growth.

Regulation and feedback

Most hormones are regulated by a feedback system, most commonly involving the pituitary gland, which is situated at the base of the brain, behind the optic chiasm, and connected to the hypothalamus by the pituitary stalk. The stalk contains a system of portal vessels that carry locally acting releasing hormones from the hypothalamus to the anterior pituitary. These stimulate the release of the relevant pituitary hormone, which in turn acts on another distant endocrine gland to stimulate the secretion of its hormone. The regulatory feedback loop is completed when the hypothalamus detects the final product hormone, and inhibits the production of its releasing hormone.

The main hypothalamic–pituitary control axes are shown in Figure 13.1, and the hormone secretion pathways are listed in Table 13.1. These feedback loops can be useful in clinical diagnosis. For example, if the thyroid gland fails to produce sufficient T_4, the plasma level of thyroid-stimulating hormone (TSH) rises in an attempt to stimulate the failing gland, and this can be measured in clinical laboratories. In the opposite situation, that is, if the thyroid produces excessive T_4, the TSH level will be suppressed.

Other endocrine systems have non-pituitary feedback loops, shown in Table 13.2. Some, such as the parathyroid gland or the insulin-secreting beta cells of the pancreatic islets,

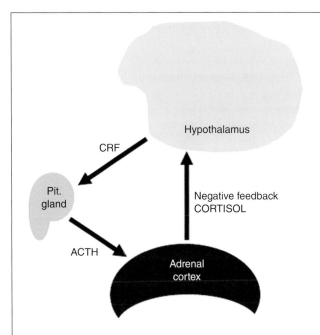

Figure 13.1 The hypothalamus–pituitary–adrenal axis. Pit. gland = pituitary gland; CRF = corticotrophin-releasing factor; ACTH = adrenocorticotrophic hormone.

Table 13.1 Hormone secretion pathways.

Hypothalamus	Pituitary	Target organ	Product
Corticotrophin-releasing hormone (CRH)	Adrenocorticotrophic hormone (ACTH)	Adrenal cortex	Cortisol (the main glucocorticoid)
Thyroid-releasing hormone (TRH)	Thyroid-stimulating hormone (TSH)	Thyroid	Thyroxine (T_4) and tri-iodothyronine (T_3)
Growth hormone–releasing hormone (GHRH)	Growth hormone (GH)	Liver	Insulin-like growth factor-1 (IGF-1)
Gonadotrophin-releasing hormone (GnRH)	Follicle-stimulating hormone (FSH) Luteinising hormone (LH)	Gonads	Testosterone Oestrogen, gametes

Table 13.2 Non-pituitary feedback loops.

Gland	Hormone	Control system
Adrenal medulla	Adrenaline	CNS
Parathyroid	Parathyroid hormone (PTH)	Plasma calcium level
Adrenal cortex	Aldosterone (a mineralocorticoid)	Plasma volume via kidneys – renin, angiotensin
Pancreatic islets of Langerhans	Insulin Glucagon	Plasma glucose

directly monitor the level of the target molecule that they regulate. Others, such as the aldosterone-secreting cells of the adrenal cortex, are involved in more complex control systems that include other organs.

Mechanisms of endocrine disease

There are three basic things that can go wrong with an endocrine gland:

- Failure to produce its hormone.
- Excessive production of hormone.
- Swelling (e.g. benign or malignant tumours).

A common cause of the failure of an endocrine gland is autoimmune destruction of the gland. Examples include type 1 diabetes, primary hypothyroidism and Addison's disease. Glands may also be removed surgically, or destroyed by other diseases such as infection, radiation or invasion by tumours. Glands involved in pituitary feedback loops can also fail secondary to pituitary disease.

Excessive production of hormones can occur independently of the normal control mechanisms with benign or malignant tumours, or due to non-neoplastic overgrowth of glands (e.g. the thyroid). It may also occur secondary to unregulated pituitary hormone secretion.

Endocrine gland tumours may be secreting or non-secreting. Problems may occur due to swelling and compression of adjacent structures. For example, a pituitary tumour can compress the portal blood supply, interrupting the regulation of normal pituitary cells. It may compress and destroy the adjacent normal pituitary cells, or it may compress the nearby optic chiasm, resulting in a visual field defect.

Important endocrine syndromes

There are a number of clinically important endocrine syndromes, some of which cause characteristic changes in the patient's general appearance, which can be recognised by the trained eye.

The adrenal glands

Cushing's syndrome

Cushing's syndrome (Figure 13.2) occurs due to glucocorticosteroid excess. This may be caused by overproduction of ACTH

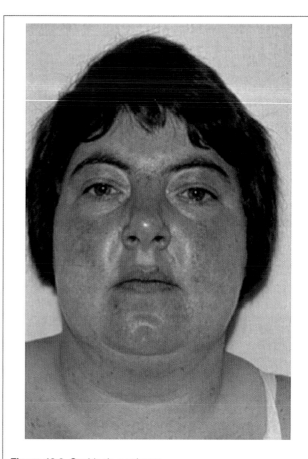

Figure 13.2 Cushing's syndrome.

from the pituitary or, more rarely, ectopic ACTH from certain other cancers. It may also be due to primary adrenal disease, such as a benign adenoma or a carcinoma. However, the commonest cause of this clinical picture is the medical use of long-term corticosteroid therapy.

It is important to realise that systemic steroid treatment suppresses the normal pituitary–adrenal axis, and results in atrophy of the normal cortisol-secreting adrenal cells. Therefore, it must never be suddenly stopped, and the dose of steroid treatment may need to be increased in severe illness.

The most common non-iatrogenic cause of Cushing's syndrome is a pituitary adenoma secreting ACTH. Primary adenomas or adenocarcinomas of the adrenal glands are less common.

Clinical features of Cushing's syndrome and disease are many and varied. The obvious clinical feature is a change in body shape. The face becomes round, the so-called 'moon face'; fat is deposited at the top of the back, referred to as a 'buffalo hump'; and there is abdominal obesity and wasting of proximal limb muscles, resulting in a 'lemon on sticks' shape.

Thinning of the skin results in abnormal bruising (purpura) and abdominal stretch marks, and thinning of the bones results in osteoporosis and increased risk of fractures. Female sufferers may develop hirsutism – that is, male type of facial hair growth due to androgen excess, particularly in adrenal tumours. Cortisol causes resistance to insulin, resulting in impaired glucose tolerance or diabetes. Mineralocorticoid effects result in salt and water retention, causing oedema and hypertension.

Suspected cases of non-iatrogenic Cushing's disease or syndrome need careful investigation in a hospital. The key biochemical test is measurement of the plasma or urine cortisol level, which will be elevated, and is not suppressed by dexamethasone, an artificial steroid analogue that normally suppresses the hypothalamic–pituitary drive to cortisol production. Measurement of plasma ACTH helps to distinguish pituitary causes (when it will be raised) from adrenal causes (when it will be suppressed). MRI of the pituitary or adrenals is needed to localise the tumour. Treatment is usually by surgical removal of the adrenal or pituitary tumour.

Addison's disease

Addison's disease occurs due to autoimmune destruction of the adrenal cortex, resulting in failure to produce cortisol and aldosterone. The term is sometimes used more loosely to include other causes of adrenal failure. The glands can also be affected by cancer, TB and surgery. Hypoadrenalism can also be secondary to a lack of ACTH due to pituitary failure.

The clinical features of Addison's disease can be nonspecific, with general tiredness, weakness and weight loss. A clinical clue is hyperpigmentation. This may occur generally over the whole skin, but is particularly prominent in the palmar creases of the hands and on the buccal mucosa. It may therefore be detected during dental examination. The hyperpigmentation is caused by an excess of melanocyte-stimulating hormone, which is a byproduct of ACTH.

If diagnosis is delayed, an 'Addisonian crisis' may occur. Features of this emergency include vomiting and loss of salt and water, resulting in severe hypotension, electrolyte disturbances and hypoglycaemia. The hypotension or hypoglycaemia may result in coma.

The basic laboratory investigations for suspected Addison's disease involve checking the plasma cortisol level, which will be low; ACTH, which will be raised unless the hypoadrenalism is due to pituitary failure; and adrenal autoantibodies. Urea, electrolytes and glucose should also be measured, especially in an Addisonian crisis.

Treatment of an Addisonian crisis requires emergency intervention with intravenous hydrocortisone, glucose, and fluid and electrolyte replacement. Long-term treatment of Addison's disease is with hydrocortisone and fludrocortisone. 'Hydrocortisone' is the pharmaceutical name for cortisol. Fludrocortisone is a synthetic analogue of aldosterone, which stimulates the retention of salt and loss of potassium via the kidneys. Replacement allows the patient to return to normal activities (and even presidency of the USA, as demonstrated by John F Kennedy, a famous patient of Addison's disease).

Patient education is important. They must never stop their treatment, and increased doses are needed during illness, since hydrocortisone is an essential stress hormone. Patients taking either hydrocortisone replacement or therapeutic steroids for inflammatory disease should always carry a steroid card to highlight this in case of emergency.

Conn's syndrome

Conn's syndrome occurs in people who suffer from a tumour or hyperplasia of the adrenal cortex. The resulting high levels of aldosterone secretion lead to potassium loss and sodium retention. The decreased potassium leads to muscle weakness and polyuria, whereas sodium retention leads to hypertension.

The thyroid gland

Hyperthyroidism

The thyroid gland secretes two iodine-containing hormones, T_4 and T_3. Although T_4 is produced in greater quantities, T_3 is the active form of the hormone, and T_4 is deiodinated to T_3 in the target cells.

Overproduction of thyroid hormones is also sometimes called 'thyrotoxicosis'. The term 'Graves' disease' applies to one specific form of hyperthyroidism, caused by an antibody that binds to the TSH receptor on the thyroid cells and stimulates it. Other causes of hyperthyroidism are thyroid adenoma and toxic multinodular goitre. The term 'goitre' applies to any swelling of the thyroid gland (Figure 13.3). One form is the multinodular goitre, which may function normally, but nodules sometimes become autonomous from TSH stimulation, resulting in thyrotoxicosis. In contrast to hyperadrenalism, which is most commonly due to an ACTH-secreting pituitary tumour, hyperthyroidism due to a TSH-secreting tumour is very rare.

The clinical features of thyrotoxicosis relate largely to an increase in the metabolic rate and to stimulation of the sympathetic nervous system (Table 13.3). The increased metabolic rate results in weight loss despite the increased appetite. The patient always feels hot, even in cold weather. Bowel activity is increased, with loose motions. Adrenergic or sympathetic activity results in tremor, most easily demonstrated in the outstretched hand, which is also warm and sweaty. Tachycardia occurs, and may develop into atrial fibrillation and heart failure (as happened in the case of George Bush Senior in 1991, during his presidency).

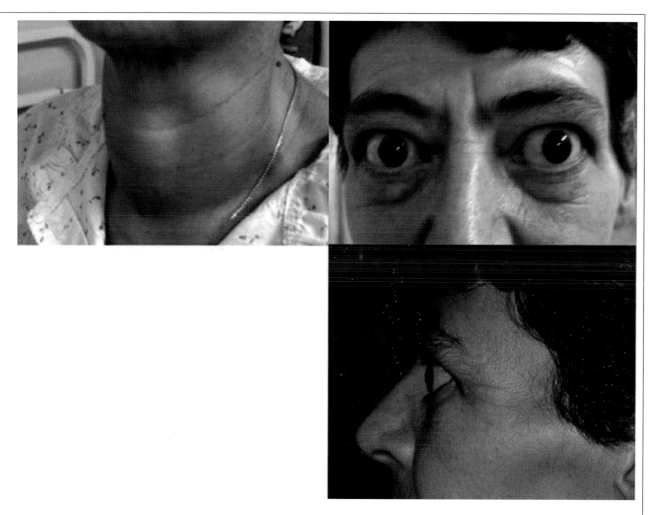

Figure 13.3 A goitre and demonstration of exophthalmos.

Table 13.3 Hyperthyroidism and hypothyroidism.

	Hyperthyroidism	Hypothyroidism
Causes	Graves' disease – antibodies against TSH receptors. Common cause in women aged 20–50 years. Toxic multinodular goitre, thyroid adenoma	Spontaneous – primary autoimmune Drug induced (e.g. antithyroid drugs, iodine deficiency)
Symptoms	Weight loss Dislike of heat Tremor, irritability Emotionally labile	Weight gain Dislike of cold Lethargy Depression
Signs	Tachycardia Atrial fibrillation Tremor Enlarged thyroid Exophthalmos Goitre	Bradycardia Goitre Dry skin and hair
Treatment	Carbimazole or propylthiouracil Beta blockers for symptom control Partial thyroidectomy Radioactive iodine	Thyroxine replacement

Many patients will have a goitre, which is visible in front of the larynx in the neck, moving upwards on swallowing. This may be smooth (in Graves' disease) or lumpy (in toxic multinodular goitre). A single toxic adenoma may cause a localised swelling of the part of the thyroid.

Graves' disease also causes certain non-thyroidal manifestations. Deposition of mucinous material in the orbit and extraocular muscles results in exophthalmos (protrusion of the eyes). Retraction of the upper eyelid, with white sclera visible above the iris, is partly due to the mechanical effects of the protrusion, and partly due to sympathetic stimulation of the muscle that raises the eyelid. Eye movements can be affected, resulting in double vision, and severe cases may even need surgical decompression of the orbit. Rare non-thyroidal manifestations of Graves' disease are 'thyroid acropachy' (a form of fingernail clubbing) and 'pre-tibial myxoedema' (skin thickening at the shins and dorsum of the foot).

The investigation of suspected hyperthyroidism involves measurement of the free plasma levels of T_4 and T_3, which will be raised, and TSH, which will be suppressed. Thyroid-stimulating antibodies can be detected in Graves' disease. Radioisotope scans, ultrasound and MRI scans are helpful in differentiating the different causes of hyperthyroidism and in planning treatment.

Surgical removal of abnormal tissue is undertaken in thyroid adenoma or multinodular goitre. Both of the latter treatments may result in permanent hypothyroidism, and patients should therefore be monitored by periodic blood tests, and T_4 replacement started if needed.

Hypothyroidism

A hallmark of a severely underactive thyroid is the deposition of mucinous material in the subcutaneous tissues – the so-called 'myxoedema'. The term 'myxoedema' is sometimes used synonymously with 'hypothyroidism'. The biochemical abnormalities found on blood thyroid function tests are the opposite of thyrotoxicosis – low levels of free T_4 and T_3, and a high TSH.

Hypothyroidism due to autoimmune destruction of thyroid can occur at any age, but is common in the elderly. Other causes are radioiodine therapy or surgery to the thyroid gland. It is occasionally secondary to pituitary failure, when the TSH will be low, and there will be evidence of failure of other pituitary hormones.

Clinical features are the opposite of hyperthyroidism, with the slowing down of metabolism and sympathetic underactivity (Table 13.3). The weight increases despite a modest appetite. The patient feels cold, mentally and physically lethargic, and constipated. The pulse slows, and the skin becomes dry. Slow and abnormal relaxation of muscles is evident on testing the tendon reflexes, such as the knee jerk. In severe cases, myxoedema causes puffy facial features, especially bags under the eyes, and the voice becomes deep and croaky.

The treatment of hypothyroidism is simple and very successful – T_4 replacement is given as a single daily tablet, with the dose adjusted to maintain a normal TSH level.

T_4 and antithyroid drugs

Hypothyroidism is normally treated with T_4, which is administered orally. T_3 may also be used, but it is mainly employed as an emergency drug for the treatment of myxoedema, where a fast-acting agent is essential.

The agents used to treat hyperthyroidism can be classified as:

- Antithyroid drugs.
- Iodide.
- Radioactive iodine.

In addition, β-adrenergic-blocking drugs can be used to control some of the symptoms of thyrotoxicosis, such as tremor and tachycardia. The antithyroid drugs are thioureylenes, carbimazole and propylthiouracil. They achieve their effect by the prevention of incorporation of iodine into the thyroid hormones T_4 and T_3.

It might seem odd that iodide, an essential component of thyroid hormones, is used to treat hyperthyroidism. The mechanism of action is by inhibition of the release of thyroid hormones caused by the presence of excessive levels of iodide. Iodide is mainly used preoperatively before thyroidectomy, or to treat thyrotoxic crisis. Radioactive iodine is administered orally as a single dose.

Impact of thyroid disease and treatment on dental management

Uncontrolled hyperthyroidism is a contraindication to the use of adrenaline in dental local anaesthetics; however, such an event is unlikely in general dental practice. Opportunistic infections such as oral candidiasis may occur in those who are hypothyroid, owing to reduced immune response.

In patients who are hypothyroid, sedation should only be provided in specialist units. The antithyroid drugs carbimazole and propylthiouracil may cause taste disturbance.

The pituitary gland

Acromegaly

Acromegaly is caused by growth hormone excess as a result of a pituitary tumour. During childhood, as its name suggests, growth hormone stimulates growth. Excessive production during adult life cannot increase the length of long bones, since the epiphyses are fused. Instead, it causes gradual widening and coarsening of bones and growth of soft tissues, producing a characteristic appearance. A patient with acromegaly is shown in Figure 13.4.

The facial features become coarse, with enlargement of the nose and brow ridges, thick lips, an enlarged tongue, prognathism and malocclusion. The hands become thick, and are often described as 'spade-like'. Patients may report an increase in the size of hats, gloves, rings and shoes. Just as prognathism results in malocclusion, growth of other bones results in joint

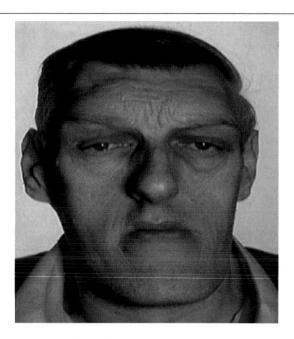

Figure 13.4 A patient with acromegaly.

deformity and arthritis, including that of the temporomandibular joint (TMJ). Insulin resistance occurs, resulting in glucose intolerance or frank diabetes. Hypertension is common, and therefore the risk of atherosclerosis is increased.

Any pituitary tumour, and not just those secreting growth hormone, may cause headaches. Compression of the optic chiasm results in a characteristic visual field defect known as 'bitemporal hemianopia'. This occurs because the nerve fibres from the nasal half of the retina (which receives the temporal half of the visual field) cross over to the other side of the brain. Damage to these crossing fibres results in loss of the temporal or lateral half of the field in both eyes.

The diagnosis of acromegaly is confirmed by measuring plasma levels of the growth hormone and IGF-1. A glucose tolerance test (see the following section titled 'Diabetes mellitus') can be undertaken with additional growth hormone measurements. Normally, growth hormone is suppressed by glucose, and suppression is absent in acromegaly. Pituitary MRI scans are needed to delineate the tumour. Treatment is ideally by transsphenoidal surgery to remove the tumour. If this is not possible, radiotherapy can be used. Octreotide and lanreotide are somatostatin analogues which, when given by injection, control the tumour and growth hormone production. New growth hormone antagonists are now available for cases in which other treatments have failed.

Other pituitary disease

Pituitary tumours causing acromegaly and Cushing's syndrome are described in the preceding text. Other pituitary tumours may produce prolactin, which results in failure to menstruate and to produce milk (in women), or they may be non-secreting. These

may still produce pressure effects – on either the pituitary itself, the stalk or adjacent structures at the base of the brain.

Pituitary failure may occur due to pituitary tumours, surgery, radiotherapy or, occasionally, other causes, such as infarction of the pituitary gland. Sudden pituitary failure is a medical emergency, but gradual onset or stable hypopituitarism is managed by the replacement of essential missing hormones.

Not all of the pituitary hormones are replaced directly. Their target organ hormones may be given instead. The basic essential replacements are T_4 and cortisol. Patients of reproductive age are given oestrogen or testosterone replacement, the latter via slow-release subcutaneous implants. Growth hormone replacement has symptomatic benefits in adults, and is essential in growing-age children. Induction of fertility requires more complex management.

On a day-to-day basis, the most important component of pituitary replacement is cortisol, which must never be omitted, and may need to be increased in illness, just as in the treatment of hypoadrenalism.

The parathyroid glands

Hyperparathyroidism

The parathyroid glands are situated posterior to the thyroid gland, and these are closely associated anatomically. They secrete PTH, which regulates calcium homeostasis. Hypercalcaemia is (usually) due to an adenoma of the parathyroid glands, which secretes excess PTH. Hyperparathyroidism is discussed in more detail in Chapter 10 (titled 'Shock').

The features are often asymptomatic. The mnemonic 'Stones, bones, abdominal groans and psychic moans' is helpful. Kidney stones (calcium); bone cysts, 'brown tumours', subperiosteal resorption; constipation, dyspepsia, pancreatitis; and confusion and depression can all occur.

The cause is usually a parathyroid adenoma. Hyperparathyroidism is investigated by testing blood for raised calcium with high PTH (which should be suppressed if the calcium level is high). Parathyroid scans are also used. Treatment is by surgical removal of the parathyroid tumours.

Hypoparathyroidism

Hypoparathyroidism produces hypocalcaemia, which causes tingling and tetany due to the excitability of nerves and muscles. The cause may be autoimmune or a complication of thyroid surgery. Treatment is by vitamin D analogues and calcium supplements (PTH replacement is not available).

Diabetes mellitus

Terminology and classification

The term 'diabetes' is derived from the Greek word for 'siphon', and 'mellitus' is Latin for 'sweet', referring to the fact that patients with diabetes mellitus pass large amounts of sweet urine. The unrelated condition described by 'diabetes insipidus' results in the production of large amounts of dilute urine. When used alone, the term 'diabetes' refers to diabetes mellitus.

In diabetes, there is a deficiency of insulin-stimulated uptake of glucose from the blood into the body's cells, resulting in elevated plasma glucose levels. The excess glucose passes through the renal glomeruli in amounts that exceed the ability of the renal tubules to reabsorb it. The presence of glucose in the urine raises the osmotic pressure, thus reducing reabsorption of water.

Types of diabetes

Type 1 diabetes develops during childhood or early adult life, and is caused by the autoimmune destruction of the beta cells of the islets of Langerhans in the pancreas that produce insulin. A complete lack of insulin is fatal if not treated. This type of diabetes is often called 'insulin-dependent diabetes'.

Type 2 diabetes usually develops in or after the middle age, and is caused by a combination of insulin resistance and relative insulin deficiency. There is still residual insulin production. The condition is often called 'non-insulin-dependent diabetes'.

Other rarer forms of diabetes mellitus include *gestational diabetes*, an important temporary condition occurring in pregnancy, and *secondary diabetes*, caused by some other condition – for example, Cushing's syndrome or surgical pancreatectomy.

Clinical features and diagnosis

Type 1 diabetes characteristically presents with polyuria, polydipsia (increased drinking due to thirst caused by dehydration) and weight loss. Patients may complain of blurred vision due to osmotic changes in the eye, or symptoms of oral or genital candidiasis. The blood glucose level will be markedly elevated, and the diagnosis is not in doubt. Immediate treatment with insulin is needed.

Type 2 diabetes may be asymptomatic for long periods, and indeed can occasionally present with long-term complications in patients not known to be diabetic. It is often associated with obesity, and may also cause thirst, polyuria and infections of the skin, oral or genital areas, or urinary tract. In some cases, the glucose levels may be only mildly elevated, and diagnostic criteria are based on the fasting blood glucose and that measured 2 hours after a 75-g glucose load given orally (the oral glucose tolerance test, see Table 13.4). It is important to realise

that diabetes, which is biochemically 'mild' and asymptomatic, can still result in serious long-term complications.

The terms 'impaired fasting glucose' and 'impaired glucose tolerance' refer to levels that are abnormal, but not diagnostic of diabetes. A proportion of these patients will go on to develop full-blown type 2 diabetes.

Measurement of glycated haemoglobin (HbA1c) is used to estimate the overall blood glucose control over the past few weeks, and thereby the success of diabetes treatment. It is also sometimes used for the diagnosis of diabetes, where a cut-off of 48 mmol/mol is recommended.

Management

The aims of diabetes management are threefold:

- Control of symptoms.
- Prevention of complications (described in the following text).
- Helping the patient to lead a normal life.

The first step is to control raised blood glucose concentrations. Factors that raise or lower the blood glucose level are given in Table 13.5.

Diabetic diet

The dietary advice for people with diabetes should not differ significantly from general advice for healthy eating, although those on insulin treatment should maintain regular meal times. Overweight patients should be advised about calorie restrictions. The glycaemic index of a carbohydrate-containing food is the area under the plasma glucose curve for the given amount of carbohydrate ingested. Foods with large particles of starch have a lower glycaemic index than soluble and easily digested sugars. Since diabetes is a risk factor for atherosclerosis, dietary factors that raise the blood pressure (particularly salt) or plasma cholesterol (especially saturated fat) should be limited.

Oral hypoglycaemic drugs

There are several classes of drugs that are used to lower blood glucose in type 2 diabetes (Table 13.6).

Metformin is a long-established drug that is widely used, since it does not cause hypoglycaemia or weight gain, and has been shown to reduce the risk of long-term complications. It can cause some gastrointestinal side effects including diarrhoea

Table 13.4 Blood glucose levels in health and disease.

	Plasma glucose (mmol/l)	
	Fasting	2 hours after 75 g glucose
Normal	<6.1	<7.8
Impaired	6.1–7 impaired fasting glucose	7.8–11.1 impaired glucose tolerance
Diabetes	>7	>11.1

Table 13.5 Factors that raise and lower blood glucose levels.

Raises glucose	Lowers glucose
Food	Starvation
Glucagon, adrenaline, cortisol, growth hormone	Insulin, antidiabetic drugs
Illness/stress	Exercise

Table 13.6 Type 2 diabetes – drugs used to lower blood glucose levels.

Mechanism	Classes	Common examples
Insulin secretagogues	Sulfonylureas Meglitinides	Gliclazide, glipizide, tolbutamide Repaglinide
Insulin sensitisers	Biguanides Thiazolidinediones ('glitazones')	Metformin Pioglitazone
Delay carbohydrate absorption	α-Glucosidase inhibitors	Acarbose
Combined actions	DPP-4 inhibitors ('Gliptins') GLP-1 agonists	Sitagliptin, saxagliptin Exenatide, liraglutide

and reduced appetite. A rare, potentially fatal, side effect is a build-up of lactic acid in the blood, and the drug should be avoided in patients with risk factors for this complication. It can produce taste disturbances.

Sulfonylureas have also been used for many years; they stimulate insulin secretion, and can therefore cause hypoglycaemia and weight gain. Repaglinide, which is not in common use, is a short-acting insulin secretagogue that is given before meals.

The glitazones, as with metformin, increase insulin sensitivity and reduce the risk of some long-term complications, but concerns about other aspects of their safety have caused a reduce in their use. Pioglitazone remains available in the UK, but is contraindicated in heart failure. Acarbose is rarely used, and can cause intestinal wind.

Two newer classes of drugs have in introduced in the recent years. Exenatide and liraglutide are agonists of the glucagon-like peptide-1 (GLP-1) receptor, stimulation of which results in increased insulin secretion, reduced glucagon secretion and delayed gastric emptying. They are injected subcutaneously, and assist with prevention of weight gain in type 2 diabetes. Sitagliptin and related 'gliptins' inhibit dipeptidyl peptidase-4 (DPP-4), which enhances insulin secretion and suppresses glucagon secretion. They are given orally in type 2 diabetes as second-line therapy for certain groups of patients.

Type 2 patients whose glucose is not controlled by diet or tablets should be treated with insulin.

Insulin treatment

All patients with type 1 diabetes need insulin replacement. Insulin is normally secreted into the blood by the beta cells of the pancreatic islets in response to a rise in plasma glucose, and stimulates uptake of glucose into cells, particularly liver, muscle and adipose tissue. The beta cells are highly responsive to changes in glucose concentration, and insulin secretion rises rapidly after a meal, falling to low basal levels during a fast.

Insulin is normally administered by a subcutaneous injection, and enters the blood from the depot under the skin. In emergency situations, it may be administered intravenously. In order to mimic the normal changes in insulin secretion, various insulin preparations are available with different speeds of absorption into the blood, and thus different time courses of action. Many patients use 'pen injectors' rather than conventional syringes and needles. The pens contain a cartridge of insulin and a fine subcutaneous needle, which can be reused by an individual patient with normal hygienic precautions, without the need to be sterilised for each use.

The main types of conventional human insulin are soluble insulin, which has a peak of action around 2 hours after injection, and isophane, which peaks at around 6 hours and has a duration of about 12 hours. There are several proprietary pre-mixed insulins available, with varying proportions of the two types.

Newer insulin analogues have been developed with different absorption characteristics. These include *lispro* and *aspart*, which have faster peak actions, more closely mimicking the physiological insulin peak after meals. Conversely, *glargine* has very prolonged absorption, and can mimic basal, fasting insulin secretion from a single injection daily. *Detemir* is another long-acting insulin analogue, but it does not achieve a full 24-hour viability.

Conventional insulin therapy depends on regular dietary habits, with three main meals per day and three snacks – at mid-morning, mid-afternoon and bedtime. With this regular pattern, a common insulin regimen comprises a twice-daily injection of a mixture of soluble and isophane insulins, given half an hour before breakfast and before the evening meal. The morning soluble insulin controls the glucose peak after breakfast, and the mid-morning snack prevents hypoglycaemia before lunch. The delayed action of the isophane peaks shortly after the mid-day meal, and takes the patient through to the next injection before the evening meal. A bedtime snack is needed to prevent glucose levels from dropping overnight.

A regimen that allows more flexibility of meal times is the 'basal-bolus' regimen. Here, an injection of a long-acting insulin is given at bedtime, and a short-acting insulin injection is given before each meal. This may be with conventional soluble and isophane insulins, but the combination of a basal injection of glargine and boluses of lispro results in a more physiological insulin profile, with improvements in control and flexibility.

A technique that gives insulin-dependent patients more flexibility and control over their food habits is 'dose adjustment for normal eating' (DAFNE). Here, patients are taught to estimate the carbohydrate content of their food and adjust their pre-prandial doses according to this, and their pre-meal blood glucose concentration.

Other treatments for selected patients include a continuous subcutaneous infusion of insulin via a small pump, and islet cell transplantation.

Complications of diabetes

The complications can be classified as *acute* or *chronic*. The acute complications are:

- Hypoglycaemia.
- Diabetic ketoacidosis (DKA).
- Hyperosmolar hyperglycaemic state.

Chronic long-term complications are:

- Microvascular – retinopathy and nephropathy.
- Macrovascular – coronary, peripheral and cerebral.
- Neuropathy.
- Mixed complications – diabetic foot, erectile dysfunction.
- Increased susceptibility to infection – skin, mouth and general.

Hypoglycaemia

Hypoglycaemia in diabetes occurs in response to treatment, usually with insulin, but sometimes with glucose-lowering drugs. A low blood glucose level can also occur in non-diabetic subjects for a variety of reasons, but this is much less common. Although levels of 2.8 mmol/L may be seen in normal fasting subjects, in the context of diabetes treatment, a level of 4 mmol/L or below is considered to be hypoglycaemic, and the slogan 'four's the floor' is a useful mnemonic. The patient's symptoms depend not only on the absolute level, however, but also on the rate of fall and the usual blood glucose level.

The symptoms (Table 13.7) are of rapid onset, appearing over a few minutes. They are divided into those caused by brain dysfunction as a result of shortage of glucose (which is the main fuel for the CNS), and symptoms caused by the rise in adrenaline (which is released in an attempt to raise the blood glucose level). Insulin is the only hormone that lowers glucose. Adrenaline, cortisol, glucagon and growth hormone are 'counter-regulatory' hormones that can raise blood glucose by stimulating the breakdown of stored glycogen (glycogenolysis) or by synthesising glucose from other sources (gluconeogenesis).

People with diabetes are taught to recognise the warning symptoms and to always carry some rapidly available glucose with them (e.g. Dextrosol® tablets). Some, for example, those with autonomic neuropathy from long-term diabetes, may lose the warning symptoms that allow them to take action before they get too confused (the so-called 'hypoglycaemic unawareness'). It is particularly important to avoid hypoglycaemia in this group.

If hypoglycaemia is suspected in a dental surgery, the diagnosis should be confirmed, if possible, by measuring blood glucose with a finger-prick test. If in doubt, the patient should be treated anyway. Inappropriate treatment of hypoglycaemia will cause a temporary rise in blood glucose, but no permanent harm is done. Failure to treat could be serious.

Treatment of hypoglycaemia

In the conscious, cooperative patient, glucose should be given orally. Three or four dextrose tablets, a carton of natural fruit juice or a warm drink with several teaspoons of sugar – any of these will suffice. In the uncooperative patient, 'GlucoGel', a glucose gel, can be squeezed into the mouth. Intramuscular glucagon (1 mg) is the preferred treatment in the unconscious patient, and this should be kept in the emergency drug cupboard. Glucose can only be given intravenously, and must be injected into a good vein using a large needle. Extravasation of concentrated glucose can cause severe skin necrosis, and a 50% solution will be viscous and difficult to inject if it is cold, or if the cannula is too small. A volume of 20–30 ml of 50% dextrose is an appropriate dose, as shown in Table 13.8.

DKA

DKA is a complication of severe insulin deficiency in type 1 diabetes. Normally, in states of starvation, the body breaks down fats to produce the 'ketone bodies' 3-hydroxybutyrate and acetoacetate, which can act as a fuel for cerebral metabolism. With severe insulin deficiency, these acids build up to excess and lower the blood pH. At the same time, the blood

Table 13.7 Signs and symptoms of hypoglycaemia.

Adrenergic warning symptoms	Neuroglycopaenic symptoms
Tremor	Confusion
Sweating	Slurred speech*
Anxiety	Aggression*
Hunger	Coma
Palpitations	Convulsions
Dry mouth	Death

*Always check glucose level in suspected alcohol intoxication.

Table 13.8 Treatment of hypoglycaemia.

Check plasma glucose if possible, but, IF IN DOUBT, TREAT	
Conscious and cooperative	Oral dextrose tablets, sugary drink, carton of sweet natural fruit juice
Uncooperative	Buccal hypostop gel (GlucoGel®)
Uncooperative or unconscious	Intramuscular glucagon (1 mg)
Unconscious	Intravenous 50% dextrose (30–50 ml)

glucose rises, resulting in osmotic diuresis and dehydration, together with losses of sodium and potassium, which leak out of cells and are lost in the urine.

New patients with type 1 diabetes can present with ketoacidosis. It can be precipitated by severe illness, most commonly infection, and also by omission of insulin intake in patients already on treatment. Symptoms include thirst, polyuria, apparent breathlessness (the low blood pH stimulates respiration), confusion and coma, and the condition usually develops over 12–24 hours. Treatment is given as an emergency in the hospital, with intravenous fluid and electrolyte replacement, and intravenous insulin. It is fatal if left untreated.

Prevention is therefore vitally important. Patients, their doctors and other healthcare professionals should know that insulin should *never* be omitted. If a type 1 diabetic patient is ill and unable to take food, there is a risk of hypoglycaemia. The patient should continue to take their insulin, monitor their blood glucose carefully and take their oral carbohydrate in liquid form. If this is failing, for example, due to vomiting, hospital admission is required to give intravenous glucose and insulin *before* full-blown ketoacidosis or hypoglycaemia develop.

Hyperosmolar hyperglycaemic state

This is also known as hyperosmolar non-ketotic coma (HONK). It occurs in type 2 diabetes, when the basal insulin secretion is enough to prevent ketoacidosis, but insufficient to control hyperglycaemia. The patient becomes severely dehydrated with marked losses of sodium and potassium. It usually occurs in older patients and builds up over several days, presenting at a severe stage when the patient may be comatose and in renal failure due to dehydration. The deep breathing stimulated by the acidosis is not seen.

Treatment is similar to that of ketoacidosis, but rapid correction of the dehydration and hyperglycaemia can cause complications, and careful treatment is hence needed.

Long-term complications of diabetes mellitus

Long-term complications occur after diabetes has been present for several years. Macrovascular disease is increased in impaired glucose tolerance, but microvascular complications are specific to diabetes. An important part of the care of the diabetic patient involves achieving as near normal glucose levels as practicable, treating additional risk factors, and monitoring to detect early complications at a stage when it can be treated.

Macrovascular

The risk of stroke in diabetes is doubled, that of MI is quadrupled, and that of gangrene requiring amputation of part of the foot is increased 50-fold. The mortality rates for diabetic patients suffering a stroke or MI are also increased. Therefore, aggressive control of the risk factors (for these, see Chapter 5A, titled 'Introduction to cardiovascular disease') is essential.

Microvascular

Damage to the microcirculation principally affects the retina, the renal glomerulus and the nerve sheaths.

Annual monitoring to detect diabetic retinopathy at an early stage enables treatment by laser photocoagulation of the retina, which greatly reduces the progression of vascular changes and the consequent risk of blindness.

Annual monitoring of renal function, including measurement of urinary albumin leaking, can help detect early nephropathy. Aggressive blood pressure control using ACE inhibitors is important in preventing progression to renal failure. Diabetes is one of the most common causes of renal failure, requiring dialysis or transplantation.

Diabetic neuropathy can occur in any peripheral nerve, but the most common pattern is the 'glove and stocking' sensory neuropathy, causing numbness of the feet and, to a lesser extent, the hands.

The combination of circulatory and sensory impairment gives rise to the 'diabetic foot', which is susceptible to several severe complications. Neuropathic ulcers develop over pressure points, particularly the metatarsal heads. Localised gangrene can occur, requiring 'ray amputation' of a toe. Infection or gangrene may spread more widely, necessitating more radical amputations. Meticulous care by a combination of diabetes physicians, specialist nurses, vascular surgeons, podiatrists and orthotists can reduce the risk of amputation.

Erectile dysfunction is another problem caused by a combination of vascular and neuropathic changes. Sildenafil (Viagra) has proved effective in many cases. Details of more advanced treatments are beyond the scope of this book.

Diabetes during surgery
Routine dental procedures

For patients with diabetes requiring dental surgery, it is important to know about the patients' usual treatment regimens and their normal degree of glycaemic control. If they are monitoring their blood glucose, review their record books. For those on insulin, ask about hypoglycaemia, and whether they get warning symptoms; also, check whether they carry any glucose. Long-term complications such as angina or heart failure may also require special consideration.

When performing procedures in patients on insulin or oral hypoglycaemic drugs, minimise any disruption to their usual routine. List them first on the morning list, and allow them to take their usual medications. Check their blood glucose before the procedure, allow a midmorning snack and check the glucose before leaving. The dentist should be prepared to diagnose and treat hypoglycaemia as discussed earlier if it does occur.

Although diabetic patients are more prone to infections, routine prophylactic antibiotics are not recommended.

For surgery requiring a period of fasting

This is seldom applicable for routine dentistry, but many hospital dental or oral and maxillofacial procedures or other medical interventions require an empty stomach – for example, gastrointestinal endoscopy or procedures requiring a general anaesthetic,.

For short procedures, the routine is 'fast and check'. Omit the morning insulin or oral hypoglycaemic drugs and breakfast. Monitor the blood glucose and perform the procedure first on the morning list. Then, give a late breakfast with normal medication.

For longer or major procedures, intravenous therapy is required. Patients who are treated by diet alone may simply require monitoring while on standard intravenous hydration. For those who take oral hypoglycaemic drugs or insulin, an intravenous infusion of insulin, together with intravenous glucose and potassium, will be needed. One way of giving this is by using a 'GKI' – an infusion bag containing 10% dextrose, potassium and insulin.

One common GKI starting dose involves the following, given at a predetermined rate:

- 10% dextrose 500 ml.
- 10 mmol KCl.
- 10 units of soluble insulin.

The patient's glucose is monitored hourly, and the aim is to keep the level in the 4–10 mmol/l range. If the glucose trend is leading outside this range, then the bag is replaced with one containing an adjusted dose of insulin, given at the same rate. Some hospitals put the insulin into a separate syringe, so that its rate can be adjusted independently of the glucose and potassium infusion.

Oral contraceptives

Many patients will be taking the *oral contraceptive pill* (OCP), which comprises varying proportions of synthetic oestrogens and progestogens. It is the oestrogen component that tends to cause complications. The major risk here is the increased threat of thromboembolic disease, especially DVT. Hypertension and diabetic tendency are other potential risks. The 'pill' is usually maintained for minor procedures but, if a prolonged general anaesthetic is being given, prophylaxis against DVT (e.g. subcutaneous heparin) should be given, due to the increased risk of venous stasis. Some surgeons recommend discontinuing the OCP for 2 months prior to a surgical procedure to eliminate the potential for these complications.

Oral contraceptives are available as:

- Combined oral contraceptive (oestrogen and progesterone).
- Progesterone-only contraceptive.
- Oestrogen only ('morning after' pill).

Many patients receive *hormone replacement therapy* (HRT), which may be given orally or as an implant, and aims to replace oestrogen, which is deficient owing to reduced secretion (e.g. after menopause or ovary removal). Osteoporosis is inhibited in patients who are on HRT, and it also appears to reduce the rate of alveolar bone resorption.

Impact on dental management

Oestrogen (and, to a lesser extent, progesterone) increases plaque-induced inflammation and gingival crevicular fluid. It may also cause gingival pigmentation. The incidence of dry socket increases with oestrogen dose in oral contraceptives.

Drug interactions

Broad-spectrum antibacterial drugs can cause the failure of contraceptive action because of their effect on gut flora, which are essential for the release of oestrogen from oestrogen glucuronide. This has been demonstrated in animals, but is probably theoretical in humans. Nevertheless, women taking oral contraceptives who are prescribed broad-spectrum antibacterials should be advised of this possibility. Drugs such as carbamazepine and phenytoin, which are enzyme inducers, can reduce the efficacy of oral contraceptives.

Pregnancy

Pregnancy is associated with physiological changes affecting the cardiovascular, endocrine and haematological systems. Pregnancy can also produce significant changes in behaviour and mood, largely owing to hormonal influences.

Many of the changes that occur during pregnancy will reverse after birth. A diabetic state may occur (gestational diabetes), which normally resolves after birth. As a result of the increase in blood volume and cardiac output, a cardiac murmur may occur, which also will resolve after birth. Occasionally, an initial fall in blood pressure may be seen in the circulation, with altered dynamics leading to syncope or postural hypotension.

Hypertension may occur in pregnancy. It may be asymptomatic, but can be associated with oedema and proteinuria, in which case it is termed 'pre-eclampsia'. This may lead to eclampsia, which comprises hypertension, oedema, proteinuria and convulsions. It can be fatal.

Pregnancy, although a physiological state, can cause situations of direct relevance to the dentist. Pregnant patients are at increased risk of DVT, and are prone to anaemia due to the expansion of blood volume.

In the later stages of pregnancy, pregnant patients may become hypotensive if laid in the supine position, owing to the gravid uterus compressing the inferior vena cava and reducing venous return to the heart.

Care should be exercised when prescribing for pregnant patients. The first trimester (3 months) is a particularly important period in foetal development as organogenesis is taking place. The *British National Formulary* should always be consulted to check for the appropriateness of drugs prescribed to pregnant patients, and prescriptions should only be given when absolutely necessary. Local anaesthetics are safe for routine dental treatment, but local anaesthetics are drugs and should therefore be treated as such.

It is important to avoid exposure to ionising radiation, particularly in the first trimester. Dental radiography is unlikely to be a significant risk, but should nonetheless be avoided if possible. If radiography is essential, the exposure should be kept to an absolute minimum.

Some drugs may pass into breast milk, and this should be borne in mind when prescribing drugs to lactating female patients.

Other endocrine conditions of relevance

A *phaeochromocytoma* is a rare cause of hypertension. It is a usually benign tumour of the adrenal medulla (usually unilateral), producing excess catecholamines (e.g. adrenaline). Symptoms are episodic and consist of headaches, palpitations and sweating, together with pallor and hypertension. Elective treatment should be delayed until the tumour has been dealt with. Local anaesthetic injections with adrenaline should be avoided. Treatment of phaeochromocytoma is surgical, and both α- and β-blockers are used to prevent hypertensive crises during such surgery.

The patient may report having been diagnosed with *diabetes insipidus* – a condition in which impaired water reabsorption occurs in the kidney as a result of either too little antidiuretic hormone (ADH) being produced by the posterior pituitary or an impaired response to ADH by the kidney. The patient will complain of drinking lots of fluids and passing lots of urine. Causes include head injury, pituitary tumour or sarcoidosis. Patients may complain of a dry mouth. The *syndrome of inappropriate ADH secretion* (SIADH) may occur secondary to some malignancies and certain benign chest disorders (e.g. pneumonia). It may occur secondary to trauma, and is characterised by a low blood sodium level and a high urinary sodium concentration.

The main pancreatic problem of relevance in an endocrine context is diabetes mellitus, which has been discussed in the preceding text. Hormone-secreting *pancreatic tumours* are rare and include the Zollinger–Ellison syndrome, in which a gastrin-secreting tumour leads to duodenal ulceration and diarrhoea. Insulinomas may also occur, leading to hypoglycaemia. Glucagonoma leads to hyperglycaemia, oral bullae and erosions.

Nelson's syndrome affects people who have had bilateral adrenalectomy, for example, to treat Cushing's syndrome, which leads to increased pituitary activity and adenoma formation. ACTH is released in great quantities, and cutaneous or oral pigmentation may result.

Dental aspects in endocrine patients

The most common endocrine condition encountered in a dental patient is diabetes mellitus. Other points to be obtained in the history of a dental patient with an endocrine disorder are given in Table 13.9. The safest mode of treatment is by using local anaesthesia. It is important to check that the patient has

Table 13.9 Points to remember in the history of a dental patient with an endocrine disorder.

- Diabetes mellitus
  - Insulin dependent?
  - Diet or tablet controlled?
  - What degree of control has been achieved?
- Thyroid disorders. Is the patient hyperthyroid or hypothyroid?
- Does the patient take oral contraceptives?
- Is the patient pregnant? If so, at what stage of pregnancy?
- History of:
  - Cushing's disease/syndrome?
  - Addison's disease?
  - Hyper- or hypoparathyroidism?
  - Conn's syndrome?
  - Phaeochromocytoma?
  - Diabetes insipidus?
  - Acromegaly?

eaten that day and taken the usual medications. When the diabetic regimen needs to be altered (e.g. to facilitate a general anaesthetic), this is best done in conjunction with the patient's physician. It is important that management in these cases be tailored to the individual patient, while bearing in mind the proposed surgical procedure. An outline of the preparation of a diabetic patient for surgery has been given earlier in this chapter.

Latest research shows that steroid supplementation in most patients who have taken therapeutic steroids is often not necessary prior to surgical dental treatment. In other endocrine patients, the use of supplemental steroids may be required. For example, after unilateral adrenalectomy for Cushing's adenoma, steroid support may be required for a period of weeks or months, and the patient's physician should be consulted.

After adrenal surgery for phaeochromocytoma, steroid supplementation may occasionally be required if the adrenal cortex has been damaged in the operation. A general anaesthetic is contraindicated in the uncontrolled patient with phaeochromocytoma. Local anaesthetics with adrenaline should be avoided in these patients. An additional complication could be dysrhythmias or hypertension. Elective treatment should therefore be carried out when the phaeochromocytoma has been treated. If emergency treatment is unavoidable, the blood pressure must first be controlled by enlisting medical help.

A general anaesthetic may precipitate a condition known as 'thyroid crisis' in the untreated patient with hyperthyroidism, resulting in a risk of cardiac dysrhythmias. A thyroid crisis is characterised by marked anxiety, dyspnoea and tremor. It is therefore critical to control hyperthyroidism before a general anaesthetic is contemplated. With appropriate management, this condition should not arise in contemporary practice. The use of general anaesthesia and sedation in patients who are hypothyroid and not controlled should be performed with great care, and is best carried out in specialist units. The use of local anaesthetics containing adrenaline is not contraindicated in patients taking thyroid replacement therapy, but should be avoided during thyroid storm, a situation in which extreme hyperthyroidism occurs secondary to thyroid surgery, trauma or infection.

In pregnant patients, general anaesthesia or intravenous sedation should be avoided during the first trimester and the last month. There is an increased tendency for vomiting, particularly in the last trimester, mainly due to pressure from the gravid uterus. It is important with all pregnant patients that appropriate liaison take place with the patients' medical practitioners.

Some drugs that can be prescribed by dental practitioners can be affected by concurrent therapy for endocrine conditions. Erythromycin may interact with diabetic medication – for example, with chlorpropamide, it may produce liver damage, and its concurrent use with glibenclamide may precipitate hypoglycaemia.

FURTHER READING

SIGN 116: Management of diabetes. Available from:
http://www.sign.ac.uk/guidelines/fulltext/116/index.html.

MULTIPLE CHOICE QUESTIONS

1. Which of the following hormones does *not* raise blood glucose levels?
   a) Growth hormone.
   b) Glucagon.
   c) Adrenaline.
   d) T_4.
   e) Cortisol.
   Answer = D

2. Type 1 diabetes:
   a) Is always treated with insulin.
   b) Is associated with obesity.
   c) Has a peak age of onset of 25 years.
   d) Is commonly asymptomatic.
   e) Is often discovered during pregnancy.
   Answer = A

3. Cushing's syndrome is most commonly caused by:
   a) Adrenal carcinoma.
   b) Pituitary tumour.
   c) Therapeutic use of glucocorticosteroids.
   d) Adrenal adenoma.
   e) Ectopic ACTH production from cancers.
   Answer = C

4. Therapeutic insulin:
   a) Is usually injected intramuscularly.
   b) Is best given after meals.
   c) Rarely causes hypoglycaemia.
   d) Should be omitted in type 1 diabetes if the patient is vomiting.
   e) Prevents ketone body formation.
   Answer = E

5. Which of the following should *not* be given in the treatment of hypoglycaemia?
   a) Intramuscular glucose.
   b) Intramuscular glucagon.
   c) A carton of fruit juice.
   d) Intravenous glucose.
   e) Dextrose tablets.
   Answer = A

6. Which of the following is an adrenergic warning symptom of hypoglycaemia?
   a) Tremor.
   b) Confusion.
   c) Coma.
   d) Convulsions.
   e) Slurred speech.
   Answer = A

7. Buccal pigmentation is a clinical sign in:
   a) Hypopituitarism.
   b) Vitiligo.
   c) Cushing's syndrome.
   d) Acromegaly.
   e) Addison's disease.
   Answer = E

8. Which of the following is *not* a feature of acromegaly?
   a) Hyperglycaemia.
   b) Malocclusion.
   c) Headache.
   d) Homonymous hemianopia.
   e) TMJ arthritis.
   Answer = D

9. Graves' disease:
   a) Is a form of insulinoma.
   b) Is a form of hypothyroidism.
   c) Is a form of hyperthyroidism.
   d) Is only seen in the immunosuppressed.
   e) Is only seen in diabetic patients.
   Answer = C

10. Conn's syndrome:
    a) May be seen in hyperplasia of the adrenal cortex.
    b) May be seen as a result of excess alcohol intake.
    c) Results in high serum potassium levels.
    d) Results in low serum sodium levels.
    e) Results in decreased urine output.
    Answer = A

CHAPTER 14
Pain and anxiety control

CC Currie, J Durham and JG Meechan

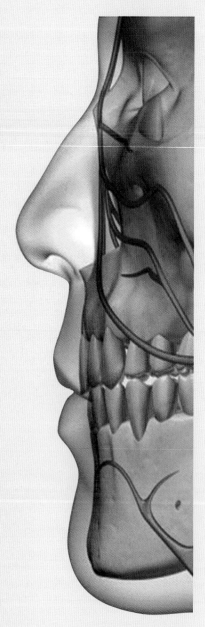

Key topics

- Local anaesthesia.
- Vasoconstrictors.
- Adverse effects of local anaesthetics.
- Commonly used analgesics, use and their pharmacology.
- Drugs used in conscious sedation.

Learning objectives

- To understand the pharmacology of local anaesthetics, their action and potential complications.
- To have knowledge of the more common analgesics used in dental practice.
- To have knowledge of the drugs used in conscious sedation.

Essentials of Human Disease in Dentistry, Second Edition. Mark Greenwood.
© 2018 John Wiley & Sons Ltd. Published 2018 by John Wiley & Sons Ltd.
Companion website: www.wiley.com/go/greenwood/human-disease-in-dentistry

Introduction

Dental treatments have the potential to be painful both peri- and post-operatively, and therefore dentists must have a good understanding of how to prevent and/or manage any pain experienced by patients. There are several methods to prevent or relieve pain related to dental procedures: removal of the peripheral stimulus, interruption of nociceptive input, stimulation of nociceptive inhibitory mechanisms, modulation of central appreciation of pain, and blocking or removing secondary factors maintaining pain. The most common methods used for the management of acute pain by dental practitioners are *local anaesthesia* and *analgesia*. Given the role of psychosocial factors in acute and chronic pain, careful consideration should also be given to the use of verbal and/or pharmacological anxiolytic techniques as adjuncts to the management of pain.

Local anaesthetics

Introduction

Local anaesthetics are the mainstay of pain control in dental practice. They are used both topically and by injection. When given by injection, they are often combined with a vasoconstrictor such as adrenaline or felypressin.

Pharmacology of local anaesthetics

The properties of the ideal local anaesthetic are listed in Table 14.1. Unfortunately, the first property of being specific for peripheral sensory nerves is not achieved by the drugs in current use. The fact that these drugs can affect any excitable membrane, such as central nervous and cardiac tissue, leads to unwanted effects (see the following text).

Local anaesthetics have a similar basic structure, consisting of three parts. These are a lipophilic terminal, an intermediate chain and a substituted amino (hydrophilic) terminus (Figure 14.1). The importance of having both lipophilic and hydrophilic components is discussed in the following text.

The intermediate chain determines the classification of local anaesthetics. The two types are *esters* and *amides*. These differ in two important respects. First, they vary in the way they are metabolised; and second, esters are more likely to produce allergic reactions as compared to amides. Table 14.2 shows the classification of common local anaesthetics.

Mechanism of action

Transmission of impulses along nerves depends on nerve cell depolarisation. Local anaesthetics act by interfering with this depolarisation, which they accomplish by blocking the entry of sodium into the cell. There are two theories for how local anaesthetics achieve this: the membrane expansion and specific receptor theories. The local anaesthetic solution can either diffuse into the nerve cell membrane, causing the membrane to expand and physically block the sodium channel, or the local anaesthetic molecule can bind to specific

Table 14.1 Properties of the ideal local anaesthetic.
A specific and reversible action
Non-irritant
Produces no permanent damage
No systemic toxicity
High therapeutic ratio
Active topically and by injection
Rapid onset
Suitable duration of action
Chemically stable and sterilisable
Combinable with other agents
Non-allergic
Non-addictive

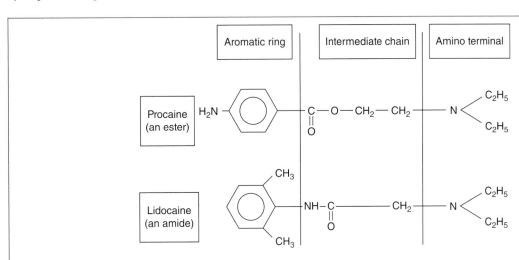

Figure 14.1 Local anaesthetic molecular structure.

Table 14.2 Classification of local anaesthetics.

Amides	Esters
Lidocaine	Benzocaine
Prilocaine	Tetracaine
Mepivacaine	Procaine
Articaine	
Bupivacaine	
Levobupivacaine	
Etidocaine	
Ropivacaine	

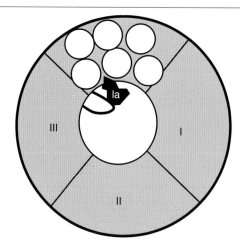

Figure 14.3 The sodium channel in the refractory configuration. A protein loop between domains III and IV extends into the channel, inhibiting the entry of sodium. The local anaesthetic molecule (Ia) binds on or close to this loop, maintaining this configuration.

$$\log \frac{ionised\ base}{unionised\ base} = pKa - pH$$

Figure 14.4 The Henderson–Hasselbach equation.

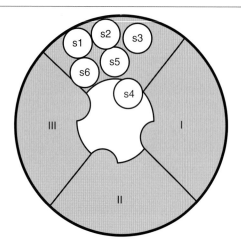

Figure 14.2 The sodium channel comprises three subunits, known as α, β 1 and β 2. The figure shows the α subunit, which contains the pore through which sodium enters the cell, in the resting configuration. The unit is made up of four domains (I–IV), each of which contains six protein helical segments (S1–6) that traverse the length of the channel. At rest, the positively charged S4 segments extend into the pore, obstructing sodium entry. When the nerve cell fires, the S4 segments retract into the wall of the pore, allowing sodium entry.

receptors in the sodium channel. Once bound, the local anaesthetic maintains the channel in a configuration that prevents the entry of sodium. This arrangement is similar to that which occurs during the refractory period, when the nerve will not transmit. Figures 14.2 and 14.3 show the different formations that the sodium channel can adopt, depending on its phase of activity.

An important point is that the local anaesthetic gains access to its binding site from within the nerve cell. This means that the local anaesthetic molecule has to enter the cell to be effective. To do this, the molecule must be lipid soluble, and uncharged. On the other hand, as the ultimate action of a local anaesthetic involves specific binding, the molecule must also have the ability to exist in a charged form. The properties of being lipid soluble and having a charged part to enable binding

are possible in local anaesthetic molecules, as they are weak bases. In solution, they exist in both charged and uncharged modes. The proportion of charged to uncharged is governed by the pH (of the solution and site of deposition) and the pKa, or the dissociation constant of the molecule. The Henderson–Hasselbach equation relates the pH and pKa to one another (Figure 14.4). Agents with a low pKa have a larger portion of uncharged molecules at a given pH. Thus, a greater proportion can enter the nerve cell, enabling a faster onset of action. Thus, several physicochemical properties govern the action of local anaesthetics, and these are described in the following text.

Physicochemical properties influencing local anaesthetic action

The following affect the action of local anaesthetics:
- pH.
- pKa.
- Partition coefficient.
- Protein binding.
- Vasodilator ability.

As mentioned in the preceding text, pH and pKa govern the proportion of charged and uncharged fractions of the agent. More uncharged molecules are available when the pH is high and the pKa low. The pKa of different local anaesthetic agents is given in Table 14.3.

The partition coefficient determines the relative solubility of a material in lipid and water – the higher the coefficient, the more fat-soluble it is. Local anaesthetics with high coefficients will enter the cell more rapidly and have a quicker onset.

Table 14.3 pKa of some local anaesthetics.

Drug	pKa
Lidocaine	7.9
Prilocaine	7.9
Bupivacaine	8.1
Procaine	9.1

Protein binding determines the duration of action of a local anaesthetic. Greater protein binding capacity provides longer-lasting anaesthesia as the molecule binds to its receptor for longer. In addition, the bound fraction acts as a reservoir for material absorbed from the site of deposition. Bupivacaine is 96% bound to protein, as compared to 64% for lidocaine; thus, the former is a longer-acting agent. Most local anaesthetics are vasodilators, but the degree varies between drugs. The more a drug's degree of vasodilatation, the more readily it is absorbed from its site of deposition, and the shorter the duration of action. Mepivacaine causes less vasodilation than lidocaine, and hence it lasts longer when used as a plain (i.e. vasoconstrictor-free) solution.

Metabolism of local anaesthetics

The metabolism of local anaesthetics differs between esters and amides. Esters are rapidly broken down in plasma by pseudocholinesterases, followed by hydrolysis in the liver. In the general population, 1 person in 2800 lack pseudocholinesterases, which impairs their ability to metabolise esters. The metabolism of amides is more complex, with their metabolites being active. Most amides are broken down in the liver in multiple stages, such as: dealkylation, hydrolysis, hydroxylation, further dealkylation, then conjugation. Exceptions to this rule are prilocaine and articaine. In addition to hepatic metabolism, prilocaine undergoes some breakdown in the lungs. Articaine, despite being an amide, is initially metabolised in the plasma by pseudocholinesterase. This early metabolism of articaine means it is less toxic systemically; thus, it can be administered in greater concentrations than lidocaine, and can also be of use in patients who are medically compromised – for instance, those with liver disease. Higher concentrations of local anaesthetics, however, may produce more localised toxicity (see the following text).

Local anaesthetics are excreted via the kidney, with very little (about 2%) being excreted unchanged in urine.

Vasoconstrictors

Vasoconstrictors are added to many local anaesthetic solutions. Vasoconstrictor-containing solutions have the following advantages as compared to vasoconstrictor-free (or plain) formulations:

- Longer-lasting anaesthesia.
- More profound anaesthesia.
- Reduced operative haemorrhage.

A disadvantage is that there may be more side effects with vasoconstrictor-containing anaesthetics. The vasoconstrictors used in dental local anaesthesia can be divided into two groups. These are:

- Catecholamines.
- Peptides.

The catecholamine most commonly used is adrenaline (epinephrine). It is present in concentrations varying from 1:50 000 to 1:400 000. The usual concentration in the UK is in the range 1:80 000–1:100 000. A standard 2.2 ml cartridge at 1:80 000 would contain 27.5 µg of adrenaline.

The peptide used as a vasoconstrictor is felypressin (Octapressin). This is a synthetic material that differs from the naturally occurring vasopressin in two of its eight amino acids.

Adrenaline causes vasoconstriction in peripheral blood vessels by its direct action on α-adrenergic receptors. In addition, it has systemic effects (e.g. increasing the rate and force of contraction of the heart). Consequently, there are patients with certain medical conditions in whom the dose of adrenaline should be reduced. It is wise to limit the dose of adrenaline to no more than two cartridges of a 1:8 00 000 solution in adults with significant cardiac disease, or to use a solution with a lower concentration of adrenaline, such as 1:1 00 000 (e.g. Articaine in the UK) or 1:2 00 000. Drug interactions with adrenaline are discussed in Chapter 15 (titled 'Adverse drug reactions and interactions').

Felypressin achieves vasoconstriction by binding to vasopressin V1 receptors to produce a phospholipase C–dependent release of intracellular calcium. The usual dose in dental local anaesthetics is 0.03 IU/ml (0.54 µg/ml).

In addition to peripheral vasoconstriction, felypressin can cause coronary artery vasoconstriction and uterine contraction. The latter effect is not apparent at the dose levels used in dentistry. As a consequence of its cardiac effects, excessive doses should be avoided in patients with compromised cardiac function.

Adverse effects of dental local anaesthesia

Adverse events following the injection of a local anaesthetic may be physical or pharmacological. Physical damage to a nerve by a needle may lead to long-lasting numbness or altered sensation, but this is likely to resolve within a couple of weeks. Touching a large artery with a needle may lead to painful arteriospasm. This is short-lived. Adverse effects due to the solution may be localised or systemic.

As with needles, the local problems caused by solutions may affect nerves or blood vessels. In vitro studies have shown that nerve damage increases with increasing local anaesthetic concentrations, so it may be more likely with more concentrated solutions. Deposition of vasoconstrictors such as adrenaline into arteries may trigger localised arterial shut down, which can cause dramatic effects such as alterations in vision. Deposition of local anaesthetics into a blood vessel can also cause increases in the risk of local anaesthetic toxicity – for example, if a standard 2.2 ml cartridge of lidocaine is injected intravascularly in a child, he or she would immediately be subjected to a toxic dose. The routine use of an aspirating technique should reduce the chances of this happening.

Systemic effects may be caused by local anaesthetics, vasoconstrictors or other components of the local anaesthetic delivery system. Systemic effects include:

- Allergy.
- Toxicity.
- Drug interactions.

Allergy

Allergy to amide local anaesthetics is very rare. The esters are more likely to cause this problem, owing to their metabolite para-aminobenzoic acid, and are no longer used routinely as injectable agents. However, they are available as topical preparations, and practitioners should therefore be aware of their allergic potential. The full range of allergic reactions, including anaphylaxis, after dental local anaesthetic injections has been described. In addition to local anaesthetics, allergic reactions may be caused by other constituents of the solution, such as preservatives or reducing agents, although most solutions are now preservative-free. Latex contained in the cartridge bungs of local anaesthetics may also cause allergy. Latex-free cartridges are available; if in doubt, practitioners should confirm this with the cartridge manufacturer.

Toxicity

Toxic reactions can be caused by:
- Injecting intravascularly.
- Injecting too much solution.
- Inability of the patient to metabolise.

The routine use of aspiration should help prevent inadvertent intravascular injection.

Knowledge of the maximum dose of different local anaesthetics is essential to prevent overdose. Maximum doses are weight dependent. The recommended maximum doses for commonly used dental local anaesthetics are given in Table 14.4.

As the main site for the metabolism of amide local anaesthetic agents is the liver, care should be taken in those with liver disease. In the case of mild disease, dose reduction is advised; alternatively, articaine may be considered for the reasons

discussed earlier. Patients who have severe liver disease should not be given local anaesthesia without first discussing with the patient's medical practitioner. Elderly patients can also have reduced liver function, so this should be considered when calculating the maximum doses that can be used.

Local anaesthetic toxicity primarily affects the central nervous and cardiovascular systems. The CNS is normally the first to manifest problems. The earliest symptoms are signs of excitation, such as restlessness. This is because the first areas of the CNS to be inhibited are inhibitory components. As the dose increases, the effect becomes depressant. At lethal doses, respiratory depression occurs. The signs and symptoms of toxicity are listed in Table 14.5, and the necessary steps for the treatment of toxicity are listed in Table 14.6.

At the doses used in dental local anaesthetic cartridges, it is easier to develop toxicity to the local anaesthetic agent rather than the vasoconstrictor. Idiosyncratic reactions to adrenaline-containing local anaesthetic agents are more common, however. The symptoms and treatment of adrenaline overdose are listed in Tables 14.7 and 14.8.

Drug interactions

Drug interactions and local anaesthetics are discussed in Chapter 15 (titled 'Adverse drug reactions and interactions').

Table 14.5 Signs and symptoms of local anaesthetic toxicity.

Plasma level	CNS effects	CVS effects
5 mg/L	Sedation Dizziness Anxiety	Increased heart rate Increased blood pressure
10–15 mg/L	Confusion Slowed speech Drowsiness Shivering	Cardiac instability
15–20 mg/L	Seizure Coma	Cardiac arrest

Table 14.6 Treatment of local anaesthetic overdose.

Stop the procedure.
Lie the patient flat.
Administer oxygen.
Give intravenous fluids.
Give intravenous anticonvulsants (e.g. midazolam).*
Perform basic life support if needed.

* To be performed by medically trained personnel.

Table 14.4 Maximum doses for commonly used dental local anaesthetics.

Drug	Maximum dose
Lidocaine	4.4 mg/kg
Mepivacaine	4.4 mg/kg
Prilocaine	6 mg/kg
Articaine	7 mg/kg

Table 14.7 Signs of adrenaline overdose.

Fear

Anxiety

Restlessness

Headache

Trembling

Sweating

Weakness

Dizziness

Pallor

Respiratory difficulties

Palpitations

Table 14.8 Treatment of epinephrine overdose.

Stop the procedure.

Place in a semi-supine or erect position to minimise the increase in cerebral blood pressure.

Reassure patient.

Administer oxygen if the patient is not hyperventilating.

Analgesia in dentistry

Analgesics can be either peripherally or centrally acting.

Peripherally acting analgesics

Peripherally acting analgesics predominately target the inflammatory cascade via the inhibition of algogenic substances at, or near to, the site of injury, and hence the name 'peripheral'. This group of analgesics include paracetamol, non-steroidal anti-inflammatory drugs (NSAIDs) and COX-2 Inhibitors. In addition to being analgesics, they all also have antipyretic and anti-inflammatory properties, although of varying degrees.

Paracetamol

Paracetamol has analgesic and antipyretic properties, and is also a weak anti-inflammatory agent. The mechanism of action of paracetamol is unknown; however, its antipyretic effect is likely to be due to prostaglandin inhibition in the hypothalamus. Paracetamol is absorbed from the small intestine and metabolised in the liver, with the vast majority being conjugated with glucuronide to produce inactive metabolites, which are then excreted in the urine. However, a small proportion of paracetamol is also metabolised by the cytochrome P450 system to produce N-acetyl-p-benzoquinone imine (NAPQI), an active metabolite. NAPQI is then inactivated by conjugation with glutathione and excreted in the urine.

The standard dental regimen of paracetamol is 500 mg–1 g, four times a day. When given at this dose, paracetamol has very few unwanted effects. However, in case of overdose, the active metabolite of paracetamol, NAPQI, can accumulate, since the stores of glutathione that conjugate with it and inactivate it are exhausted. NAPQI is hepatotoxic, and the increased levels of NAPQI present in a paracetamol overdose lead to hepatocellular injury and death. A dose of >150 mg paracetamol per kg body weight is defined as being an overdose, and this limit is lowered to 75 mg/kg in those with risk factors such as pre-existing liver disease, alcohol abuse and malnourishment. A significant problem with paracetamol overdose is that symptoms only emerge 2–6 days following overdose. This means that the patient can often feel well after an overdose, and therefore continue to take paracetamol, thereby causing more liver damage. It is, therefore, important to carefully examine the history of those who have used paracetamol for acute dental pain for any indication of accidental overdose, even if the patient feels well and has no immediate clinical manifestations. If in doubt, the patient should be discussed with, and potentially referred to, the local accident and emergency department for further investigation and treatment as required. Treatment is with acetylcysteine (a precursor of glutathione).

NSAIDs

Examples of NSAIDs include aspirin, ibuprofen, naproxen, mefenamic acid and diclofenac. Dental practitioners will most commonly encounter and prescribe ibuprofen for its analgesic properties. NSAIDs have a number of beneficial effects, including analgesic, antipyretic and anti-inflammatory properties. In addition, aspirin has a much more profound antiplatelet action as compared to other NSAIDs. Unfortunately, NSAIDs can also have several unwanted effects, as discussed in the following text.

This group of analgesics achieve their effect, and also their side effect profile, by nonselective blockage of cyclooxygenase (COX) enzymes (Figure 14.5). They achieve their therapeutic effect by inhibition of COX-2, thereby decreasing production of the eicosanoids that cause acute pain. The unwanted effects associated with their use are via the inhibition of COX-1, which causes the inhibition of prostaglandin synthesis, in turn reducing the production of gastric mucus and increasing gastric acid production, thereby increasing the risk of gastric ulceration. NSAIDs are also highly protein bound, and therefore have several potential drug interaction possibilities (discussed in Chapter 15, titled 'Adverse drug reactions and interactions'). Finally, due to their nonselective blocking of prostaglandin production, NSAIDs can reduce renal prostaglandin synthesis, which results in decreased renal afferent arteriole vasodilation and, consequently, decreased glomerular filtration rate in those with pre-existent risk factors (e.g. renal disease, chronic hypertension and atherosclerosis) – thereby potentially contributing to acute kidney injury

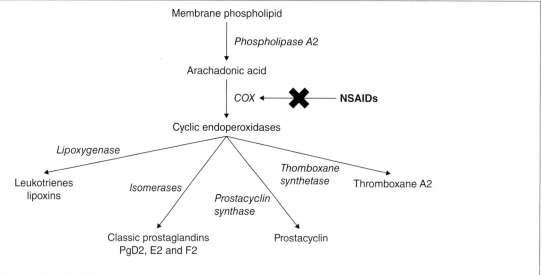

Figure 14.5 Mechanism of action of NSAIDs.

in the 'at-risk' group. NSAIDs can also produce an immunological reaction (acute interstitial nephritis), which causes an acute kidney injury.

Aspirin (acetylsalicylic acid) is a weak organic acid and a prodrug. It is rapidly absorbed from the gastrointestinal tract, and then metabolised by esterase enzymes to salicylic acid (salicylate), which undergoes conjugation in the liver before being excreted as salicyluric acid and glucuronides in the urine. Aspirin has mild analgesic actions, being most effective against pain associated with inflammation, owing to its anti-inflammatory ability. It is also an effective antiplatelet agent, and is therefore useful in the prevention of thromboembolic disorders. This effect is achieved by the inhibition of COX-1, decreasing the production of thromboxane A$_2$ and thereby, ultimately, inhibiting platelet aggregation. Aspirin's main use in the dental setting is in the treatment of suspected myocardial infarction (Chapter 20, titled 'Haematology'). Due to the risk of Reye's syndrome, aspirin (or products containing Aspirin) should not be prescribed to paediatric patients.

Ibuprofen is a propionic acid derivative, and is rapidly absorbed following oral administration, metabolised in the liver and excreted in the urine. It has better analgesic effect than aspirin and paracetamol, and is therefore useful in the treatment of dental pain. The usual adult dental regimen is 400 mg orally, three times a day with food. The maximum total daily dose is 1.2–2.4 g.

Due to their side effect profile, NSAIDs should be avoided in patients with gastric ulceration, asthma, pre-existent coagulopathies and renal disease.

Ibuprofen and paracetamol can be used in combination for treatment of acute dental pain. Patients should be advised to stagger the two drugs at the doses described. Should this not relieve their pain, then the medications can be taken combined, increasing their analgesic effect, and a weak opioid added between doses if required.

COX-2 Inhibitors

COX-2 inhibitors include celecoxib and parecoxib. These classes of drugs have similar mechanisms of action as NSAIDs. However, they selectively block COX-2, thereby reducing their side effect profile in relation to COX-1 in comparison to NSAIDs. They also, however, block vascular prostacyclin synthesis, thereby decreasing vasodilation and inhibition of platelet aggregation. However, at the same time, COX-2 inhibitors do not affect thromboxane A2. This upsets the homeostatic equilibrium between thromboxane and prostacyclin (Figure 14.6), and predisposes to platelet aggregation and vasoconstriction, inducing the patient to a prothrombotic state, and thereby increasing the risk of myocardial infarction. Hence, COX-2 inhibitors are sparingly used, and are not a first-line treatment for acute dental pain.

Centrally acting analgesics

Opioids are centrally acting analgesics, since they modify neural activity within the CNS to exert their effects. An opioid is any drug that exerts its effect at opioid receptors, and whose effects are antagonised by naloxone. Examples include morphine, codeine, tramadol, dihydrocodeine and fentanyl. They can be classified by their analgesic strength – as *weak, intermediate* or *strong*; and by their action – as *pure* or *partial agonists* of opioid receptors. Opioids bind to opioid receptors centrally to produce activation of descending inhibitory control over nociception, and peripherally to cause peripheral afferent hyperpolarization, inhibiting neurotransmitter release, and therefore stopping propagation of nerve impulses.

A major disadvantage of opioids is the number of unwanted effects associated with their use. They can cause respiratory depression, nausea, emesis, constipation, urinary retention and dependence.

Opioid use is indicated for the treatment of terminal illness and severe post-operative pain from highly invasive procedures

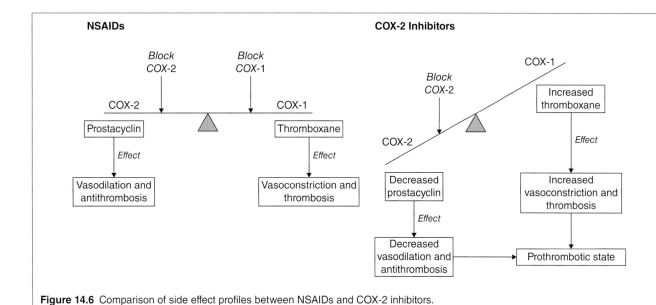

Figure 14.6 Comparison of side effect profiles between NSAIDs and COX-2 inhibitors.

(e.g. abdominal surgery, and some extensive oral and maxillo-facial surgery procedures). They have little effect on acute inflammatory dental pain. This, combined with the many unwanted effects associated with their use, means they have very limited use in dentistry, and will not be indicated in a primary dental care setting.

Morphine

Morphine exerts it effect on the μ and κ opioid receptors. It is most effective on pain that has a major component of suffering – for example, cancer pain. In addition to its analgesic effect, it also produces euphoria, drowsiness and sedation, which can be beneficial to patients suffering from terminal illnesses.

Morphine undergoes extensive first-pass metabolism in the liver if given orally, and is therefore normally given intravenously or intramuscularly. It can also be given via patient-controlled analgesia (PCA), such that patients can titrate the dose according to their pain levels, and is locked out once the maximum dose is reached. Morphine is metabolised in the liver to form both active and inactive metabolites, and then excreted via the kidney. As morphine is a prodrug, care must be taken in those with liver and renal diseases.

Codeine

Codeine is also known as '3-methylmorphine'. It achieves its effect at the μ opioid receptors, being only a weak agonist. It is one of the few opioids that is effective when given orally. It has weak analgesic properties, but is a very effective antitussive, so is often added to cough medicines. The main unwanted effect associated with its use is constipation, and there is minimal risk of respiratory depression and dependence. The usual dosing regimen is 30–60 mg orally, four times a day. Its use in acute dental pain is limited, and it is better used as part of multimodal analgesia.

Codeine is also metabolised in the liver, with one of its metabolites being morphine.

Tramadol

Tramadol is a weak agonist at the μ opioid receptors. In addition to this, it inhibits noradrenaline and serotonin reuptake. It has similar unwanted effects to the other opioids; however, it causes less constipation, dependence and respiratory depression. It can, however, lower the seizure threshold, and therefore may be best avoided in individuals with previous history of seizures. As tramadol inhibits serotonin reuptake, concomitant administration with other serotonergic agents can risk the development of serotonin syndrome. The normal dosing regimen is 50–100 mg, four times a day.

Tramadol undergoes some first-pass metabolism when given orally – however, to a lesser extent as compared to morphine. It is also a prodrug, producing active metabolites in the liver, before being excreted via the kidneys.

Drug interactions with analgesics are discussed in Chapter 15 (titled 'Adverse drug reactions and interactions').

Drugs used in conscious sedation

Introduction

Conscious sedation for dentistry is defined by the General Dental Council as 'A technique in which the use of a drug or drugs produces a state of depression of the central nervous system enabling treatment to be carried out, but during which the verbal contact is maintained throughout the period of sedation. The drugs and techniques used to provide conscious sedation for dentistry should carry a margin of safety wide enough to render unintended loss of consciousness unlikely'.

The drugs used to produce conscious sedation can be administered in several routes. These include:

- Intravenous.
- Inhalational.
- Oral.
- Transmucosal.

Intravenous sedation

Modern intravenous conscious sedation in dentistry relies on the use of two types of drugs – *benzodiazepines* and *propofol*. The drug most commonly used at present is benzodiazepine midazolam. In addition to providing excellent sedation, this drug also produces amnesia.

Benzodiazepines

Mechanism of action of benzodiazepines

Benzodiazepines exert their effects at the GABA receptor–chloride channel complex. GABA is an inhibitory neurotransmitter that stabilises excitable membranes. It achieves this by binding to a receptor at the chloride channel, causing an increase in chloride influx, which results in hyperpolarisation (stabilisation). The chloride channel contains binding sites for several drugs, including benzodiazepines, which can act as agonists and antagonists. Binding of a benzodiazepine agonist such as diazepam or midazolam increases the affinity of GABA for its binding site, thus promoting chloride influx. Binding of the benzodiazepine antagonist flumazenil, which is used to reverse sedation, reduces the affinity of GABA for its binding site.

There are many different receptor sites for benzodiazepines in the brain – including the reticular activating system (which governs consciousness and alertness), the limbic system in the cortex (which controls emotions) and other sites in the cerebral cortex – that account for the anticonvulsant effects of benzodiazepines (see Chapter 21, titled 'Medical Emergencies').

Unwanted effects of benzodiazepines

The most important adverse effect of benzodiazepine sedation is respiratory depression. Effects on the cardiovascular system are minimal, although benzodiazepines can cause a small fall in blood pressure.

Drug interactions are discussed in Chapter 15 (titled 'Adverse drug reactions and interactions'), but it is important to mention here the additive effect when administered with other CNS depressants that could expedite respiratory depression.

One of the metabolites of diazepam has sedative properties, and this can lead to a prolonged recovery to the normal state.

As benzodiazepines affect the limbic system, they have the potential to produce sexual fantasies in recipients, and this has certainly been described in dental patients receiving conscious sedation. This effect appears to be dose related, with doses of <0.1 mg/kg appearing not to produce this phenomenon.

Benzodiazepines used for intravenous sedation

Two benzodiazepines have been used in intravenous sedation for dentistry. These are diazepam and midazolam. The latter drug is currently the agent of choice, as it offers a number of advantages over diazepam. These include water solubility, which makes injection more comfortable, and a shorter half-life, which ensures more rapid recovery.

Technique of intravenous sedation with midazolam

Midazolam is presented in solution as 5 mg of the drug in a 5 ml solution. There is no standard dose, and the drug is injected via an indwelling cannula in increments (e.g. 1 mg/min) until the desired end point is reached. There is no fixed sign of the end point, and it is often determined by clinical experience; however, unconsciousness should not be produced, the aim being to establish a relaxed but communicative patient. Most patients will reach the end point with <10 mg of midazolam. A working time of around 45 min is achieved using this method. During sedation, the patient's oxygen saturation is monitored continuously with a pulse oximeter; availability of emergency oxygen supply must be ensured, since supplemental oxygen may be required. If inadvertent oversedation occurs, an injection of intravenous flumazenil will reverse the actions of midazolam. The reversal agent is supplied as a 5-ml aqueous solution containing 100 µg/ml of flumazenil. It is administered intravenously as a 200 µg bolus, and then incrementally at the rate of 100 µg/min until reversal occurs.

When providing intravenous sedation, it is imperative that a suitable chaperone be present, since, as mentioned earlier, sexual fantasy is a side effect of this treatment.

Propofol

Propofol is a general anaesthetic induction agent that can be used to provide conscious sedation. The technique is different from that with benzodiazepines, as this drug is continually infused to maintain a level of sedation. The infusion can be controlled by the operator, on demand by the patient or automatically using effect-site concentration. Propofol is metabolised very quickly, allowing rapid reversal. It achieves its sedative effect in a similar manner as benzodiazepines – that is, by agonist action at the GABA receptor–chloride channel complex.

Inhalational sedation

Although general anaesthetic agents such as sevoflurane have been employed as inhalational sedation agents, the main drug used in this regard is nitrous oxide (N_2O), in a technique known as 'relative analgesia'.

N_2O

Physical properties

N_2O is a colourless gas at room temperature and atmospheric pressure. It is supplied under pressure in blue cylinders as a liquid. It is poorly soluble in blood, and is a weak anaesthetic. The minimum alveolar concentration required to produce general anaesthesia in 50% of the population (MAC_{50}) is 110%.

Pharmacological actions

Inhalation of N_2O produces two useful actions, namely sedation and analgesia. The analgesic effect is particularly useful in the management of ischaemic muscle pain – for example, that occurring during myocardial infarction.

Sedation is achieved because N_2O acts as a CNS depressant; however, its exact mode of action is not clearly understood. The analgesic effect is probably due to action at the opioid receptors, and the sedation may be the result of an agonist effect at the GABA receptors and antagonistic action at the NMDA receptors.

Unwanted effects

N_2O has several unwanted effects; however, these mainly affect dental staff rather than the patient. This is because most adverse effects are the result of chronic exposure. The main problems in the patient are the result of hypoxia, which happens when insufficient oxygen is administered during inhalational sedation (see the following text). Adverse effects occur because N_2O oxidises reduced vitamin B_{12}. Among other consequences, this interferes with the action of the enzyme methionine synthetase, which is involved in the synthesis of DNA. Effective scavenging of waste gases and monitoring of staff exposure levels should be performed to combat the problems described in the following text.

Reproductive problems

Chronic exposure to N_2O can lead to miscarriage and decreased fertility.

Neurological effects

Chronic exposure to N_2O has been reported to increase neurological problems fourfold.

Haematological problems

N_2O can cause bone marrow suppression, which interferes with red cell production. At high doses, white cell production is impaired.

Liver and kidney problems

The incidence of both renal and hepatic disease is increased in those chronically exposed to N_2O.

Malignancy

It has been reported that the incidence of cervical cancer is increased in dental nursing staff exposed to high levels of N_2O.

Relative analgesia

The technique of relative analgesia relies on the inhalation of a mixture of N_2O and oxygen via a nasal hood. The machinery used to deliver relative analgesia limits the maximum dose of N_2O to 70% of the inhaled mixture. Most patients are sedated at well below this level. The patient begins by inhaling 100% oxygen, and then N_2O is introduced in 10% increments at intervals of about 1 min until 20% N_2O is being administered; if this is not sufficient for adequate sedation, then further 5% increments per minute are added. At the end of sedation, the patient is allowed to breathe 100% oxygen for a couple of minutes to prevent diffusion hypoxia, which is the result of the rapid loss of N_2O from the blood into the lungs.

Oral sedation

Oral sedation is not as predictable as the methods described in the preceding text, as there is variable absorption and latency of onset. The drug of choice is benzodiazepine temazepam. It is normally administered in a dose of 10–40 mg, around 45 min prior to dental treatment.

Transmucosal sedation

There are three routes for transmucosal sedation. These are sublingual, intranasal and rectal. The drug of choice is midazolam. Doses higher than those administered intravenously are used, and the onset time is 10–15 min.

FURTHER READING

Australian and New Zealand College of Anaesthetists and Faculty of Pain Medicine. Acute pain management: scientific evidence; 2015. pp. 329–331. Available from: http://asp-au.secure-zone.net/v2/index.jsp?id=522/2055/8212&lng=en.

Bailey E, Worthington HV, van Wijk A, Yates JM, Coulthard P, Afzal Z. Ibuprofen and/or paracetamol (acetaminophen) for pain relief after surgical removal of lower wisdom teeth (Review). *Cochrane Database Systematic Review*. 2013; **12**: p. CD00.4624. Available from: http://www.cochrane.org/CD004624/ORAL_ibuprofen-versus-paracetamol-acetaminophen-for-pain-relief-after-surgical-removal-of-lower-wisdom-teeth.

E-Den. Module 3 Anxiety and Pain Control in Dentistry. Available from: http://www.e-lfh.org.uk/programmes/dentistry/.

Meechan JG. Local anaesthesia: risks and controversies. *Dent Update*. 2009; **36**: 278–80, 282–3.

National Institute for Health and Care Excellence. Analgesia – mild-to-moderate pain; 2015. Available from: http://cks.nice.org.uk/analgesia-mild-to-moderate-pain.

Royal College of Surgeons of England. Standards for Conscious Sedation in the Provision of Dental Care; 2015. Available from: https://www.rcseng.ac.uk/fds/publications-clinical-guidelines/standards-for-conscious-sedation-in-the-provision-of-dental-care-2015.

Segev G, Katz RJ. Selective COX-2 Inhibitors and Risk of Cardiovascular Events. *Hospital Physician*. 2004; **40**: 39–46.

MULTIPLE CHOICE QUESTIONS

1. A patient who suffers from stable angina attends a dental practice for the extraction of a lower first molar tooth. Which of the following local anaesthetic regimens would be the most appropriate to use?
   a) Inferior alveolar nerve block and buccal infiltration with 2% lidocaine, 1:80 000 adrenaline (total 4.4 ml).
   b) Inferior alveolar nerve block and buccal infiltration with 4% articaine, 1:100 000 adrenaline (total 4.4 ml).
   c) Inferior alveolar nerve block with 2% lidocaine, 1:80 000 adrenaline and buccal infiltration with 4% articaine, 1:100 000 adrenaline (total 4.4 ml).
   d) Buccal and lingual infiltrations with 2% lidocaine, 1:80 000 adrenaline (total 2.2 ml).
   e) Buccal and lingual infiltrations with 4% articaine, 1:100 000 adrenaline (total 2.2 ml).
   Answer = C

2. A medically fit patient who weighs 70 kg attends a dental surgery for root canal treatment on the upper first molar. Which of the following is the maximum local anaesthetic dose that can be used?
   a) 15.4 ml/308 mg, 2% lidocaine, 1:80 000 adrenaline.
   b) 17.6 ml/352 mg, 2% lidocaine, 1:80 000 adrenaline.
   c) 13.2 ml/264 mg, 2% lidocaine, 1:80 000 adrenaline.
   d) 11 ml/110 mg, 2% lidocaine, 1:80 000 adrenaline.
   e) 19.8 ml/396 mg, 2% lidocaine, 1:80 000 adrenaline.
   Answer = A

3. Which of the following local anaesthetics would be the most appropriate for prolonged pain relief following a general anaesthetic for lower wisdom tooth removal?
   a) 2% Lidocaine, 1:80 000 adrenaline.
   b) 4% Articaine, 1:100 000 adrenaline.
   c) 3% Mepivacaine.
   d) 3% Prilocaine with Octapressin.
   e) 0.25% Bupivacaine, 1:200 000 adrenaline.
   Answer = E

4. Which of the following local anaesthetics would have the fastest onset of action?
   a) pKa 9.1, pH 4.
   b) pKa 7.9, pH 9.
   c) 96% protein bound, pH 4.
   d) 96% protein bound, pKa 9.
   e) 63% protein bound, pKa 7.9.
   Answer = B

5. A dentist has extracted a lower second molar in practice, and is giving the patient, who is medically fit, post-operative advice regarding analgesia. Which of the following is the most appropriate regimen to advise?
   a) 1 g paracetamol four times a day, 400 mg ibuprofen three times a day, staggered.
   b) 500 mg paracetamol four times a day, 400 mg ibuprofen three times a day, staggered.
   c) 1 g paracetamol four times a day, 30 mg codeine four times a day, staggered.
   d) 500 mg paracetamol four times a day, 400 mg ibuprofen three times a day, 30 mg codeine four times a day, staggered.
   e) 400 mg ibuprofen four times a day, 60 mg codeine three times a day, staggered.
   Answer = A

6. A patient attends an emergency appointment, complaining of toothache for the previous 2 weeks. On questioning, the patient admits having taken 5 g paracetamol daily for the past 5 days. What is the best course of action?
   a) Carry out the necessary dental emergency treatment, and advise the patient to stop taking paracetamol.
   b) Refer the patient to the local oral and maxillofacial surgery department for treatment.
   c) Carry out the necessary dental treatment, and refer the patient to a general medical practitioner for investigation.
   d) Ring the local accident and emergency department for advice and referral.
   e) None of the above.
   Answer = D

7. Which of the following patients should not be prescribed ibuprofen?
   a) Paediatric patients.
   b) Patients with liver disease.
   c) Asthmatic patients.
   d) Elderly patients.
   e) All of the above.
   Answer = C

8. A patient is being treated under intravenous sedation. During the procedure, the patient's oxygen saturation drops to 95%. Which is the best course of action?
   a) Reverse the sedation with intramuscular flumazenil.

b) Give supplemental oxygen via a nasal cannula, and reassess the oxygen saturation.
c) Give supplemental oxygen via a face mask, and reassess the oxygen saturation.
d) Reverse the sedation with intravenous flumazenil.
e) None of the above.
Answer = B

9. A dentist has finished a restorative procedure on a patient undergoing inhalation sedation, and now needs to reverse the sedation. What actions should be taken?
a) Give 100% oxygen for 2–3 min.
b) Remove the nose mask, and ask the patient to take deep breaths of room air.
c) Titrate the N_2O levels to 0% by 10% increments over 2–3 min.
d) Titrate the N_2O levels to 0% by 5% increments over 2–3 min, and then give the patient 100% oxygen for 2–3 min.
e) Give the patient flumazenil.
Answer = A

10. During intravenous sedation, which of the following should be monitored?
a) Respiratory rate, oxygen saturation, blood pressure.
b) Heart rate, respiratory rate, blood pressure.
c) Respiratory rate, heart rate, oxygen saturation.
d) Respiratory rate, oxygen saturation, temperature.
e) All vital signs.
Answer = A

CHAPTER 15

Adverse drug reactions and interactions

RA Seymour and M Greenwood

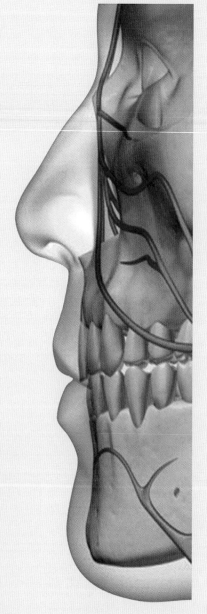

Key topics

- Adverse drug reactions
- Drug interactions

Learning objectives

- To be aware of the nature and types of drug interactions.
- To be aware of some of the more common adverse drug reactions of relevance to dental practice.

Adverse drug reactions

Adverse drug reactions are the unwanted effects arising from a patient's medication. Such reactions can be conveniently classified as type A (*A*ugmented reactions) or type B (*B*izarre reactions).

Type A reactions are the result of an exaggerated but otherwise normal pharmacological action of a drug given in the usual therapeutic dose. An example would include prolonged bleeding due to the antiplatelet action of aspirin. These reactions are largely predictable based on a drug's known pharmacology.

In contrast, type B reactions have totally aberrant effects that are not to be expected from the known pharmacological actions of a drug when given in the usual therapeutic doses to a patient whose body handles the drug in the normal way. Examples include hypersensitivity reactions to penicillin, angioedema arising from ACE inhibitors and drug-induced gingival overgrowth.

Oral and dental structures are frequently the sites of adverse drug reactions. Targets include salivary glands, oral mucosa, periodontal tissues, teeth and alveolar bone.

Salivary glands

Systemic drug therapy can have a profound effect on salivary gland function. Drug-induced xerostomia is perhaps the most widespread oral adverse drug reaction seen in dentistry. Other adverse drug reactions impacting on salivary glands and function include sialorrhoea, gland swelling, and pain and taste disturbances.

Drug-induced xerostomia

The salivary glands are under the control of the autonomic nervous system, and hence their function can be affected by a variety of drugs. Most of the drugs that reduce salivary flow do so by competing with acetylcholine release at the parasympathetic effector junction. Some 400 drugs have been implicated in causing xerostomia, and a list of the different categories with examples is shown in Table 15.1.

Oral problems associated with xerostomia include impaired speech, and difficulty in eating and swallowing. Patients become more susceptible to oral infections, especially those caused by *Candida albicans*. For dentate patients, the reduced salivary flow rate and hence its reduced buffering capacity increases the risk of dental caries, especially root caries. Other oral problems associated with xerostomia include an increased risk of angular cheilitis, mucosal ulceration and development of leukoplakia. For the edentulous patient, drug-induced xerostomia produces significant problems with denture retention.

Management of drug-induced xerostomia

For the most part, patients learn to adapt and cope with their reduced salivary flow. Local measures such as frequent sips of water or chewing sugar-free gum may help to alleviate some of

Table 15.1 Categories of drugs and examples that can cause xerostomia.

Category	Example
Tricyclic antidepressants	Amitriptyline
Muscarinic receptor antagonist	Oxybutynin
α-Receptor antagonist	Terazosin
Antipsychotics	Phenothiazines Lithium
Diuretics	Furosemide
Histamine H_1 receptor blockers	Chlorphenamine
Histamine H_2 receptor blockers	Cimetidine
Central antihypertensives	Moxonidine
Angiotensin-converting enzyme inhibitors	Lisinopril
Serotonin antagonists	Fluoxetine
Noradrenaline re-uptake inhibitors	Reboxetine
Dopamine re-uptake inhibitors	Bupropion
Appetite suppressants	Fenfluramine Phentermine
Systemic bronchodilators	Tiotropium
Opioids	Morphine
Proton pump inhibitors	Omeprazole
Cytotoxic drugs	5-Fluorouracil
Retinoids	Isotretinoin
Anti-HIV drugs	Didanosine and HIV protease inhibitors
Antimigraine drugs	Rizatriptan
Decongestants	Pseudoephedrine

the problems. A variety of salivary substitutes are commercially available, but one that contains fluoride would be beneficial in reducing the risk of root caries.

Pilocarpine (50 mg), a muscarinic antagonist, has been shown to be useful in the management of xerostomia. The drug does have unwanted effects, including increased sweating, headache, nausea, urinary frequency and palpitations. Such unwanted effects may affect compliance.

Many of the xerogenic drugs are taken once a day, and patients may prefer to take such medications first thing in the morning. This allows the maximum xerogenic effect to occur during the day, and has maximum impact on eating and swallowing. Switching the timing of the medication, if appropriate, to night time will reduce the impact of the drug's xerostomic effect.

Drug-induced sialorrhoea

Hypersalivation or sialorrhoea is often recognised as drooling. The latter is caused either by an increase in saliva flow that cannot be compensated by swallowing, or by impaired swallowing that cannot manage normal or even reduced amounts of saliva. The drug most frequently associated with sialorrhoea is clozapine, the antipsychotic agent. This drug is one of the first-line agents in the management of schizophrenia; thus, switching medications may not be an option for the management of this unwanted effect.

Drug-induced pain and swelling of the salivary glands

Several drugs have been cited as causing pain and swelling mainly in the parotid gland, especially drugs that can either concentrate in the gland or be accidentally aspirated into it. Iodine, which is used as a radiographic contrast medium, concentrates in the parotid gland up to 100-fold the levels in plasma. Parotid swelling is a rare unwanted effect arising from chlorhexidine mouthrinsing. The swelling appears to subside spontaneously within a few days after discontinuing use. The clinical features have the appearance of mechanical obstruction of the parotid duct. It is suggested that over-vigorous mouthrinsing may create a negative pressure in the parotid and aspiration of chlorhexidine into the gland. Patients should be instructed to be less vigorous with their mouthrinsing, so as to avoid this unwanted effect.

Drug-induced taste disturbances

Many drugs induce abnormalities of taste, either via reducing serum zinc levels (zinc is essential for taste acuity) or by direct interaction with proteins or taste bud receptors. The alteration in taste may be simply a blunting or decreased sensitivity in taste perception (hypogeusia), a total loss of the ability to taste (ageusia) or a distortion in perception of the correct taste of a substance – for example, sour for sweet (dysgeusia).

Drugs that contain a sulphhydryl group (e.g. penicillamine and captopril) are common causes of taste disturbances. The sulphhydryl group binds with proteins on taste buds and reduces taste acuity. Loop diuretics (e.g. furosemide) and, to a lesser extent, thiazide diuretics (e.g. bendroflumethiazide) are causes of taste disturbances. Both types of diuretics deplete the body of a variety of metallic salts, including zinc. Of particular concern to the dental profession is the relationship between chlorhexidine and taste disturbances. Following a chlorhexidine rinse, the appreciation of sweetness is affected first, followed by saltiness and bitterness. This unwanted effect is compounded by repeated use. The mechanism of chlorhexidine-induced taste disturbances may be related to the drug's ability to bind to proteins on the taste buds.

Oral mucosa and tongue

A variety of drugs can cause or exacerbate well-recognised conditions of the oral mucosa and tongue. Such conditions can be classified by specific lesions, and include drug-induced vesiculobullous conditions, oral ulceration, lichenoid eruptions and other white lesions of the oral mucosa, and discoloration of the oral mucosa.

Drug-induced vesiculobullous lesions

Such conditions include erythema multiforme (which also includes Stevens–Johnson syndrome), mucous membrane, pemphigoid and pemphigus vulgaris (see Chapter 11, titled 'Musculoskeletal disorders'). Drugs that are frequently cited as causal in these various vesiculobullous conditions are listed in Table 15.2.

Lichen planus

Oral lichen planus is a chronic inflammatory oral mucosal disease of unknown aetiology. The term 'lichenoid drug eruptions' can be used in two senses – first, drug eruptions similar or identical to lichen planus and, second, drug eruptions that do not necessarily appear like lichen planus, but have histological features very like this condition. A list of drugs that have been associated with lichenoid eruptions are shown in Table 15.3.

In addition to systemic medication, lichenoid reactions can be associated with dental materials. Amalgam, especially mercuric chloride, is the material most frequently cited. For some patients, replacing their amalgam restorations may result in an improvement of their oral lesions.

Table 15.2 Categories of drugs that have been cited as causing vesiculobullous lesions.

Category	Example
Analgesics	Aspirin, diclofenac, diflunisal, mefenamic acid, piroxicam, ibuprofen
Antibiotics	Clindamycin, streptomycin, tetracyclines, vancomycin, co-trimoxazole
Calcium channel blockers	Diltiazem, nifedipine, verapamil, amlodipine
Antiepileptic	Carbamazepine, phenytoin
Antifungals	Fluconazole, griseofulvin
Diuretics	Hydrochlorothiazide, furosemide
Antidiabetics	Chlorpropamide, tolbutamide
Hormones	Mesterolone, progesterone
Miscellaneous	Quinine, retinol, mercury, omeprazole, zidovudine

Table 15.3 Drugs that have been associated with lichenoid reactions.

ACE-1 inhibitors (e.g. captopril)	Mercury (amalgam)
Antimalarials	Metronidazole
Beta-adrenoreceptor blockers (e.g. propranolol)	NSAIDs
Carbamazepine	Oral contraceptives
Chloral hydrate oral	Penicillins
Chlorpropamide	Phenytoin
Cinnarizine	Quinine
Dipyridamole	Rifampicin
Furosemide	Streptomycin
Ketoconazole	Sulfonamides
Lincomycin	Tetracyclines
Lithium	Thiazide diuretics
Lorazepam	Tolbutamide

Other drug-related white lesions of the oral mucosa

Such lesions include candidiasis, hairy leukoplakia and leukoplakia. Many of these conditions arise in immunosuppressed organ transplant patients, and are secondary to a combination of ciclosporin, azathioprine and prednisolone.

It should also be emphasised that these types of lesions can be found in HIV patients, further underlining the aspect of immunosuppression in their pathogenesis.

Drug-induced discoloration of the oral mucosa

Many food substances and beverages can stain the oral mucosa, albeit temporarily. Apart from food, the most common discoloration of the tongue is known as black hairy tongue. This results from hypertrophy of the filiform papillae, which may grow up to 1 cm in length. Oral penicillins and other topical antimicrobials can cause black hairy tongue. Brushing the tongue may reduce this unwanted effect.

A common cause of drug-induced discoloration of the oral mucosa relates to the drug enhancement of melanogenesis. Hormones are the main drug implicated in this unwanted effect. Other details of drug-induced discoloration of the oral mucosa, together with possible underlying mechanisms, are listed in Table 15.4.

Drug-induced oral ulceration

Several drugs can cause a wide range of ulcerative lesions of the oral mucosa. These range from local irritants that cause oral burns to drug-related aphthous-type ulcerations and fixed drug eruptions. It is always worth bearing in mind that medication might have a bearing in cases of oral ulceration.

Nicorandil, used in some patients for prophylaxis and the treatment of stable angina, is a potassium channel activator that has increased in use in recent years. It is a drug that can sometimes produce quite severe and debilitating oral ulcerations as an unwanted side effect. In some cases, these ulcers can be so severe and persistent that incisional biopsy becomes necessary. Other areas of the gastrointestinal tract may also be affected by ulceration in patients taking nicorandil.

Methotrexate, a chemotherapeutic agent sometimes used orally in the treatment of rheumatoid arthritis, is also well known for sometimes causing troublesome oral ulceration as an unwanted side effect.

Local irritants

The best-known example is the so-called 'aspirin burn', arising from patients placing an aspirin tablet against a tooth for relieving their pain. This has no benefit in the management of toothache, and the corrosive action of the acidic aspirin can result in a large area of ulceration. Similar burns have been reported following the use of proprietary toothache solutions.

Cocaine abusers have been reported to suffer from extensive oral ulceration when the drug is applied topically. Cocaine abusers or 'drug pushers' often rub the cocaine powder into the attached gingivae, often in the upper premolar area. Since cocaine is a powerful topical anaesthetic, this local application onto the oral mucosa is used to 'test' the purity of the substance. The ulceration is probably due to the intense vasoconstrictive properties of cocaine.

Other drugs can act as local irritants, including potassium chloride, isoprenaline, pancreatin and ergotamine tartrate. Damage results when the drug is retained in the mouth for too long – for example, sucking the tablets, as opposed to swallowing them.

Drug-related aphthous-type ulceration

Aphthous ulceration, often referred to as 'recurrent aphthous ulceration' (RAU), is a common condition that is characterised by multiple, recurrent, small, and round/ovoid ulcers (Figure 15.1). The aetiology of RAU is, for the most part, unknown, but several risk factors have been identified.

Systemic medication can cause RAU, and the drugs implicated include certain NSAIDs, β-adrenoceptor blockers, captopril (an ACE-1 inhibitor), nicorandil (a potassium channel activator), protease inhibitors and tacrolimus, the new immunosuppressant agent.

Diagnosis of drug-induced RAU can be problematic. The ulcers usually occur and then disappear with discontinuation of the drug. It is necessary to dose the patient again with the same drug to confirm the cause and effect, and this raises ethical issues. The mechanisms of drug-induced RAU remain uncertain.

Table 15.4 Drugs that can cause discoloration of the oral mucosa.

Blue	Brown (hypermelanosis)	Black	Grey
Amiodarone	Aminophenazone	Betel nut	Amodiaquine
Antimalarials	Betel nut	Bismuth	Chloroquine
Bismuth	Bismuth	Methyldopa	Fluoxetine
Mepacrine	Busulphan	Minocycline	Hydroxychloroquine
Minocycline	Clofazimine		
Phenazopyridine	Contraceptives		
Quinidine	Cyclophosphamide		
Silver	Diethylstilbestrol		
Sulphasalazine	Doxorubicin		
	Doxycycline		
	Fluorouracil		
	Heroin		
	Hormone-replacement therapy		
	Ketoconazole		
	Menthol		
	Methaqualone		
	Minocycline		
	Phenolphthalein		
	Propranolol		
	Smoking		
	Zidovudine		

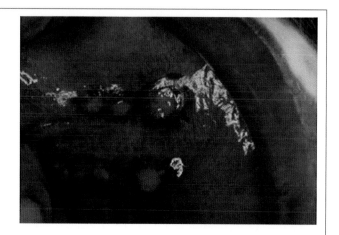

Figure 15.1 Drug-related aphthous ulceration.

Table 15.5 Some drugs commonly cited as causing fixed drug eruptions.

Lidocaine
Chlorhexidine
Penicillamine
Salicylates
Sulphonamides

Fixed drug eruptions

Such eruptions often occur as repeated ulcerations at the same site in response to a particular drug or other compound. They are essentially type IV or delayed hypersensitivity reactions. When the ulceration is due to a systemic medication, then the term 'fixed drug eruption' is appropriate. If the ulceration is from local contact, then it is more appropriate to refer to this as 'contact stomatitis'. Table 15.5 lists the drugs commonly cited as causing fixed drug eruptions.

Many compounds have been cited as causing contact stomatitis. These include cosmetics, chewing gum, ingredients of toothpaste and certain dental materials. Metals are frequently implicated, especially nickel-containing alloys. The increasing fashion of tongue and lip piercing has resulted in a rise in contact dermatitis, since many of the lip and tongue decorations contain nickel.

Dental structures

Systemic drug therapy can affect the dental structures, although this is mainly an indirect effect mediated by a drug-induced alteration in the oral environment. The following discussion concerns drugs that affect dental structures, and the problems of sugar-based medicines.

Tooth development

Phenytoin, the antiepileptic drug, can cause abnormalities in the roots of the teeth. Defects include shortening of the root, root resorption and an increased deposition of cementum. The mechanism of phenytoin-induced root abnormalities is uncertain, but may be related to the drug inhibiting vitamin D metabolism or PTH production.

Intraligamentary injections of lidocaine and prilocaine are cytotoxic to the enamel organ, and will interfere with amelogenesis. Chemotherapeutic agents used in treatments of childhood malignancies can interfere with the formation of dental tissues. Such drugs can disrupt the development of the enamel organ and produce several dental abnormalities, including failure of tooth to develop, microdontia, hypoplasia, enamel opacities and impaired root development.

Drug-induced staining of the dental structures

Chlorhexidine

Staining of the teeth, restorations and dentures is the most common problem associated with chlorhexidine usage. The extent and severity of the staining appear to be related to the drug's concentration. Less staining is reported to occur with the use of 0.12% solution as compared to the 0.2% solution.

Chlorhexidine-induced staining is enhanced by dietary factors, especially foods and drinks that contain high levels of tannins (e.g. red wine, tea and coffee). The primary site of discoloration appears to be the acquired pellicle, which suggests that salivary proteins (the source of the pellicle) play an important role in the chlorhexidine-induced staining process. Removal of chlorhexidine staining can be problematic, and often requires professional cleaning.

Tetracyclines and other antibiotics

The possible effects of tetracyclines on the developing teeth are well established. Immediately after absorption, tetracyclines are incorporated into the calcifying tissues, which become a permanent feature in the teeth. For the most part, the discoloration is grey, but brownish-yellow discoloration can occur with certain tetracycline preparations. Tetracycline-induced discoloration only occurs during the formative stages of tooth development, and hence these drugs should be avoided during this period. Ciprofloxacin has also been reported to cause a greenish discoloration of the teeth.

Sugar-based medicines

Sugars (sucrose, glucose and fructose) are widely used in the formulation of liquid medicines. Long-term use of such medicines is associated with increased caries, and the term 'medication caries' has been used to describe this condition. Plaque pH studies have shown that medicines sweetened with sucrose cause prolonged pH depression. The effects of this are more pronounced in such medicines when given at night, as reduced salivary flow decreases further resistance to caries.

Sugar has many advantages as a constituent of medicines. It is cheap, nontoxic and soluble. In liquid form, sugars provide important diluent, preservative and viscosity-modifying properties. These, together with the sweetening properties of sugar, improve palatability and compliance, and make the replacement of sugars with non-sugar-based alternatives difficult.

Over 50% of prescriptions dispensed for potential long-term use in children are sugar based. Children taking these medications are most likely to be suffering from epilepsy, cystic fibrosis, chronic renal failure and asthma. The detrimental effects of sugar-based medicines on the dental health of these children are relevant since certain dental procedures can carry greatly increased morbidity in these medical conditions. While there is a trend to increase the availability of sugar-free medicines, the climate of increasing drug bills does restrict this option. Wherever possible, practitioners should try and find a sugar-free alternative, especially for long-term use.

Periodontal tissues

Systemic medication can have three main effects on periodontal tissues – (1) a direct adverse effect on the periodontium; (2) reducing the rate of periodontal breakdown; and (3) increasing the response of the periodontal tissues to bacterial plaque. The two more frequently recognised adverse effects on the periodontal tissue are drug-induced gingival overgrowth and drug-induced desquamative gingivitis.

Drug-induced gingival overgrowth

Three drugs have been implicated in causing this unwanted effect – notably, the antiepileptic phenytoin, the immunosuppressant ciclosporin and the calcium channel blockers (e.g. nifedipine and amlodipine). Approximately 50% of patients medicated with phenytoin experience drug-induced gingival overgrowth (Figure 15.2). The figures for ciclosporin and calcium channel blockers are 30% and 10%, respectively.

Risk factors for drug-induced gingival overgrowth

The risk factors for this unwanted effect include age, drug variables, concomitant medication and periodontal variables.

1. *Age.* Young patients are more susceptible to drug-induced gingival overgrowth. This would suggest a hormonal factor. Increased levels of circulating sex hormones do increase

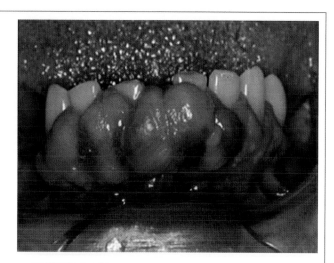

Figure 15.2 Gingival overgrowth in a patient taking nifedipine, a calcium channel blocker.

the response of the gingival tissues to bacterial plaque. Any increase in inflammation will compound the expression of gingival overgrowth.

2. *Drug variables.* There is no clear picture on the relationships between several drug variables and the expression of gingival overgrowth. Despite these findings, there must be a baseline or threshold drug concentration to induce such gingival changes. Such a threshold concentration may vary from drug to drug, and from individual to individual.

3. *Concomitant medication.* The three major drugs implicated in gingival overgrowth are seldom the only medications prescribed to the patient. Nifedipine and other calcium channel blockers are used extensively in organ transplant patients medicated with ciclosporin. As these drugs also cause gingival overgrowth, it is not surprising that the prevalence of this unwanted effect increases significantly in transplant patients. In contrast, other immunosuppressants taken to prevent graft rejection in such patients may also provide them with a degree of protection against the development of gingival overgrowth. Other antiepileptics can affect the hepatic metabolism of phenytoin, which in turn could increase the expression of gingival overgrowth.

4. *Periodontal variables.* Any plaque-induced inflammatory changes within the tissues exacerbate the expression of drug-induced gingival overgrowth. This finding suggests causality, with a patient's oral hygiene being a significant risk factor for both the development and the expression of drug-induced gingival overgrowth.

A patient's underlying periodontal condition may also be a significant risk factor for drug-induced gingival overgrowth. Of particular concern is the extent of inflammation present in the gingival tissues prior to dosing. The importance of periodontal risk factors does impact upon how drug-induced gingival overgrowth is managed. Improving a patient's oral hygiene and reducing the inflammatory component in gingival tissues by nonsurgical means have an impact on this unwanted effect, especially in reducing the risk of recurrence after surgical correction.

Pathogenesis of drug-induced gingival overgrowth

The main histopathological feature of drug-induced gingival overgrowth is a fibrotic or expanded connective tissue with various levels of inflammation and an enlarged gingival epithelium. Thus, the main feature in the pathogenesis of this unwanted effect is a drug-induced alteration in connective tissue homeostasis. This is possibly mediated via a reduction in collagen breakdown. A key factor in the pathogenesis is the role of inflammatory cytokines, as plaque-induced gingival inflammation enhances the expression of the overgrowth. While the precise mechanism of drug-induced gingival overgrowth remains uncertain, it is plausible that inflammatory cytokines could inhibit the action of certain collagenases. This process is potentiated or stimulated by local concentrations of the implicated drugs. It is hoped that a greater understanding of the pathogenesis of this unwanted effect will lead to improved management strategies for both its prevention and treatment.

Treatment of drug-induced gingival overgrowth

Gingival surgery (invariably gingivectomy) remains the main treatment of choice for correcting drug-induced gingival overgrowth. In addition to surgery, various treatments have been investigated either to prevent this unwanted effect or to reduce the incidence of recurrence. Such treatments include rigorous nonsurgical management, and the use of plaque-inhibitory agents and systemic antibiotics.

Plaque control, removal of plaque retentive factors and treatment of any underlying periodontal condition will reduce gingival inflammation, and hence the severity of any drug-induced gingival overgrowth. In some patients, these measures alone will not reduce the occurrence or recurrence of overgrowth, and surgical excision remains the only option.

One obvious solution in the management of drug-induced gingival overgrowth is to change the medication. For many years, this was not an option for ciclosporin. New immunosuppressant medication is now available (e.g. tacrolimus). Converting from ciclosporin to tacrolimus does reduce the severity of the overgrowth and the need for corrective surgery.

Although phenytoin usage is declining and there are more antiepileptics available, changing the medication for these patients can be a challenge. Carbamazepine, ethosuximide and sodium valproate are alternatives to phenytoin. If a change in anticonvulsant therapy is being considered, this should be accomplished gradually over a period of 2–3 months. During this time, the serum levels of the antiepileptics and the occurrence of seizures should be monitored.

Drug-induced desquamative gingivitis

Several drugs can cause oral lichenoid reactions, which can present as desquamative gingivitis (see Figure 15.3). The drugs most commonly implicated include β-adrenoceptor blockers (e.g. atenolol), antidiabetic drugs (e.g. chlorpropamide) and some NSAIDs. The diagnosis of drug-induced desquamative gingivitis can be problematic, and often involves stopping the suspended drug and re-challenging the patient. Most of the drugs frequently implicated can be substituted by an alternative medication with the same therapeutic goal.

Drugs that can increase the expression of periodontal disease

Drug therapy alone cannot cause periodontal disease. Certain drugs can enhance plaque-induced gingivitis. Sex hormones are the group of drugs most frequently associated with this unwanted effect. The oral contraceptive pill can mimic the gingival and periodontal changes observed in pregnancy. In contrast, hormone replacement therapy does afford a patient some degree of protection against periodontal breakdown, possibly mediated by their beneficial effects in the management of osteoporosis. The latter is now considered to be a significant risk factor for periodontal breakdown.

A further mechanism whereby systemic drug treatment can increase the rate of periodontal breakdown is via suppression of the bone marrow. Many drugs can cause this unwanted effect, and gingival tissues can often be the first manifestation of drug-induced bone marrow suppression. Thrombocytopaenia is one of the first manifestations of bone marrow suppression, and this can cause extravagant and often spontaneous bleeding from the gingivae.

An increase in periodontal breakdown following drug-induced bone marrow suppression will be mediated by a reduction in white blood cells, especially polymorphonuclear cells.

The latter provide the 'first line of defence' in periodontal tissues, and any impairment in either function or numbers will render the periodontal tissues more susceptible to bacterial plaque and its products.

Alveolar bone

Bisphosphonate-induced osteonecrosis

Bisphosphonates are used in the treatment of osteoporosis and to treat osteolytic tumours. These drugs bind to and accumulate in bone, and remain there for months after therapy is discontinued. Bisphosphonates have a variety of actions on bone homeostasis, resulting in an inhibition of bone resorption and an increase in bone mass.

As a consequence of their action on bone, osteoclastic function is severely impaired. Therefore, osteocytes are not replaced, and the capillary network in the bone is not maintained. This results in avascular necrosis (Figure 15.4).

Several case reports and studies have now confirmed the association between bisphosphonate therapy and osteonecrosis of the jaw. This particularly follows the use of intravenous preparations of bisphosphonates, and frequently occurs after dental extractions.

Prevention of bisphosphonate-induced osteonecrosis

Before starting on bisphosphonate therapy, patients should be counselled regarding the possible occurrence of jaw osteonecrosis. If possible, invasive dental procedures, including tooth extraction, should be avoided while patients are taking the medication. A thorough soft tissue and dental examination should be performed before a patient starts bisphosphonate therapy. If bisphosphonate therapy can be briefly delayed, then dental treatment should be completed

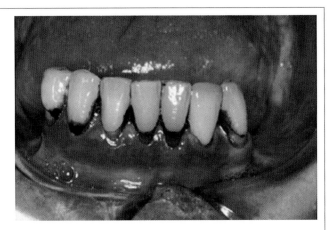

Figure 15.3 Drug-induced desquamative gingivitis.

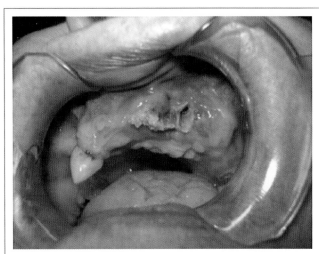

Figure 15.4 Osteonecrosis induced by bisphosphonates and a dental extraction.

before dosing. Once bisphosphonate therapy has started, patients should receive regular dental care and screening. If extractions are required, it is important to protect the tooth socket, and to try and achieve healing by getting primary closure of the soft tissues.

Treatment of bisphosphonate-induced osteonecrosis

Treatment of this condition remains problematic. Aggressive surgical intervention (e.g. bone resection) appears counter-productive, and often produces further bone exposure. Hyperbaric oxygen may be of some use. Other conservative approaches successfully used include a combination of wound irrigations using povidone-iodine, daily rinsing with 0.12% chlorhexidine mouthrinse, and systemic antibiotics.

Dry socket (alveolar osteitis)

The use of oral contraceptives has been associated with a significant increase in the frequency of dry sockets after the removal of impacted third molars. The magnitude of this increased risk is two- to threefold. Oral contraceptives, especially the oestrogen component, induce increased fibrinolysis, a key factor in dry socket formation. This unwanted effect can be minimised in patients taking oral contraceptives by carrying out the extractions during days 23–28 of the tablet cycle.

Cleft lip and palate

From time to time, several different drugs have been tentatively suggested as predisposing to the development of cleft lip, with or without cleft palate, in the offspring of mothers who have taken the drug during pregnancy. Few drugs can be firmly categorised as teratogenic in humans, except chemotherapeutic agents and some hormones. Drugs that have been significantly implicated include benzodiazepines, antiepileptics, vitamin A analogues and sulphasalazine. Wherever possible, all drugs should be avoided during pregnancy, especially in the early part of the first trimester.

Miscellaneous oral adverse drug reactions

Angioedema and ACE inhibitors

Examples of ACE inhibitors include enalapril and lisinopril, which are both used in the management of hypertension and heart failure. Several case reports have identified the problem of angioedema arising from the usage of these drugs.

The precise mechanism whereby these drugs cause angioedema remains uncertain. The most plausible explanation for the development of this unwanted effect relates to the pharmacodynamics of ACE inhibitors. ACE, also known as kinase II, is responsible for converting angiotensin I to the more powerful angiotensin II. In addition, the enzyme is also responsible for the metabolism of the peptide bradykinin. This peptide is an important mediator of inflammation, causing vasodilation and increased vascular permeability. Following the administration of an ACE inhibitor, bradykinin levels are raised, and its action is prolonged. This may account for the troublesome cough that many patients experience while on these drugs.

The prime concern in the management of angioedema is protection of the airway. Surgical intervention is rarely needed. It is tempting to recommend antiallergic therapy in cases of angioedema secondary to ACE inhibitors. Drugs such as adrenaline, corticosteroids and antihistamines (H1 receptor blockers) may be of limited value, because the mechanism of angioedema does not appear to be mediated by an antibody–antigen reaction. Case reports have documented the use of these drugs in the management of angioedema, but it is difficult to ascertain whether the reduction in swelling was the natural sequence of events or the result of the emergency drug treatment.

Angioedema is a serious, distressing and potentially life-threatening condition. A change in the patient's medication may be required, because angioedema can be recurrent. It is important to discuss such episodes with the patient's physician.

Drug-induced dyskinesias

The muscles of facial expression and mastication can be affected by systemic drug therapy. Such effects will result in dyskinesias or dystonia (involuntary movement of the facial muscles, resulting in lip smacking, facial grimaces and tongue protrusions). The drugs that have been implicated for this are predominantly the antipsychotics (e.g. phenothiazines and butyrophenones).

Summary

The mouth and associated structures are frequent targets for unwanted effects arising from systemic drug therapy. These range from troublesome xerostomia to a potentially life-threatening angioedema. As drug development and therapy are likely to increase, all members of the dental team should be alert to potential oral adverse reactions. If an oral adverse drug reaction becomes troublesome and affects the quality of life, then consideration should be given to a change in medication. Such changes can only be implemented after consultation with the patient's physician.

Drug interactions

If a medication is prescribed or administered to a patient who is already receiving drug therapy, then a drug interaction may occur. Some drug interactions are beneficial – for example, the combination of a local anaesthetic and a vasoconstrictor offers several advantages over a vasoconstrictor-free solution (see Chapter 14, titled 'Pain and anxiety control'). The number of possible drug interactions is large and impossible to commit to memory. Fortunately, there are good reference sources available, and Appendix 1 of the *British National Formulary* is an excellent example. The interactions described in this chapter are restricted to those that might occur between drugs administered or prescribed in dental practice and concurrent medication that dental outpatients may be receiving.

Mechanisms of drug interactions

There are three categories of drug interactions. These are pharmacokinetic, pharmacodynamic or pharmaceutical interactions. Pharmaceutical interactions are not relevant to outpatient dental practice.

Pharmacokinetic interactions

A pharmacokinetic interaction occurs when the presence of one drug affects the concentration of another drug at its site of action. The following aspects can be affected:

- *Absorption:* For example, local anaesthetics and adrenaline.
- *Distribution:* For example, warfarin and aspirin (aspirin displaces warfarin from protein-binding sites, thereby increasing the effective warfarin free plasma concentration).
- *Metabolism:* For example, β-adrenergic-blocking drugs and local anaesthetics (the reduction in hepatic blood flow produced by the former may increase the toxicity of the latter).
- *Excretion:* For example, probenecid inhibits the excretion of penicillin.

Pharmacodynamic interactions

A pharmacodynamic interaction is one where the drug effect is modified without its concentration at the site of action being affected. When interacting in this way, the drugs may act as agonists or antagonists, and the effects may be beneficial or adverse, as illustrated in the following examples.

- *Beneficial agonists:* The antibacterial drug co-trimoxazole relies on the combined action of two drugs (sulphamethoxazole and trimethoprim) that interfere at two different stages in bacterial folic acid production.
- *Adverse agonists:* The sedative agents used in dental practice combine with other CNS depressants such as alcohol, and this can lead to respiratory depression.
- *Beneficial antagonists:* Flumazenil antagonises the effects of midazolam, and can be used to reverse sedation.
- *Adverse antagonists:* The action of salbutamol, a β_2-adrenergic agonist used in the routine and emergency management of asthma, is antagonised by β-adrenergic-blocking drugs.

Relevance of drug interactions in dental practice

The clinical relevance of drug interactions can be classified by using the 'ACT' system. This is an acronym for *Avoid/Caution/T* heoretical. 'A' indicates that this combination should be avoided, as the adverse interaction is clinically important. 'C' implies that caution should be exercised, as an adverse interaction may occur. 'T' denotes that an interaction is theoretically possible, but unlikely to occur at the doses used in clinical dentistry.

Drug interactions that are relevant to dental practice are classified in Table 15.6 using the ACT system. Interactions in the A and C categories are discussed in the following text.

Agents that interfere with local anaesthetics and vasoconstrictors

There are very few drugs that interact with local anaesthetics and vasoconstrictors at normal clinical doses. There are some theoretical interactions that may occur if amounts reaching the higher end of the maximum dosage are employed.

Interactions with local anaesthetics

Other local anaesthetics

The toxic effects of local anaesthetics are additive; hence, when deciding the maximum dose, the total amount of the drug must be considered in cases where different local anaesthetic formulations (including topical application) are used in the same patient. The maximum doses for healthy patients are described in Chapter 14 (titled 'Pain and anxiety control').

Antimicrobials

Methaemoglobinaemia is a side effect of some local anaesthetics, especially prilocaine. Methaemoglobinaemia is caused by the iron in haemoglobin being in the ferric rather than the ferrous form, which reduces the oxygen-carrying capacity of haemoglobin. It presents as cyanosis. It can also be caused by other drugs such as sulphonamide antibacterials, and combined therapy has been reported to produce methaemoglobinaemia.

The protease inhibitor drugs that are used in the management of HIV may increase the plasma levels of lidocaine, and therefore may increase toxicity of the local anaesthetic.

Benzodiazepines

There is a beneficial interaction between midazolam and lidocaine. Benzodiazepine reduces the CNS toxicity of the local anaesthetic. Not all benzodiazepine–local anaesthetic interactions are helpful, however, as diazepam increases the toxicity of bupivacaine by raising the serum levels of the local anaesthetic.

Cardiovascular drugs

The pharmacokinetic effect of β-adrenergic-blocking drugs increasing local anaesthetic toxicity was mentioned in the preceding text. Large doses of local anaesthetics should be avoided in patients receiving β-blockers; one or two cartridges should not cause a problem in adults.

Similarly, the calcium channel blocker verapamil increases lidocaine toxicity, but this should not be a concern when one

Table 15.6 Drug interactions relevant to dental practice.

Drugs	Analgesics	Anti-abuse/abuse/social drugs	Antiasthma drugs	Anticoagulant drugs	Anticonvulsants	Antidiabetic drugs	Antihistamine drugs	Antimetabolites	Antimicrobials	Benzodiazepines	Cardiovascular drugs	Cations	CNS drugs	Corticosteroids	GI tract drugs	Drugs used in gout	Immunosuppressants	Lipid-lowering drugs	Local anaesthetics	Muscle relaxants	Oral contraceptives	Retinoids
LA	C				T				C	C	C								C	T		
Vasoconstrictors	C	C									C		C						C	C		
Benzodiazepines	A	A	C						A	C	C		A		C				C	T	T	
Aspirin	C			A	A	A		A			C			A	T	T						
Ibuprofen	C			C		C		A			A		A	A						C		
Paracetamol				C											T							
Penicillins	T			C				A	A		T					C					C	
Erythromycin	A	A	C	C		C	A	A			C		A	T	A	C	A	C			C	
Metronidazole	A	A		A	C	C		C	C				A	C	C	C	C	C			C	
Tetracyclines			C	C		A		C	A		C	C	C		C						C	
Clindamycin									T		C	C			C							
Antifungals	A		C	A		C	A		C	C	C	C	C	C	C		C				C	C

A = some drug combinations produce important interactions and should be avoided (see text for specific drugs involved); C = interactions that can occur in dental practice, and thus caution is required (see text for specific drugs involved); T = theoretical interaction unlikely in dental practice at normal clinical doses; LA = local anaesthetic.

or two cartridges are used in adults. Calcium channel blockers increase the cardiotoxicity of bupivacaine, the long-acting local anaesthetic.

Anticonvulsants

Phenytoin and lidocaine depress cardiac activity. This is unlikely to be a problem at the doses used in dentistry.

Interactions with vasoconstrictors

Cardiovascular drugs

Antihypertensive drugs can interact with adrenaline. When the β-adrenergic effects of the catecholamines are inhibited by concurrent use of β-adrenergic-blocking drugs, the unopposed α-adrenergic effects, which increase systolic blood pressure, could cause a cerebrovascular accident. One or two cartridges in adults should be safe; if more than that is required, an adrenaline-free solution is recommended. A helpful interaction with β-adrenoreceptor blockers is protection from the increase in heart rate produced by adrenaline.

Adrenaline decreases plasma potassium levels. This effect is exaggerated in dental patients receiving non-potassium-sparing diuretics. This interaction is not an absolute contraindication to the use of adrenaline-containing local anaesthetics; however, it is recommended that a limit of one or two cartridges be set in adults taking these diuretics.

Adrenaline-induced reductions in plasma potassium may also be exaggerated by calcium channel-blocking drugs; however, this has not been demonstrated during dental treatment.

Drugs acting on the CNS

The initial enzyme involved in the metabolism of adrenaline is catechol-*O*-methyltransferase (COMT). Entacapone, which is a drug used to treat Parkinson's disease, is a COMT inhibitor (the enzyme that initiates exogenous adrenaline metabolism). There is no evidence of a clinical interaction between adrenaline in dental local anaesthetic cartridges and entacapone; however, it would seem wise to limit the total dose of the vasoconstrictor. Monoamine oxidase inhibitors exert their action at a later stage in exogenous adrenaline breakdown, and are thus of little concern.

Tricyclic antidepressants decrease the re-uptake of adrenaline into nerve cells. This results in the pressor effects of adrenaline being increased. This is only a concern at high doses, and should not affect the administration of one or two cartridges in adult patients.

Drugs of abuse

Amphetamines, cannabis and cocaine have sympathomimetic actions that can increase adrenaline toxicity. It is wise to avoid or limit the amount of adrenaline-containing local anaesthetics in patients who have abused such drugs in the previous 24 hours.

Drugs that interact with oral and intravenous sedation

Other sedative agents

The sedative effects of midazolam and propofol are more than additive.

Analgesics

The NSAIDs aspirin and diclofenac increase the sedative effect of midazolam, and this can lead to a reduction in the onset time of sedation. Paracetamol reduces diazepam excretion, but this is of no clinical importance.

Antiasthma medication

Aminophylline can antagonise the actions of benzodiazepines and may reduce their effectiveness.

Antimicrobials

Antimicrobials can have quite different effects on the actions of benzodiazepines – for example, the metabolism of diazepam is decreased by ciprofloxacin and isoniazid, but increased by rifampicin. Erythromycin inhibits the metabolism of midazolam, and combined therapy can produce profound sedation. The antifungal drugs itraconazole, ketoconazole, miconazole and fluconazole, and the antiviral drugs efavirenz, indinavir, nelfinavir, ritonavir and saquinavir, increase the effect of midazolam. The interaction with these antiviral drugs is such that concurrent therapy should be avoided.

The effect of midazolam is also increased by probenecid, a drug used to increase the effect of penicillins.

Cardiovascular drugs

As with local anaesthetics, β-adrenergic-blocking drugs reduce diazepam metabolism; however, concurrent therapy seems to be safe. Diltiazem and verapamil increase the effect of midazolam, which can lead to a prolonged recovery time.

Drugs that act on the CNS

The combination of sedation with other CNS depressant agents (including alcohol) should be avoided, as oversedation that might lead to respiratory depression may ensue.

The effects of anticonvulsant medication on diazepam are variable and inconsistent. Diazepam both raises and reduces the plasma levels of phenytoin, varying between patients. Carbamazepine can inhibit the action of diazepam, whereas sodium valproate increases the sedative action.

The antidepressant drugs fluoxetine and fluvoxamine increase the effects of diazepam. The combination of diazepam and clozapine is contraindicated, as it can produce severe hypotension and respiratory depression.

The efficacy of levodopa is reduced by diazepam, and prolonged therapy can lead to a reduction in the control of Parkinson's disease.

Drugs acting on the gastrointestinal tract

The sedative effects of diazepam and midazolam can be increased by cimetidine and omeprazole, as these drugs inhibit benzodiazepine metabolism. This means that sedation may occur at lower than normal doses. Concurrent therapy with metoclopramide can enhance the action of oral diazepam.

Local anaesthetics

Beneficial and adverse effects of combined therapy with local anaesthetics were discussed in the preceding text.

Muscle relaxants

The effects of diazepam and midazolam are increased by the muscle relaxant baclofen.

Drugs that interfere with analgesics prescribed by dentists

Aspirin

Other analgesics

The combined use of aspirin with other NSAIDs increases adverse effects such as gastric irritation.

Anticoagulants

Aspirin increases the risk of bleeding when administered to patients receiving anticoagulants. Combined therapy should be avoided.

Anticonvulsants

Aspirin increases the anticonvulsant effects of phenytoin and sodium valproate.

Antidiabetic drugs

The urinary excretion of the oral hypoglycaemic drug chlorpropamide is decreased by aspirin. Combined therapy may cause hypoglycaemia.

Antimetabolites

Aspirin increases methotrexate toxicity as a result of the inhibition of renal excretion. This is only a concern when the antimetabolite is prescribed at large doses during the

management of malignancy; at the lower doses used to treat arthritis, this is not such a problem.

Cardiovascular drugs

The diuretic action of acetazolamide and spironolactone is reduced by aspirin. The plasma levels of digoxin can be increased by aspirin, and this can be problematic in elderly patients or in those with renal disease.

Corticosteroids

Both corticosteroids and aspirin produce gastrointestinal ulceration. Combined therapy should not be used, particularly in patients with a history of peptic ulceration.

Ibuprofen

Antihaemostatic drugs

The combination of ibuprofen with warfarin increases the chances of haemorrhage. Ibuprofen increases the risk of gastrointestinal bleed if administered to patients receiving antiplatelet therapy with drugs such as clopidogrel.

Antimetabolites

As with aspirin, ibuprofen reduces the excretion of methotrexate, which might result in toxic levels of the antimetabolite.

Cardiovascular drugs

The hypotensive action of β-adrenoceptor blockers and ACE inhibitors can be antagonised by ibuprofen. Ibuprofen reduces the renal clearance of digoxin, and this can result in digoxin toxicity.

Corticosteroids

Combined therapy with corticosteroids and ibuprofen should be avoided, as both may cause peptic ulceration.

Drugs that act on the CNS

Ibuprofen reduces lithium excretion. This might lead to toxicity of the latter drug, and combined use is contraindicated.

Muscle relaxants

Baclofen excretion is reduced by ibuprofen.

Paracetamol

Anticoagulants

The prolonged use of paracetamol can damage liver cells. This can interfere with the production of clotting factors, and may increase the chances of haemorrhage in patients receiving anticoagulants. As this adverse effect only occurs with prolonged use of the analgesic, a short-term course to manage dental pain is not a concern.

Drugs that act on the gastrointestinal tract

The absorption of paracetamol is enhanced by combined therapy with drugs that reduce gastric emptying.

Drugs that interfere with antimicrobials prescribed by dentists

Penicillins (including amoxicillin) and other antimicrobials

The action of the penicillins is decreased by tetracyclines. Plasma levels of penicillin V are reduced during combined therapy with neomycin, and doubling of the dose is required.

Anticoagulants

Penicillins may increase the anticoagulant effects of warfarin. This is only a concern during prolonged therapy, and frequent testing of the International Normalised Ratio (INR) (see Chapter 5, titled 'Cardiovascular disorders', and Chapter 13, titled 'Endocrinology and diabetes') is needed in such instances.

Antimetabolites

Penicillins increase the toxicity of methotrexate as a result of decreased excretion of the antimetabolite. This can be a serious adverse interaction, particularly in older patients or in those with decreased renal function.

Drugs used in the treatment of gout

Probenecid and sulphinpyrazone both increase the half-life of penicillin G. This interaction with probenecid is used to increase the efficacy of penicillin. The combined use of amoxicillin and allopurinol increases the production of skin rashes.

Oral contraceptives

There is a potential interaction between antibacterial drugs and oral contraceptives. Interference with gut flora inhibits absorption of the drug. This might lead to failure of contraception and, although the evidence for this is scarce, it is sensible to advise on other methods of contraception during antibiotic therapy.

Erythromycin

Antiasthma drugs

Erythromycin increases the plasma levels of theophylline. The dose of the latter drug may have to be lowered during combined use.

Anticoagulants

Erythromycin reduces the metabolism of warfarin and nicoumalone, and this might increase the risk of haemorrhage.

Combination therapy is not absolutely contraindicated; however, monitoring of the INR is required during prolonged administration of the antibacterial drug.

Antidiabetic drugs

Combined use of erythromycin with chlorpropamide may damage the liver, and concurrent therapy with glibenclamide can induce hypoglycaemia.

Antihistamines

The serum level of loratadine is raised by erythromycin. This does not appear to produce the severe cardiac effects reported with other antihistamines such as astemizole and terfenadine, which have been removed from the *British National Formulary*.

Antimetabolites

Erythromycin increases vinblastine toxicity, and combined use should be avoided.

Cardiovascular drugs

The metabolism of digoxin is reduced by erythromycin therapy, and this can lead to toxicity of the former drug. Erythromycin increases the plasma levels of other cardiovascular drugs, including disopyramide, quinidine, nadolol and felodipine.

Drugs acting on the CNS

Erythromycin increases the plasma levels of many drugs that affect the CNS. These include carbamazepine, ergotamine, alfentanil, clozapine, midazolam, triazolam, alprazolam, zopiclone, bromocriptine and cabergoline. The interactions with carbamazepine and ergotamine can be serious, and combined therapy is best avoided.

Drugs acting on the gastrointestinal tract

Cimetidine increases the plasma concentration of erythromycin, increasing the toxicity of the latter drug.

Immunosuppressants

Erythromycin increases the plasma levels of the immunosuppressant drugs tacrolimus and ciclosporin. The interaction with ciclosporin can be serious, and combined therapy is not recommended. If erythromycin therapy is crucial, then ciclosporin doses may have to be lowered.

Oral contraceptives

Erythromycin may interfere with the oral contraceptive pill, and other methods of contraception should be recommended during combined use.

Metronidazole

Alcohol and anti-abuse medication

Metronidazole (similar to the anti–alcohol abuse drug disulphiram) inhibits the metabolism of alcohol. It causes an accumulation of aldehydes that cause nausea and vomiting. Similarly, metronidazole interacts with disulphiram, which may lead to confusion and psychosis.

Other antimicrobials

A disulphiram-like reaction may occur when metronidazole is administered with the antiviral agent ritonavir. Rifampicin increases metronidazole loss, but the importance of this is unknown.

Anticoagulants

Metronidazole inhibits the metabolism of warfarin, resulting in a significant increase in anticoagulation. If treatment with metronidazole is critical, then the dose of warfarin may have to be lowered.

Anticonvulsants

Metronidazole may increase the toxicity of carbamazepine and phenytoin. Combined therapy with barbiturates increases metronidazole loss, and higher doses of the antimicrobial may be needed.

Antimetabolites

Metronidazole increases the toxicity of 5-fluorouracil.

Drugs acting on the CNS

Lithium toxicity is increased by metronidazole. This is an important interaction, and combined therapy should be avoided. If metronidazole is essential, then patients must be monitored for signs of lithium toxicity, such as confusion and renal damage.

Drugs that act on the gastrointestinal tract

As aluminium hydroxide reduces the absorption of metronidazole, dosing should be separated.

Immunosuppressants

Ciclosporin levels are increased during therapy with metronidazole, and patients on such a combination need to be closely monitored for signs of toxicity, such as severe gastrointestinal upsets. Corticosteroids increase metronidazole loss, and increased dosing of the latter may be required.

Lipid-lowering drugs

Colestyramine reduces the absorption of metronidazole, so dosing should be separated.

Oral contraceptives

As with the other antibacterials used in dentistry, metronidazole may decrease the efficacy of oral contraceptives, and other means of contraception should be advised.

Tetracyclines

Other antimicrobials

Tetracyclines reduce the efficacy of penicillins and cephalosporins, but may increase the serum levels of the antimalarial medication mefloquine.

Anticoagulants

Tetracyclines may increase the anticoagulant action of warfarin and the other coumarin anticoagulants.

Antiasthma drugs

Tetracyclines can increase the toxicity of theophylline by increasing the plasma concentration of the latter drug.

Antidiabetic drugs

As tetracyclines have a hypoglycaemic action, their administration to patients receiving insulin or oral hypoglycaemic medications should be avoided.

Antimetabolites

Tetracyclines may increase the risk of methotrexate toxicity, although this is not as severe as that seen with the penicillins. Patients on this combination should be monitored for signs of toxicity, such as haemorrhage and oral ulceration.

Cardiovascular drugs

Tetracyclines can increase the serum levels of digoxin. This is an important effect. If tetracycline is essential, patients should be monitored for signs of digoxin toxicity, such as arrhythmias, weakness and severe gastrointestinal upsets. Tetracyclines can increase blood urea levels. This effect is exacerbated in combined therapy with diuretics. The absorption of tetracyclines is reduced by quinapril.

Cations

Tetracyclines form chelates with calcium and other cations. Several drugs (such as calcium and zinc salts) and foods (such as dairy products) contain cations, and these reduce absorption of the antibacterial. By the same mechanism, tetracyclines inhibit the absorption of iron and zinc.

Drugs that act on the CNS

Combined therapy with ergotamine can produce ergotism. This is potentially serious, as it can cause gangrene.

Drugs that act on the gastrointestinal tract

As with cations, antacids and ulcer-healing drugs, such as sucralphate and the ion-exchange resin colestipol, all reduce the absorption of tetracyclines.

Oral contraceptives

Tetracyclines, similar to the other antibacterials mentioned earler, may reduce the efficacy of oral contraceptives, and alternative methods of birth control should be recommended during combined therapy.

Retinoids

Cranial hypertension that can cause headache and dizziness may result when tetracyclines are taken in combination with retinoids.

Antifungals

Amphotericin

Combined therapy with other antifungals reduces the action of amphotericin. Combination therapy with pentamidine (a drug used to treat *Pneumocystis* pneumonia in patients with AIDS) can lead to acute renal failure. Amphotericin increases the toxicity of the antiviral agent zalcitabine, which is used in the management of HIV. Amphotericin can produce potassium loss, and this is exaggerated during simultaneous treatment with corticosteroids. Similarly, the risk of hypokalaemia is increased during treatment with non-potassium-sparing diuretics.

Miconazole

Miconazole has a potentially life-threatening interaction with warfarin as a result of increased anticoagulation. It is important to realise that this can occur even after topical application of miconazole, and combined therapy is contraindicated. Miconazole increases the anticonvulsant action of phenytoin and increases the plasma concentrations of ciclosporin and midazolam, and the sulphonylurea oral hypoglycaemic medications.

Summary

Several interactions can occur with drugs that dentists prescribe. A thorough drug history and access to a reference source of drug interactions, such as the *British National Formulary*, are important.

FURTHER READING

British National Formulary. Available from: www.bnf.org/bnf/index.

UK Medicines Information. Available from: http://www.ukmi.nhs.uk.

MULTIPLE CHOICE QUESTIONS

1. Drug-induced gingival overgrowth may be seen in:
   a) Treatment with ACE inhibitors.
   b) Treatment with carbamazepine.
   c) Treatment with nicorandil.
   d) Treatment with calcium channel blockers.
   e) Treatment with thiazide diuretics.
   Answer = D

2. Which of the following drugs can cause a blue discolouration of the oral mucosa?
   a) Amiodarone.
   b) Betel nut.
   c) Methyldopa.
   d) Fluoxetine.
   e) Hydroxychloroquine.
   Answer = A

3. Which of the following drugs has been implicated in the aetiology of sialorrhoea?
   a) Amitriptyline.
   b) Oxybutynin.
   c) Fluoxetine.
   d) Lisinopril.
   e) Clozapine.
   Answer = E

4. Which of the following has traditionally been recognised as a potential side effect of (or has drug interactions with) the oral contraceptive pill?
   a) Protection against deep vein thrombosis.
   b) Increased risk of dry socket (alveolar osteitis).
   c) Decreased risk of dry socket (alveolar osteitis).

d) Osteonecrosis.
e) The prescription of ibuprofen.
Answer = B

5. Which of the following is *not* a risk factor for drug-induced gingival overgrowth?
   a) Age.
   b) Concomitant medication in transplant patients.
   c) Impaired oral hygiene.
   d) Use of electric toothbrush.
   e) Drug variables.
   Answer = D

6. Which of the following drugs has angioedema as a well-recognised potential side effect?
   a) Chlorhexidine 0.12%.
   b) Chlorhexidine 0.2%.
   c) Atenolol.
   d) Bismuth.
   e) Captopril.
   Answer = E

7. Which of the following antibiotics can cause defects in the tooth enamel in the developing dentition?
   a) Phenoxymethylpenicillin.
   b) Tetracycline.
   c) Metronidazole.

d) Clindamycin.
e) Flucloxacillin.
Answer = B

8. Which antibiotic forms a chelate with calcium and other cations?
   a) Erythromycin.
   b) Penicillin.
   c) Flucloxacillin.
   d) Clindamycin.
   e) Tetracycline.
   Answer = E

9. Ibuprofen:
   a) Is only available on prescription.
   b) Is steroid based.
   c) Is generally contraindicated in diabetic patients.
   d) Is generally contraindicated in asthmatic patients.
   e) Has no interaction with warfarin.
   Answer = D

10. Which of the following is *not* true of miconazole?
    a) It has no interaction with warfarin.
    b) It is an anti-fungal medication.
    c) It increases the plasma concentration of ciclosporin.
    d) It increases the action of phenytoin.
    e) It increases the plasma concentration of phenytoin.
    Answer = A

CHAPTER 16
General oncology

CM Robinson and PJ Thomson

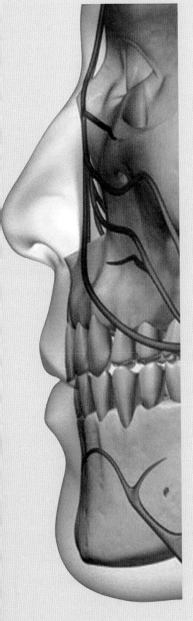

Key topics

- Disorders of growth and differentiation.
- Neoplasia.
- Tumour identification and diagnosis.
- Oral complications of malignancy.

Learning objectives

- To have knowledge of the pathology of disorders of growth and differentiation.
- To have knowledge of the pathological basis of cancer.
- To be familiar with tumour classification.
- To have knowledge of oral complications of malignancy and its treatment.

Essentials of Human Disease in Dentistry, Second Edition. Mark Greenwood.
© 2018 John Wiley & Sons Ltd. Published 2018 by John Wiley & Sons Ltd.
Companion website: www.wiley.com/go/greenwood/human-disease-in-dentistry

Introduction

Oncology is the branch of medicine that deals with the management of tumours, literally meaning the science of new growths, while the term 'cancer' is applied somewhat more loosely to malignant tumours in general. Cancer is caused by the accumulation of damage to cellular DNA. The multistage theory of carcinogenesis is based on the sequential acquisition of critical alterations in DNA that underpin the hallmarks cancer. There is a close correlation between cancer incidence and increased age, reflecting the time required to accumulate the necessary genetic abnormalities to form a viable cancer cell.

Malignant tumours defy the normal growth control mechanisms of the body, leading to excessive cell proliferation; loss of differentiation; and, ultimately, local tissue invasion, destruction and metastasis (spread of the primary tumour to other organs and tissues). Death may result from tumour deposition within vital organs such as the liver (Figure 16.1), lungs or brain, and from the generalised effects of cancer (e.g. uncontrolled disease at the primary tumour site or metabolic effects of the tumour).

Cancer may affect any organ or tissue in the body, but it arises commonly from epithelia of the skin, lungs and gastrointestinal tract, which are directly affected by carcinogens (cancer-inducing agents) such as UV radiation, tobacco smoke, alcohol and chemicals in foodstuff.

In order to appreciate the nature and significance of malignant disease in the body, it is necessary to understand how the normal physiological control of cell proliferation, tissue growth and differentiation becomes disrupted during tumourigenesis.

Disorders of growth and differentiation

Introduction

Coordinated cell proliferation, differentiation and tissue morphogenesis are essential for the successful development and maintenance of a large complex multicellular organism. The process of embryogenesis starts with a single cell, the fertilised ovum. The genetic information encoded within this cell is the blueprint of life. During cell division, the genetic information is precisely copied and disseminated to the daughter cells. It is the coordinated expression of this genetic information (genotype) that determines the fate of the cell and its role in the organism (phenotype).

The progeny of stem cells are destined to become specialised cells with specific functions in the organism (differentiation). There is accumulating evidence that sets of genes (e.g. homeobox genes) are important in determining the movement and physical positioning of cells (morphogenesis). The process of apoptosis (programmed cell death) is also essential in development and tissue maintenance, to counterbalance excessive proliferation and delete unwanted cells.

In addition to the increase in cell numbers, termed 'multiplicative growth', individual cells can also increase in size, which is called 'auxetic growth'. Skeletal muscle increases in size by auxetic growth. In some tissues (e.g. bone), growth is mainly achieved by deposition and remodelling of the extracellular matrix, which is called 'accretionary growth'.

When considering multiplicative growth, cells in the adult can be classified by their potential to proliferate. This determines the ability of different tissues to respond to environmental changes and tissue damage. Labile cells are continuously lost and replaced. They include the haemopoietic cells of the bone marrow, and epithelial cells that constitute the epidermis and line the mucous membranes. Stable cells are not continuously replaced, but can be induced to proliferate in certain conditions – for example, hepatocytes of the liver and renal tubular cells of the kidney. Non-dividing cells cannot be stimulated to proliferate, and include cardiac myocytes and neurons. Intuitively, labile cells are the most susceptible to disorders of growth, whereas non-dividing cells are unaffected.

Disorders of growth

Within specific tissues and organs, alteration in growth takes place as an adaptive response following a change in demand (physiology) or underpins part of a disease process (pathology). Growth as a consequence of increased cell number is termed *hyperplasia*. Hyperplasia is mainly a consequence of increased mitosis, but reduction of apoptosis will also result in accumulation of cells. In contrast, growth as a result of increased cell size, without cell division, is termed *hypertrophy*. In most tissues, increased growth is a combination of hyperplasia and hypertrophy.

A good example of physiological hyperplasia is the increase in the number of erythrocytes when an individual moves to a high-altitude location. The reduced partial pressures of oxygen at high altitudes stimulates the body to produce more erythrocytes in order to optimise oxygen delivery to the tissues. Athletes sometimes use 'altitude training' as a performance-enhancing strategy. Following a period of training at high altitudes, which results in erythrocyte hyperplasia, when the athlete competes at sea level, the body has an increased

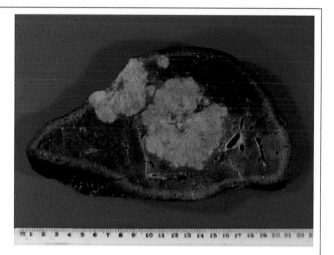

Figure 16.1 A section of a liver showing metastatic deposits.

oxygen-carrying capacity, with greatly increased delivery of oxygen to the peripheral tissues. The illegal use by athletes of erythropoietin (EPO), a hormone that stimulates the production of erythrocytes, is another method of inducing erythrocyte hyperplasia. Another example of physiological hyperplasia is the increase in the amount of breast tissue observed during the development of the mammary glands in puberty, and the increase in breast size during pregnancy in preparation for lactation. Hyperplasia is also characteristic of some diseases – for example, a generalised increase in the size of the thyroid gland is called *goitre*. In some circumstances, the hyperplasia is a consequence of inappropriate stimulation of the thyroid gland by an autoantibody that simulates the action of a thyroid-stimulating hormone, which is called *Graves' disease*. The hyperplastic thyroid tissue produces excess thyroxine (hyperthyroidism), and the patient develops clinical symptoms that include weight loss, tremor, sweating, tachycardia and heat intolerance.

Physiological hypertrophy of skeletal muscle occurs following increased usage and physical demand. Muscle hypertrophy observed in 'body builders' and athletes is a striking example. Hypertrophy of the cardiac muscle fibres in the left ventricle is an adaptive response to sustained peripheral resistance (hypertension), and is also a feature of hypertrophic cardiomyopathy, a cause of unexpected death in young adults (see Chapter 5A, titled 'Introduction to cardiovascular disease').

Terms used to describe inadequate growth include 'aplasia', 'hypoplasia' and 'atrophy'. *Aplasia* is the complete failure of an organ or tissue to develop. Aplasia of organs is uncommon, and, in most cases, it is incompatible with life. Examples of viable infants with aplasia include unilateral aplasia of a kidney and thymic aplasia in DiGeorge syndrome, which results in severe immunodeficiency. Cleidocranial dysostosis is an inherited skeletal defect characterised by abnormalities of the skull and clavicles. Some of these individuals have aplasia of the clavicles and are able to adduct the shoulders to the midline (Figure 16.2).

Hypoplasia is used to describe the partial failure of development of an organ or tissue, such that the normal size is not attained. Hypoplasias are more common than aplasia, and are seen in a variety of inherited diseases – for example, hypoplastic left heart syndrome, testicular hypoplasia in Klinefelter syndrome, segmental renal hypoplasia and optic nerve hypoplasia.

The term 'atrophy' is used to describe a decrease in size of an organ or tissue. Atrophy may be the result of a reduction in cell size or cell number, or a combination of both. Confusingly, the terms 'hypoplasia' and 'atrophy' are often used synonymously. However, 'hypoplasia' should be used to indicate a failure in attainment of normal size in the context of development, whereas 'atrophy should be used to indicate a reduction in the size of an organ or tissue following complete development. Examples of physiological atrophy include atrophy of the ductus arteriosus in the neonate, and thymic atrophy following T cell development in early adulthood. Disuse atrophy of muscles and osteoporosis can occur during prolonged

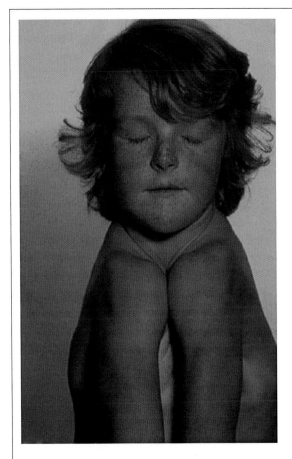

Figure 16.2 Cleidocranial dysostosis.

Table 16.1 Disorders of growth.
Hyperplasia – increase in cell numbers
Hypertrophy – increase in cell size
Aplasia – complete failure of an organ or tissue to develop
Hypoplasia – partial failure of an organ or tissue to develop
Atrophy – a decrease in size of an organ or tissue
Cachexia – 'wasting syndrome' seen in chronic disease states, especially cancer

periods of immobility, and in cases where the use of a limb is lost following a fracture or denervation of a muscle group. Disuse atrophy is usually reversible following a return to normal activity. Cachexia is a 'wasting syndrome' seen in chronic disease, particularly cancer, which is typified by weight loss and attendant muscle atrophy. A summary of growth disorders is given in Table 16.1.

Disorders of differentiation

Differentiation is the process whereby cells become specialised and are assigned specific functions within the organism. Disorders of differentiation and morphogenesis are important when considering abnormalities that arise during embryogenesis. In the adult, changes in the differentiation of cells are classified as *metaplasia* and *dysplasia*.

Metaplasia is a change from the normal pattern of differentiation to another type. Metaplasia is usually an adaptive response to changes in the environment. Changes in the differentiation of specialised epithelia are common. For example, squamous metaplasia can be induced in respiratory-type epithelium (ciliated pseudostratified epithelium) during chronic exposure of the respiratory tract to tobacco smoke. Squamous metaplasia of ductal epithelium is seen in chronic sialadenitis and sialolithiasis (salivary gland stones). Squamous epithelium can be induced to undergo glandular metaplasia, sometimes called 'mucous metaplasia'. Chronic gastric reflux into the lower part of the oesophagus causes the original squamous epithelium to be replaced by specialised columnar epithelia that contains mucus-secreting goblet cells, which resembles the lining of the colon. These changes are called 'Barrett's oesophagus', which is associated with an increased risk of developing oesophageal adenocarcinoma.

Metaplasia can also occur in mesenchymal tissues. For example, the development of bone in anatomical structures composed of cartilage – such as the larynx, trachea and bronchi – is called 'osseous metaplasia'. Osseous metaplasia may also develop in the complicated plaque of atherosclerosis.

'Dysplasia' is a term used to describe disordered tissue architecture. It develops because of increased cell growth and altered cellular differentiation. The term is most frequently used to describe the histological changes in the epithelia that comprise skin and mucous membranes – called 'epithelial dysplasia'. The term is also used to describe changes in other tissues – for example, the myelodysplastic syndromes of the haemopoietic system and fibrous dysplasia of bone. Epithelial dysplasia is commonly detected in biopsy material from the mucosa of the upper aerodigestive tract and uterine cervix. In the upper aerodigestive tract, there is strong correlation between epithelial dysplasia and chronic exposure to tobacco smoke, whereas, in the cervix, infection with oncogenic human papilloma virus (HPV) is the strongest risk factor (Table 16.2).

Pathologists grade epithelial dysplasia based on assessment of the architectural and cytological changes (Table 16.3). Grading systems vary, but the changes are most commonly classified into low- and high-grade dysplasia, or termed *mild*, *moderate* and *severe dysplasia*. It is known that lesions with epithelial dysplasia have an increased risk of developing into cancer; this has led to a variety of terms for dysplastic lesions that include 'potentially malignant lesions', 'pre-malignant lesions', 'precursor lesions' and 'pre-cancer'.

Table 16.2 Disorders of differentiation.

Metaplasia – change in the normal pattern of differentiation
Dysplasia – disordered tissue architecture

Table 16.3 Parameters used to render a diagnosis of epithelial dysplasia.

Architecture	Cytology
Irregular stratification of the epithelium	Abnormal variation in cell size (anisocytosis)
Loss of basal cell polarity	Abnormal variation in cell shape (cellular pleomorphism)
Drop-shaped rete processes	Abnormal variation in nuclear size (anisonucleosis)
Increased number of mitotic figures	Abnormal variation in nuclear shape (nuclear pleomorphism)
Suprabasal mitotic figures	Increased nuclear:cytoplasmic ratio
Single-cell dyskeratosis	Increased nuclear size
Keratin pearls within rete processes	Hyperchromasia Increased number and size of nucleoli Atypical mitotic figures

Neoplasia

Definitions and terminology

Neoplasia means 'new growth' (Greek: *neo* = 'new', *plassein* = 'to form'). The most widely cited definition is that devised by RA Willis, the eminent British pathologist, in the 1950s: 'A neoplasm is an abnormal mass of tissue, the growth of which exceeds and is uncoordinated with that of the normal tissues, and that persists in the same excessive manner after the cessation of the stimulus which evoked the change'. This precise definition separates neoplasia from the other abnormalities of growth and differentiation, described in the preceding text, and emphasises the inherent growth potential of a neoplasm. Perhaps a contemporary definition should also take account of the genetic basis of neoplasia – for example, a *neoplasm* is a growth disorder characterised by genetic alterations that lead to loss of the normal control mechanisms that regulate cell growth and differentiation.

The term 'tumour' is used synonymously with 'neoplasm', but literally means 'swelling', and was originally used to describe swellings caused by inflammation (tumour: one of the cardinal signs of inflammation). Hamartomas can also produce a tumour-like mass of tissue that mimics neoplasia. Hamartomas represent an overgrowth of tissue that is typically indigenous to the anatomical site, grows with the individual and has a limited growth potential. A common hamartoma is the melanocytic naevus or 'mole'. Another example is the pulmonary hamartoma, which appears as a coin-shaped radiodensity on chest radiography and is composed of respiratory-type epithelium admixed with mature cartilage. The vascular abnormalities such as *haemangioma* and *lymphangioma* are also best considered as hamartomas rather than true neoplasms.

Neoplasms are classified as benign or malignant, depending on their clinical presentation, histological appearance and biological behaviour. A general term for malignant neoplasia is 'cancer', which is an emotive term that patients associate with suffering and death.

General features of neoplasia

Benign neoplasms tend to be small; however, occasionally, large benign neoplasms develop, but they do not usually cause any significant symptoms (depends on their anatomical location). In other circumstances, a patient may not have sought treatment or been able to access appropriate healthcare services (e.g. in underdeveloped countries). Benign tumours are invariably well circumscribed and often delineated by a rim of compressed fibrous tissue, called a 'capsule' (encapsulated). Benign tumours are composed of mature tissue that resembles the tissue of origin. The growth rate is slow, and mitotic figures are infrequent. Most benign tumours do not show any evidence of local tissue invasion, although there are a few exceptions to this rule, most notably *ameloblastoma*, which is a benign odontogenic tumour that shows bone invasion. By definition, benign tumours remain localised and do not spread to form new neoplasms at other sites (Table 16.4).

The majority of malignant neoplasms tend to be rather large at diagnosis. They invade and destroy local tissues and, as a consequence, have ill-defined borders and are fixed to the adjacent tissues (Figure 16.3). Malignant neoplasms show varying degrees of resemblance to the tissue of origin, and are graded depending on the degree of differentiation, namely: *well differentiated*, *moderately differentiated* and *poorly differentiated*. The growth rate is variable, but usually more rapid than

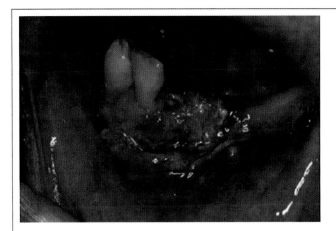

Figure 16.3 A squamous cell cancer of the oral cavity. Note the ulceration and irregular margins. The soft tissue component is usually hard to palpation (indurated) and fixed to the underlying tissues.

that of benign neoplasms. Mitotic figures are usually easily identified, and some may look abnormal. In rapidly growing neoplasms, the growth may exceed the development of an adequate blood supply, leading to necrosis. Malignant neoplasms invade and destroy the surrounding tissues. There may be invasion along peripheral nerves, termed 'neural invasion'.

Malignant cells may invade blood vessels or lymphatic channels, which is called *vascular invasion*. Vascular invasion is associated with the dissemination of malignant cells to other parts of the body (metastasis). Spread by lymphatic channels usually results in the development of regional lymph node metastases, whereas dissemination via the haematogenous route (blood vessels) results in metastases to other tissues or organs (e.g. the lungs, liver, brain and bones).

Some malignant neoplasms spread across body cavities, which is called *transcoelomic spread*. The classical example is the Krukenberg tumour, which is a primary adenocarcinoma of the stomach that metastasises to the surface of the ovary. Erosion of the stomach wall by an adenocarcinoma causes an effusion (leakage of fluid) into the peritoneal cavity. The effusion contains malignant cells that seed on the peritoneal surfaces of the abdominal cavity and, in the case of Krukenberg tumour malignant cells, seed on to the surface of the ovary and grow to produce metastases. Transcoelomic spread is also a feature of pleural and pericardial effusions caused by breast and lung cancers. In some circumstances, malignant cells are able to spread through epithelial-lined conduits. In Paget's disease of the nipple, malignant cells derived from an underlying breast adenocarcinoma spread throughout the epithelium of the ductal system and eventually reach the epidermis of the nipple, which produces an eczematous appearance on the skin surface. Occasionally, the latter may be the initial clinical presentation of an occult breast cancer. Melanoma cells can also disseminate through the epidermis by Pagetoid spread, particularly in superficial spreading malignant melanoma.

Table 16.4 Typical features of benign and malignant neoplasms.

	Benign	Malignant
Size	Small	Large
Borders	Circumscribed/ encapsulated	Ill defined
Differentiation	Resembles tissue of origin	Variable
Growth rate	Slow	Rapid
Mitotic figures	Rare	Common
Necrosis	No	Yes
Invasion	No	Local structures Vascular and neural Bone and cartilage
Metastasis	No	Yes

Metabolic effects of neoplasia

Benign neoplasms of the endocrine system may result in excess hormone production. For example, a thyroid adenoma may cause thyrotoxicosis, and a patient with an adrenocortical adenoma may develop Cushing's syndrome. Some malignant neoplasms, particularly those that show neuroendocrine differentiation, produce unexpected hormones. For example, small-cell carcinoma of the lung may produce ACTH and ADH; however, the hormone levels rarely cause clinically significant symptoms. Humoral hypercalcaemia of malignancy is thought to be caused by malignant cells that secrete PTH-related protein (PTHrP). The latter causes similar clinical features to those seen in hyperparathyroidism. Furthermore, cachexia, a 'wasting syndrome' seen in cancer, is also considered to be mediated by metabolically active factors produced by malignant cells.

It is well recognised that cancer is capable of producing a general set of potential complications. These are shown in Table 16.5.

Classification of neoplasms

Neoplasms are classified according to their behaviour and the tissue that they most resemble (histogenesis). All neoplasms have the suffix 'oma'. Benign epithelial neoplasms are either *papillomas* (derived from surface epithelium) or *adenomas* (derived from glandular epithelium). Benign mesenchymal neoplasms have a prefix to denote the histogenesis (e.g. a benign neoplasm of fibrous tissue is called a 'fibroma'). Malignant epithelial neoplasms are called *carcinomas*, and malignant mesenchymal neoplasms are called *sarcomas* (Table 16.6). There are notable rule breakers in this system. The term 'lymphoma' suggests a benign neoplasm; however, they are malignant neoplasms of the lymphoreticular system. Furthermore, melanoma has a 'benign' sounding name, but is a highly aggressive malignant neoplasm. These diseases are sometimes qualified by preceding the entity with 'malignant' (e.g. malignant lymphoma, malignant melanoma).

Biological characteristics of cancer

The biological characteristics of malignant neoplasms or cancers have been described. There are six hallmarks of cancer, namely (1) self-sufficiency in growth signals; (2) insensitivity

Table 16.6 Histogenetic classification of benign and malignant neoplasms.

	Benign	Malignant
Epithelium		
Squamous	Squamous cell papilloma	Squamous cell carcinoma
Transitional	Transitional cell papilloma	Transitional cell carcinoma
Glandular	Adenoma	Adenocarcinoma
Mesenchyme		
Fibrous tissue	Fibroma	Fibrosarcoma
Smooth muscle	Leiomyoma	Leiomyosarcoma
Striated muscle	Rhabdomyoma	Rhabdomyosarcoma
Adipose tissue	Lipoma	Liposarcoma
Blood vessels	Haemangioma	Angiosarcoma
Cartilage	Chondroma	Chondrosarcoma
Bone	Osteoma	Osteosarcoma

to antigrowth signals; (3) evasion of apoptosis; (4) limitless replicative potential; (5) sustained angiogenesis; and (6) tissue invasion and metastasis. It is important to emphasise that the acquisition of these capabilities is a multistep process. A single cell must acquire multiple, non-lethal and stable genetic abnormalities, which are conserved during cell division and propagated to daughter cells. In some cancers, the recognition of pre-malignant lesions has facilitated the characterisation of a genetically defined step-wise progression towards cancer. The prototype for this concept is the pathogenesis of colon cancer (adenocarcinoma).

The best described genetic changes in cancer are the abnormalities in two classes of genes, namely *oncogenes* and *tumour suppressor genes* (TSGs). An *oncogene* is a mutated or overexpressed version of a normal gene (called a 'proto-oncogene') that promotes the development of cancer. In most cases, oncogenes encode proteins that increase cell proliferation. For example, the mutant gene may produce an altered version of a protein that is abnormally active (constitutively active), which promotes uncontrolled cell growth. Alternatively, the cell may simply produce increased amounts of a normal protein with a similar oncogenic effect. Oncogenes are considered to have a dominant effect, because the alteration of only one copy of the gene (allele) produces the additive effect required for uncoupled cell proliferation. There are >60 different oncogenes, and they are generally classified according to the main function of the gene product or protein (Table 16.7).

TSGs encode proteins that are normally involved in inhibiting cell proliferation or promoting apoptosis (programmed cell death), and can be considered as exerting a 'braking effect' on cell proliferation. Both copies of a TSG must be inactivated to

Table 16.5 General complications of cancer.

- Cachexia, wasting and malaise
- Anaemia, infection and pyrexia
- Nutritional deficiencies
- Cutaneous manifestations – infections, pruritus, ichthyosis, purpura
- Endocrine disorders – Cushingoid, hypercalcaemia, diuresis
- Rare manifestations – neuromyopathies, acanthosis nigricans, dermatomyositis

Table 16.7 Classification of oncogenes with examples.

Protein function	Proto-oncogene
Growth factor	c-*sis* (platelet-derived growth factor, PDGF)
Growth factor receptor	c-*erbB* (epidermal growth factor receptor, EGFR)
Tyrosine kinase	c-*src*
G protein	c-H-*ras*
Transcription factor	c-*myc*

exert an adverse effect on the cell, and this is often referred to as 'Knudson's two-hit hypothesis'. It was Knudson's observations of patients with retinoblastoma that led to this seminal discovery. Retinoblastoma is a malignant neoplasm of the retina, generally occurring in children. There are inherited and sporadic cases of the disease. Hereditary retinoblastoma is characterised by a germline deletion of part of the long arm of chromosome 13 that encodes the retinoblastoma gene (Rb). Subsequent inactivation of the remaining normal allele (e.g. by somatic mutation) causes retinoblastoma. In the sporadic form of the disease, the individual has two normal copies of Rb, and both copies need to be inactivated before the disease can develop – that is, the normal cell must acquire 'two hits' at the Rb chromosomal locus in order to transform into a cancer cell. Rb is involved in controlling the cell cycle, and inactivation of Rb in other cells, at other sites of the body, contributes to the development of neoplasia. p53 is another well-characterised TSG, and is considered to be the most common molecular defect in human cancers. p53 is important because it is involved in triggering the repair of damaged DNA and is capable of inducing apoptosis if the DNA damage is excessive. Inactivation of p53 (e.g. by mutation of one copy of the gene and deletion of the other allele) results in the loss of p53 function, such that cells with damaged DNA are able to propagate unchecked; for this reason, p53 is sometimes referred to as the 'guardian of the genome'.

Clinical oncology

It is estimated that one in four people develop cancer. Cancer is generally a disease of old age, and the majority of patients are diagnosed in the seventh and eighth decades of life. Living with cancer can have profound physical and psychological effects. The suffering associated with the disease is referred to as 'morbidity', and one in five die as a consequence of the disease, termed 'mortality'. There are >100 distinct types of cancer, and there are innumerable histological subtypes. In the UK, the most common cancers are those of the lung, colon, breast, and prostate. These four cancers account for over half the new cases each year.

The types of cancer vary with age. The most common cancers are: in children, leukaemias and brain tumours; in males, testicular tumours (in 20–30-year-olds), carcinoma of the bronchus (45–65-year-olds), and prostatic cancer (aged above 70 years); in females, carcinomas of the breast and uterine cervix predominate throughout adulthood (especially between 25 and 65 years of age).

Tumour identification and diagnosis

Tumours arising from easily accessible epithelial surfaces such as the skin and oral mucosa are readily diagnosed by clinical examination and direct palpation, but many may arise in deeper body cavities, requiring endoscopic examination or imaging techniques such as CT, MRI or ultrasound scanning to visualise primary tumour masses. Other techniques include radioisotope bone scanning and PET CT scans to locate metastatic or recurrent disease at other sites in the body.

Tumour diagnosis requires a biopsy and histopathological examination to identify the type of tumour, and grade of differentiation, which guides treatment planning and patient prognosis. Many immunohistochemical and genetic profiling techniques are available in modern clinical practice to aid tumour classification and predict treatment outcome.

The principal clinical features of the most common cancers are summarised in Table 16.8.

Management of malignant disease

In general, malignant neoplasms are treated using one or a combination of the following treatment modalities: surgery, radiotherapy, chemotherapy and hormonal manipulation. The selection, timing and prescription of these anticancer treatments are now the remit of highly specialised multidisciplinary oncology teams, and vary considerably depending on the tumour type and site. As a general principle, the earlier a tumour is diagnosed and treated, the better the prognosis will be.

Unfortunately, metastases often develop before primary tumours are diagnosed, and improved survival depends on more effective and earlier detection of potentially malignant disease. Indeed, this is the basis of cancer-screening programmes – to target widespread examination of asymptomatic patients at risk of cancer. While screening has not proved efficacious for all malignancies, breast screening with mammography and cervical smear testing have helped reduce female death rates from both breast and cervical cancer in recent years.

Surgery

The principal aim of surgical treatment is the complete excision of the malignancy, ideally with a wide margin of normal tissue surrounding the tumour in anticipation of local microscopic spread, together with removal of the channels of metastatic spread, especially lymphatics and blood vessels. Good surgical access is fundamental in cancer surgery to allow effective exposure and ensure complete tumour removal. The surgical approach must facilitate repair, produce minimal scarring, preserve function and minimise deformity.

Surgical excision of primary tumours may also be indicated to alleviate local tumour effects such as pain, bleeding and

Table 16.8 Clinical details of common human cancers.

Site (aetiology/ predisposing factors)	Pathology	Patients	Clinical features	Identification	Treatment
Lung (tobacco)	Squamous cell carcinoma Adenocarcinoma Small-cell carcinoma	Older males	Cough Dyspnoea Haemoptysis	CXR CT scan	Chemotherapy Radiotherapy Lobectomy Pneumonectomy
Colorectal (familial, polyps, colitis, low-fibre diet)	Adenocarcinoma	Middle aged	Rectal bleeding Pain/obstruction Altered bowel habit Right iliac fossa mass	Sigmoidoscopy	Colectomy Chemotherapy Radiotherapy
Breast (familial, sporadic)	Adenocarcinoma	Females	Breast lump Skin tethering Paget's disease of nipple Axillary lymphadenopathy	Mammogram FNAB Core biopsy	Surgery Radiotherapy Chemotherapy Tamoxifen Herceptin
Prostate (unknown)	Adenocarcinoma	Elderly males	Impaired micturition	PR exam	Prostatectomy Radiotherapy Stilboestrol LHRH Cyproterone

CXR = chest X-ray; FNAB = fine needle aspiration biopsy; LHRH = luteinising hormone-releasing hormone; PR = rectal examination.

obstruction; indeed, in advanced disease, surgery may serve an important palliative role in combating distressing symptoms from ulcerating, fungating or bleeding tumours, and in airway preservation in head and neck cancers.

Radiotherapy

Radiotherapy refers to the therapeutic application of localised ionising radiation (X-rays, β-rays or γ-rays) to destroy malignant cells. Cells exposed to radiation form free radicals in their intracellular water and, because of DNA damage, undergo mitotic death when stimulated to divide. Radiotherapy is thus particularly effective against rapidly proliferating tumour cells, which are killed more efficiently than slowly growing or normal cells. While this is a considerable advantage in cancer treatment, it does not spare normal cells with high replication rates – such as in epithelium of skin and mucous membranes, highly specialised cells in neurological tissue, salivary gland secretory tissue or osteoblasts in bone – which, when damaged, are unable to regenerate.

Radiotherapy is especially indicated if patients are unfit for major surgical procedures, if tumours are inaccessible or technically unresectable, or where surgery may produce severe deformity or functional morbidity.

Chemotherapy

The use of chemotherapeutic agents (anticancer drugs) is most often employed systemically in the treatment of widespread malignancies (such as leukaemia or lymphoma), although more recent recognition of early systemic spread of solid tumours (such as breast cancer and even head and neck malignancy) has resulted in greater use of chemotherapy in modern treatment protocols. Chemotherapy agents target actively dividing cells to eliminate tumours, while allowing normal cells to recover and repair. Drugs are usually administered in high doses intermittently, and often in combination to achieve synergy and overcome the development of cancer cell resistance. Newer head and neck regimes utilise chemotherapy agents administered as radiosensitisers prior to radiotherapy to increase treatment efficacy, but this may also enhance treatment side effects.

Chemotherapy agents are inevitably highly toxic, and risk important systemic effects such as infections and bleeding due to bone marrow involvement and resultant neutropenia and thrombocytopenia. It is important to liaise with an individual patient's oncologist to ensure that dental or oral surgical treatments are timed to avoid periods of maximum bone marrow depression. Table 16.9 lists examples of chemotherapy drugs, their mechanisms of action and different modes of administration.

Hormonal manipulation

The growth of certain carcinomas, such as prostate and some breast cancers, is partly dependent on sex hormones. Consequently, drugs blocking or antagonising these hormones may inhibit tumour growth – for example, luteinising hormone-releasing hormone (LHRH) and cyproterone acetate in prostate cancer, and tamoxifen in breast cancer.

Table 16.9 Chemotherapy drugs and regimens.

Drug classification	Mode of action	Examples
Alkylating agents	Cross-linkage of DNA	Cisplatin
		Bleomycin
Antimetabolites	Impaired DNA synthesis	Methotrexate
		Fluorouracil
Mitotic inhibitors	Disrupt cell division	Vincristine
Treatment regimen	**Administration**	**Aim**
Induction	Prior to other treatments	Reduce tumour size
Sandwich	Between treatments	Reduce risk of metastases
Adjuvant	After treatment	Improve disease-free survival
Concurrent	With other treatments	Sensitise tumour cells
Palliative	After other treatments	Shrink residual tumours/pain relief

Prognosis

Prognosis is the prediction of the outcome of a disease process. When considering cancer, prognosis is dependent on the type of cancer, the amount of disease (stage) and the effectiveness of available treatments. Prognosis is usually presented to patients as the likelihood of cure and chances of survival. The latter is usually described as the proportion of patients with the disease that survive a period of 5 years.

Type of cancer

The histogenetic classification of neoplasia facilitates the separation of neoplasms into groups that have similar biological behaviour and respond to specific treatment regimens. It is incumbent on the pathologist to provide an accurate tissue diagnosis, which is initially based on the morphological assessment of haematoxylin and eosin (H&E) stained sections by light microscopy. Additional information may be provided by using different staining techniques, immunohistochemistry to identify specific antigens, and electron microscopy. In addition, cytogenetics (the study of chromosomes) and molecular biology techniques (e.g. polymerase chain reaction and *in situ* hybridisation) are being increasingly employed to refine diagnoses. Pathologists usually grade malignant neoplasms. Grading criteria differ for individual cancers, but the major determinates are the degree of differentiation, number of mitotic figures, cytological abnormality and necrosis. Grading systems may simply describe the degree of differentiation – well differentiated, moderately differentiated or poorly differentiated. Other grading systems are more complex. The most common type of breast cancer, ductal carcinoma, a type of adenocarcinoma, is graded by assessing the percentage of the neoplasm that is composed of tubular elements, the number of mitoses per ten high-power fields, and nuclear pleomorphism.

Numerical values are assigned to these three parameters, which are added together to derive a final score. The latter is then converted into one of three grades (I, II, III), where grade III represents high-grade adenocarcinoma.

Stage

Cancer staging is a method of recording the amount of cancer a patient has. Staging information can be used in treatment planning, and is a useful way of assessing the effectiveness of treatment outcome for groups of patients. Staging may form part of the clinical assessment (clinical staging). If the cancer is surgically removed, a thorough assessment of the specimen by a pathologist will allow formulation of the pathological stage. In most cases, the clinical and pathological stages correlate; however, occasionally, a detailed pathological assessment reveals subclinical disease, which alters the overall stage.

The most commonly used staging system is the tumour, node and metastasis (TNM) classification of malignant tumours. The classification is divided into regions of the body and by types of cancer. There are three parameters: the T, N and M categories. The T category encodes the size of the primary tumour and its extent of local invasion. The N category represents cancer spread to local (regional) lymph node groups, and the M category records the presence of distant metastasis to other organs or tissues. To illustrate the concept of staging, a version of the TNM classification of carcinomas of the oral cavity is shown in Tables 16.10 and 16.11. Patients with stage I cancer have early disease, which is potentially curable, whereas those with stage IV cancer have advanced disease and poor prognosis. Survival figures quoted for various cancers are usually qualified by stating the stage – for example, the 5-year survival for stage I oral cancer is about 90%, whereas for stage IV it is around 40%.

Table 16.10 TNM classification of carcinomas of the oral cavity.

T category	
T1	Tumour ≤2 cm in greatest dimension
T2	Tumour 2–4 cm in greatest dimension
T3	Tumour >4 cm in greatest dimension
T4a	Tumour invades through cortical bone into the deep/extrinsic muscle of tongue, maxillary sinus or skin of face
T4b	Tumour invades masticator space, pterygoid plates or skull base; or encases internal carotid artery
N category	
N0	No lymph node metastasis
N1	Metastasis in a single ipsilateral lymph node, ≤3 cm in dimension
N2	Metastasis in a single ipsilateral lymph node, 3–6 cm in greatest dimension Metastasis in multiple ipsilateral lymph nodes Metastasis in bilateral or contralateral lymph nodes
N3	Metastasis in a lymph node >6 cm in dimension
M category	
M0	No distant metastasis
M1	Distant metastasis

Table 16.11 Stage grouping.

Stage	T category	N category	M category
I	T1	N0	M0
II	T2	N0	M0
III	T1, T2	N1	M0
	T3	N0, N1	M0
IVA	T1, T2, T3	N2	M0
	T4a	N0, N1, N2	M0
IVB	Any T	N3	M0
	T4b	Any N	M0
IVC	Any T	Any N	M1

Introduction to head and neck oncology

In modern clinical practice, dental practitioners will be expected to advise and treat many patients with cancer at various stages of their disease who require oral healthcare. As a consequence of their malignancy, patients with cancer suffer from a number of general physical, medical and emotional problems, and it is important that dental practitioners have an understanding, not only of the effects of malignant disease on their patients, but also of the specific problems consequent upon their individual cancer treatments.

Of particular relevance to dentists, however, are those patients with head and neck cancer. Many of these patients may present first to their dental practitioner with signs and symptoms of an occult head and neck malignancy, and it is important that dental clinicians have a sound understanding of the type and nature of these tumours (Table 16.12).

Oral complications of malignancy

A number of signs and symptoms may present in the orofacial region as a consequence of malignant disease, due to both local tumour manifestations and systemic features of tumours (Table 16.13).

The orofacial region contains one of the highest concentrations of specialised tissues and sensory organs in the body, and it is hardly surprising that the effects of cancer treatment exert particularly severe effects here. Cellular damage following radiotherapy and chemotherapy produce similar effects on oral tissues, although more widespread and systemic complications occur following chemotherapy. Table 16.14 lists the oral complications of radiotherapy and chemotherapy.

Mucositis is a particularly distressing condition arising from damage to the oral mucosal lining, involving widespread oral erythema, pain, ulceration and bleeding. It may arise during localised head and neck radiotherapy, or as a consequence of systemic chemotherapy. Although an acute and usually relatively short-lived problem, it can significantly impair quality of life and prevent oral dietary intake, leading to hospitalisation; if especially severe, it may cause interruption to therapeutic regimes, and can act as a portal for septicaemia. Management of established mucositis includes systemic analgesia, the use of intraoral ice and topical analgesics such as benzydamine hydrochloride, 2% lidocaine lollipops or mouthwash.

Xerostomia is responsible for the most common and long-standing problems following head and neck radiotherapy. Salivary gland function rarely recovers following secretory cell damage. While newer computerised radiotherapy techniques help to spare full salivary gland irradiation, it remains difficult to avoid gland damage. Permanent mouth dryness, glutinous phlegm in the posterior oral cavity and pharynx, reduced or altered taste, as well as fragile and sensitive oral mucosa are significant post-radiotherapy sequelae impairing patients' quality of life. Xerostomia also increases the risk of rapidly destructive dental caries (radiation caries) and advanced periodontal disease. Artificial saliva preparations may be helpful, while oral administration of pilocarpine may help increase flow in patients with some residual salivary gland function.

Infections are common due to immunosuppression, especially candidal infection. Appropriate use of antifungal agents

Table 16.12 Head and neck cancers.

Site	Aetiology	Pathology	Clinical appearance	Treatment
Lip	UV radiation	SCC	Ulcer Plaque Fissure	Radiotherapy Surgery
Oral cavity	Tobacco Alcohol	SCC	Ulcer Leukoplakia Erythroplakia Neck lump	Surgery Radiotherapy
Tonsil and oropharynx	Tobacco Alcohol HPV	SCC	Ulcer Trismus Neck lump	Radiotherapy Chemotherapy Surgery
Nasopharynx	EBV	SCC	Epistaxis Deafness Cranial nerve palsies Neck lump	Radiotherapy
Nasal cavity and paranasal sinuses	Dust inhalation	SCC	Nasal obstruction/bleeding Cheek/palatal swelling Diplopia/proptosis/numbness Trismus	Surgery Radiotherapy
Larynx and hypopharynx	Tobacco	SCC	Hoarseness Cough Dyspnoea Dysphagia	Radiotherapy Surgery
Thyroid	Unknown	Thyroid carcinoma	Neck lump	Surgery Radiotherapy
Salivary glands	Unknown	Adenocarcinoma	Facial/neck lump	Surgery

EBV = Epstein–Barr virus; SCC = squamous cell carcinoma; HPV = human papilloma virus.

Table 16.13 Orofacial manifestations of cancer.

Primary tumour in orofacial tissues

- Oral squamous cell carcinoma
- Salivary adenocarcinoma

Metastases in jaws or oral soft tissues

- From breast, lung and prostate

Effects of tumour metabolites

- Facial flushing
- Pigmentations
- Amyloidosis –(disorder characterised by extracellular deposits of an abnormal protein called 'amyloid')
- Oral erosions

Functional disturbances

- Purpura
- Bleeding
- Infections
- Anaemia

Table 16.14 Oral complications of cancer therapy.

Radiotherapy

- Mucositis/ulceration
- Radiation caries/dental hypersensitivity/periodontal disease
- Xerostomia/loss of taste
- Dysphagia
- Candidiasis
- Osteoradionecrosis
- Trismus
- Craniofacial defects (children)

Chemotherapy

- Mucositis/ulceration/lip cracking
- Infections
- Bleeding
- Orofacial pain

such as miconazole or systemic fluconazole may be necessary to treat severe oral candidiasis.

Osteoradionecrosis arises due to the death of irradiated and lethally damaged bone cells, and is compounded by radiation-induced endarteritis obliterans, which compromises the blood supply. The mandible is particularly susceptible, as it has an end artery supply and minimal co-lateral blood supply. The osteoradionecrotic process usually starts as ulceration of the alveolar mucosa, with brownish dead bone exposed at the base (Figure 16.4). Pathological fracture may occur in weakened bone, and secondary infection leads to severe discomfort, trismus, foetor oris and general malaise. Radiographically, the earliest changes are a 'moth-eaten' appearance of the bone, followed by sequestration.

Treatment should be predominantly conservative, with long-term antibiotic therapy and careful local removal of sequestra when necessary. In intractable cases, extensive surgical resection and reconstruction, with free tissue transfer of compound muscle and bone flaps, may be necessary. Hyperbaric oxygen and ultrasound therapy to increase tissue blood flow and oxygenation have also been recommended.

Osteonecrosis is a recently recognised complication of bisphosphonate treatment. Bisphosphonates are a group of drugs, including alendronic acid and disodium etidronate, which are adsorbed onto hydroxyapatite crystals, thus slowing their rate of growth and dissolution. They have been used in the treatment of bony metastases and the hypercalcaemia of malignancy, as well as in the management of osteoporosis in post-menopausal women (see Chapter 15 titled 'Adverse drug reactions and interactions').

Management of head and neck radiotherapy patients

Table 16.15 summarises the important management principles for patients undergoing radiotherapy for head and neck malignancy.

Table 16.15 Management of patients receiving head and neck radiotherapy.
Before radiotherapy
• Oral hygiene/preventive and restorative dentistry
• Risk/benefits of retaining teeth
• Dental extractions
During radiotherapy
• Discourage smoking and alcohol
• Eliminate infections (using antibiotics/antifungals/antivirals)
• Relieve mucositis
• Saliva substitutes
• TMJ physiotherapy for trismus
After radiotherapy
• Oral hygiene/preventive dentistry
• Specialist OMFS for dental extractions/oral surgery
• Topical fluorides
• Avoidance of mucosal trauma
• Saliva substitutes
OMFS = oral and maxillofacial surgery; TMJ = temporomandibular joint.

Management of patients on chemotherapy

Table 16.16 lists the principles of management of patients receiving chemotherapy.

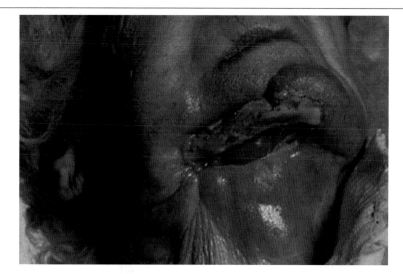

Figure 16.4 A case of osteoradionecrosis. This patient had radiotherapy in her head and neck region. There is also a poor blood supply to the soft tissues, which led to breakdown.

Table 16.16 Management of patients receiving chemotherapy.

Before chemotherapy

- Oral/dental assessment
- Oral hygiene/preventive dentistry

During chemotherapy

- Folic acid to reduce ulceration
- Ice to cool oral mucosa
- Chlorhexidine mouthwashes
- Eliminate infections (using antibiotics/antifungals/antivirals)

After chemotherapy

- Oral hygiene/preventive dentistry
- Risk of anaemia/bleeding/infection

Palliative care

Despite significant advances in diagnostic and therapeutic sciences, many patients with malignant disease will eventually die from progression of their primary tumours, or from uncontrolled and widespread metastatic disease.

Palliative care refers to the provision of treatment, which may be medical, surgical or radiotherapeutic, administered in the realisation that, while curing of disease is not possible, prolongation of symptom-free life may be achievable. Medical care should include attention to general well-being and morale, and the provision of optimal nutritional intake.

Patients with disseminated disease deteriorate until they reach a terminal stage, leading ultimately to organ system failure and death. Attention to alleviating pain, constipation, nausea and vomiting, abdominal symptoms, dysphagia and dyspnoea becomes paramount during this phase. This aspect of care is termed 'terminal care'.

Provision of specialist palliative care services for cancer patients at their homes, in hospital or at hospices is an integral part of modern cancer care.

The future

Extensive scientific and clinical research is ongoing into the biology of tumours and the mechanisms of carcinogenesis. Future developments in cancer treatment will focus on prevention, early diagnosis and 'personalised' treatment of disease (based on genetic profiling), along with the development of more effective anti-cancer drugs.

FURTHER READING

Cross S. *Underwood's Pathology: S Clinical Approach*, sixth edition. London: Churchill Livingstone; 2013.

MULTIPLE CHOICE QUESTIONS

1. A benign neoplasm of the parotid gland may present with:
   a) Bell's palsy.
   b) Xerostomia.
   c) Fusiform swelling.
   d) Cervical lymphadenopathy.
   e) Paraneoplastic syndrome.
   Answer = C

2. A malignant neoplasm of the parotid gland may present with:
   a) Lower motor neuron palsy of the facial nerve.
   b) Upper motor neuron palsy of the facial nerve.
   c) Hearing loss.
   d) Generalised lymphadenopathy.
   e) Paraneoplastic syndrome.
   Answer = A

3. Cigarette smoking greatly increases the risk of developing:
   a) Prostate cancer
   b) Malignant lymphoma
   c) Non-small-cell lung cancer
   d) Mesothelioma
   e) Malignant melanoma
   Answer = C

4. Human papilloma virus type 16 is the main cause of:
   a) Genital warts.
   b) Squamous cell papilloma.
   c) Squamous cell carcinoma of the uterine cervix.
   d) Focal epithelial hyperplasia (Heck's disease).
   e) Laryngeal cancer.
   Answer = B

5. Tumour suppressor genes are:
   a) Located mainly on chromosomes 13 and 21.
   b) Inactivated during carcinogenesis.
   c) Activated during carcinogenesis.
   d) Growth promoting.
   e) Used in gene therapy.
   Answer = B

6. Oncogenes are:
   a) Amplified in retinoblastoma.
   b) Inactivated in breast cancer.
   c) Amplified in breast cancer.
   d) Immune-regulatory genes.
   e) Used in gene therapy.
   Answer = C

7. Cancer stage is a measure of:
   a) The time taken to reach a diagnosis.
   b) The 'amount' of cancer a patient has.
   c) The rate of growth of the cancer.
   d) The likelihood of developing metastasis.
   e) The response to treatment.
   Answer = B

8. A patient receiving radiotherapy for oral cancer is most likely to experience:
   a) Hearing loss.
   b) Acute mucositis.
   c) Radiation caries.
   d) Generalised lymphadenopathy.
   e) Osteoradionecrosis.
   Answer = B

9. What is the most likely complication following extraction of a mandibular molar tooth in a patient who has received head and neck radiotherapy?
   a) Fracture of the roots.
   b) Fracture of the mandible.
   c) Osteoradionecrosis.
   d) Damage to the inferior alveolar nerve.
   e) Excessive bleeding.
   Answer = C

10. A patient with multiple myeloma has an extraction and develops a non-healing socket. Which of the following medications are associated with this post-surgical complication?
    a) Lidocaine.
    b) Anti-fungal medication.
    c) Amoxicillin.
    d) Alendronic acid.
    e) Ibuprofen.
    Answer = D

CHAPTER 17
Child health

FE Hogg and RR Welbury

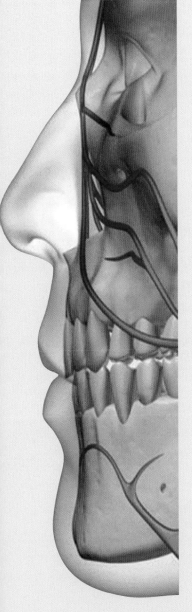

Key topics

- Child development.
- Infections in childhood.
- Cleft lip and palate.
- Child abuse.

Learning objectives

- To be familiar with normal child development and possible anomalies.
- To be aware of the issues in relation to safeguarding.

Essentials of Human Disease in Dentistry, Second Edition. Mark Greenwood.
© 2018 John Wiley & Sons Ltd. Published 2018 by John Wiley & Sons Ltd.
Companion website: www.wiley.com/go/greenwood/human-disease-in-dentistry

Development

A child's development represents the interaction of hereditary and environmental factors. Hereditary factors determine the potential of the child, and the environment influences if that potential is achieved. For optimal development, the environment must meet and provide for the child's intellectual and psychological needs. Such needs will naturally vary with the age of the child and the chronological state of development. For example:

- Infants will be physically dependent on parents, and requires a limited number of carers to meet its psychological needs.
- Primary school children can usually meet some of their own physical needs, as well as cope with social relationships.
- Teenagers are able to meet most of their physical needs, but have increasingly complex emotional needs.

Children whose development is delayed, or who have not reached standard chronological 'milestones', need medical assessment to determine the cause and work out how best the children and their families can be helped. Development can be disrupted by a direct medical disorder (e.g. cerebral palsy); indirectly through chronic ill-health (e.g. severe congenital cardiac disease); owing to physical or psychological needs not being met (environmental factors); or because of reduced inherited potential.

Development is most rapid in the first 4 years of life, which can conveniently be split into five periods, as shown in Table 17.1. There is considerable individual variation in the age at which a child passes from one period to another.

Specific areas of development

Development can be divided into eight functional skills. These can provide a framework for detailed assessment and surveillance in developmental paediatrics:

- Gross motor skills.
- Fine motor skills.
- Language comprehension.
- Expressive language.
- Hearing.
- Vision.
- Social skills.
- Behaviour and emotional development.

It is possible for a child to have a deficiency in one skill area that can impact on other areas – for example, hearing impairment can result in poor language development and social skills.

Table 17.1 The five periods of the first 4 years of life.
The newborn
The supine infant (6–8 weeks of age)
The sitting infant (6–9 months of age)
The mobile toddler (18–24 months of age)
The communicating infant (3–4 years of age)

Range of normality and individual variation

Rate of development

Although there is a variation in the rate at which children attain milestones, all normally developing children may come within normally accepted limits.

Pattern of development

Development is not straightforward and uniform. Motor milestones can be attained in different ways by different children. There is even more variation in the areas of social skills and behaviour.

Eventual level of attainment

This depends on heredity and environment.

Key milestones

In assessing milestones, it is essential to appreciate that both attainment and quality are important. Table 17.2 lists some developmental 'age limits'.

Child health surveillance

In the UK, child health surveillance examinations occur at regular intervals, which correspond to the stages outlined in Table 17.1. At each of these reviews, the individual areas of developmental skills are considered. Equally important is the child's overall development. How well are individual skills integrated, and what is the quality of development? At these reviews, the child's health and growth are also checked. Immunisation is another important part of health that is also addressed in the first 5 years of life. The standard UK immunisation schedule is shown in Table 17.3.

Table 17.2 Some developmental 'age limits'.	
Age	**Developmental sign**
8 weeks	Responsive smiling
3 months	Good eye contact
5 months	Reaches for objects
10 months	Sits unsupported
18 months	Walks unsupported
18 months	Says single words with meaning
30 months	Speaks in phrases

Further assessment is indicated if these skills have not been acquired by this age.

Table 17.3 UK immunisation schedule.

Age	Vaccination type
8 weeks	5-in-1 Vaccine (DTP, polio, Hib), PCV, rotavirus, MenB
12 weeks	5-in-1 Vaccine, rotavirus
16 weeks	5-in-1 Vaccine, PCV, MenB
1 year	Hib/MenC vaccine, MMR, PCV, MenB
2–7 years	Annual flu vaccine
3 years, 4 months	4-in-1 Preschool booster (DTP, polio), MMR
12–13 years (girls)	HPV vaccine
14 years	3-in-1 Teenage booster (DTP), MenACWY

DTP = diphtheria, tetanus, pertussis; Hib = *Haemophilus influenzae* type b; PCV = pneumococcal vaccine; Men = meningococcal; MMR = measles, mumps, rubella.

Language and speech

Language and *speech* are different entities. In a language disorder, the speech sounds are perfect, but a child is unable to communicate because of language difficulty. Alternatively, they may use the underlying rules for speech, but cannot communicate, because no one can understand what they say.

Language can be further subdivided into *language comprehension* and *expressive language*, and a deficit may occur in either. Both these elements go through a developmental progression.

Language problems are recognised first by parents and health professionals. Diagnosis and treatment are specialist areas requiring speech and language therapists or paediatricians.

Language and speech delay

Common causes include hearing loss, environmental deprivation or general developmental delay. Once a cause is identified and hearing checked, a therapy programme may be initiated under the therapist's direction.

Language and speech disorders

These are more serious and require specialist diagnosis and treatment – for example, stammering, incomprehensible speech (dysarthria), receptive aphasia (inability to comprehend language) and expressive aphasia (inability to speak). Some conditions related to speech and language problems include *autism* and *Asperger's syndrome*.

Hearing

The early detection of deafness is very important because, if untreated, the child will have impaired speech, language and learning, and behavioural problems because of communication difficulty.

Hearing loss

This can be divided into *sensorineural* and *conductive* (see Chapter 9, titled 'Neurology and special senses').

Sensorineural loss is uncommon (1 in 1000 of all births). It is usually present at birth, or develops in the first few months of life. It is caused by damage to the cochlea or central neural pathways. Screening occurs at birth (otoacoustic emission), 6–9 months (distraction test), 15 months to 4 years (threshold audiometry), and 4 years and above at school entry if hearing loss is suspected (threshold audiometry).

Sensorineural loss is irreversible. Early amplification with hearing aids is necessary for optimal speech and language development. Cochlear implants may be required where aids give insufficient amplification. Intensive peripatetic specialist teaching support is required.

Children with hearing impairment can be educated either in mainstream schools or in specialist hearing units attached to mainstream schools. If the need is unmet with these measures, then schools for children with severe hearing impairment can play a vital role.

Conductive hearing loss from middle ear disease can be up to 60 dB, but is usually less. It is more common than sensorineural hearing loss. It is often acquired in the early years of life, and may be recurrent. In most children, there are no risk factors; however, children with cleft palate are prone to Down syndrome and atopy.

Children with delayed or poor speech or language must have their hearing checked. Detection is generally by the same methods as detailed for sensorineural loss, with the exception of electrical stimulation tests, which are not useful. Impedance audiometry tests whether the middle ear is functioning normally. If decongestants and long-course antibiotics do not improve the condition, then surgery with the insertion of tympanoplasty tubes (grommets) with or without adenoid removal may be considered. The role of surgery is controversial.

Intervention should be based on functional disability rather than absolute hearing loss.

Vision

Most newborns can fix and move their eyes horizontally. There is a preference for looking at faces. Initially, there may be an apparent squint when looking at near objects, owing to overconvergence. By 6 weeks, the eyes should move together with no squint. Babies slowly develop the ability to focus at distances, and visual acuity improves until adult-level acuity is achieved at 3 years. Visual impairment may present in infancy with:

- Lack of following and fixation.
- Random eye movements.
- Nystagmus.
- Not smiling responsively by 6 weeks post-term.
- Delayed development and visual inattention.
- Squint.

- Photophobia.
- Loss of red reflex from a cataract.
- A white reflex in the pupil (from retinoblastoma, cataract, retinopathy of immaturity, etc.).

Respiratory infections in childhood

Upper respiratory tract infections (URTIs) account for almost half of children's visits to their GPs. Up to 15% of children in the UK have asthma, and this figure is rising.

URTIs

Most are viral, but it may be hard to distinguish viral from bacterial infections.

Otitis media (OM)

OM is an acute infection of the middle ear. In bacterial infections, the tympanic membrane may be bulging. In viral infections, there is an appearance of dilation of blood vessels around the circumference of the drum and over the handle of the malleus. Viral OM is usually bilateral, and associated with viral pharyngitis. Rarely, bacterial infection may spread to mastoiditis and meningitis. The most frequent complication is a persistent middle ear effusion (glue ear), with loss of hearing and a potential detrimental effect on language development.

Tonsillitis

White exudate on the tonsil does not distinguish viral from bacterial infection. Viral tonsillitis (often adenovirus) is more common in preschool children. Bacterial infection with *Streptococcus* is more common in school-age children. EBV (glandular fever) causes florid tonsillitis, and petechial haemorrhages may be seen on the palate. All children should have a throat swab for culture and blood screening for glandular fever (monospot test) where appropriate.

A β-haemolytic streptococcal infection may be complicated by glomerulonephritis or rheumatic fever, although this is more common in developing countries.

Rarely, a peritonsillar abscess (quinsy) may require surgical treatment. All children should have symptomatic treatment with paracetamol, and antibiotics should be given when the throat swab results are available.

Acute lower respiratory tract infection

Worldwide, this is the most common cause of death in children under 5 years. Mortality is low in the UK, and is largely confined to children with pre-existing cardiac and respiratory disease.

Bacterial pneumonia

Worldwide, *Streptococcus pneumoniae* and *Haemophilus influenzae* are common causes. In the UK, atypical organisms such as *Mycoplasma pneumoniae* are responsible for a large number

of cases. It is important to identify the organism responsible, and a nasopharyngeal aspirate should be collected if possible for bacterial culture and viral immunofluorescence, together with samples for blood culture and serology. Antibiotics and follow-up chest radiographs are required to ensure effective treatment.

Measles

This is uncommon now in the UK owing to immunisation, but it is still a common cause of death in the developing world. Measles may be followed by croup, OM or bronchopneumonia.

Croup

Laryngotracheobronchitis is commonly caused by the parainfluenza virus in spring or autumn. A cough with no respiratory distress or stridor requires no treatment. Steroids with or without intubation may be necessary in more severe cases.

Epiglottitis is now rare, owing to Hib immunisation. The affected children have high temperature, and are unable to drink or swallow secretions. They should be seen urgently by an experienced anaesthetist for intubation and prompt antibiotic treatment.

Bronchiolitis

This is an acute viral infection of airways that are <1 mm in diameter, and chiefly affects children under 1 year of age. The respiratory syncytial virus (RSV) is the most common cause, but parainfluenza, influenza and adenoviruses can also be responsible. The illness largely occurs in winter epidemics, is mostly mild and self-limiting, and is treated symptomatically. RSV is highly infectious, and cross-infection in hospital is common. Children with chronic respiratory and cardiac diseases are particularly at risk.

Pertussis

Full immunity to *Bordetella pertussis* does not develop in infants until the third triple vaccine is given at 5 months of age. Diagnosis depends on isolation of the bacteria from a pernasal swab from the nasopharynx. Antibiotic treatment may be effective in early stages; otherwise, treatment is supportive.

Cystic fibrosis (CF)

In developed countries, CF is responsible for the majority of deaths from lung disease in childhood. It is an inherited autosomal recessive condition with an incidence of 1 in 2500 live births. It is a multisystem disorder affecting the lung, gastrointestinal tract, sweat glands, hepatobiliary system, pancreas and reproductive system. Most deaths are from respiratory failure.

There is a failure of chloride transport into the lumens of the affected exocrine organs. Water is drawn into the cell by osmosis from the lumen, leaving the mucus dehydrated. This interrupts ciliary action and leads to bacterial colonisation of the mucus.

Diagnosis is performed using a dried blood spot sample collected on the 'Guthrie card' at 5 days after birth. This screening test is taken at the same time as tests for phenylketonuria and hypothyroidism. Management consists of physiotherapy, daily pancreatic enzyme supplements, vitamin supplementation with fat-soluble vitamins (usually A and E), dietary supplementation and, in some cases, nasogastric or gastrostomy feeds. Early treatment of chest infections may prevent chronic damage and the need for regular intravenous antibiotics.

As CF-affected children survive longer, complications in the biliary system may lead to biliary cirrhosis, portal hypertension and oesophageal varices. An older CF patient who does not gain weight may have diabetes and require regular insulin.

The only definitive treatment for end-stage respiratory failure is a lung or heart–lung transplant.

Asthma

Asthma is a reversible airways obstruction that causes intermittent wheezing (see Chapter 6, titled 'Respiratory disorders'). The symptoms occur owing to spasm of smooth muscles in the bronchial wall, and mucosal inflammation with oedema and increased secretions. In many primary school children, a viral respiratory infection triggers an attack. Other important allergens include the faeces of the house dust mite, pollens, fungal spores and, occasionally, pets. Inhaled irritants, including cigarette smoke, can act as triggers. The British Thoracic Society and Scottish Intercollegiate Guidelines have been devised to encourage a stepwise approach to the management of asthma in children over 12 months of age:

- *Step 1*: Inhaled short-acting β_2-agonist bronchodilators as required. If these are needed more than once per day, move to step 2.
- *Step 2*: Add inhaled corticosteroids as a regular preventer medication.
- *Step 3*: Add long-acting β_2-agonist bronchodilators. Assess the patient's control. If there is persistent poor control, move to step 4.
- *Step 4*: Higher-dose inhaled corticosteroids. If continuous frequent use of steroids is required, move to step 5.
- *Step 5*: Use of daily steroid tablets in addition to high-dose corticosteroids. Refer patient to respiratory physician.

There is no proven link to dental caries with the inhaled drugs used in the management of asthma. Asthmatic patients are at risk of developing dental erosion for the following reasons:

- Inhaled drugs cause drying of the oral mucosa. If an acidic drink is taken to relieve the dryness, then this predisposes to dental erosion.

- β_2-agonists may cause relaxation of the lower oesophageal sphincter, predisposing to greater gastric acid reflux.
- Poorly controlled asthma with night time coughing fits may result in an increased gastric acid reflux.
- Patients on oral corticosteroids are predisposed to oral candidiasis as a result of drug deposition in the mouth.

Oral infections

Viruses, bacteria, fungi or protozoa may cause infections of the oral mucosa.

Viral

Primary herpes simplex infection

This condition usually occurs in children between the ages of 6 months and 5 years. A degree of immunity is transferred to the newborn from circulating maternal antibodies, so an infection in the first 12 months of life is rare. Almost all adults in urban populations are carriers of, and have neutralising antibodies to, the virus. This acquired immunity suggests that the majority of childhood infections are subclinical. Transmission is by droplet infection, and the incubation period is about 1 week. The child develops a febrile illness with a raised temperature of 37.8–38.9 °C. Headaches, malaise, oral pain, mild dysphagia and cervical lymphadenopathy are the common symptoms that accompany the fever, and they precede the onset of a severe, oedematous marginal gingivitis. Characteristic fluid-filled vesicles appear on the gingiva and other areas, such as the tongue, lips, and buccal and palatal mucosa. The vesicles, which have a grey membranous covering, rupture spontaneously after a few hours, and leave painful yellowish ulcers with red inflamed margins. The clinical episode runs a course of about 14 days, and the oral lesions heal without scarring. Rare and severe complications include aseptic meningitis and encephalitis. If doubts exist about the diagnosis, then smears from the newly ruptured vesicles should be checked to see if they reveal degenerating epithelial cells with intranuclear inclusions. The virus protein also tends to displace nuclear chromatin to produce enlarged and irregular nuclei.

Herpetic gingivostomatitis does not respond well to active treatment. The child should be kept well hydrated during the febrile stage and advised to take bed rest and a soft diet. Sugar-free paracetamol suspension should be used to reduce the pyrexia. Secondary infection of ulcers may be prevented using chlorhexidine. A 0.2% mouthwash may be used two or three times daily in older children; in children under 6 years of age, a chlorhexidine spray can be used twice daily, or the solution applied using a swab. In severe cases of herpes simplex, systemic aciclovir can be prescribed as a suspension (200 mg) and swallowed, five times daily for 5 days. In children under 2 years of age, the dose is halved. Aciclovir is active against the virus, but is unable to eradicate it completely. The drug is most effective when given at the onset of the infection.

Secondary herpes simplex infection

The herpes virus remains dormant in the epithelial cells of the host. Reactivation of the latent virus or reinfection in subjects with acquired immunity occurs in adults. Recurrent disease presents in an attenuated form of the infection at the labial mucocutaneous junction as a vesicular lesion that ruptures and forms a crusting, producing the common 'cold sore'. Cold sores are treated by applying aciclovir cream (5%, five times daily for about 5 days).

Varicella zoster

The varicella zoster virus causes shingles, which is much more common in adults than in children, and is highly contagious. The vesicular lesion develops within the peripheral distribution of a branch of the trigeminal nerve. Chickenpox, a more common presentation of varicella zoster in children, produces a vesicular rash on the skin. The intraoral lesions of chickenpox resemble those of primary herpetic infection.

Mumps

Mumps is a contagious condition that produces a painful enlargement of the parotid glands. It is usually bilateral, and the associated complaints include headache, vomiting and fever. Symptoms last for about a week. The causative agent is a myxovirus.

Measles

The intraoral manifestation of measles occurs on the buccal mucosa. The lesions appear as white speckling surrounded by a red margin, and are known as 'Koplik's spots'. The oral signs usually precede the skin lesions, and disappear early in the course of the disease. The skin rash of measles normally appears as a red maculopapular lesion. Fever is present, and the disease is contagious.

Herpangina

This is caused by a Coxsackie A virus infection, and it can be differentiated from primary herpetic infection by the different location of the vesicles, which are found in the tonsillar or pharyngeal region. Herpangina lesions do not coalesce to form large areas of ulceration. The condition is short-lived.

Hand, foot and mouth disease

This Coxsackie A virus infection produces a maculopapular rash on the hands and feet, which lasts for 10–14 days. The intraoral vesicles rupture to produce painful ulceration. The condition is common in nurseries and primary schools.

Infectious mononucleosis

The Epstein–Barr virus (EBV) causes this condition, which is not uncommon among teenagers. The usual form of transmission is by kissing. Oral ulceration and petechial haemorrhage may occur at the hard–soft palate junction. There is lymph node enlargement and associated fever. There is no specific treatment. It should be noted that the prescription of ampicillin and amoxicillin can cause a rash in those suffering from infectious mononucleosis. These antibiotics should be avoided during the course of the disease.

The treatment of the preceding viral illnesses is symptomatic, and relies on analgesia and maintenance of fluid intake. Aspirin should be avoided in children under 12 years of age.

Human papillomavirus

This is associated with several warty tumour-like lesions of the oral mucosa.

Bacterial

Staphylococcal infections

Staphylococci and streptococci may cause impetigo. This can affect the angles of the mouth and the lips. It presents as crusting vesiculobullous lesions. The vesicles coalesce to produce ulceration over a wide area. Pigmentation may occur during healing. The condition is self-limiting, although antibiotics may be prescribed in some cases. Staphylococcal organisms can cause osteomyelitis of the jaws in children. Although the introduction of antibiotics has reduced the incidence of severe forms of the condition, it can still be devastating. Surgical intervention is often required to remove bony sequestra.

Streptococcal infection

Streptococcal infections in children vary from a mucopurulent nasal discharge to tonsillitis, pharyngitis and gingivitis. Scarlet fever is a β-haemolytic streptococcal infection consisting of a skin rash with maculopapular lesions of the oral mucosa. It is associated with tonsillitis and pharyngitis. The tongue shows characteristic changes – from a strawberry appearance in the early stages to a raspberry-like form in the later stages.

Congenital syphilis

Congenital syphilis is transmitted from an infected mother to the foetus. Oral mucosal changes such as rhagades, which is a pattern of scarring at the angle of the mouth, may occur. In addition, this disease may cause characteristic dental changes in the permanent dentition. These include Hutchinson's incisors (the teeth taper towards the incisal edge rather than the cervical margin) and mulberry molars (globular masses of enamel over the occlusal surface).

Tuberculosis

Tuberculous lesions of the oral cavity are rare; however, tuberculous lymphadenitis affecting submandibular and cervical lymph nodes is occasionally seen. These present as tender, enlarged nodes, which may progress to abscess formation with discharge through the skin. Surgical removal of infected glands produces a much neater scar than that caused by spontaneous rupture through the skin if the disease is allowed to progress.

Cat-scratch disease

This is a self-limiting disease that presents as an enlargement of the regional lymph nodes. The nodes are painful, and enlargement occurs up to 3 weeks following a cat scratch. The nodes become suppurative and may perforate the skin. Treatment often involves incision and drainage.

Fungal

Candida

Neonatal acute candidiasis (thrush) contracted during birth is not uncommon. Likewise, young children may develop the condition when resistance is lowered or after antibiotic therapy. Easily removed white patches on an erythematous or bleeding base are found. Treatment with miconazole or fluconazole is effective. Compliance with nystatin has been found to be poor due to its taste. Miconazole oromucosal gel, 24 mg/ml can be prescribed in children aged 2–6 years – that is, a pea-size amount applied twice daily after food. Fluconazole, a systemic antifungal, is available as an oral suspension, and can be used to treat oropharyngeal candidiasis.

Actinomycosis

Actinomycosis can occur in children. It may follow intraoral trauma, including in dental extractions. The organisms spread through the tissues, and can cause dysphagia if the submandibular region is involved. Abscesses may rupture on to the skin, and long-term antibiotic therapy is required. Penicillin should be prescribed and maintained for at least 2 weeks following clinical cure.

Protozoal

Infection by *Toxoplasma gondii* may occasionally occur in children, the principal reservoir of infection being cats. Glandular toxoplasmosis is similar in presentation to infectious mononucleosis, and is found mainly in children and young adults. There may be a granulomatous reaction in the oral mucosa, and there can be parotid gland enlargement. The disease is self-limiting, although an antiprotozoal such as pyrimethamine may be used in cases of severe infection.

Clefts of the lip and palate

Cleft teams in the UK record all babies born with a cleft lip and palate, including variations in the lip, alar, nostril floor, palate and uvula. They also record the shape of the cleft and any respiratory problems. These data are sent to the Craniofacial

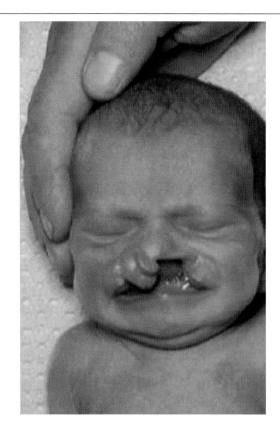

Figure 17.1 A baby with a CLP.

Anomalies Register, the aim of which is to record every case of cleft in the UK.

The simple nomenclatures that are universally used are: 'cleft lip' (CL), 'cleft palate' (CP), and 'cleft lip and palate' (CLP), with the prefixes 'U' and 'B' for 'unilateral' and 'bilateral', respectively (Figure 17.1).

Aetiology of clefts

In the majority of cases, a cleft will be the only defect, but it may also be found associated with other congenital anomalies, and may occur as part of a syndrome. A *non-syndromic* (NS) *cleft* is defined as a cleft that occurs in the absence of any other disabilities. The aetiology of clefts is thought to be multifactorial, with possible genetic and environmental contributory factors.

Genetic factors

Several genes may be involved in the aetiology of NS clefts. It does not follow Mendelian inheritance; however, family and twin studies show the evidence for genetic predisposition to NS CLP. It is thought that twin pregnancy does not change the risk of cleft anomaly. While no specific disease-causing gene mutations have been identified in NS clefting, several candidate genes have been isolated through both linkage and association studies.

Environmental factors

It has been recognised for some time that teratogens play a role in the aetiology of CLP.

Socioeconomic status

In Scotland, a higher incidence of clefts was observed in areas with higher proportions of local authority housing involving young families, high unemployment and a preponderance of unskilled workers. The converse was found in affluent areas with high proportions of professional and non-manual workers in large owner-occupied housing.

Smoking

Maternal smoking during pregnancy has been suggested as a risk factor for having a child with CLP. It has been suggested that incorporating information regarding the effects of maternal smoking on oral clefts into public health campaigns might be useful.

Alcohol consumption

The association between maternal alcohol consumption during pregnancy and oral clefts in offspring remains unclear. There is conflicting evidence regarding the association between alcohol consumption and oral clefts, although CP has been described as an associated defect in 10% of severe foetal alcohol syndrome cases.

Nutrition

There have been many studies demonstrating the evidence of the protective effect of folic acid on neural tube defects. Nevertheless, it is not known why a neural tube defect resulting from folic acid deficiency does not occur in combination with facial clefts.

Folic acid supplements reduce the incidence of cleft. Other factors, such as vitamin B_6 deficiency, can more often cause malformations. The exact association remains unclear, and, globally, there has been no reduction in the birth prevalence of orofacial clefting despite considerable improvements in nutrition.

Drugs

Evidence of the association of maternal drug use with orofacial clefting is conflicting. Corticosteroids and antiepileptic drugs have been implicated, and further research is required.

Birth order

There is no obvious association between birth order and the development of clefts.

Child physical abuse

Introduction

In the middle of the last century, reports appeared in the USA of unexplained skeletal injuries in children, sometimes associated with subdural haematoma. When Kempe *et al.* published their paper titled 'The battered-child syndrome' in 1962, the full impact of the physical maltreatment of children was brought to the attention of the medical community and, subsequently, the general public. Within a few years, the majority of states in the USA had introduced laws that made it mandatory for physicians, dentists and other health-related professions to report suspected cases.

Prevalence

Every week, children die because of abuse or neglect. It is estimated that about 10% of all children aged less than 5 years who are admitted in hospital accident and emergency departments will have injuries that are wilfully inflicted. In the UK, at least 1 child per 1000 under 4 years of age per year suffers severe physical abuse – for example, fractures, brain haemorrhage, severe internal injuries or mutilation. In the USA, >95% of serious intracranial injuries during the first year of life are the result of abuse.

Aetiology

Child abuse encompasses all social classes, but more cases have been identified in the lower socioeconomic groups. Many cases of child abuse are perpetrated by the child's parents, or by persons known to the child. Young parents, often of low intelligence, are more likely to be abusers. Abuse is thought to be 20 times more likely if one of the parents was abused as a child.

Identification

The following list constitutes ten points that should be considered when suspicions arise. None of them is pathognomonic on its own, and neither does the absence of any of them preclude the diagnosis of child abuse.

1. Could the injury have been caused accidentally, and, if so, how?
2. Does the explanation for the injury fit the child's age and the clinical findings?
3. If the explanation of the cause is consistent with the injury, is this itself within normally acceptable limits of behaviour?
4. Has there been a delay in seeking medical help, and are there good reasons for this?
5. Is the story of the 'accident' vague or lacking in detail, and does it vary with each telling and from person to person?
6. The relationship between parent and child.
7. The child's reaction to other people and any medical/dental examination.

8. The general demeanour of the child.
9. Any comments made by the child and/or parent that give cause for concern about the child's lifestyle or upbringing.
10. History of previous injuries.

Types of orofacial injuries in child physical abuse

At least 60% of cases diagnosed as child physical abuse involve orofacial trauma. Although the face often seems to be the focus of impulsive violence, facial fractures are not frequent. Soft tissue injuries, most frequently bruises, are the most common types of injury. In addition, it is common for a particular child to have more than one injury. It is very important to state that there are no specific single injuries that are diagnostic or pathognomonic of child physical abuse.

Bruising

Accidental falls rarely cause bruises to the soft tissues of the cheek, but instead involve the skin overlying bony prominences such as the forehead or cheekbone. Bruises cannot be accurately dated, but bruises of widely differing vintages indicate more than one episode of abuse. Bruises on the ear are commonly due to being pinched or pulled by the ear, and there will usually be a matching bruise on the posterior surface of the ear. Bruises or cuts on the neck are almost always due to being choked or strangled by a human hand, cord or some sort of collar. Accidents to this site are extremely rare, and should be looked upon with suspicion.

Bruising and laceration of the upper labial fraenum of a young child can be produced by forcible bottle feeding, and may remain hidden unless the lip is carefully everted. A fraenum tear is not uncommon in the young child who accidentally falls while learning to walk (generally between 8 and 18 months). A fraenal tear in a very young non-ambulatory patient (<1 year) should arouse suspicion (Figure 17.2).

Human hand marks

The human hand can leave various types of pressure bruises: grab marks or finger-tip bruises, linear marks or finger-edge bruises, hand prints, slap marks (Figure 17.3) and pinch marks. Grab mark bruises can occur on the cheeks if an adult squeezes a child's face in an attempt to aid feeding. Linear marks are caused by pressure from the entire finger. In slap marks to the cheek, parallel linear bruises at finger-width spacing will be seen to run through a more diffuse bruise. These linear bruises are due to the capillaries rupturing at the edge of the injury (between the striking fingers), as a result of being stretched and receiving a sudden influx of blood.

Bizarre bruises

Bizarre-shaped bruises with sharp borders are nearly always inflicted in physical abuse cases. If there is a pattern on the inflicting implement, this may be duplicated in the bruise – the so-called 'tattoo bruising' (Figure 17.4).

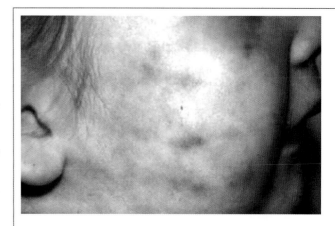

Figure 17.3 Slap marks.

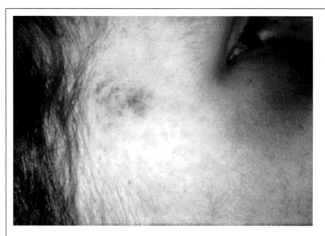

Figure 17.4 Tattoo bruising – note the pattern of the inflicting implement that has been duplicated in the bruise.

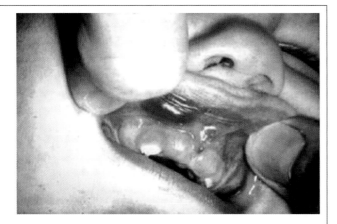

Figure 17.2 A torn labial fraenum.

Abrasions and lacerations

Penetrating injuries to the palate, vestibule and floor of the mouth can occur during forceful feeding of young infants, and are usually caused by the feeding utensil. Abrasions and lacerations on the face may be caused by a variety of objects, but are most commonly due to rings or fingernails on the inflicting hand.

Burns

Approximately 10% of physical abuse cases involve burns. Burns of the oral mucosa can be the result of enforced ingestion of hot or caustic fluids in young children. Burns from hot solid objects applied to the face are usually without blister formation, and the shape of the burn often resembles its agent. Cigarette burns give circular, punched-out lesions of uniform size.

Bite marks

Human bite marks are identified by their shape and size. When necessary, serological techniques are available that may assist in identification. Teeth marks that do not break the skin only last up to 24 hours (Figure 17.5).

Tooth trauma

Injury to either the primary or permanent dentition in children can be due to blunt trauma. A similar range of injuries to those found in accidental trauma is seen in such cases.

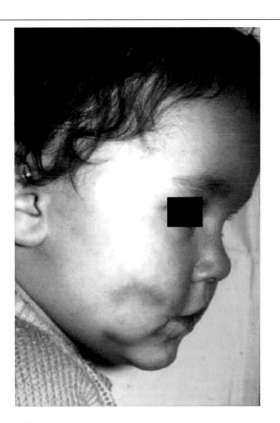

Figure 17.5 A bite mark.

Eye injuries

Most periorbital bruises caused by child abuse involve both sides of the face. Ocular damage in child abuse includes acute hyphaema, dislocated lens, traumatic cataract and detached retina. More than half of these injuries result in permanent impairment of vision affecting one or both eyes.

Fractures

Fractures are among the most serious injuries sustained in child abuse. They may occur in almost any bone, and may be single or multiple, clinically obvious, or occult and detectable only by radiography. Most fractures in physically abused children occur under the age of 3 years. In contrast, accidental fractures occur more commonly in children of school age.

Facial fractures are relatively uncommon in children. The presence of a fracture of the facial skeleton in a case of child abuse is an indication for a full skeletal radiographic survey, which may show evidence of multiple fractures at different stages of healing.

Other forms of child abuse

Emotional abuse, sexual abuse and neglect can impact as severely on a child's well-being as physical abuse. The National Institute of Clinical Excellence has produced guidelines on child maltreatment. These guidelines clearly summarise the clinical features of child maltreatment and emphasise the importance of sharing information among health and social care professionals in order to protect the child. Dental neglect is now a recognised form of child abuse, and can be defined as the persistent failure to meet a child's basic oral health needs, likely to result in serious impairment of the child's oral or general health or development. All clinicians should become familiar with the British Society of Paediatric Dentistry Policy Statement on Dental Neglect in Children. Local protocols for safeguarding children should be followed when sharing a concern for a child's well-being.

Conclusions

- The variety of orofacial injuries that may be sustained in child physical abuse is wide.
- Use the checklist of ten items provided earlier in text – five questions to ask yourself, and five observations to make – whenever there are doubts or suspicions of abuse.
- Every Primary Care Trust in the UK should have coordinated guidelines for dental practitioners. These should be available from designated doctors or nurses in the Child Protection units in every Primary Care Trust. Guidelines throughout the country should be largely generic, and the contact person should either be a named doctor or a named nurse. These persons should be there for both advice and referral.

FURTHER READING

Arduino PG and Porter SR. Herpes Simplex Virus Type 1 infection: overview on relevant clinico-pathological features. *Journal of Oral Pathology & Medicine* 2008; 37: 107–121.

British Society of Paediatric Dentistry. 2009. A policy Document on Dental Neglect in Children. Available from http://bspd.co.uk/Portals/0/Public/Files/PolicyStatements/Dental%20Neglect%20In%20Children.pdf (accessed 28.12.16).

British Thoracic Society/Scottish Intercollegiate Guideline Network British Guideline on the Management of Asthma. 2016. SIGN 153. Available from: https://www.brit-thoracic.org.uk/document-library/clinical-information/asthma/btssign-asthma-guideline-2016/ (accessed 28.12.16).

Chi D. Dental caries prevalence in children and adolescents with cystic fibrosis: a qualitative systematic review and recommendations for future research. *International Journal of Paediatric Dentistry* 2013; 23: 376–386.Child development timeline (NHS). Available from: http://www.nhs.uk/tools/pages/birthtofive.aspx (accessed 28.12.16).

CleftSiS. Cleft Pathway Scotland Cleft Care Scotland Managed Clinical Network. Available from: http://www.knowledge.scot.nhs.uk/media/CLT/ResourceUploads/4054342/UCLP%20Patient%20Pathway%20-%20Final%20website.pdf (accessed 28.12.16).

National Deaf Children's Society: Resources for Professionals. Available from: http://www.ndcs.org.uk/professional_support/our_resources/health_resources.html (accessed 28.12.16).

National Institute for Health and Care Excellence CG 89. When to Suspect Child Maltreatment. Available from: https://www.nice.org.uk/guidance/cg89 (accessed 28.12.16).

NHS immunisation schedule (UK). Available from: http://www.nhs.uk/conditions/vaccinations/pages/vaccination-schedule-age-checklist.aspx (accessed 28.12.16).

Scottish Dental Clinical Effectiveness Programme. Drug Prescribing for Dentistry. *Dental Clinical Guidance*, third edition. Available from: http://www.sdcep.org.uk/wp-content/uploads/2016/03/SDCEP-Drug-Prescribing-for-Dentistry-3rd-edition.pdf (accessed 28.12.16).

The Cleft Registry and Audit Network. Available from: https://www.crane-database.org.uk/ (accessed 28.12.16).

Welbury et al. Child protection and the dental team: an introduction to safeguarding children in dental practice. Published by COPDEND, 2006–15. Hosted by the British Dental Association from 2016. Available from: https://www.bda.org/childprotection (accessed 28.12.16).

MULTIPLE CHOICE QUESTIONS

1. A parent is concerned that his or her child's 'tongue-tie' might interfere with speech development. By what age can most children speak in phrases?
   a) 8 months.
   b) 12 months.
   c) 22 months.
   d) 30 months.
   e) 36 months.
   Answer = D

2. A mother brings in her 7-month-old child who has avulsed his or her lower left primary central incisor. She tells you that the child fell against a coffee table and bumped his or her mouth while moving about. By what age will most children have become ambulant?
   a) 5–9 months.
   b) 7–10 months.
   c) 9–12 months.
   d) 12–18 months.
   e) 18—24 months.
   Answer = D

3. A 24-month-old child presents to you with lip lacerations and an intruded tooth, sustained in a muddy playing field, and wound debridement is required. At what stage in the tetanus immunisation course would you expect the child to be at if he or she were born in the UK?
   a) Had first three doses of tetanus; two boosters still required at a later stage.
   b) Not commenced tetanus doses yet.
   c) Had first two doses; three doses remain.
   d) Completed full course of vaccination.
   e) Had first schedule of doses; one booster required.
   Answer = A

4. A 10-year-old patient with dental caries in upper permanent central incisors presents with a medical history revealing asthma, and reports to be using daily inhaled corticosteroids and daily inhaled β_2-agonists. What is most likely to have contributed to the dental disease?
   a) Dry mouth due to inhalers.
   b) Relaxation of the lower oesophageal sphincter.
   c) Increased gastro-oesophageal reflux.
   d) Drug deposition in mouth.
   e) Frequent consumption of soft-drinks.
   Answer = E

5. Which of the following statements are true of CF in developed countries?
   a) It occurs in 1:250 children, and has an autosomal recessive pattern of inheritance.
   b) It occurs in 1:2500 children, and has an autosomal dominant pattern of inheritance.
   c) It occurs in 1:25 000, children, and has an x-linked recessive pattern of inheritance.
   d) It occurs in 1:2500 children, and has an autosomal recessive pattern of inheritance.
   e) It occurs in 1:1000 children, and has an autosomal recessive pattern of inheritance.
   Answer = D

6. A mother is concerned about bleeding and ulceration from her 15-month-old child's mouth. On examination, the gingivae and soft tissues are erythematous, with ulcerations present. The child has been refusing food, and sleep has been disturbed. What virus is most likely to have contributed to these symptoms?
   a) Herpes simplex virus.
   b) Varicella zoster virus.
   c) Rhinovirus.
   d) Coxsackie A virus.
   e) Paramyxovirus.
   Answer = A

7. Which of the following conditions are treated with antibiotics?
   a) Hand, foot and mouth disease.
   b) Primary herpetic gingivostomatitis.
   c) Scarlet fever.
   d) Glandular fever.
   e) Mumps.
   Answer = C

8. Which of the following is not an environmental factor implicated in the aetiology of CLP patients?
   a) Multiple births.
   b) Maternal smoking.
   c) Maternal alcohol use.
   d) Maternal epilepsy medication.
   e) Maternal exposure to toxins.
   Answer = A

9. What percentage of physical child abuse cases will present with signs of abuse to the oral–facial region?
   a) 20%.
   b) 100%.
   c) 60%.
   d) 40%.
   e) 5%.
   Answer = C

10. Who has the responsibility to record and report concerns regarding potential child abuse?
    a) The child's health visitor.
    b) The child's medical practitioner.
    c) The child's dentist.
    d) The child's teacher.
    e) All of the above.
    Answer = E

CHAPTER 18
Medicine for the elderly

RH Jay

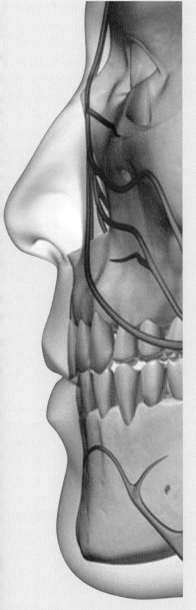

Key topics

- Ageing.
- Illness in old age.
- General principles of management of the elderly patient.
- Prescribing for elderly patients.

Learning objectives

- To be familiar with the specific potential problems in relation to patient management in the elderly.
- To have knowledge of prescribing for elderly patients.

Essentials of Human Disease in Dentistry, Second Edition. Mark Greenwood.
© 2018 John Wiley & Sons Ltd. Published 2018 by John Wiley & Sons Ltd.
Companion website: www.wiley.com/go/greenwood/human-disease-in-dentistry

Introduction

Geriatric medicine and psychiatry of old age are specialties that deal with the physical and mental problems associated with later life. All general dental practitioners will see large numbers of elderly patients, and they need to have an understanding of the effects of ageing, illness and disability that will impact on the delivery of dental care to this group.

Our population is ageing, and the survival curve in developed countries has changed markedly in the past century. In the nineteenth century (and in many developing countries even now), there were high death rates in childhood. Death rates levelled off in adult life, but rose steeply again after middle age, such that survival to what we would now consider to be old age was uncommon. Nowadays, deaths in childhood and young adult life are few, and survival rates fall more steeply in old age.

Life expectancy at birth continues to rise, despite repeated predictions over the years that it may be reaching a ceiling. In the UK, over the next 20 years, the population aged 65–84 years will rise by 39%, and those over 85 years of age by 106%. It is the >80 years age group that suffers the greatest burden of illness and disability, and which therefore needs the most care and consideration when delivering all aspects of health care.

Ageing

Ageing is a process we all recognise, but often find hard to define. One attempt at a definition of *ageing* is: 'the gradual development of changes in structure and function that are not due to preventable disease or trauma, and that are associated with decreased functional capacity and an increased probability of death'. This definition satisfies the bio-gerontologist who studies the molecular and cellular process of ageing itself, and considers them separate from the effects of disease or injury. The fact remains that older people suffer from multiple health problems that add to the burden of ageing, and some of the more common medical problems of old age are listed in Table 18.1.

Features of illness in old age

Although the conditions listed in Table 18.1 are not the exclusive preserve of the elderly, there are certain features of illness in old age that necessitate a different approach as compared to that used for the younger patient.

Non-specific presentations

Older people often present with atypical symptoms, or non-specific presentations of illness. For example, loss of appetite and weight may have many potential causes, including physical illness such as cancer, mental illnesses including depression, and oral conditions affecting the ability to eat. It is therefore important to obtain as clear a picture as possible of the presenting complaint, including a corroborative history from someone who knows the patient well. A range of investigations may be required to make a clear diagnosis.

Table 18.1 Some common medical conditions of old age.

Cardiovascular
- Ischaemic heart disease (angina/myocardial infarction)
- Heart failure
- Atrial fibrillation

Respiratory
- Chronic obstructive pulmonary disease
- Respiratory infections

Gastrointestinal
- Gastro-oesophageal reflux
- Peptic ulceration
- Constipation

Genitourinary
- Incontinence
- Urine frequency
- Bladder outflow obstruction due to prostate disease

Musculoskeletal
- Osteoarthritis
- Osteoporosis and fractures
- Muscle weakness ('sarcopenia')

Neurological/psychiatric
- Poor vision (cataracts, glaucoma and macular degeneration)
- Deafness
- Dementia
- Depression
- Parkinson's disease
- Strokes

Metabolic/endocrine
- Diabetes mellitus (type 2, non-insulin-dependent)
- Hypothyroidism

Neoplastic
- Common cancers in old age include breast, lung, gastrointestinal tract and prostate

Multiple pathology, and consequent polypharmacy

Many older people have several chronic medical conditions, and therefore require multiple medications. Both the conditions and the drugs can interact in the way they affect the patient. For example, many of the drugs used to treat heart disease can lower the blood pressure. The autonomic cardiovascular reflexes, which maintain a constant blood pressure during changes in posture, deteriorate with age. Therefore, drug treatment of angina or heart failure may cause a major drop in the blood pressure on standing up, known as 'orthostatic hypotension', resulting in faints or falls and consequent injury.

Impaired homeostasis, resistance to disease and recovery

Older people's resistance to a whole range of insults is reduced. They will fall more easily if pushed; develop hypothermia in a cold environment; display diminished resistance to infection; and are more prone to metabolic disturbances as a result of, for example, dehydration. Similarly, their processes of healing and recovery are also diminished, resulting in prolonged effects of illnesses.

Loss of functional independence

Many of the chronic diseases of old age, such as arthritis or glaucoma, have permanent effects on the patient's ability to undertake the basic activities of daily living, such as preparing meals, shopping, or even dressing and using the toilet. Relatively minor acute illnesses in a frail older person can result in complete loss of ability to cope at home, requiring emergency hospital admission. A respiratory infection, for example, may cause confusion and fatigue, such that the patient takes to bed, stops eating and drinking, and becomes seriously dehydrated.

With their burden of chronic illness, together with the reduced functional capacity of ageing itself, many older people suffer long-term incapacity. The ungainly term 'giants of geriatrics' has been used for a list of common problems that afflict the elderly:

- Incontinence.
- Instability (falls).
- Immobility.
- Intellectual impairment (dementia and delirium).

Each of these problems has multiple underlying causes or contributory factors, and they often co-exist and interact with each other. Consider the example of a patient admitted with a stroke who develops urinary incontinence. The stroke may have had a direct effect on the neurological control of the bladder, leading directly to incontinence. Even in the absence of this, the combined effects of the stroke and the unfamiliar environment may have robbed the patient of the ability to find, reach or ask for the toilet, through effects on mobility, vision, speech or cognitive function. Pre-existing prostatic hypertrophy in a man or pelvic floor weakness in a woman may have already caused difficulties in bladder control that, together with the effects of the stroke, the patient can no longer overcome.

An additional problem that older people suffer is isolation. As a result of their disabilities, they cannot get out. Their spouses and other peers are either dead or disabled themselves.

Even in a social setting, the effects of deafness and poor vision result in sensory isolation, for which the patient cannot compensate, since their mental adaptability is also reduced.

These problems all have obvious practical consequences for the delivery of dental care. Older patients may present late with advanced disease, owing to the difficulties in accessing care or in recognising the need for attention at an earlier stage. When they do finally attend, the practitioner should enquire whether any special consideration needs to be given, for example, assistance with mobility or toilet use. In some cases, essential dental care needs to be delivered in the patient's own environment or in a hospital setting.

Care settings for older people

A range of facilities are available to meet the needs of frail older people with functional disabilities. Some are designed for short-term assessment, treatment and rehabilitation, while others cater to the long-term needs of people with permanent disabilities.

Assessment and rehabilitation

Older people requiring assessment of complex and disabling problems need attention from a multidisciplinary team, which should include doctors, nurses, physiotherapists, occupational therapists and social workers. Additional input may be required from dietitians, podiatrists, speech therapists, psychiatric nurses, psychiatrists and psychologists. These teams may be based in a hospital ward; a day hospital where the patient may attend weekly for several weeks; in a residential rehabilitation unit; or in a community team that visits them in their own home.

The process of rehabilitation aims to restore patients to their fullest potential of physical, psychological and social function. Interventions may include medical treatment, exercise therapy, the use of aids and appliances, and the provision of carers to assist patients with tasks they cannot undertake themselves. For example, a patient with Parkinson's disease may receive medical treatment from the doctor, balance exercises from the physiotherapist, walking and bathroom aids from the occupational therapist, and the provision of visiting carers to help with meal preparation from the social worker.

The term 'carer' refers both to the relative or friend who provides voluntary assistance, and to the paid carer provided through social services or other organisations. The former type of carers may find themselves under considerable physical or mental strain, and the burden put upon such people should always be considered and minimised.

Long-term care

If, after full assessment, the patient cannot be supported to live independently at home, even with carers visiting to assist with essential activities, there is a range of long-term care settings where they can be cared for. The term 'sheltered housing' applies to purpose-designed block of flats or bungalows, often with a warden and a communal sitting area. Some newer 'sheltered extra-care' schemes now provide in-house carers, rather than relying on external agencies. In a residential home, each resident has a room of his or her own, but all meals are provided, and carers are present round the clock to assist with tasks such as washing and dressing, toileting and mobility. A nursing home caters to more dependent residents in the same way; nursing home residents may be immobile, doubly incontinent and need physical help with feeding. For patients with mental problems that result in difficult behaviour, 'elderly mentally infirm' (EMI – a term in declining use) homes are available to provide an appropriate level of supervision.

Temporary respite care, whether at a day centre or for a period of time in an institution, is an important way of allowing caring friends or relatives who maintain older persons in their own homes to lead their own lives for part of the time, and to recharge their physical and mental batteries.

It is important to remember that these frail, institutionalised older people need the same general medical and dental care as anyone else – indeed, usually more. A particular point for older people in institutions, especially in hospitals, is the problem of losing their dentures, which should therefore always be labelled indelibly with the patient's name to aid in identifying and returning them to the correct owner.

History taking

It is essential to know an older person's medical background when assessing or treating any new health problem, and many of the conditions listed in Table 18.1 have a direct effect on the delivery of dental treatment. To take the example of common cardiovascular disorders, angina may be brought on by the stress of dental treatment, and may need to be treated in the surgery with sublingual nitrates. Laying the patient flat may aggravate breathlessness in heart failure patients.

Those with atrial fibrillation are likely to be on anticoagulants, and may have ischaemic heart disease or heart failure.

Obtaining a clear and full history from an older person can be difficult. The complexity of their medical history itself may result in omission or misunderstanding on the patient's part. Communication may be impeded by visual impairment or deafness. The patient may suffer from dementia. Therefore, it is important to recognise these problems, seek a corroborative history from a relative or carer, and to confirm medical details and a drug history with the patient's general medical practitioner.

Social circumstances and support are an important consideration for older people with reduced physical or mental function. The ability to cooperate with some aspects of dental treatment, such as maintaining hygiene or taking prescribed medications, may be impaired. Therefore, dentists will need to establish whether the patients themselves can follow the necessary instructions, or whether extra help is required.

Some simple aids may help independence. Older people can be helped to remain independent using a wide range of aids and appliances – from glasses and hearing aids to walking frames and incontinence devices. In the context of dental treatment, toothbrushes with large handles for weak or arthritic hands may be helpful, and written instructions and reminders may be helpful for those with impaired memory.

Actual physical help or supervision from carers is needed when other measures fail. It is therefore essential to ascertain the details of the support that is available to patients – for example, whether they live with able relatives, have carers visiting them in their homes, or live in protected institutions with 24-hour care. Over 20% of those over 85 years of age live in residential or nursing homes or sheltered housing.

Examination

Specific points in the examination of patients with the medical conditions listed in Table 18.1 have been covered in other chapters. This section will therefore concentrate on the more general features in older people, and on assessment of their functions and abilities.

General observation can give important clues to an older person's health and well-being. Do they appear well nourished? Is their gait strong and steady, or do they use walking aids? Do they appear breathless on walking? Are there obvious bone or joint deformities from arthritis or osteoporotic fracture? How is their manual dexterity when removing their coats or signing forms? Can they see and hear adequately when dealing with the receptionist?

Likewise, their mental function can be deduced informally. Do they appear orientated to their surroundings, able to concentrate and converse appropriately? Are they clean and appropriately dressed? Are their answers to questions clear and plausible? Apparent mental impairment in conversation may actually be due to deafness or a speech disorder such as dysphasia following a stroke. Conversely, a patient may be able to conceal significant dementia by maintaining social graces and giving plausible answers to questions. It may therefore be useful to check a patient's basic orientation by asking them their age and address, the date and time.

General principles of management

Some important principles of management of both health and social care set out in the UK government's National Service Framework for Older People in 2001 remain applicable today. Three standards that are particularly relevant to dental care are given in the following text.

1. *Standard 1: Rooting out age discrimination* – 'NHS services will be provided, regardless of age, on the basis of clinical need alone'.

2. *Standard 2: Person-centred care* – 'NHS and social care services treat older people as individuals and enable them to make choices about their own care'.

3. *Standard 8: The promotion of health and active life in older age* – 'The health and well-being of older people is promoted through a co-ordinated programme of action…'.

An example of overt age discrimination found during work for standard 1 was a national guideline restricting conscious sedation for outpatient dental procedures to those under 70 years of age. It is perfectly true that certain co-morbidities in older patients put them at increased risk of harm from sedation: it may cause respiratory suppression in patients with chronic lung disease, confusion in those with underlying chronic brain conditions or falls in those with postural instability. However, it is not appropriate to introduce a blanket ban on sedation for all patients over 70 years of age. Each case should be considered on its own merits, and provision should be made for inpatient treatment where sedation is warranted but increased risk is anticipated.

Covert age discrimination is also common, and takes three main forms.

- Health professionals may wrongly assume that an older person has a short life expectancy and therefore has limited capacity to benefit from certain interventions. The average life expectancy of an 80-year-old is 8–9 years.
- Services required by older people may be underprovided, and have long waiting lists. The problem may be compounded if younger patients jump the queue. This was once seen in the case of cataract surgery, where some ophthalmic surgeons prioritised patients of working age with driving licences, and assumed that older patients with equivalent or worse impairments of vision could sit uncomplainingly on their waiting lists.
- Services may be inconvenient or inaccessible to frail or disabled people who require assistance and transport. They may not know who to ask or how to seek the help required.

Furthermore, inappropriate staff attitudes to older people – for example, impatience, patronising language or dismissive behaviour – may rob older patients of the dignity and respect they deserve.

A key requirement for standard 2, relevant to dental health care, is the need to provide information to older people in a way that they can understand. For the cognitively impaired, this may involve patient and careful explanation in simple language. For the visually impaired, information leaflets should be made available in large print. Special effort is also needed to communicate effectively with hearing-impaired older people. When care is taken, the majority of older people can make appropriate choices themselves and give valid consent. Where this is not possible, it is the doctors' duty to act in the patients' best interests and involve their relatives and carers in the decision-making process.

Standard 8 should include dental health promotion, including screening programmes, routine checks and preventive treatment.

Mental capacity

In England and Wales, the Mental Capacity Act governs how we should approach decision-making in people with 'an impairment of mind or brain', such as dementia. This includes consent or refusal for treatment. The basic principle is that people should have autonomy to make their own decisions, even if these may seem unwise – for example, a Jehovah's Witnesses follower refusing a blood transfusion. If the patient has mental impairment, information relevant to the decision should be presented in a way that they can understand, and their ability to use this information is judged by four steps:

- Can they understand the information?
- Can they retain it long enough to use it to make a decision?
- Can they weigh up the information to come to a decision?
- Can they communicate that decision?

Note that the capacity assessment is specific to that decision and that point of time: mental function can fluctuate, and may be sufficient for some decisions and insufficient for others. Also, a person with dementia who subsequently forgets the discussion may still have the capacity to make the decision at the time, but does also have the right to change his or her mind. Where capacity is lacking, a 'best interests' decision must be made on behalf of the patient by the professionals, in discussion with a relative or friend who knows the patient. If such a person is lacking, and the patient is 'unbefriended', then an 'independent mental capacity advocate' is engaged to act on behalf of the patient if there are important or far-reaching decisions to be made.

Prescribing for older dental patients

Because older people are possibly already taking multiple medications, there is increased likelihood of drug interactions. Their impaired homeostasis and multiple comorbidity put them at increased risk of unwanted effects. It is therefore essential to take a full treatment history and document a patient's known medical conditions before prescribing.

Altered pharmacokinetics often result in increased sensitivity of older people to drug actions. Renal function deteriorates with age, even in the absence of known renal disease, resulting in reduced drug excretion. Liver function also declines, slowing elimination of hepatically metabolised drugs. Low serum albumin in chronic ill health may increase free concentrations of protein-bound drugs. Absorption of drugs is often relatively normal, so the result of these changes is that older people often need lower doses, particularly of drugs with a narrow therapeutic window.

Of the medications listed in the 'Dental Practitioners' Formulary' section of the *British National Formulary*, most antibiotics can be prescribed at the standard doses. Many older patients take iron or calcium preparations, which can impair the absorption of tetracyclines. NSAIDs should be used with caution, particularly in patients with dyspepsia; renal disease; or heart disease requiring treatment with ACE inhibitors. Older patients are particularly prone to side effects from drugs acting on the CNS, which can cause confusion, drowsiness and falls. This is especially true of benzodiazepines and other sedatives such as promethazine, but can also be a problem with opioid analgesics, including pethidine.

Difficulty in dealing with multiple medications in the context of impaired vision, mental function or dexterity results in poor compliance. It is therefore important to consider some means of enabling patients to take their medications correctly. Careful explanation of the reason for prescribing the drug should be given, including whether it is to be taken as prescribed or 'as required'. It is useful to write down the main points, and to explain them to a relative or carer. The print on bottle labels may be invisible to the visually impaired patient, and child-proof containers should be avoided, since considerable grip strength and manual dexterity may be needed to open them.

Other means of enhancing compliance include supervision by a carer and the use of dosing boxes. These contain the medications set out in compartments labelled with the time and the day of the week. They can be set up by a relative or, commonly, by the community pharmacist. If the patient already uses one of these, and an additional prescription is needed, then liaising with the pharmacist or carer is necessary to ensure correct administration.

Practical tips on prescribing

- Never prescribe without knowing the patient's current treatment regimen and medical conditions.
- Use lower doses, particularly of drugs affecting the CNS.
- Consider the practicalities of compliance, and take steps to overcome any barriers.
- Further advice on prescribing in older people is given in the *British National Formulary*.

FURTHER READING

BMA mental capacity assessment toolkit. Available from: http://www.bma.org.uk/support-at-work/ ethics/mental-capacity/mental-capacity-tool-kit.

BDA evidence summary: access to dental care for frail elderly people. Available from: https://www.bda.org/dentists/ education/sgh/Documents/Access%20to%20dental%20 care%20for%20frail%20elderly%20people%20V2.pdf.

MULTIPLE CHOICE QUESTIONS

1. Which of the following is not a feature of natural ageing?
   a) Increased probability of death.
   b) Reduced functional capacity.
   c) Impaired homeostasis.
   d) Increased cell division.
   e) Increased susceptibility to disease.
   Answer = D

2. Which of the following is one of the 'giants of geriatrics'?
   a) Iatrogenic illness.
   b) Isolation.
   c) Instability.
   d) Impotence.
   e) Irritability.
   Answer = C

3. Which of the following is necessary to be considered as having the mental capacity to make a decision, such as consent or choice of medical treatment?
   a) Clear hearing.
   b) Ability to weigh information.
   c) Ability to remember the decision later.
   d) Clear speech.
   e) No impairment of mind or brain.
   Answer = B

4. Drug compliance in older patients is not affected by:
   a) Dementia.
   b) Lack of dexterity.
   c) Polypharmacy.
   d) Reduced drug absorption.
   e) Poor vision.
   Answer = D

5. Which of these is unlikely to cause visual impairment in older people?
   a) Cataracts.
   b) Background diabetic retinopathy.
   c) Glaucoma.
   d) Macular degeneration.
   e) Strokes.
   Answer = B

CHAPTER 19
Psychiatric disorders

SJ Brown, M Greenwood and JG Meechan

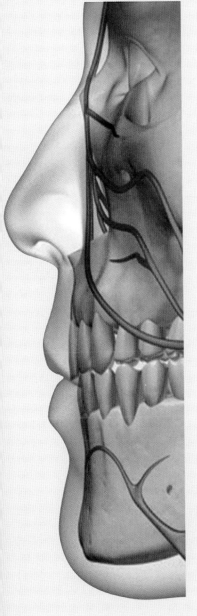

Key topics

- Common psychiatric disorders.
- Capacity and consent.
- Drug abuse.
- Anxiolytic and hypnotic drugs.

Learning objectives

- To be familiar with the more common psychiatric disorders and how they may impact on the provision of dental care.
- To be familiar with the concept of drug abuse and its potential implications.

Essentials of Human Disease in Dentistry, Second Edition. Mark Greenwood.
© 2018 John Wiley & Sons Ltd. Published 2018 by John Wiley & Sons Ltd.
Companion website: www.wiley.com/go/greenwood/human-disease-in-dentistry

19A GENERAL PSYCHIATRY

Introduction – what is psychiatry?

Psychiatry: Origin from the Greek words *psukhe* (meaning 'soul' or 'mind') and *iatreia* (meaning 'healing').

Psychiatry is the medical specialty concerned with the assessment, diagnosis and treatment of mental illness and related disorders.

Mental illness is common, affecting up to one in four people in the UK at some point in their lives. However, psychiatrists see only the tip of the iceberg, with many presenting to other medical and paramedical specialties, remaining in primary care, or seeking no help at all.

It is therefore extremely helpful for all healthcare workers to have some understanding of the basic concepts of psychiatry, and the nature of psychiatric disorders.

Relevance to dental practitioners

Dentists see patients from all ages, cultures and backgrounds, and may see them in a range of settings. A degree of dental anxiety appears to be present in the general public, and this can sometimes interfere with management.

There is also a range of psychiatric conditions that could cause problems in a consultation. These can be avoided if the dentist has an understanding of the most common psychiatric conditions, and how they may present.

Along with doctors and lawyers, dentists are recognised to be a group of professionals at a high risk of mental health problems, including drug and alcohol misuse and suicide. For dentists to recognise and understand problems in themselves or their colleagues is just as important as recognising and understanding it in their patients.

The nature and diagnosis of psychiatric disorders

Psychiatry can seem a confusing specialty – how do we define the conditions treated, and how are they distinguished from normality? There are no diagnostic tests, so how is a diagnosis made? If the cause cannot be determined, how can treatment be planned?

There are some conditions for which diagnosis may be aided by investigations – for example, psychosis due to temporal lobe epilepsy might have the diagnosis confirmed by EEG and a relevant lesion defined on MRI. CT and MRI brain scans can aid the diagnosis of Alzheimer's and other dementias, and these can be verified pathologically at post-mortem. The majority of diagnoses, however, are syndromal – that is, based on the recognition of a characteristic cluster of symptoms and signs over a defined period of time, sometimes involving the exclusion of underlying physical conditions.

Sometimes, a psychiatric illness may in fact be caused by a physical process, such as hypothyroidism. Depression is a recognised feature of hypothyroidism, and, in the presence of other symptoms and signs of thyroid disease and abnormal thyroid function tests, a new-onset depression would be considered as part of the physical illness, and thus 'organic' in nature. It would be expected to respond to correction of the underlying endocrine abnormality. A patient with hypothyroidism could also suffer from depression when euthyroid, however, or may have had a pre-existing diagnosis of depression that deteriorated with the decline in function of the thyroid gland. The distinction between these three cases would be made on the basis of the history, in conjunction with thyroid function tests.

Since physical disorders are more reliably diagnosed, organic conditions take precedence in the diagnostic hierarchy of psychiatry.

In the absence of a demonstrable physical cause, however, it must be ensured that syndromal diagnoses are reliable and reproducible. To ensure this, international classification guidelines and schedules have been developed, of which two are in common usage. These are:

- *International Classification of Diseases (ICD-10)*: World Health Organization (1992).
- *Diagnostic and Statistical Manual of Mental Disorders (DSM-IV)*: American Psychiatric Association (1994). Now revised to DSM-5.

ICD-10 was designed for use internationally, and is generally preferred in the UK; DSM-5 was developed in the USA. Both systems share predominantly common ground, but have some differences. ICD-10 is an aetiological classification with a single axis (see Table 19A.1); DSM-IV is multi-axial, taking account of psychiatric illness, personality, physical illness, psychosocial stressors and level of functioning. In DSM 2015, the number of axes in DSM-IV was reduced, by combining some of the subtypes into single categories, or axes.

Psychiatric presentations encountered by dentists

As one in four people will experience mental ill-health during their lifetimes, dentists will invariably come across this in both professional and personal spheres. This could occur in the form of one of the following scenarios:

- The underlying psychiatric condition (e.g. anxiety disorder) is exacerbated by the visit to the dentist.
- A psychiatric illness (e.g. psychogenic pain, eating disorders or substance abuse) may be detected by the dentist.
- A patient may have a psychiatric illness, which may or may not be directly related to the dental presentation.
- The dentists themselves, or someone they know personally, may be affected by a mental illness.

Table 19A.1 Diagnostic categories from ICD-10 Chapter V (titled 'Mental and behavioural disorders').

Category	Example
Organic mental disorders	Dementia Delirium Organic mood disorders (e.g. depression due to hypothyroidism)
Psychoactive substance use	Acute intoxication Dependence syndromes Withdrawal states
Schizophrenia, schizotypal and delusional disorders	Schizophrenia Persistent delusional disorders Schizoaffective disorder
Mood disorders	Bipolar affective disorder (manic depression) Recurrent depressive disorder Dysthymia
Neurotic, stress-related and somatoform disorders	Specific phobias (e.g. dental phobia) Obsessive compulsive disorder Hypochondriasis Atypical facial pain
Behavioural syndromes associated with physiological disturbances and physical factors	Anorexia nervosa Bulimia nervosa
Disorders of adult personality and behaviour	Dissocial personality disorder Histrionic personality disorder
Mental retardation (learning disability)	Down syndrome Fragile X syndrome
Disorders of psychological development	Autism Dyslexia
Behavioural and emotional disorders with onset usually occurring in childhood and adolescence	Hyperkinetic disorder Tic disorder

An overview of commonly encountered psychiatric presentations follows, with a summary of other relevant psychiatric conditions, including special mention of children, the elderly and people with learning disabilities.

Anxiety disorders

Anxiety is a normal experience in response to a perceived threat or danger. A degree of anxiety is adaptive, and can be useful as it serves to mobilise energy reserves for action and enhances performance by increasing arousal (see Figure 19A.1).

When anxiety becomes too intense, frequent or persistent, and, as a consequence, interferes with a person's general ability to function, it becomes a problem. It is then said to be 'pathological', and part of an anxiety disorder.

Some people are naturally more anxious than others, and can be said to have a high level of 'trait' anxiety, but certain circumstances will induce a 'state' of anxiety in all of us.

Anxiety symptoms can be divided into *physical* (due to motor tension and autonomic hyperactivity) and *psychological* (see Table 19A.2).

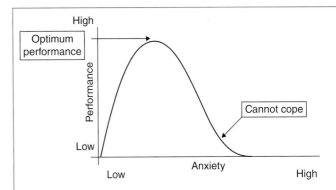

Figure 19A.1 The relationship between anxiety and performance.

From a psychiatric point of view, there are several different subtypes of the anxiety disorder. These share many common features, but vary according to the intensity and frequency of symptoms and the situations in which they occur.

ICD-10 groups anxiety disorders under the heading of 'neuroses, stress related and somatoform disorders'. Anxiety is

Table 19A.2 Symptoms of anxiety.

Psychological	Physical
Worry	*Gastrointestinal*
Sense of dread	Dry mouth
Irritability	Nausea
Poor concentration	Swallowing difficulties
Restlessness	Disturbance of bowel habit
	Cardiovascular/respiratory
	Shortness of breath
	Chest pain
	Palpitations/tachycardia
	Neuromuscular
	Headache
	Light-headedness
	Weakness
	'Jelly legs' tremor
	Muscle aches
	Other
	Sweating

Table 19A.3 Dental anxiety – typical patient characteristics.

Young adult
Female
Previous traumatic dental experience

Table 19A.4 ICD-10 diagnostic categories for anxiety relevant to dentistry.

Generalised anxiety disorder
Panic attacks
Phobias
Obsessive compulsive disorder (OCD)
Dissociative or conversion disorders of movement and sensation
Somatoform disorder
Somatisation disorder
Hypochondriasis

probably the psychiatric symptom most likely to be evident in a dental consultation, and relevant conditions will be discussed in more detail in the text that follows.

Dental anxiety – anxiety related to visiting the dentist

Some estimates suggest that up to 90% of people experience significant levels of anxiety prior to visiting the dentist, with 40% of adults delaying visits because of anxiety. People with dental anxiety tend to be naturally more anxious individuals, although they may be experiencing dental anxiety as part of a generalised anxiety disorder. People with dental anxiety tend to be younger adults, and are more likely to be female (see Table 19A.3). Perhaps understandably, it has been reported that, in early-onset dental anxiety, a previous traumatic dental experience is a major causative factor.

Anticipatory anxiety is common and may be so severe as to prevent attendance at the dentist, with 5% of people avoiding dental appointments completely because of anxiety. This may be a true dental phobia (termed 'odontophobia'), and there may be panic attacks in severe cases.

Although dental anxiety is common (Table 19A.4), it does not usually cause significant disruption to other areas of daily life, and thus does not commonly present to the psychiatrist; indeed, the dentist may rarely see this group of people if their avoidance is great enough.

Dental phobia

A *phobia* is a fear or anxiety that is out of proportion to the stimulus, and which cannot be reasoned away. The fear occurs only in specific circumstances and usually in response to a specific stimulus, which can be used to designate the type of phobia – for example, spider phobia (termed 'arachnophobia'). Anticipatory anxiety and avoidance of the feared stimulus or situation is typical.

In psychiatric practice, phobic anxiety disorders are divided into three main syndromes – *simple phobia* (fear of a specific thing), *social phobia* (fear of social situations) and *agoraphobia* (a complex phobia frequently associated with panic).

Dental phobia (odontophobia) is a simple phobia and, although common, it is not usually encountered in psychiatric practice.

Anxiety and avoidance

Avoidance of the feared stimulus or situation is one of the central features of a phobic disorder, and indeed of all anxiety disorders. It is understandable that we might wish to avoid situations that make us anxious. In the case of a phobic disorder, it is the phobic stimulus that is avoided, although generalisation to related situations is common; thus, the spider phobic will avoid spiders, but their fear may generalise, leading to the avoidance of places where spiders may be encountered. A severe dental phobic may avoid visiting the dentist, even when suffering from advanced and painful conditions, and may broaden avoidance to include hospitals and other similar places.

Avoidance results in a reduction of anxiety, but the relief experienced is transient, resurfacing again when confronted with the phobic stimulus or situation, or merely the anticipation of it. Unfortunately, the relief experienced serves to reinforce this pattern of avoidance, increasing the likelihood of anxiety being experienced in similar situations in the future. Further avoidance behaviour becomes more likely, and the range of situations avoided may broaden.

Management of dental anxiety

As with many conditions, prevention is better than cure. Management should thus be aimed at preventing the condition developing. Generally speaking, the likelihood of attendance at the dentist is not determined by the degree of anxiety experienced during the appointment, but by the degree of anticipatory anxiety prior to it.

Thinking of anxiety as a conditioned response (see Figure 19A.2), a traumatic experience while visiting the dentist is likely to result in a greater degree of anticipatory anxiety prior to the next visit, thus reducing the likelihood of future attendance.

Pre-existing dental anxiety can be managed using various measures, ranging from simple modification of the environment and clinical approach to more complex psychological techniques. Occasionally, medication may be necessary to alleviate anxiety symptoms.

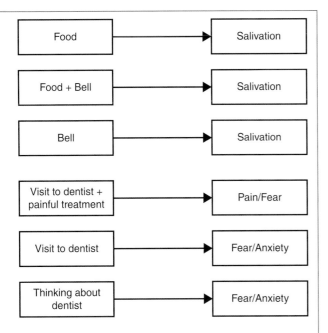

Figure 19A.2 Classical 'Pavlovian' conditioning, in which the repeated association of a bell with food leads to a salivation response to the bell alone. In a clinical situation, the pairing of an aversive stimulus (pain) with an otherwise innocuous experience (visit to a dentist or other health professional) leads to an association of that environment with pain.

Preventative measures

- Dental health education.
- Relaxed, welcoming atmosphere (lighting, pictures, music, etc.)
- Calm, sympathetic, paced approach.
- Honest, tactful and appropriate explanation of procedures.
- Confident and professional manner.

Treatment

- Education regarding anxiety (for patient and dentist!).
- Relaxation techniques/tapes aimed at teaching the subject how to relax.
- Desensitisation (graded exposure to the feared stimulus).
- Medication – anxiolytics such as midazolam may be necessary to facilitate essential dental treatment. Use should be restricted due to potential for dependency.
- Alternative therapies such as hypnosis or homeopathic remedies may also alleviate anxiety in some individuals.

Obsessive compulsive disorder (OCD)

Obsessions are recurrent, intrusive and distressing thoughts, impulses or images. The patient recognises them as coming from his or her own mind, but regards them as absurd or unpleasant, and tries to suppress or ignore them.

Compulsions are the motor responses to obsessions, and they typically take the form of ritualised and often stereotyped patterns of behaviour, such as repeated checking, handwashing or reciting lists or prayers. Patients typically try to resist carrying out the compulsive behaviours, but completion of the behaviour reduces the anxiety associated with the obsessional thought. The sense of relief associated with this reduction in anxiety acts as a powerful reinforcer, making the compulsive behaviour more likely to be carried out the next time the obsessional thought occurs.

Obsessions and compulsions are the primary features of OCD, although they can also be symptoms of other conditions, such as depression.

A typical example of an obsessional thought is the recurrent idea that one's hands are dirty. This often results in repetitive hand washing that can become so severe that patients have been known to scrub their hands in bleach for hours at a time, until the skin is raw and bleeding.

Occasionally, patients will present with obsessional ideas regarding their health, including oral and dental hygiene. This can be difficult to distinguish from hypochondriasis, which is discussed in the following text.

Management of OCD

OCD is less common than other anxiety disorders, but the symptoms are frequently disabling and usually require treatment within psychiatric services. Obsessional thoughts often respond to treatment with antidepressants; and compulsions respond to behavioural therapy. Often, a combination of psychological and pharmacological approaches is required.

Hypochondriasis

Hypochondria is one of the oldest concepts in medicine, originally describing disorders thought to arise from disease of the organs lying in the hypochondrium – that is, beneath the lower ribs.

In current usage, the term describes an abnormal preoccupation with one's state of health or bodily functions. Patients are typically convinced of the presence of an underlying disease, despite the absence of physical signs or positive investigations, and multiple minor symptoms may be presented as evidence. This is in contrast to somatisation disorders (psychogenic pain, see the text that follows), in which the focus is on the symptoms themselves, rather than on the underlying disease.

Although people presenting with hypochondriacal states may be suffering purely from hypochondriasis, it is important to remember that they often have another underlying mental disorder (e.g. depression, anxiety disorder or personality disorder). Hypochondriasis is somewhat more common in the lower socioeconomic classes, and can be a frequent cause of attendance at general medical clinics.

Hypochondriacal ideas regarding the head and neck are common. Patients may present with ideas that they have a specific illness (e.g. cancer) or with a single symptom such as pain, which they present as evidence of illness. Hypochondriasis can present at any age, although the development of these symptoms for the first time in middle or later life would increase the possibility of an underlying depressive or organic disorder.

Sufferers tend to observe and interpret normal bodily experiences in an abnormal manner, with a hypersensitivity to otherwise normal bodily sensations (e.g. noticing a dry mouth and interpreting this as indicating the presence of kidney failure).

Management of hypochondriasis

It is often very difficult to persuade people that their symptoms might have a psychological component. Such suggestions are frequently met with hostility from patients, who feel that appropriate care is not being offered, and they may choose to visit other practitioners, seeking further opinions on their conditions.

The foundation of good management is therefore in establishing a reliable diagnosis, although it is unlikely that this diagnosis will be made at the first contact.

As people present with physical rather than psychological complaints, their symptoms must be taken seriously, and physical examination and investigations should be undertaken to exclude physical disease. A degree of caution is advised, however, as inappropriate investigations conducted at the patient's request are often inadvisable, since they may merely reinforce the patient's idea that he or she is physically ill.

If hypochondriasis is suspected, it is advisable to seek psychiatric help from an early stage, as the nature of the condition is such that prolonged investigations and repeated assessments reinforce the patient's illness beliefs, and may in fact exacerbate the condition. Hypochondriasis can be difficult to treat, but treatment aims to address any underlying disorder, and may include pharmacological as well as behavioural and psychological measures. Cognitive behavioural therapy (CBT) has been shown to be useful.

Treatment outcome is better in those with an underlying, treatable psychiatric disorder such as depression or anxiety, and in those whom the symptoms are of most recent onset. Chronic cases have a poor prognosis, and management options may be limited to minimising any harm that might inadvertently be caused as a result of unnecessary investigations.

Psychogenic pain

Psychogenic pain is pain in which the cause is psychological rather than physical, although this may not be evident to the patient. It can be thought of as a physical manifestation of unarticulated psychological distress (Table 19A.5). For the sufferer, however, the perception and sensation of pain is very real, may be severe and excruciating, and should not be dismissed.

Many medical practitioners imagine that pain of psychological origin is likely to be bizarre in character and unlike the 'real' pain of identifiable organic origin. Unfortunately, this view is inaccurate, and may be unhelpful.

A psychological origin may, however, be suggested by the presence of certain characteristics. While these may arouse suspicion, diagnosis requires clear evidence of a psychological cause in conjunction with exclusion of any underlying organic process.

Perhaps up to 50% of psychogenic pain is experienced as occurring in the head, and as such it is highly pertinent to the practice of dentistry. Psychogenic pain syndromes present four to five times more commonly in females, and typically present in middle age, often postmenopausally.

Management of psychogenic pain – general principles

Correct diagnosis is very important. It should follow appropriate investigation, and be based on the absence of organic pathology in the presence of evidence of a possible psychological cause. It may take some time to establish this diagnosis.

Table 19A.5 Features suggestive of psychogenic pain.

Inconsistency with known anatomical landmarks/nerve distribution
Bilateral
Continuous with little fluctuation
May prevent from falling asleep, but does not wake up the patient
History of repeated negative investigations
Analgesia has a very limited effect
Association with emotional factors
Nature of the pain may have a symbolic significance for the patient

Table 19A.6 Dental psychogenic pain syndromes.
Atypical facial pain
Temporomandibular joint (TMJ) dysfunction syndrome (facial arthromyalgia)
Atypical odontalgia
Oral dysaesthesia

Once the diagnosis has been made, the underlying psychiatric conditions should be treated appropriately. Anxiety and depression are recognised causes of psychogenic pain, but it is important to be aware that both may actually be secondary to chronic pain.

There are at least four pain syndromes pertinent to dentistry that may have a significant psychological component. They may present as distinct syndromes or coexist in the same patient (Table 19A.6).

Atypical facial pain

Atypical facial pain is a syndrome of often poorly localised pain, which is typically described vaguely as a deep, dull ache, and does not fit a classical anatomical distribution. The exact nature of the psychological component of this disorder is unclear, but it is commonly associated with other recurrent symptoms such as back ache and features of depression.

Atypical facial pain is best treated according to the general principles of psychogenic pain management, outlined in the preceding text. There is evidence that antidepressant medication can be effective, particularly tricyclic antidepressants (TCAs). TCAs such as amitriptyline should be used with caution, however, owing to the high incidence of side effects and toxicity in overdose. Newer, selective serotonin reuptake inhibitor (SSRI) antidepressants may also be useful, particularly if there is an underlying depressive illness. Also, there is an increasing body of evidence for the effectiveness of CBT in the management of chronic pain syndromes.

TMJ dysfunction syndrome

TMJ dysfunction syndrome is a heterogeneous syndrome that may be the final common pathway for several other conditions. It presents most commonly in young female adults. Frequently reported symptoms include prolonged dull ache in the muscles of mastication, with associated tenderness, earache and/or TMJ pain. It may be bilateral or unilateral, and can be associated with joint 'sticking'/clicking/popping, trismus, bruxism and tinnitus. There would appear to be a subgroup of people with significant psychological disorders, typically anxiety or depression, which may sometimes precede the onset of the pain by 6 months or more.

Management is similar to that for atypical facial pain, and depends on the relative balance of psychological and physical components.

Atypical odontalgia

Atypical odontalgia may be considered as the dental variant of atypical facial pain. The pain may be aching, burning or throbbing, and tends to affect the molar and premolar teeth, the jaw, and the maxilla (more often than the mandible).

A proportion of such cases may be attributed to deafferentation and may be neuropathic, but many are felt to be idiopathic and unrelated to dental procedures or trauma.

Depression is commonly associated with this condition, and may be detected in up to two-thirds of patients, but may be as much a cause as a consequence. Patients are also more likely to be female, especially in their fifth decade, and are more likely to have abnormal personality traits or personality disorders.

This condition is treated according to the general principles for psychogenic pain outlined earlier. The majority of patients will respond to antidepressant medication.

Oral dysaesthesia

Patients with this condition present with abnormal and distressing oral sensations. Presentations include glossodynia (painful tongue) and glossopyrosis (burning tongue), and may include a metallic taste in the mouth. Unlike organic conditions, symptoms may be relieved by eating. Depression and anxiety may also be present.

As some of these symptoms can be associated with physical problems such as iron deficiency, routine investigations should be undertaken. In the absence of such treatable causes, education and reassurance may suffice. If present, depression and anxiety may require treatment independently.

Eating disorders

There are two main types of eating disorders: anorexia nervosa and bulimia nervosa. These are thought to be subgroups of a larger group of eating disorders with varied presentations and associated degrees of disability. These are referred to as 'eating disorders not otherwise specified' (EDNOS), and may share many of the diagnostic features of anorexia nervosa and bulimia nervosa (see Figure 19A.3). A single eating disorder may present in different ways in the course of time and meet different diagnostic criteria as it evolves.

Anorexia nervosa

Anorexia nervosa is characterised by a refusal to maintain body weight at or above a minimal weight appropriate to one's age and height. Weight loss is deliberate and may be sustained, with some patients becoming severely emaciated. There is an intense fear of becoming fat, and patients have a distorted body image, feeling and perceiving themselves to be fat even when others see them as clearly underweight. Food intake is restricted, and laxatives, diuretics and other purgatives may be abused in their attempts to lose weight. Excessive exercise may be seen, and other 'slimming' drugs may be misused.

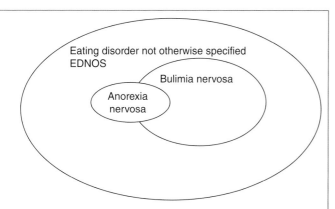

Figure 19A.3 The relationship between anorexia nervosa, bulimia nervosa and EDNOS.

Table 19A.7 A comparison of anorexia nervosa and bulimia nervosa.

Anorexia nervosa	Bulimia nervosa
Body weight maintained 15% below that expected/BMI <17.5	Weight tends to be within normal range
Weight loss by avoidance of 'fattening' foods	Recurrent episodes of binge eating with a sense of loss of control
Body image distortion with dread of fatness	Recurrent compensatory behaviours to counteract the fattening effect of food
Endocrine disorder with amenorrhoea in women, and loss of potency or sexual interest in men	Morbid fear of fatness, but without distorted body image
Puberty may be delayed or arrested	

In women, amenorrhoea is a cardinal diagnostic feature of anorexia nervosa and forms part of a broader endocrine disorder involving the hypothalamic–pituitary–gonadal axis. Men may experience loss of potency and libido.

Anorexia nervosa most commonly affects young women (up to 95% of cases), but the number of cases in young men is rising. The age of onset is typically in adolescence or early adulthood. It is more common in the higher socioeconomic classes. Patients are often described pre-morbidly as 'model children', and may be subject to high parental expectations.

However, the aetiology is complex and often multifactorial. Use of extremely thin models in fashion magazines is thought to contribute to this problem. Also, the culture of thinness among celebrities seems to create a perilous model of perfection to which young people aspire.

Anorexia nervosa can result in significant physical and psychological complications. Depression is common in this group of patients, and may be a direct consequence of malnutrition. Suicide can be a significant risk. The level of emaciation and dehydration may threaten life, and the mortality rate may be as high as 15%. Physical findings include oedema, lanugo hair (soft, downy hair on face and body), hypothermia, dehydration, bradycardia, muscle wasting and anaemia. Patients can develop profound electrolyte disturbances, including calcium and fluoride deficiency. Vitamin and mineral deficiencies can result in poor oral health and dental complications.

Management of anorexia nervosa

Patients with anorexia nervosa require referral to specialist psychiatric services. Subsequent assessment involves identification and exclusion of associated psychiatric and physical illnesses, and an evaluation of family relationships.

The goals of treatment include:
- *Restoration of adequate nutrition.* This may be urgent and require hospital admission, but is usually best managed in the community. Firm measures are occasionally needed, since patients may secretly dispose of food or induce vomiting. Nasogastric feeding is sometimes required, and, in

extreme cases, this can be done against a patient's wishes under the Mental Health Act (1983).
- *Treatment of complications.* Physical complications may require urgent hospital treatment and close monitoring while restoring the state of health. Anxiety and depression may require pharmacological interventions, which may not be safe to consider until physical health is sufficiently improved.
- *Resolution of underlying psychological issues.* Intervention is only really possible once a satisfactory weight has been achieved, and physical health stabilised. Supportive psychotherapy and family therapy are often required, and cognitive therapy has an increasing role.

Bulimia nervosa

Bulimia nervosa is characterised by recurrent binge eating (Table 19A.7). During an episode of binge eating, large quantities of high-calorie foods are eaten in a short space of time. Episodes are accompanied by a sense of lack of control, and may be followed by compensatory behaviours to avoid weight gain, such as self-induced vomiting, laxative abuse or vigorous exercise. Although the binge itself may be a pleasurable experience, patients often feel guilty afterwards. Patients tend to be preoccupied with thoughts of food and body weight, but their weight is generally within normal limits. The distortion of body image that is seen in anorexia nervosa is not present.

Bulimia nervosa is more common in women, and usually begins in late adolescence or early adult life. It tends to follow a chronic, intermittent course, and depressive symptoms may be more prominent than in anorexia nervosa.

Complications are largely due to repeated vomiting and include:
- Electrolyte imbalance – particularly potassium depletion, which can lead to cardiac arrhythmias.

- Dehydration.
- Parotid gland swelling.
- Erosion of dental enamel – may have characteristic pitting.
- Calluses on the dorsal surface of fore/middle fingers (from induced vomiting; Russell's sign).
- Depression (with/without suicidal ideation).
- Acute gastric dilatation – rare but life-threatening consequence of binge eating.

Management of bulimia nervosa

Treatment is usually conducted as an outpatient, focusing on the use of food and behaviour diaries.

There is an increasing evidence base for psychological treatments, particularly CBT. Specific programmes of CBT aim to educate and normalise eating habits, and to modify concerns about shape and weight, as well as emotional and environmental triggers for binge eating.

Other therapies include interpersonal therapy (IPT), a short-term, structured form of psychotherapy that focuses on interpersonal relationships, and is primarily used to manage depression, as well as various CBT-based, guided self-help techniques.

Antidepressant medication may be useful to treat any underlying depression, but may also independently reduce the frequency of binge eating.

The current NICE guidelines for eating disorders also recommend regular dental reviews when vomiting is a prominent feature.

The prognosis of eating disorders depends on many factors, including age of onset and duration of symptoms. Hence, early detection is desirable. In anorexia nervosa, around one-fifth of patients recover completely, and one-fifth remain ill, with the remainder tending towards a chronic, fluctuating pattern.

In bulimia nervosa, the outlook is generally better, with two-thirds making substantial improvements. Unfortunately, the nature of the illness makes it likely that symptoms have been present for a long time before they come to the attention of health professionals, making treatment more challenging and reducing the likelihood of a full recovery.

Substance misuse

It is not only the patients who are at risk of substance misuse. Drug and alcohol problems are high among medical and dental professionals. It is therefore advisable for dentists to remember that both themselves and their colleagues are also at risk. It is important to be alert to the signs of problematic substance use that, if left untreated, can be devastating on personal, social and professional levels.

Alcohol abuse

Alcohol abuse should be suspected if a patient smells of alcohol or has a tremor, which could be due to withdrawal. Attention should be paid to the time of day, as many alcohol-dependent patients drink early in the morning to overcome withdrawal

phenomena. The CAGE questionnaire is a simple and useful screening tool to detect alcohol dependency. Patients scoring 2 or more are highly likely to have alcohol problems, but a negative CAGE response does not rule out alcohol misuse.

The CAGE questionnaire

C: Have you ever felt you should *C*ut down the amount you drink?
A: Are you *A*nnoyed if people comment on the amount you are drinking?
G: Do you ever feel *G*uilty about the amount you are drinking?
E: Have you ever had a drink early in the morning as an '*E*ye-opener'?

The amount of alcohol contained in most common drinks is shown in Table 19A.8, with current guidelines for safe drinking shown in Box 19A.1.

The effects of alcohol on the oral structures and the practice of dentistry are discussed in Chapter 19B (titled 'Drug abuse').

Management of drug and alcohol misuse

Prevention is undoubtedly better than cure, and education and availability of information are key to this.

Most drug and alcohol programmes offer a combination of psychological and pharmacological approaches in a community setting. They typically take a motivational approach to move people through the 'stages of change' model with adjunctive prescribing of appropriate medication to support withdrawal, abstinence or safe use. This may occur in a variety of settings, most usually in the community, but inpatient management may occasionally be necessary. Principles of treatment include:

- Prevention.
- Education.
- Withdrawal (with/without detoxification).
- Maintenance therapy when withdrawal is not possible.
- Harm reduction or minimisation.
- Psychological treatments.
- Rehabilitation.

Table 19A.8 Number of units of alcohol in common drinks.

A pint of ordinary strength lager – 2 units
A pint of strong lager – 3 units
A pint of ordinary bitter – 2 units
A pint of best bitter – 3 units
A pint of ordinary strength cider – 2 units
A pint of strong cider – 3 units
A 175 ml glass of red or white wine – around 2 units
A pub measure of spirits – 1 unit
An alcopop – around 1.5 units

Box 19A.1 Safe drinking levels (UK guidelines)

The UK limit for legal driving is 80 mg/100 ml.

The Department of Health recommends that adult males should drink no more than 3 units of alcohol a day (21 units per week); adult females should drink no more than 2 units of alcohol a day (14 units per week); and women who are pregnant or trying to conceive should consume no alcohol at all, because of risks to the foetus.

Schizophrenia

Schizophrenia is a serious psychiatric condition with a lifetime risk of approximately 1%. The age of onset is usually early/middle adulthood, although early- and late-onset cases are not uncommon. Men and women are affected in equal numbers.

Schizophrenia is a heterogeneous disorder, the precise definition of which is still under debate. The term 'schizophrenia' was proposed by Eugen Bleuler to describe the 'splitting' of psychic functions, which he felt to be of fundamental importance, in contrast to previous descriptions of the condition as a form of dementia. It does not mean 'split personality' in a 'Jekyll and Hyde' sense, although the term is frequently misused in this way.

The presentation of schizophrenia is highly variable. Core features include abnormal, often bizarre, thoughts and experiences. These may be associated with, or may progress to, a reduction in drive and social function, and an alteration in emotion.

Typically, there is an acute syndrome in which florid psychotic symptoms (delusions and hallucinations) are present. This may relapse and remit, or progress into a more chronic syndrome of social impairment. Occasionally, there is a more insidious presentation, with a chronic deterioration in function without psychotic symptoms ever developing.

Symptoms may be categorised in several different ways, but are generally described as 'positive' (a presence of abnormal thoughts and experiences) and 'negative' (an absence of drive, emotion, social interaction and activity). Positive symptoms are more common in acute presentations, and negative symptoms predominate in chronic presentations. Both may be present at different times.

Positive symptoms of schizophrenia

Delusions

These are false beliefs that are fixed and not amenable to reason, and are out of keeping with the person's social, cultural and educational backgrounds. In schizophrenia, delusions are often of being persecuted, or that one's thoughts and actions are being controlled by someone else. The delusional systems that develop may be quite bizarre.

Hallucinations

These are perceptual experiences in the absence of an external stimulus, and may occur in any sensory modality. In schizophrenia, this is most commonly auditory – that is, patients typically hearing voices discussing themselves, their thoughts or their actions.

Passivity phenomenon

This is probably a type of delusion, in which people feel they are passive bystanders in their own thoughts or actions. They may believe their thoughts and bodily movements are under the control of someone or something other than themselves.

For example, they may feel that thoughts are being inserted into their head (different from a hallucination), and that their own thoughts are being withdrawn by an outside influence or broadcast to others.

Negative symptoms of schizophrenia

Social withdrawal

This may be driven by persecutory delusions, or apathy, or be part of an increasing 'oddness' as the illness progresses.

Emotional blunting

Patients do not experience the same range of emotional experiences as before the illness. At interview, they may appear emotionally unresponsive or 'flat'.

Apathy

This is a lack of drive, motivation and volition.

Slowing

Slowing of thought and action (psychomotor retardation or bradyphrenia/bradykinesia) may occur.

Impairment of social functioning

Social interaction and work may become increasingly difficult, because of positive or negative symptoms, leading to isolation and alienation.

Management of schizophrenia

Management of all psychiatric illness aims to address physical, psychological and social aspects. Drug therapy is central to the treatment of schizophrenia.

Antipsychotics

Also known as major tranquillisers or 'neuroleptics', these drugs are used in the treatment of psychotic illnesses, bipolar disorder and, less commonly, OCD. Antipsychotic drugs are classified into 'typical' and 'atypical' agents according to their pharmacodynamic profiles, although their shared action in blocking dopamine is thought to be of paramount importance.

Most antipsychotics can cause QT prolongation on ECG and predispose to cardiac dysrhythmias. Cardioactive drugs should therefore be used with caution after checking for interactions. Antipsychotics also enhance the action of sedative drugs.

'Typical' antipsychotic drugs, such as haloperidol and chlorpromazine, are potent antagonists of dopamine receptors. They are effective in treating positive symptoms of schizophrenia, but have numerous unpleasant and dose-limiting side effects. They are available in oral form and as intramuscular slow-release 'depot' preparations for injection. Depot preparations should always be enquired about, as patients may forget that their regular injections may be of relevance to other health professionals.

Extrapyramidal side effects (EPSEs: Parkinsonism, dystonia, oculogyric crisis, bradykinesia, etc.) are common, and acute dystonic reactions do occur. Tardive dyskinesia, a serious and distressing side effect, can occur with prolonged use, particularly in elderly and female patients. Tardive dyskinesia most often affects the face, and presents with 'lip-smacking' and protrusion or rolling of the tongue. The patient may attribute this to ill-fitting dentures, and thus present to dental services.

'Atypical' antipsychotic drugs, such as olanzapine, risperidone and quetiapine, are newer and have actions on both dopaminergic and serotonergic receptors. They are as effective as typical agents in treating positive symptoms but also improve negative symptoms. Side effects include restlessness, weight gain and diabetes in some cases, particularly with olanzapine. They may still cause extrapyramidal side effects (particularly risperidone), but are less likely to do so and tend to be better tolerated.

Clozapine is the archetypal atypical antipsychotic agent and has superior efficacy to the other atypical medications, particularly in treating negative symptoms. It can cause neutropaenia in 2–5% of patients, however, and requires regular blood testing for monitoring. As such, it is reserved as a third-line agent in the UK. Patients may present to dentists with oral infections or hypersalivation.

Other treatments

Other therapies are increasingly being employed for patients with schizophrenia. Psychological approaches such as CBT can be effective in the management of delusions. Family therapy and psycho-education are also helpful. Psychodynamic psychotherapy is not effective in the treatment of psychotic symptoms.

Physical health problems, as well as housing and other social difficulties, may develop as a consequence of illness, and can exacerbate symptoms; hence, these needs should also be addressed.

Schizophrenia and the dentist

Many people with schizophrenia or other psychotic illness will not advertise this fact to the dentist, and indeed it is not always relevant. There may be clues in the medication list, but many psychiatric drugs also have other indications. A diagnosis of schizophrenia should be considered in all patients presenting with bizarre complaints (e.g. the belief that one's teeth are being dissolved by rays from the television, or that a microchip has been inserted to control them), and psychiatric advice sought or suggested.

Patients with schizophrenia may lack motivation, or may become socially withdrawn. As a consequence, they are less likely to attend to their dental health on a regular basis. In many cases, when combined with poor self-care and inadequate nutrition, dental hygiene can become problematic.

Patients taking clozapine are at increased risk of dental infections and abscesses.

Mood disorders

Mood disorders, also known as the 'affective' disorders, have disturbance of mood as their core feature. Moods can be either lowered (as in depression) or elevated (as in mania). The disturbance of mood is accompanied by alterations in energy levels and other biological processes. At their extremes of presentation, mood disorders may be accompanied by psychotic symptoms (hallucinations and delusions).

Depression

Mood may be depressed as a normal experience or in response to difficult experiences in everyday life, such as bereavement or the breakdown of an important relationship. In a depressive illness, the symptom of 'low mood' becomes part of a syndrome of depression, which is abnormal in severity and duration, in the presence of other abnormal features and significant impairment of function (Table 19A.9).

The term 'unipolar affective disorder' is used to describe recurrent depressive episodes, and to differentiate it from 'bipolar affective disorder' (or 'manic-depression'), in which episodes of elevation of mood (mania or hypomania) and depression of mood alternate.

Depressive illness is very common, affecting up to 10% of men and 20% of women at some point in their lives. More severe types of depression will affect 1–3% of the population.

Depressive illness is categorised as mild, moderate or severe, according to the number and severity of symptoms present. Psychotic symptoms are only seen in severe episodes, although they are not always present. In contrast, suicidal thoughts and actions may be seen in all degrees of severity, and can also occur in the absence of psychiatric illnesses.

Table 19A.9 Depression.

Core features of depression	Additional features
Depressed mood 　Most days 　For most of the day 　For 2 weeks or more	Diurnal variation of mood Poor appetite and weight loss Sleep disturbance Poor concentration
Lack of energy (anergia)	Psychomotor retardation or agitation
Loss of enjoyment (anhedonia)	Feelings of guilt and worthlessness
Hopelessness and suicidal ideation	
Loss of libido	
Delusions and hallucinations if severe	

Management of depression

Treatment should be holistic, aiming to address the biological, psychological and social difficulties that a patient is experiencing. Exercise, self-help, an increased level of support and psychotherapy may sometimes be sufficient to improve mild–moderate episodes of depression, but medication is often indicated.

Antidepressants

Antidepressants are effective in the treatment of depression, although it can take 2–6 weeks for their therapeutic effects to become apparent; this may be longer in the elderly. There are many different antidepressants available, in several main classes according to their mode of action.

- *SSRIs* – for example, fluoxetine, paroxetine, citalopram and sertraline – are modern antidepressants commonly prescribed in primary and secondary care. They are effective in most types of depression, and are therapeutic even at their lowest doses. Side effects include gastrointestinal upset and restlessness. Serotonin syndrome can occur at higher doses, or in combination with other serotonergic drugs (e.g. amitriptyline).
- *TCAs* – for example, amitriptyline – are older drugs with many side effects, including cardiac dysrhythmias, which make them particularly dangerous in overdose. There are also several important drug interactions, including with various anaesthetic and sympathomimetic agents, and they may potentiate the effects of sedatives. They are a useful and effective treatment for depression.
- *Monoamine oxidase inhibitors (MAOIs)* – for example, phenelzine – are not commonly used now. Their main indication is 'atypical' depression (with a tendency to increased sleep and appetite). MAOIs have numerous important drug interactions. Dietary restrictions are necessary due to their

interaction with the amino acid tyramine, which is commonly found in foods such as mature cheeses, pickled herring, broad bean pods, fermented soya bean extract and yeast extract (e.g. Bovril, Oxo, Marmite and most alcoholic or low-alcohol drinks). Tyramine-containing foods and some over-the-counter cold and flu remedies containing sympathomimetics can lead to catastrophic hypertensive reactions if taken with MAOIs. In addition, they interact with opioid analgesics, causing CNS depression or excitation, and should not be co-administered or given within 2 weeks of discontinuation.

- *Other antidepressants.* Other newer antidepressant drugs include venlafaxine and duloxetine, which act on both noradrenergic and serotonergic systems, as does mirtazapine, although via a different mechanism. These drugs tend to be reserved for third-line treatment.

Augmentation

Standard antidepressant treatment can also be augmented with several different drug treatments, as well as other non-pharmacological measures such as exercise or psychotherapy. Lithium is commonly used as an adjunct to antidepressants in treatment-resistant depression. Various combinations of antidepressant drugs and other psychoactive drugs also have augmenting properties, but should be prescribed by specialists only.

Electroconvulsive therapy (ECT)

ECT is now reserved for severe cases of psychiatric illness. It is useful in severe depression with psychosis. Contrary to popular media depiction, it is not a barbaric procedure! Carefully controlled electric current at the minimum voltage required to cause a seizure is applied to the brain, while a patient is under a short-acting general anaesthetic, given with a muscle relaxant. Each episode of treatment takes only a few minutes, and the tonic–clonic convulsions observed are usually very subtle, visible only on EEG. The main risks are from the anaesthetics, and patients may occasionally complain of some impairment of recent memory, although it can be difficult to determine whether this is due to the ECT or the illness itself.

Psychological therapies

Psychological therapies such as CBT are effective in mild–moderate depression, and in the recovery stages of severe depression. Psychodynamic psychotherapy has a growing evidence base for its use in depression (although not in the acute stages, or if psychosis is present). Social, occupational and family support measures are all useful, and exercise has also been shown to be beneficial in treating mild depression.

Dental aspects of depression

Depressive illness is often associated with hypochondriacal ideas and delusions, and may worsen pre-existing dental anxiety. In severe depression, appetite is reduced, and patients may ascribe their reluctance to eat to physical causes, such as a delusion that one's teeth are too weak to allow eating. Alcohol excess may be a cause or a consequence of depression, and can lead to numerous dental presentations. Oral hygiene may deteriorate in the presence of self-neglect.

Bipolar affective disorder (mania)

Elevated mood may also be a normal experience in response to exciting and enjoyable life events. If the change in mood is sustained and pervasive, and there are associated features that affect a person's function, then this may be deemed abnormal. Patients who experience mania (Table 19A.10) will almost invariably also suffer from episodes of depression, and are therefore said to have 'bipolar' affective disorder, or 'manic-depression' as it is also commonly known.

Bipolar affective disorder will affect approximately 1% of the population at some point in their lifetime. Men and women are equally at risk. Less severe elevation of mood is termed 'hypomania', episodes of which are less disruptive and, by definition, do not result in hospital admission.

Management of bipolar affective disorder

Mania is a very disruptive illness, with financial, social and personal consequences as a result of the uncharacteristic behaviours that may occur. Sufferers usually lack insight into their condition and the consequences of their behaviour. Hospital admission is usually required for stabilisation.

Treatment aims to reduce the severity and impact of the current episode of illness and to reduce the likelihood of further episodes. Episodes of depression in a person with bipolar affective disorder can be difficult to treat. Antidepressants may be effective, but should be combined with a mood stabiliser to prevent a possible switch to mania.

The general principles of management of acute episodes of mania are outlined here.

- *Safety* of the patient (and other people). Mania can be very damaging socially, psychologically and physically, as the patient must live with the consequences of whatever risky or extravagant behaviour he or she may have engaged in. Hospital admission is frequently necessary, and may be against the patient's will.
- *Tranquillisation* is required. Initial treatment is usually with *sedatives* and *antipsychotic* medication (even if not psychotic), which patients frequently resist, and medication may have to be administered intramuscularly.
- *Mood stabilisation* is needed. Stabilisation of mood is key to preventing relapse and further episodes of either mania or depression. There are a several drugs that can be used to achieve this. The most commonly used *atypical antipsychotics* have mood-stabilising properties, but the body of evidence and experience is greatest with *lithium* and anticonvulsants such as *sodium valproate*.

Lithium

Lithium can be effective in acute episodes as an antimanic agent. It has a narrow therapeutic window and requires regular serological monitoring, which is rarely practical in the acute phase of mania. Sodium valproate may be more easily administered and monitored.

Lithium has several side effects, and causes a characteristic syndrome of toxicity in excess. Side effects include a metallic taste in the mouth and polydipsia. Goitre, with or without overt thyroid disease, may also be seen.

Severe toxicity results in a coarse tremor, ataxia, confusion and coma, and should never be ignored. Toxicity can occur with dehydration, possibly because of a painful or protracted dental condition. Of particular note, lithium interacts with the

Table 19A.10 Features of mania.

Core features	Additional features
Elevated or irritable mood for >1 week, or resulting in hospital admission	Overactivity
Distractibility	Disinhibited behaviour (sexualised/aggressive)
Reduced need for sleep	Risk-taking behaviour, including overspending
Inflated self-esteem	
Speech rapid, loud and difficult to interrupt, often punctuated with puns and rhymes	
Racing thoughts (flight of ideas)	
Delusions (typically grandiose, but may be persecutory)	
Hallucinations	

antibacterial agent metronidazole and several anti-inflammatory drugs, all of which impair the renal excretion of lithium, increasing the risk of toxicity.

Relapse prevention and rehabilitation

Episodes of mania can be very disruptive to all aspects of a person's life, and adequate rehabilitation and support during recovery is important. Education regarding the illness and identification of 'relapse indicators' form a key part of longer-term management, and is also useful for those involved in the care and support of someone with bipolar affective disorder.

Dental aspects of bipolar affective disorder

Dentists are unlikely to experience acute episodes of mania in patients, but may see people with residual symptoms, who can appear a little disinhibited and may have difficulty in retaining the advice given, owing to poor concentration. It is more likely that they will present in a depressed state, as described in the preceding text.

Specific groups for special consideration: children

Children generally benefit from a little special consideration when they visit the dentist, but those with psychiatric difficulties may need a more understanding approach. Childhood psychiatric disorders are listed in Table 19A.11. In ICD-10, childhood psychiatric disorders are broadly divided into two groups.

- *Disorders of psychological development* (specific developmental disorders of scholastic, motor and/or speech/language skills, or pervasive developmental disorder).
- *Behavioural and emotional disorders with onset usually occurring in childhood and adolescence* (hyperkinetic, emotional and conduct disorders).

Many of these problems will be of little relevance to the dental practitioner, but some are worthy of mention, particularly *autistic spectrum disorders* (within the pervasive developmental disorders group), and *hyperkinetic disorders*.

Autistic spectrum disorders

Autism and related disorders are part of a group of pervasive developmental disorders, characterised by abnormalities of communication and social interaction and a restricted range of interests and activities. The current view is that these disorders are best viewed as a spectrum, owing to the range of difficulties and disabilities seen in this diagnostic group.

Boys are affected four times more commonly than girls, and the prevalence is approximately 5.2 per 10 000 children. Problems usually emerge before the age of 3 years, and may be evident from early infancy.

Table 19A.11 Childhood psychiatric disorders.

ICD-10
Disorders of psychological development
Specific developmental disorders of scholastic skills
Specific developmental disorders of motor function
Specific developmental disorders of speech and language
Pervasive developmental disorders
Behavioural/emotional disorders with onset usually occurring in childhood/adolescence
Hyperkinetic disorders
Conduct disorders
Childhood-onset emotional disorders
Tic disorders
Childhood- and adolescent-onset social-functioning disorders
Other childhood- and adolescent-onset behavioural/emotional disorders

Speech and language may be late to develop, or may never develop, and may be part of a broader cognitive deficit. Speech, when present, may be appear to be a monologue rather than conversational.

Social interaction and development problems can occur. Children with autism lack warmth and affection and may appear indifferent in their relationships. They may avoid eye contact and generally avoid social interaction.

There is a *restricted range of interests and activities*. Children with autism may demonstrate an obsessive desire for things to be the same, and can appear very distressed by perceived changes in their environments.

A large proportion of children with autism will be intellectually impaired, and behavioural difficulties are more common in this group. Some will have no significant intellectual impairment, and a small number may excel in a restricted area of intellectual function.

Asperger's syndrome is a condition with similar characteristics as childhood autism. It may be considered as the high-functioning end of the autistic spectrum, where children have better language skills and express a greater degree of interest in others, although still lacking friends and close relationships.

Aetiology

It is likely that the autistic spectrum disorders are multifactorial in aetiology. Genetic factors have been implicated in twin studies, but there is no clear line of inheritance. Abnormal parenting is not felt to be a causal factor, although problematic patterns of behaviour will undoubtedly arise in the families of some affected children. Although the reported figures for autism vary widely, so does diagnostic practice. It is likely that any recently reported increase in incidence is due to variations in diagnosis rather than any other factor. In particular, the MMR (measles, mumps, rubella) vaccine has been cited widely in the media as being a causal factor in autism. However, this has not rigorously been demonstrated scientifically, and the original study proposing this has been largely discredited. According to current advice, the safest course of action is to ensure that children are adequately protected against childhood illnesses, with the MMR vaccine being integral to this.

Management

There is no specific treatment for autistic spectrum disorders. A holistic approach embracing the whole family unit should be taken, with recognition of the difficulties experienced in various settings (home, school, other social settings), and offering support to the family and the individual to overcome these difficulties.

In a dental setting, sensitive preparation may be required, with particular awareness that children with autistic spectrum disorders may find the close proximity of dentists and their tools exceedingly distressing. Simple measures to make the environment less threatening, such as using music and pictures and avoiding white coats, may be useful. Specific advice is available for dentists and other health professionals from the National Autistic Society.

Autism is a lifelong condition, for which there is no cure at present. Children with autism grow into adults with autism. For the dentist, the principles of management of an adult with autism are the same as for a child, although the degree of resistance to treatment and, indeed, to more general oral hygiene measures may be much greater. Similar principles apply to people with a learning disability, discussed in the following text.

Hyperkinetic disorder (or 'attention-deficit hyperactivity disorder', ADHD)

Strictly speaking, in the UK, the term 'hyperkinetic disorder' is preferred, but the American term ADHD is widely used synonymously, although the diagnostic criteria are less strict.

Many children may seem overactive in certain situations, and many parents find children's greater levels of activity a challenge. About one-third of children are described as 'overactive' by their parents, compared with only around one-fifth of school children, when described by their teachers. Hyperactivity disorders may be diagnosed when the overactivity is severe and there are associated features that impact on a child's function.

The core features are impaired attention, hyperactivity and impulsiveness. ICD-10 requires that both impaired attention and hyperactivity be present.

Again, the prevalence varies according to the diagnostic criteria employed. It is likely that there are many aetiological factors – ranging from mild neurodevelopmental delay or impairment to possible genetic factors, as well as an array of social factors. Food additives and various other nutritional and environmental toxins have previously been put forward as possible causal factors, but there is no convincing evidence to support this idea.

Management

This management needs to take a broad view of the child and family, and recognise and support the child's needs in a range of settings. Behavioural techniques may be useful to improve the situation, but medication is frequently required. Medication is usually a mild stimulant, such as methylphenidate (Ritalin) or dexamphetamine, which works by increasing dopamine and noradrenaline activity in the brain, enhancing attention.

These treatments seem to be quite effective but are not without side effects. They impair appetite and growth, and cause depression in some children; hence, they require regular monitoring. A common side effect is dry mouth.

Anxiety disorders and phobias

Anxiety is a common symptom in children, particularly during visits to dentists. As a disorder, however, anxiety is less common in children, although, when it is present, the principles of management are largely psychological rather than pharmacological.

It should be borne in mind that many simple phobias (such as dental phobia) originate in childhood, stemming from a traumatic experience, and steps should be taken with all children to make their experience at the dentists as unthreatening as possible.

Specific groups for special consideration: the elderly

Some psychiatric disorders diagnosed earlier in life may recur (such as depression) or persist (such as schizophrenia and autism) in later life, and thus the same range of disorders already discussed may be seen. New diagnoses of depression or late-onset schizophrenia may be made in this group, and the dental practitioner may be in a position to detect these. Of specific relevance in the ageing population, however, are dementia and delirium.

Dementia

Dementia is defined as an acquired impairment of global cognitive function, which is generally progressive and largely irreversible. Although confusion may be a prominent feature, there is usually no clouding of consciousness. There are several subtypes of dementia, divided according to the main features and aetiology, as well as based on the regions of the brain affected (see Table 19A.12).

Some dementias have treatable causes, and thus a thorough assessment including physical factors is essential. The two major causes of dementia are Alzheimer's disease and vascular disease, which will be considered in more detail in the following text.

Table 19A.12 Subtypes of dementia.

Cortical – prominent memory impairment an early feature, with impaired word-finding and visuospatial processing

Alzheimer's disease

Frontotemporal dementias

Creutzfeldt–Jakob disease

Subcortical – slowness of thought, impairment in complex sequential tasks and personality, with relative preservation of language and learning skills

Normal-pressure hydrocephalus* (triad of abnormal gait, progressive confusion and urinary incontinence)

Huntington's disease

Parkinson's disease

Focal lesions in thalamus and basal ganglia*

Multiple sclerosis

AIDS–dementia complex*

Hypothyroidism*

Dementia pugilistica

Mixed

Multi-infarct (vascular) dementia

Dementia with Lewy bodies (triad of fluctuating confusion, visual hallucinations and features of Parkinsonism)

Corticobasal degeneration

Neurosyphilis*

*May be treatable if cause identified.

Clinical features

The central feature of most dementias is deterioration in memory. Changes in social function, personality and behaviour are also frequently observed. The decline is usually gradual, and dementia may only present as a problem when a change in circumstances (such as death of a spouse, moving home, or intercurrent illness) disrupt an individual's ability to cope.

Alzheimer's disease

Alzheimer's disease is the most common cause of dementia. The prevalence increases significantly with age, with approximately 1% of 65-year-olds, 5% of 75-year-olds and 20% of 85-year-olds affected.

There is a gradual progression from forgetfulness, which might initially be considered a part of normal ageing, to a more significant memory disturbance, and the development of social difficulties associated with the broader decline in cognitive function, affecting many aspects of behaviour. Mood symptoms are common, and hallucinations may occur in the advanced stages of Alzheimer's disease.

There are characteristic neuropathological changes seen in the brain in Alzheimer's disease, with generalised cerebral atrophy greater than that expected in normal ageing, and widespread deposition of neurofibrillary tangles and amyloid plaques. Most cases are sporadic, but an autosomal dominant form of inheritance has been described in a subgroup of cases with a strong pedigree.

In general, first-degree relatives of a sufferer are three times more likely than the general population to develop Alzheimer's disease.

Vascular dementia

Vascular dementia (or multi-infarct dementia) is due, as the name suggests, to vascular disease, usually atherosclerosis. It is a little more common in men and, as with Alzheimer's, the prevalence increases significantly with age, typically presenting towards the end of the seventh decade. The presentation may be more dramatic, with a history of stroke and the presence of several cardiovascular risk factors such as hypertension, diabetes, obesity and smoking. As might be expected, patients frequently suffer from ischaemic heart disease, which is the cause of mortality in approximately 50% of cases.

Classically, the history is that of step-wise deterioration, interspersed with periods of slight improvement. The memory deficit may not be evident until after a deterioration in personality is noted.

Diagnosis

Diagnosis of the dementias requires a detailed assessment to establish any reversible causes or the presence of other treatable neurological and psychiatric conditions. Assessment is usually multidisciplinary; takes place in a range of settings, with collateral history from family and other relevant informants; and includes cognitive assessment, physical investigations and, increasingly, neuroimaging.

Management of dementia

As yet, there is no cure for dementia, although a number of pharmacological, psychological and social measures can improve the outcome. A depletion of neurotransmitters, particularly acetylcholine, occurs in Alzheimer's disease, owing to neuronal loss in key nuclei. Drugs have been developed to correct this deficit, and acetylcholinesterase inhibitors can delay the progression of symptoms. These drugs have also been used with some degree of success in dementia with Lewy bodies.

Treatment of any intercurrent physical illness is essential, since pain, infection and depression may all exacerbate confusion. The self-neglect frequently seen in dementia may lead to numerous health complications, including dental problems, which may not present until quite advanced.

In the early stages, simple measures to aid memory may be useful, and environmental modifications and social support for both patient and carer are also essential in the management of dementia.

As the disease advances and cognitive function declines, communication may become impaired and behaviour may deteriorate, with aggression or neurological deficits rendering personal care difficult. Medication frequently used in the elderly may cause dry mouth or bruxism. Damaged or decaying teeth, periodontal disease, ill-fitting dentures and ulceration may all cause pain and poor nutrition in the elderly, both of which can exacerbate confusion.

At the different stages of dementia, different advice regarding oral hygiene may be appropriate, both for the patient and for the carer. Similarly, management of dental problems will vary according to the extent of the disease. Dental extractions to prevent pain and further deterioration may be more relevant in the later stages.

Delirium

Delirium is a reversible state characterised by an impairment of consciousness, with associated disturbances in attention, perception, thinking, memory, psychomotor behaviour, emotion and the sleep–wake cycle. Symptoms may fluctuate throughout the day, but are usually short-lived, with many cases lasting only days, and most resolving within a month. Delirium is commonly associated with physical illness or prescribed medication. It is common in hospital patients, occurring in 5–15% of general medical and surgical inpatients, and in up to 30% of patients in surgical intensive care units.

Delirium is more common in those over 60 years of age, and may be superimposed upon dementia, exacerbating any existing cognitive impairment. There are many causes of delirium, some of which are shown in Table 19A.13.

Management of delirium

Management of delirium depends on identification and treatment of the underlying cause. Additional measures may also be necessary to reassure the patient, prevent distress and avoid accidents. These include general environmental measures such as calm and consistent nursing from familiar staff, a quiet room and adequate lighting (including at night). Medication should be minimised as far as possible, and any drug that may further impair consciousness should be avoided.

With adequate treatment, the prognosis for delirium is good, with most cases resolving quickly. Untreated, however, there is a significant mortality.

Specific groups for special consideration: people with learning disabilities

'Learning disability' is the term used to describe the presence of an intellectual deficit present from childhood. Current diagnostic criteria use the term 'mental retardation', but 'learning disability' is preferred in practice. Terms such as 'feeble-minded', 'mentally deficient', 'mentally subnormal' or 'mental handicap' are outmoded, carry stigma and should not be used.

People with learning disabilities are a heterogeneous group (Table 19A.14) with intellectual impairment stemming from early childhood, in contrast to that developing later in life (dementia) or due to an acquired brain injury. It should be remembered that people with learning disabilities are as susceptible as the rest of us to dementia and brain injury, as well as a range of physical conditions that may impair cognitive function. In some cases, those with learning disabilities may be more vulnerable. The presentation of these problems may not be as straightforward as in the general population.

Presentation

People with learning disabilities vary enormously in their ability to function in a range of environments. A mild degree of impairment may go unnoticed, and those with moderate impairment may function well in the community with adequate support, while those with profound learning disabilities usually have significant physical disabilities and require constant care and supervision.

Table 19A.13 Causes of delirium.

Drug intoxication (opiates, sedatives, digitalis, L-dopa, anticonvulsants, poisons)
Drug withdrawal (alcohol, anxiolytic sedatives)
Metabolic causes (liver failure, respiratory failure, cardiac failure, electrolyte imbalances)
Endocrine causes (hypoglycaemia)
Infectious causes (pneumonia, septicaemia, encephalitis, meningitis)
Head injury
Nutritional deficiencies (thiamine, vitamin B_{12})
Epilepsy

Table 19A.14 Diagnosis of learning disabilities.

- A significant impairment of intellectual functioning (IQ<70).
- A significant impairment of adaptive functioning.
- Onset in childhood (i.e. before the age of 18 years).

Learning disability is further classified according to standardised IQ scores and may also be described by the presence and extent of any impairment of behaviour.

- Mild: IQ 50–69
- Moderate: IQ 35–49
- Severe: IQ 20–34
- Profound: IQ<20

Aetiology

There are many causes of learning disability. The frequency of these varies according to the populations studied. Genetic abnormalities, some of which may be inherited, are important in many cases, but neurological damage may be sustained at all stages of foetal development – during pregnancy, delivery and postnatally – due to a range of causes.

Some common causes are listed in Table 19A.15, and Down syndrome is discussed in more detail in the following text.

Dental aspects

Psychiatric illness is three to four times more prevalent in people with a learning disability. Epilepsy is common, and can exacerbate the neurological deficits and other psychiatric conditions. People with learning disabilities may misinterpret information, so careful and patient explanation and simple instructions are important.

Dental hygiene problems are common for those with severe or profound difficulties. Supervision is typically required, such as in young children, but it may be vigorously resisted, which can be a problem, particularly in adults with learning disability.

Diet is often poor and high in refined sugar, and sugar-free medication may be poorly tolerated. Bruxism is common in this group.

Down syndrome (trisomy 21)

Down syndrome is the most common specific cause of learning disability. It occurs in 1 in 650 live births, the incidence increasing with maternal age – from approximately 1 in 2000 for mothers aged 20–25 years, to 1 in 30 at 45 years of age. In 95% of cases, individuals have an extra copy of chromosome 21, with a few cases due to another translocation or mosaicism. There are several typical features that remain relevant to clinical diagnosis, however, and include a flattened face and occiput; eyes sloping upwards and outwards; small ears, mouth and teeth; large tongue; and single transverse palmar crease. Associated abnormalities are common, including heart disease and intestinal problems, and there are increased risks of infection, leukaemia and dementia, to name a few.

Learning disability is almost invariably present, although a wide variation is seen. Typically, IQ is between 20 and 50 (a mental age of under 10), but it may be >50 in around 15% of cases. Some potential causes of learning disability are listed in Table 19A.15.

Behaviour problems are less frequent, however, and children with Down syndrome are frequently described as warm and loveable.

Dental aspects

Development of dentition may be delayed, with a range of abnormalities in size, shape and alignment of teeth. Dental hygiene may be poor due to mouth-breathing or medication, in addition to poor diet and the more general resistance to regular brushing typical of many children.

Special care in manipulation of the head and neck may be necessary, as there is a higher risk of atlantoaxial instability.

Usually a patient with a significant learning disability will be accompanied by a relative or carer, who may be able to help make the experience easier for all involved. While the carer may be useful in supplementing the history and facilitating treatment, it is important to respect the patient's autonomy, address the patient directly and involve him or her in decision-making as far as possible.

Specific issues regarding capacity and consent may arise in this group. This is addressed in the following text.

Capacity and consent

It is easy to assume that patients suffering from significant psychiatric illnesses, dementia, learning disability or other impairments may not have the capacity to make their own decisions about treatment or to give consent. Indeed, at times, relatives and carers may apply pressure on clinicians to accept the decisions they make on behalf of patients.

The Mental Capacity Act (2005) (introduced into practice in 2007) is an important piece of legislation designed to protect the rights of individuals to make their own decisions, and provides guidelines to address this.

It sets out guidance for decision-making on behalf of people who lack decision-making capacity. It applies to all people aged

Table 19A.15 Causes of learning disability.

Genetic	Antenatal	Perinatal	Postnatal
Fragile X syndrome	Infection	Birth asphyxia	Injury
Down syndrome (trisomy 21)	Intoxication	Prematurity	Intoxication
Metabolic disorders	Trauma	Kernicterus	Infection
Neurofibromatosis	Placental dysfunction	Intraventricular haemorrhage	Autism
Tuberous sclerosis	Endocrine disorders		
	Brain malformations		

16 years and above in England and Wales. Scotland has separate legislation, the Adults with Incapacity (Scotland) Act 2000. Decision-making capacity is considered to be task specific, relevant only to a specific decision at a given time, and should not be generalised to other situations and decisions.

The five basic principles are as follows, and are guided by principles of medical ethics and good practice:

- *Autonomy.* Presumption of capacity. People are presumed to have capacity until proven otherwise.
- *Decision-making capacity* must be maximised by all practicable means.
- An individual has *the right to make an unwise decision.*
- *Best interests.* Decisions or acts taken on behalf of a person who is found to lack capacity must be taken in their best interests.
- *Least restrictive.* Where an individual is found to lack decision-making capacity, the least restrictive decision or action should be taken.

Assessment of capacity

Capacity should be assessed by the person who is proposing treatment and seeking consent. The initial question is in two parts:

- Is there an impairment of, or a disturbance in the functioning of, the mind or brain?
- If so, does its presence impair the person's ability to make a particular decision?

A four-stage test adapted from common law must then be applied, looking at the decision-making process itself.

> A person is unable to make a decision for himself or herself if he or she is unable to:
>
> *A:* Understand the information relevant to the decision.
> *B:* Retain that information.
> *C:* Use or weigh that information as part of the process of making the decision.
> *D:* Communicate the decision (by talking, using sign language or any other means).

The information should be provided in a manner appropriate to the needs of the patient, involving an interpreter, where relevant; similarly, the patient should be supported in communicating the decision.

The amount of time the information can be retained need only be as long as is necessary for the actual making of the decision.

If an individual is found to be lacking the capacity to make a particular decision, the course of action taken must satisfy the five basic principles set out in the preceding text. 'Best interests' must be determined on an individual basis, taking into account all possible sources of information.

Most routine dental consultations will be relatively straightforward regarding consent, but there may be some situations in which carers or other health professionals may seek treatment for patients with learning disabilities or dementia, for example, and for which the patient may not be able to consent. When concerns such as these arise, there are several avenues to pursue following an assessment of capacity as laid out in the preceding text.

Problems are more likely to arise when a patient is refusing treatment. In cases where a decision may have serious consequences, it may occasionally be necessary to seek further advice. There are several avenues that could be pursued following an initial assessment of capacity as laid out earlier. These include seeking a second opinion from a psychiatrist; requesting an independent mental capacity advocate (IMCA) to represent the patient and ensure decisions are made in his or her best interests; or applying to the Court of Protection to make a decision on someone's behalf or to appoint a deputy to do so.

Health professionals should also take steps to determine whether a lasting power of attorney (LPA) exists. LPAs replace the existing system of enduring power of attorney (EPA), and enable a person to appoint someone to act on his or her behalf in relation to health and welfare decisions, as well as in relation to property and affairs, should they lose capacity in the future. This may be relevant to people with relapsing psychiatric illness, as well as to people who lose capacity through a neurological injury or dementia.

Further information is contained within the Mental Capacity Act and its Code of Practice, and guidance is available specifically for healthcare professionals through organisations such as the British Medical Association.

Referral to psychiatric services

On occasion, dentists will encounter patients suffering from psychiatric illness that require further assessment and intervention. Dentists are not expected to do this themselves, and it is thus important to have an understanding of the indications for and the appropriate routes of referral.

Indications and routes of referral

There are no hard and fast rules about who should and should not be referred for further assessment. Many scenarios may arise in dental practice:

- If a new presentation of psychiatric illness is suspected, encourage the patient to speak to a medical GP about whatever symptoms have been noticed.
- If deterioration of existing illness is occurring, encourage the patient to speak to a medical GP or existing psychiatric services (Table 19A.16).
- If there is overt suicidal ideation (either as new or altered presentation), then advise the patient to speak to a GP or connect to accident and emergency services, or contact on-call psychiatric services or the police directly.
- If the patient is presenting an immediate danger to others, then call the police.

New presentations of psychiatric illness likely to be encountered by dentists have already been discussed. The most likely presentations are those of anxiety disorders, psychogenic pain

Table 19A.16 Core details of the presentation.

Details of current symptomatology

- Nature of symptoms
- Severity of symptoms
- Impact on functioning

History of the presenting complaint

- Nature of the change in presentation
- Chronological development
- Rapidity of development
- Likely triggers

Relevant past psychiatric history

- Known to psychiatric services
- Key worker details
- Next scheduled appointment

Relevant medical history

Current medication and estimate of compliance

Risk assessment

- Risk to self from suicide or neglect
- Risk to others

Table 19A.17 High-risk characteristics for suicide.

Male > female

- Age >40 years (increasing in young men)
- Evidence of planning
- Undertakes act when alone
- Social classes I and V
- Living alone
- Unemployed
- Not married
- Loss events: bereavement, shifting residence, financial, immigration

Table 19A.18 Mental state examination.

Appearance and behaviour

- Dishevelled/unkempt, flamboyant dress, odd clothing
- Withdrawn/retarded, overactive/intrusive, on-edge/jumpy
- Odd mannerisms, aggression/violence, etc.

Speech

- Rate
- Rhythm
- Volume
- Intonation
- Spontaneity

Thought

- Form
- Content (including delusions)

Mood

- Objective and subjective
- Reactivity

Abnormal sensory experiences

- Hallucinations and misperceptions

Cognitive functioning

- Orientation
- Memory
- Concentration

Insight

- Understanding of the problem
- Willingness to receive help/treatment

and substance abuse. Depression may also be detected. In many cases, sharing your concerns with the patient and recommending a consultation with a GP will suffice. In situations in which the dentist is more concerned, direct consultation with a GP may be indicated to ensure that an appointment is made and followed up, usually with consent from the patient.

It is rare for referrals to secondary care to come straight from dental practitioners. Handing over of care to a GP who can make a secondary care referral if required is often more appropriate.

Deterioration of an existing illness can be difficult to detect without experience of psychiatry and prior knowledge of the patient. It is important to establish if there has been a genuine deterioration, and if this requires further intervention. Generally, patients with mild–moderate illnesses will be known to their GP, and a simple liaison with the practice in question will suffice. Patients under secondary psychiatric care will usually have an appointed key worker, such as a community nurse or social worker, who will be aware of the patient and have access to full case details. Arrangements can usually be made for an earlier review of the patient if the key worker feels it is appropriate.

Overt suicidal ideation is unlikely to present to dental practitioners. The assessment of suicidality is best performed by experienced, trained mental health workers. In the absence of experience and support, all patients voicing ideas of suicide should be referred for further assessment (although, again, contact with primary care or a known key worker is the appropriate route) (Table 19A.17). Details of a basic risk assessment are provided in the following text, with the goal of facilitating referral, and *not* replacing it.

These characteristics define those at greatest risk, but are not intended to substitute a referral for specialist assessment when presented with a patient expressing suicidal intent.

Basic psychiatric assessment

A comprehensive psychiatric assessment requires time and experience, and covers all aspects of symptomatology, past presentation, development and function. In general terms, such an assessment is not required for a dental referral. It is important, however, for all healthcare professionals who are in a position to refer to other services to be able to provide basic, core information that will allow prioritisation of the referral in question.

In addition to history and physical assessment, psychiatrists undertake a mental state examination during assessment and subsequent interviews. This serves to objectively describe the patient's presentation in several domains.

Non-psychiatrists are not expected to complete a formal mental state examination, but a description of what has been observed can be very helpful when making a referral (Table 19A.18).

19B   DRUG ABUSE

Dental problems such as caries and periodontal disease are common among drug abusers. This is a result of the combined effect of a poor diet – for example, an increased carbohydrate intake as a result of stimulation of energy, carbohydrate additives to drug formulations and side effects of the abused drug, such as dry mouth. In addition, treatment may not be sought at an early stage as the drug of abuse may mask the discomfort caused by the oral disease.

The impact on general health created by drug abuse will also affect dental management. Cardiac and hepatic disease may result from the intravenous use of illicit drugs, and blood-borne viral infections may result from the sharing of needles. Illicit drugs may interact with the drugs prescribed by dentists.

The impact of drugs of abuse on dental management is discussed in the following text, and is summarised in Table 19B.1.

Alcohol

Effects on orodental structures

Alcohol abuse can cause loss of dental hard tissues. Enamel may be dissolved by alcohol or any mixers added to it. In addition, alcohol can cause an increase in regurgitation of acidic gastric contents, resulting in loss of tooth tissue, especially on the lingual/palatal surfaces. Traumatic loss of dental hard tissue may be the result of alcohol-fuelled violence.

Alcohol is a risk factor for oral cancer. Other mucosal changes caused by the abuse of alcohol, such as glossitis and stomatitis, are the result of nutritional deficiencies and anaemia. Alcohol may also produce a painless swelling of the salivary glands known as 'sialosis'.

Effect on management

Chronic abuse of alcohol can lead to hepatic dysfunction. This impacts on dentistry in two ways. First, the handling of drugs may be impaired, and second, blood clotting may be affected, leading to excess bleeding after surgical procedures. It is therefore advised that clotting studies be performed before engaging in surgery in patients who abuse alcohol.

Drug interactions

Aspirin should be avoided due to the increased bleeding in the alcoholic patient. Metronidazole, tinidazole, some cephalosporins and the antifungal drug ketoconazole can all cause the so-called disulfiram reaction when taken with alcohol. This unpleasant reaction is characterised by flushing, hyperventilation and feelings of panic.

Smoking

Effects on orodental structures

Females who smoke >20 cigarettes a day appear to be at a greater chance of developing dry socket as compared to non-smokers. Smoking is a risk factor for adult periodontitis. In addition, it can discolour the teeth and alter the appearance of the oral mucosa. The soft tissue changes can be keratotic or

Table 19B.1 The impact of drugs of abuse on dentistry.

	Teeth	Oral mucosa	GA/ sedation	LA with adrenaline	Bleeding	Cardiac effects	HIV/hepatitis	Drug interactions
Alcohol	+	+	+		+	+		+
Nicotine	+	+	+					
Cannabis		+	+	+				
Opioids			+		+	+	+	+
CNS depressants		+	+		+			+
CNS stimulants		+	+	+	+	+	+	+
Hallucinogens								+
Solvents			+	+		+		
Anabolic steroids/ performance enhancers			+	+	+	+	+	+

+ = an interaction between the drug and the structure/function indicated.

melanotic. Nicotinic stomatitis appears as a grey discoloration of the palate, with red spots that correspond to the minor salivary gland ducts. These soft tissue changes are reversible on smoking cessation. More serious conditions such as leukoplakia do not disappear when smoking stops. The most serious complication of smoking in the mouth cavity is the production of oral cancers.

Effect on management

In some patients, the successful treatment of periodontal disease depends on smoking cessation.

Drug interactions

Smoking induces hepatic enzymes and thus interferes with the action of concurrent drug therapy. Smokers may require larger doses of sedatives and postoperative analgesics than non-smokers.

Cannabis

Effects on orodental structures

Smoking cannabis can cause gingival enlargement and oral leukoplakia.

Effect on management

Cannabis has a sympathomimetic action, and this could, in theory, exacerbate the systemic effects of adrenaline in dental local anaesthetics.

Heroin and methadone

Heroin and methadone are opioids. Dentists are more likely to deal with patients receiving methadone, which is widely used in rehabilitation programmes.

Effects on orodental structures

Oral methadone has a high sugar content, which can cause rampant caries.

Effect on management

Heroin can cause thrombocytopaenia, which can cause post-extraction haemorrhage. Some of those addicted to heroin have a low pain threshold, and may demand excessive postoperative analgesics. Heroin interacts with some drugs that dentists may prescribe. The absorption of paracetamol and orally administered diazepam is delayed and reduced due to delayed gastric emptying.

Drug interactions

Carbamazepine reduces serum methadone levels. Methadone increases the effects of TCAs. Barbiturates and benzodiazepines, both central nervous system depressants, are also subjected to abuse. Cocaine, amphetamines and ecstasy are all central nervous system stimulants.

Cocaine

Effects on orodental structures

The vasoconstrictor action of cocaine can cause ischaemia, resulting in loss of tissue. The common practice of testing the quality of the illicit drug by rubbing it on the oral mucosa (to test for numbing) can lead to loss of gingivae and alveolar bone. Similarly, dental caries may occur, since the drug may be bulked out with carbohydrates.

Children of mothers who abuse cocaine have a higher incidence of ankyloglossia (tongue-tie) than control populations.

Effect on management

Cocaine is one of many drugs that can produce thrombocytopaenia, and a pre-surgical platelet count is therefore advised.

Drug interactions

Carbamazepine reduces the cocaine 'high'. This makes the illicit drug less pleasurable. Cocaine and the intravenous sedative propofol can produce grand mal seizures when used concurrently. As is the case with cannabis, the sympathomimetic action of cocaine can increase the systemic effects of adrenaline in dental local anaesthetic solutions.

Amphetamines and ecstasy

Effects on orodental structures

Amphetamines and ecstasy can produce dry mouth. These drugs have been implicated in the production of TMJ dysfunction as they increase bruxism.

Effect on management

These drugs can produce thrombocytopaenia and interfere with blood clotting.

Drug interactions

Both MAOIs and TCAs should be avoided in those taking amphetamines. Combined therapy can precipitate a hypertensive crisis.

Hallucinogens

Lysergic acid diethylamide (LSD), mescaline and phencyclidine (angel dust) are hallucinogenic drugs.

Effects on orodental structures

The use of hallucinogens increases the risk of maxillofacial injury and dental trauma. Hallucinogens can increase bruxism, resulting in TMJ dysfunction.

Effect on management

Stressful situations, such as dental treatment, can precipitate flashback and cause panic attacks.

Drug interactions

Opioids can interact with phencyclidine to precipitate respiratory depression.

Solvent abuse

Effects on orodental structures

The circumoral erythema known as 'glue-sniffer's rash' may be apparent in solvent abusers. Oral frostbite can be caused by aerosols. As mentioned in the preceding text, with alcohol and hallucinogens, orofacial injuries may occur during periods of intoxication.

Effect on management

Reduction in the dose of adrenaline-containing anaesthetics is recommended in those who chronically abuse solvents, as these agents can sensitise the myocardium to the actions of catecholamines. As solvent abuse increases the risk of convulsions, status epilepticus is a risk in those who abuse these substances.

Anabolic steroids and performance enhancers

Effects on orodental structures

Anabolic steroids and performance enhancers can precipitate excessive carbohydrate consumption, which can increase the incidence of caries.

Effect on management

The systemic effects of adrenaline in dental local anaesthetics can be exacerbated by performance-enhancing drugs that possess sympathomimetic actions. As with many illicit drugs, anabolic steroids interfere with blood clotting.

19C ANXIOLYTIC AND HYPNOTIC DRUGS

Anxiolytic drugs

Anxiolytic drugs have several uses. These include:

- As a premedication prior to general anaesthesia.
- As sedation agents (see Chapter 14, titled 'Pain and anxiety control').
- As muscle relaxants (e.g. to treat TMJ dislocations).
- As anxiolytics during severe pain (e.g. myocardial infarction).
- As emergency drugs (e.g. in the treatment of status epilepticus (see Chapter 21, titled 'Medical Emergencies').
- As producers of amnesia.

Not all agents produce all the effects mentioned in the preceding text. There are several ways of administering anxiolytics, including the oral, transmucosal and intravenous routes, and also via inhalation. The drugs used as anxiolytics can be classified as follows:

- Alcohol.
- Benzodiazepines.
- Nitrous oxide.
- Buspirone.
- β-Adrenergic blocking drugs.

Although alcohol was used in the past as a sedative, it is not used these days as an agent prescribed by the dentist. Patients may self-prescribe this treatment, however, for controlling anxiety prior to dental treatment. The mechanism of action of benzodiazepines and the use of nitrous oxide are described in Chapter 14 (titled 'Pain and anxiety control'). The anxiolytic effect of benzodiazepines is achieved as a result of their action on the limbic system of the cerebral cortex.

Buspirone is an azapirone. It is a potent agonist at serotonin receptors; however, its exact mechanism of action is not totally understood, since it takes weeks to exert a clinical effect. Although an anxiolytic, it does not produce sedation. Buspirone can impact on dental management, since it can produce a dry mouth.

β-Adrenergic-blocking drugs are used to treat somatic anxiety when sympathetic overstimulation can produce physical effects such as tremors and palpitations. They are not used to treat anxious dental patients. The impact of β-adrenergic-blocking drugs on dentistry was discussed in Chapter 5 (titled 'Cardiovascular disorders').

Hypnotic drugs

Hypnotic drugs are used to treat insomnia. There are two types of insomnia, namely *initial insomnia* and *early-morning wakening*. Different drugs are used to treat the two types. A drug with a quick onset of action and short half-life is best for the treatment of initial insomnia (e.g. temazepam). Early-morning wakening is better managed by a drug such as nitrazepam, which has a longer half-life.

Unfortunately, the type of sleep induced by hypnotics is not the same as physiological sleep. Drug-induced sleep has a reduced rapid eye movement (REM) component. On withdrawal of hypnotics, there can be overcompensation in REM sleep, leading to nightmares.

The drugs used as hypnotics can be classified as:

- Benzodiazepines.
- Barbiturates.
- Antihistamines.
- Miscellaneous.

The benzodiazepines were discussed comprehensively in Chapter 14 (titled 'Pain and anxiety control').

Barbiturates are not the first-choice drugs these days, since they have several unwanted effects. They have a high suicide risk, a low safety margin, produce respiratory depression and have no chemical antidote. In addition, they can cause automatism – this is a state of drug-induced confusion where patients cannot remember taking their medications, and hence takes more drugs. Amobarbital is a barbiturate used as a hypnotic, and it is only prescribed for those who have intractable insomnia and are already taking these drugs. Barbiturates achieve their effect in a manner similar to benzodiazepines. They act at the chloride ion channel and enhance the affinity of the inhibitory neurotransmitter GABA for its binding site at the chloride channel, resulting in prolongation of chloride influx, which causes hyperpolarisation. Barbiturates are enzyme inducers, and are therefore involved in drug interactions. Carbamazepine, doxycycline and warfarin are some of the drugs whose metabolism is enhanced by barbiturates. Amobarbital can cause dry mouth and fixed drug eruptions on the oral mucosa.

Some of the H_1-blocker group of drugs that are used in anti-allergy therapy can produce drowsiness as a side effect. They are therefore useful as hypnotics that are only used in children, the drug used is promethazine. This agent can produce dry mouth, and, as with all central nervous system depressants, it will enhance the effects of other such drugs when used in combination.

The miscellaneous hypnotics include chloral hydrate, triclofos, clomethiazole, zaleplon, zolpidem and zopiclone. Chloral hydrate was the original hypnotic, synthesised in 1832. It is metabolised to its active form of trichloroethanol, although its exact mechanism of action is unknown. It is used mainly in children and the elderly, since it produces little post-hypnotic confusion. As with barbiturates, chloral hydrate is an enzyme inducer. It can produce a disulfiram-like reaction when taken with alcohol.

Triclofos is an ester of chloral hydrate and shares its properties, although it is less potent. Clomethiazole increases the action of GABA, and may be used during alcohol withdrawal. A side effect of therapy is the development of nasal congestion, which might make the use of rubber dams difficult during dental treatment.

Zaleplon, zolpidem and zopiclone, although not benzodiazepines, act at benzodiazepine receptors. As they can produce dizziness, amnesia and lack of coordination, their use may impact on dental management.

FURTHER READING

BMJ. Available from: http://www.bmj.com/specialties/psychiatry.

Royal College of Psychiatrists. Available from: http://www.rcpsych.ac.uk.

MULTIPLE CHOICE QUESTIONS

1. Which one of the following is *not* a core feature of mania?
   a) Distractibility.
   b) Decreased need for sleep.
   c) Risk-taking behaviour.
   d) Racing thoughts.
   e) Hallucinations.
   Answer = C

2. Which one of the following is *not* a core feature of depression?
   a) Loss of libido.
   b) Lack of energy.
   c) Loss of enjoyment.
   d) Poor concentration.
   e) Delirium and hallucinations if severe.
   Answer = D

3. Which one of the following is a TCA?
   a) Amitriptyline.
   b) Fluoxetine.
   c) Paroxetine.
   d) Citalopram.
   e) Sertraline.
   Answer = A

4. The correct number of units of alcohol in a pub measure of spirits is:
   a) 2.
   b) 0.25.
   c) 0.5.
   d) 1.
   e) 1.5.
   Answer = D

5. Which of the following is a feature suggestive of possible psychogenic pain?
   a) Unilateral pain.
   b) Bilateral pain.
   c) Easily identified on testing.
   d) Analgesia is usually effective.
   e) No association with emotional factors.
   Answer = B

6. In the term 'CAGE questionnaire', used for assessing alcohol dependency, the 'A' stands for:
   a) Amount.
   b) Alcohol.
   c) Assessment.
   d) Annoyed.
   e) Accusatory.
   Answer = D

7. Positive symptoms of schizophrenia include:
   a) Social withdrawal.
   b) Emotional blunting.
   c) Apathy.
   d) Slowing.
   e) Delusions.
   Answer = E

8. 'Atypical' antipsychotic drugs include:
   a) Olanzapine.
   b) Amitriptyline.
   c) Sertraline.
   d) Haloperidol.
   e) Chlorpromazine.
   Answer = A

9. SSRIs include:
   a) Haloperidol.
   b) Risperidone.
   c) Citalopram.
   d) Quetiapine.
   e) Clozapine.
   Answer = C

10. Which of the following is *not* an anxiolytic?
    a) Midazolam.
    b) Nitrous oxide.
    c) β-adrenergic antagonists.
    d) Alcohol.
    e) Caffeine.
    Answer = E

CHAPTER 20
Haematology

J Hanley, A Lennard and S Mathia

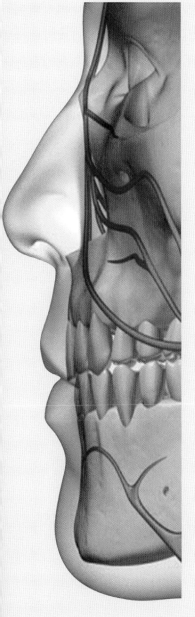

Key topics

- General aspects of haematology.
- Haemostasis.
- Principles of transfusion medicine.

Learning objectives

- To be familiar with the more common disorders encountered by the haematologist.
- To have knowledge of anticoagulants and their impact on the practice of dentistry.

Essentials of Human Disease in Dentistry, Second Edition. Mark Greenwood.
© 2018 John Wiley & Sons Ltd. Published 2018 by John Wiley & Sons Ltd.
Companion website: www.wiley.com/go/greenwood/human-disease-in-dentistry

20A   GENERAL HAEMATOLOGY, HAEMATO-ONCOLOGY

Normal haemopoiesis

Haemopoiesis is the term referring to the formation of blood cells. In humans, it occurs in different sites during foetal development and following birth. During the first 8 weeks of gestation, the yolk sac is the main site of haemopoiesis. During 2–7 months of gestation, the liver and spleen take over blood production; from 7 months, the bone marrow is the major site. The bone marrow remains the chief source of haemopoiesis throughout adulthood, with haemopoietic tissue found within the central skeleton and proximal long bones of adults.

All blood cells originate from a common pluripotential stem cell that is capable of self-renewal. Stem cells undergo differentiation to produce the early progenitor cells of each of the cell lineages. As further differentiation and maturation occur, cells become haemopoietic progenitors committed to a single cell lineage, ultimately resulting in the formation of granulocytes, erythrocytes, monocytes, macrophages, megakaryocytes, eosinophils, basophils, and T and B lymphocytes (Figure 20A.1).

The bone marrow stroma

Bone marrow stromal cells form a specialised microenvironment for stem cell growth and differentiation. Adipocytes, fibroblasts, macrophages and other cells secrete substances such as collagen, glycoproteins and glycosaminoglycans, which form an extracellular matrix on which stem cells can grow. The stromal cells also secrete haemopoietic growth factors, which stimulate differentiation and maturation of blood cells. Adhesion molecules produced by the stromal cells fix the marrow precursor cells to the extracellular matrix, enabling them to mature under the influence of the growth factors.

Erythropoiesis

The stem cell differentiates to form the early mixed myeloid progenitor cell, followed by BFU-E (burst-forming unit erythroid) and then CFU-E (colony-forming unit erythrocyte), from which the pronormoblast arises. This large cell has a basophilic (blue) cytoplasm and a large

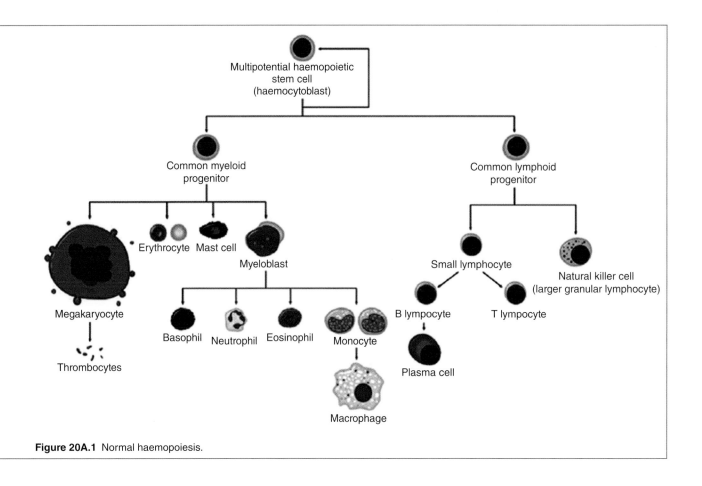

Figure 20A.1 Normal haemopoiesis.

central nucleus with clumped chromatin. Successive smaller normoblasts develop within the marrow. These contain increasing amounts of haemoglobin in the cytoplasm, and therefore stain increasingly pink. Finally, in the marrow, the nucleus is extruded from the late normoblast to form a reticulocyte. The reticulocyte contains ribosomal ribonucleic acid (rRNA), and is released into the peripheral blood for 1–2 days before losing its RNA to form a mature erythrocyte. Red cells are non-nucleated biconcave discs that survive for 120 days in the peripheral blood before they are broken down by macrophages belonging to the reticuloendothelial system.

The haemopoietic growth factor that controls erythropoiesis is erythropoietin, a hormone produced by the kidney. In anaemia, oxygen levels in the renal tissue fall, stimulating erythropoietin production. This in turn increases erythropoiesis within the bone marrow. Conversely, in states of increased red cell mass (polycythaemia), the increased oxygen tension in the kidneys reduces erythropoietin production, and reduces erythropoiesis.

Haemoglobin

The primary role of red blood cells is to transport oxygen to the body tissues via the systemic arterial system, and to carry carbon dioxide from the tissues to the lungs in the venous system. Red cells transport oxygen and carbon dioxide via the specialised protein that they contain – called *haemoglobin* (Hb).

A normal Hb molecule is composed of two pairs of polypeptide chains, each of which encloses an iron-containing porphyrin called *haem*, which can bind reversibly with oxygen. The relationship between the four globin chains is known as the *quaternary structure*, and can change depending on whether or not the haemoglobin molecule is oxygenated. When oxygen is released from Hb, the globin chains slide on each other, allowing 2,3-diphosphoglycerate (2,3-DPG) to enter the Hb molecule, reducing its affinity for oxygen. Oxygenation of Hb pulls the β-chains together, and 2,3-DPG is extruded from the Hb molecule.

Changes in the quaternary structure are responsible for the sigmoid shape of the Hb–oxygen dissociation curve (Figure 20A.2). Hypoxia increases synthesis of 2,3-DPG, pushing the Hb–oxygen dissociation curve to the right, resulting in increased offloading of oxygen to the tissues. Acidosis, pyrexia and high carbon dioxide concentrations also push the curve to the right (the Bohr effect).

The predominant Hb produced during foetal life is 'foetal haemoglobin' (HbF), which contains two α-globin chains and two γ-globin chains. At 3–6 months of age, infants switch to producing 'adult haemoglobin' (HbA; two α- and two β-chains).

Although HbA is the predominant Hb after 6 months of age, small quantities of HbF and HbA$_2$ (two α- and two δ-chains) persist into adulthood.

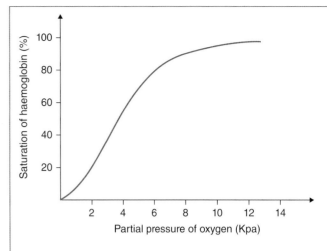

Figure 20A.2 The Hb–oxygen dissociation curve.

Red cell metabolism

The *Embden–Meyerhof pathway* is an anaerobic glycolytic pathway within the red cell that generates energy in the form of adenosine triphosphate (ATP). ATP helps to maintain red cell volume, shape and flexibility. Reduced nicotinamide adenine dinucleotide (NADH) is also formed during glycolysis and is needed to convert functionally inactive metHb, containing oxidised iron (Fe^{3+}), to functionally active Hb, which contains ferrous iron (Fe^{2+}).

Red cells generate reduced nicotinamide adenine dinucleotide phosphate (NADPH) via the hexose monophosphate pathway. NADPH is used to generate reduced glutathione, which protects the cell from oxidant stress. 2,3-DPG is also produced by the red cell to regulate the oxygen affinity of haemoglobin.

Anaemia

Anaemia is a reduction in the Hb concentration of the blood. Although normal reference ranges for Hb concentration vary between laboratories, a Hb < 11.5 g/dl in females and < 13 g/dl in males is considered low in general.

Anaemias may be classified according to red cell indices (Table 20A.1). The *mean corpuscular volume* (MCV) is the volume of the average red blood cell, and the *mean corpuscular haemoglobin* (MCH) is the Hb content of the average red cell.

General features of anaemia

A fall in Hb concentration leads to a reduction in the oxygen-carrying capacity of the blood, resulting in tissue hypoxia. The body attempts to compensate by increasing the stroke volume and heart rate, thereby increasing cardiac output. Young, fit patients may experience few symptoms and signs apart from pallor (due to vasoconstriction of blood vessels in the skin), fatigue, tachycardia and, occasionally, development of heart

Table 20A.1 Classification of anaemias according to red cell indices.

Hypochromic microcytic	Normochromic normocytic	Macrocytic
Iron deficiency	Anaemia of chronic disease (some cases)	Megaloblastic anaemias
Thalassaemia	Renal failure	Liver disease
Lead poisoning	Acute blood loss	Alcohol excess
Hereditary sideroblastic anaemia	Haemolysis	Pregnancy
Anaemia of chronic disease (some cases)	Bone marrow infiltration	Hypothyroidism
	Mixed deficiencies	Myelodysplasia
		Aplastic anaemia
		Multiple myeloma
		Reticulocytosis

murmur due to hyperdynamic circulation. Older patients may not tolerate the anaemia, however, and can develop additional features such as palpitations, dyspnoea, ischaemic symptoms such as angina, and signs of cardiac failure.

Iron deficiency anaemia

Iron absorption and distribution

A normal diet contains approximately 10 mg of elemental iron, but usually only 10% of the iron is absorbed. Dietary iron is converted from the ferric form (Fe^{3+}) to the ferrous form (Fe^{2+}) by acid in the stomach. Fe^{2+} binds to transferrin, which is produced by duodenal epithelial cells. Bound iron is absorbed mainly in the duodenum, but also in the jejunum. Absorbed iron is used to form the haem part of haemoglobin, and is also found in myoglobin in muscles and in liver enzymes. The remainder is stored in the liver, bone marrow and spleen as ferritin and haemosiderin.

Causes of iron deficiency

The most common cause of iron deficiency is chronic blood loss, which may occur from any site. A common site is the gastrointestinal (GI) tract, where inflammation, ulceration or malignancy may be the source of blood loss. Menorrhagia and haematuria may also cause iron deficiency. Other causes are listed in Table 20A.2.

Clinical features of iron deficiency anaemia

In addition to the general features of anaemia, patients with iron deficiency may also develop specific signs such as koilonychia (concave nails), generalised pruritus, pica (cravings for unusual foods), angular stomatitis and painless glossitis. In children, psychomotor delay and cognitive decline can occur. Rarely, adults may present with dysphagia and iron deficiency due to the presence of a pharyngeal web, which is associated

Table 20A.2 Causes of iron deficiency.

Chronic blood loss – may be from any site, but commonly in the uterus, gut or urinary tract.

Malabsorption of iron – seen in patients with coeliac disease (villous atrophy in the jejunum), atrophic gastritis and those who have undergone gastric or duodenal surgery.

Dietary deficiency – common in children, but is rarely the sole cause of iron deficiency in adults.

Increased physiological demands – growth during infancy and adolescence; menstruation and pregnancy; and lactation – all increase the risk of iron deficiency occurring.

with oesophageal cancer (Plummer–Vinson or Paterson–Kelly syndrome).

Laboratory investigation of suspected iron deficiency

- In the full blood count (FBC), a low Hb, MCV and MCH are seen. The platelet count may be moderately raised, especially if there is ongoing blood loss.
- In the blood film, hypochromic, microcytic red cells are seen. Anisocytosis (variation in red cell size), pencil-shaped red cells and target cells are also present.
- Iron studies show low serum iron, raised total iron-binding capacity (TIBC), low serum ferritin, transferrin saturation (serum iron/TIBC) <10%, and raised serum transferrin receptor level.
- Anti-endomysial antibodies are assayed to screen for coeliac disease.

Treatment

Iron replacement (oral or parenteral) is required, and the underlying cause should be investigated.

Megaloblastic anaemias

Megaloblastic anaemia results from the deficiency of vitamin B_{12} or folic acid. Vitamin B_{12} and folate are needed for the synthesis of deoxyribonucleic acid (DNA) within the nucleus of maturing erythroblasts. Deficiency of either causes delayed maturation of the nucleus as compared to the cytoplasm, resulting in the formation of megaloblasts in the marrow.

Absorption of vitamin B_{12}

Vitamin B_{12} is found in foods of animal origin and binds to the intrinsic factor, which is produced by gastric parietal cells. The intrinsic factor–B_{12} complex is absorbed in the terminal ileum. B_{12} binds to transcobalamin I in the blood, but it is transcobalamin II that is responsible for the delivery of B_{12} to the peripheral tissues. Table 20A.3 highlights the common causes of vitamin B_{12} deficiency.

Folate deficiency

Folic acid is found in leafy vegetables and is absorbed mainly in the duodenum. The common causes of folate deficiency are listed in Table 20A.4.

Clinical features of megaloblastic anaemia

Both B_{12} and folate deficiency can cause angular stomatitis, painful glossitis and mild jaundice. In severe cases, infertility may occur. Specifically, vitamin B_{12} deficiency can cause demyelination of the dorsal columns and corticospinal tracts in the spinal cord, along with peripheral nerve damage. This is known as 'subacute combined degeneration of the cord'.

Table 20A.3 Causes of vitamin B_{12} deficiency.

Pernicious anaemia – caused by the formation of autoantibodies directed against the intrinsic factor; more common in females and Northern Europeans, and can be familial.

Malabsorption of B_{12} – may occur in patients with Crohn's disease, or in those who have undergone gastric or ileal surgery; other ileal disease, such as the presence of blind loops, may also result in B_{12} malabsorption.

Dietary deficiency of B_{12} – rare, except in vegans.

Table 20A.4 Causes of folate deficiency.

Dietary deficiency – common.

Increased physiological demands – for example, during pregnancy.

Malabsorption of folate – seen in patients with Crohn's disease and following duodenal surgery.

Use of antifolate drugs – such as trimethoprim, methotrexate and anticonvulsants.

Patients may present with ataxia due to loss of proprioception and vibration sense. Corticospinal tract lesions in combination with a peripheral neuropathy classically cause extensor plantar responses, brisk knee reflexes and absent ankle reflexes. Rarely, cognitive decline and visual loss also occur.

Laboratory investigations

- FBC shows low Hb, high MCV.
- Blood film shows typically oval macrocytes, and hypersegmented neutrophils are seen.
- Measurement of serum B_{12} and red cell folate shows one or both to be low.
- Intrinsic factor antibodies should be checked if vitamin B_{12} deficiency is found.
- Bone marrow aspirate (not usually required for diagnosis) demonstrates a hypercellular marrow. Megaloblasts and giant metamyelocytes are seen in the marrow.
- Schilling test – radiolabelled B_{12} is ingested and, if absorbed, is excreted in the urine. Unlabelled B_{12} is given as an intramuscular injection to saturate tissue stores. In malabsorptive states, <5% of the radiolabelled B_{12} will be detected in the urine. The test is then repeated with the addition of the intrinsic factor. If the addition of the intrinsic factor results in normal B_{12} levels in the urine, the malabsorption must be due to pernicious anaemia rather than an intestinal cause.

Treatment

Replacement with folic acid and/or vitamin B_{12} is required. If folate deficiency is detected, B_{12} deficiency must always be excluded and, if present, corrected before folate replacement is given, since folate replacement alone may precipitate subacute combined degeneration of the cord. The reticulocyte count, which begins to rise 2–3 days after commencing treatment and peaks at 6–7 days, may be used to monitor response to treatment. B_{12} replacement in patients with dorsal column involvement can partly improve the peripheral neuropathy, but the spinal cord damage is irreversible.

Anaemia of chronic disease

A normochromic, normocytic anaemia (occasionally hypochromic, microcytic) can be seen in patients with chronic inflammatory and malignant conditions. Serum iron is low despite adequate iron stores in the bone marrow. TIBC is also low, and serum ferritin may be normal or raised, since ferritin is an acute-phase protein that rises in response to inflammation. Increases in cytokines such as tumour necrosis factor and interleukin-1 lead to blunted marrow response to erythropoietin, impaired iron uptake into erythroid precursors and reduced red cell survival. In addition, hepcidin released from the liver in response to inflammation inhibits the release of iron from macrophages into the plasma. Treatment of the underlying condition may improve the anaemia. Patients with renal failure and some malignant conditions may also benefit from treatment with recombinant erythropoietin.

Haemolytic anaemias

Haemolysis is the increased destruction of red cells. Red cell destruction may be:

- *Intravascular* – lysis of red cells within blood vessels owing to complement activation.
- *Extravascular* – antibodies bind to red cells; antibody-coated red cells are then removed from circulation by macrophages within the liver and/or the spleen.

If haemolysis is mild, the marrow is able to compensate by increasing red cell production. Erythroid hyperplasia in the marrow causes reticulocytosis. Reticulocytes are visible as polychromatic erythrocytes (larger than normal red cells, which stain slightly blue) on the blood film. In severe haemolysis, the marrow cannot compensate fully, and the patient becomes anaemic.

In addition to the general features of anaemia, patients with haemolysis become jaundiced owing to the release of unconjugated bilirubin from lysed red cells. Extravascular haemolysis often causes splenomegaly.

All patients with haemolytic anaemia are at risk of developing acute marrow aplasia if they become folate deficient or develop parvovirus B19 infection. Marrow production of red cells is switched off, causing profound anaemia with reticulocytopaenia, often requiring red cell transfusion.

Classification of haemolytic anaemias

Haemolytic anaemias may be hereditary or acquired (see Table 20A.5).

Laboratory investigation of haemolysis

- FBC shows low Hb; the MCV is often raised due to the presence of large numbers of reticulocytes in the blood.

- In the blood film, red cell fragments are seen in intravascular haemolysis. Spherocytes (small, densely staining red cells with no central pallor) are seen in extravascular haemolysis.
- A raised lactate dehydrogenase (LDH) reflects high cell turnover.
- There is raised unconjugated bilirubin.
- There are low serum haptoglobins – haptoglobins are plasma proteins that bind the polypeptide chains released from the breakdown of Hb. Bound haptoglobin is then taken up by cells of the reticuloendothelial system.
- The direct antiglobulin test (DAT) detects antibodies bound to the surface of red cells. A positive DAT is seen in *autoimmune haemolytic anaemia* (AIHA).

Red cell membrane defects

The red cell membrane is made up of a phospholipid bilayer, integral proteins and a cytoskeleton located on the inner aspect of the lipid bilayer (see Figure 20A.3). The cytoskeleton is composed of proteins such as α- and β-spectrin, actin and protein 4.1, which maintain red cell shape and flexibility. These structural proteins connect to the transmembrane protein band 3 via ankyrin and protein 4.2. The most common hereditary haemolytic anaemia in Northern Europe is HS, and it is caused by defects in these 'vertical connections'.

Hereditary spherocytosis (HS)

HS is usually inherited as an autosomal dominant condition. The majority of patients with HS have mutations of spectrin and ankyrin genes, resulting in defects in the ankyrin–spectrin complex. About 25% of patients have deficiency of band 3 protein. A smaller number have deficiency of protein 4.2, or the defect is unknown. Disruption of these 'vertical connections' in the red cell membrane results in the formation of spherocytes, which are destroyed early by the spleen. The clinical severity of the condition varies from mild to severe, and patients with moderate or severe haemolysis usually require splenectomy.

Table 20A.5 Causes of haemolytic anaemias.

Hereditary	Acquired
Red cell membrane abnormalities (e.g. hereditary spherocytosis, hereditary elliptocytosis)	Autoimmune
	Alloimmune (e.g. haemolytic transfusion reaction)
Defects in red cell metabolism (e.g. glucose-6-phosphate dehydrogenase deficiency)	Red cell fragmentation syndromes (e.g. thrombotic thrombocytopaenic purpura – TTP)
Haemoglobinopathies (e.g. sickle cell anaemia)	Renal and liver disease
	Burns
	Drugs causing oxidative haemolysis (e.g. dapsone)
	Paroxysmal nocturnal haemoglobinuria
	Infection (e.g. malaria)

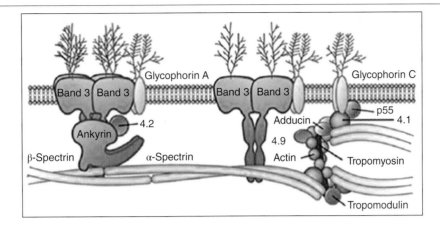

Figure 20A.3 Structure of the red cell membrane.

AIHA

AIHA is an acquired form of haemolysis in which autoantibodies directed against red cell antigens attach to red cells, resulting in increased erythrocyte destruction. If the autoantibody attaches at body temperature, it is classed as a warm-acting antibody. These antibodies are usually polyclonal IgG antibodies and cause a strongly positive DAT.

First-line treatment of warm AIHA is high-dose oral prednisolone. Red cell transfusion is only given if the Hb is dangerously low, or if the patient's cardiovascular system is compromised by the anaemia.

Cold-acting autoantibodies are usually IgM antibodies that bind to erythrocytes in the peripheral circulation at lower temperatures and may cause red cell agglutination. Cold haemagglutinin disease (CHAD) is the most common form of cold AIHA. The idiopathic form of CHAD is more common in older patients, and often runs a chronic course. CHAD may also occur following an infection when polyclonal IgM forms as a response to the infection but cross-reacts with red cell antigens. Mild haemolysis usually develops 2–3 weeks after the infection, and is self-limiting. Rarely, severe intravascular haemolysis occurs following *Mycoplasma pneumoniae* infection. CHAD may also be associated with lymphoproliferative disorders.

Haemoglobinopathies

Mutation of globin genes or the genes that control their expression can result in changes in the amino acid sequence of globin, resulting in the synthesis of structurally abnormal or 'variant' Hb. A variant Hb may possess altered oxygen affinity, solubility or stability as compared to normal Hb. Globin gene mutation can also result in a reduced rate of synthesis of globin chains (thalassaemia). Mutation of the α- and β-globin genes causes α- and β-thalassaemia, respectively. The clinical severity of the condition corresponds to the number of genes affected.

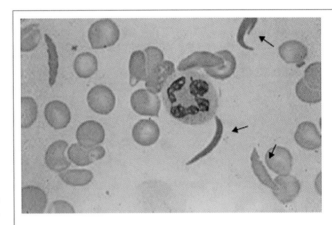

Figure 20A.4 Sickle cells.

Sickle cell disease (SCD)

Sickle cell haemoglobin (HbS) is an example of a β-chain variant in which mutation of the β-globin gene results in substitution of valine for glutamic acid at position 6 of the β-globin chain. On deoxygenation, the solubility of HbS is reduced, and polymerisation occurs. This distorts the red cell into a 'sickle' shape (Figure 20A.4). The deformed red cells occlude capillaries, leading to tissue hypoxia.

The sickle mutation is prevalent in Africa, the Mediterranean, the Americas and Asia. Homozygosity for haemoglobin S (HbSS) results in SCD. Heterozygosity (HbAS) is known as 'sickle cell trait', and is asymptomatic, but the mutated β-gene may be inherited by children. Sickle cell trait affords some protection against infection with *Plasmodium falciparum*. The mutated β-globin gene may also be co-inherited with other β-chain variants, causing the clinical features of SCD.

Clinical features of SCD

Dehydration, hypoxia or exposure to the cold or infection precipitates painful sickling of red cells, leading to vascular occlusion. Renal infarction can occur, with eventual progression to renal failure. Retinal ischaemia can jeopardise vision. Avascular necrosis or osteomyelitis can result from bony infarcts, and infarction of the skin can lead to ulceration. Recurrent pulmonary infarcts may lead to the development of pulmonary hypertension. In children, pooling of red cells in a rapidly enlarging spleen causes acute anaemia, and is known as 'splenic sequestration'. A life-threatening complication of SCD is the 'acute chest syndrome'. It is characterised by acute hypoxia, fever, chest pain and pulmonary infiltrates on the chest radiograph. The hypoxia can cause widespread sickling, leading to organ failure. Cerebral haemorrhage and infarction are also significant causes of morbidity. All patients are at increased risk of infection as they become functionally hyposplenic following recurrent splenic infarction. In addition, chronic haemolysis leads to the formation of pigment gallstones, and symptomatic patients should undergo cholecystectomy.

Acute management of a painful crisis

Painful sickling requires rehydration with intravenous fluids, oxygen support, opiate analgesia and antibiotics if infection is suspected. Prophylactic-dose low-molecular-weight heparin (LMWH) is given to prevent thrombotic events. Red cell transfusion or exchange transfusion may be required.

α-Thalassaemia

Reduced rate of production of α-globin is usually caused by deletions of one or more of the four α-genes on chromosome 16. Occasionally, α-thalassaemia may be non-deletional, due to point mutations causing gene dysfunction, or due to mutation in genes controlling α-gene expression.

Pathophysiology

Reduced production of α-globin results in an excess of γ- or β-chains that form tetramers (HbH and Hb Barts). HbH is unstable and precipitates out in red cells, forming red cell inclusions. Chronic extravascular haemolysis ensues as red cells are removed from the circulation by the spleen. In addition, HbH has a very high affinity for oxygen, resulting in reduced offloading of oxygen to the tissues.

'α-Thalassaemia trait' is caused by the deletion of either one or two of the α-genes. Patients often have a normal blood count or a mild hypochromic, microcytic anaemia and raised red cell count. Loss of three genes causes HbH disease, characterised by a moderate hypochromic, microcytic anaemia and splenomegaly. HbH comprises tetramers of β-chains. Loss of all four genes leads to total failure of α-chain synthesis, so that no synthesis of HbF, A or A_2 can occur. Hb Barts forms in the foetus, and is composed of four γ-chains. A severe anaemia develops, causing cardiac failure and a hydropic foetus. Death usually occurs *in utero* or shortly after birth.

β-Thalassaemia

Pathophysiology

Reduced or absent β-chain production results in an excess of α-chains, which form complexes with γ- or δ-chains to form HbF and HbA_2, respectively. The remaining α-chains precipitate out in developing erythroblasts, causing them to undergo apoptosis within the marrow, resulting in 'ineffective erythropoiesis'. Some mature red cells do enter the peripheral blood but, as they contain α-chain inclusions, they are removed by the spleen. The combination of ineffective erythropoiesis and haemolysis leads to anaemia. Anaemia, along with the high level of HbF, stimulates erythropoietin production and the marrow expands to compensate.

There are two allelic β-globin genes on chromosome 11. β-Thalassaemia results from the mutation of one or both β-genes, or the mutation of a gene controlling the β-gene expression. β-Thalassaemia heterozygosity (or 'β-thalassaemia trait') is symptomless, and carriers have a mild hypochromic, microcytic anaemia, raised red cell count and raised HbA_2.

Homozygosity or compound heterozygosity for β-thalassaemia (or 'β-thalassaemia major') produces a clinically severe phenotype. At 3–6 months of age, the switch from γ- to β-chain synthesis cannot occur, and anaemia develops. If untreated, marrow expansion causes bony deformity, such as bossing of the skull. Chronic haemolysis causes hepatosplenomegaly. These features can be largely avoided by regular red cell transfusion. Repeated transfusion leads to iron overload, however, and iron deposition in the liver, heart and endocrine organs. Without long-term iron chelation therapy, patients die young of cardiac failure or cardiac arrhythmias.

Red cell fragmentation syndromes

Fragmentation of red cells can occur when they come into contact with abnormal surfaces or turbulent blood flow. Common causes of physical damage to red cells are prosthetic cardiac valves, arterial grafts and arteriovenous malformations. Red cell fragmentation is often visible on a peripheral blood film (Figure 20A.5).

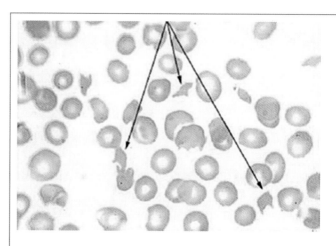

Figure 20A.5 Red cell fragmentation.

Microangiopathic haemolytic anaemia (MAHA) refers to the fragmentation of red cells due to an abnormal microcirculation. The pathological changes to the microvasculature that cause red cell damage include the deposition of fibrin strands in small vessels, vasculitis, and platelet adherence and aggregation. MAHA develops in conditions such as disseminated intravascular coagulation (DIC). In pregnancy, MAHA may be seen in preeclampsia and the associated haemolysis, elevated liver enzymes, low platelets (HELLP) syndrome.

Multiple myeloma

Multiple myeloma is a neoplastic proliferation of the bone marrow plasma cells. The condition has an annual incidence of approximately 50 per million in the UK, with a median age of presentation of 70 years.

Clinical presentation

Myeloma may present with a normochromic, normocytic (occasionally macrocytic) anaemia. The ESR is raised, and rouleaux (stacking of red cells on top of each other) formation is seen on the blood film (Figure 20A.6). Renal impairment and hypercalcaemia may develop. Osteolytic lesions cause bone pain, and recurrent infections may also be a feature. Occasionally, patients will present with symptoms of hyperviscosity (visual loss, haemorrhagic tendency, neurological symptoms and cardiac failure), spinal cord compression or have features of amyloidosis.

Investigations

Monoclonal protein is often detectable in serum and/or urine. An IgG paraprotein is detected in approximately two-thirds of cases, and an IgA paraprotein in one-third. IgD and IgM myeloma are rare. Normal serum immunoglobulins may be reduced, increasing the risk of infection. Free κ or λ light chain may be detectable in the urine (Bence–Jones protein).

Rare cases of non-secretory myeloma may be difficult to diagnose, as there is no detectable serum or urine paraprotein. Serum free light chain assay is abnormal (showing an abnormal ratio of κ:λ light chain in the serum), and a plasma cell infiltrate can be demonstrated in the marrow. Bone marrow biopsy is required to confirm a clonal plasma cell infiltrate. Skeletal survey (plain X-rays of the skeleton) can demonstrate lytic lesions. CT and MRI are useful for detailed images of the skeleton or soft tissue masses, and to investigate suspected spinal cord lesions.

Tables 20A.6 and 20A.7 highlight the diagnostic criteria for asymptomatic and symptomatic multiple myeloma.

Prognosis

Poor prognostic markers include high serum levels of β-2-microglobulin, low serum albumin and poor risk cytogenetic abnormalities within the neoplastic clone.

Treatment

Prior to commencing chemotherapy, acute renal failure can often be improved with intravenous fluids, although some patients may require renal replacement therapy. Hypercalcaemia also requires intravenous rehydration and, occasionally, treatment with a bisphosphonate. Urgent radiotherapy is used to treat impending cord compression, and can also help to control bone pain.

Patients under the age of 65 years with an adequate performance status are eligible to undergo intensive chemotherapy followed by autologous haemopoietic stem cell transplantation. Autologous transplantation involves the harvesting of stem cells from the patient and storing them. Myeloablative conditioning

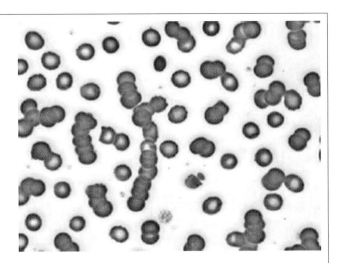

Figure 20A.6 Rouleaux formation.

Table 20A.6 Diagnostic criteria for myeloma.

Asymptomatic myeloma	Symptomatic myeloma
Serum paraprotein >30 g/l and/or bone marrow clonal plasma cells >10%	Paraprotein detected in serum and/or urine
No myeloma-related end-organ damage	Bone marrow clonal plasma cells or biopsy-proven plasmacytoma
	Any myeloma-related end-organ damage

Table 20A.7 Myeloma-related end-organ damage.

Hypercalcaemia.
Renal insufficiency.
Anaemia.
Bone lesions.
Other – symptomatic hyperviscosity, amyloidosis, recurrent bacterial infections.

chemotherapy is then given, which results in marrow aplasia. The patient is then 'rescued' by stem cell infusion, allowing the marrow to repopulate.

Myeloma is currently incurable, with a median survival varying between 3 and 6 years. The only potentially curative procedure is allogeneic stem cell transplantation, but this option is only available to selected younger patients. Reduced-intensity allogeneic transplants for older patients are not widely performed (see the section on allogeneic transplantation in acute leukaemia).

Osteonecrosis of the jaw

Bisphosphonates are given to all patients with symptomatic myeloma to prevent the progression of bone disease. They act mainly by inhibiting osteoclast activity. Oral preparations (clodronate) and intravenous preparations (pamidronate and zoledronic acid) are available. In recent years, there have been increasing reports of a complication of bisphosphonate therapy called 'osteonecrosis of the jaw' (ONJ). Lesions develop in the maxilla and/or mandible. Osteonecrosis is discussed in Chapter 15 (titled 'Adverse drug reactions and interactions').

Bone marrow failure syndromes

Acute leukaemias

Acute leukaemias are aggressive disorders characterised by the accumulation of malignant white cells in the bone marrow and blood. The malignant cells are early bone marrow haemopoietic progenitors called *blast cells* (Figure 20A.7). In a normal marrow, <5% of the nucleated cells are blasts. However, in acute leukaemia, by definition, the percentage of blasts in the marrow or peripheral blood is ≥20%. Without treatment, the median survival of acute leukaemia is only a few months.

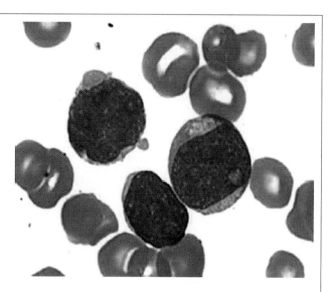

Figure 20A.7 Blast cells in the peripheral blood.

Acute leukaemia is broadly subdivided into 'acute myeloid leukaemia' (AML) and 'acute lymphoblastic leukaemia' (ALL), depending on whether the blasts are myeloid or lymphoid in origin. This is determined from blast cell morphology, and from whether myeloid or lymphoid cell markers are detected on the blasts (immunophenotyping). AML is subtyped according to cytogenetic abnormalities within the blasts, the presence of multilineage dysplasia, whether the leukaemia is therapy related, and by blast cell morphology. ALL is subtyped according to the blast cell immunophenotype (whether the lymphoid blasts are B-cells or T-cells), and their stage of differentiation. AML is predominantly a disease of adulthood, with a median age of presentation of 60 years. ALL commonly occurs in children.

Clinical presentation

Blast cell infiltration of the marrow causes bone marrow failure, leading to peripheral blood cytopaenias. Patients present with symptoms of lethargy and dyspnoea due to anaemia, and may have recurrent infections and mouth ulcers due to neutropaenia. Severe thrombocytopaenia results in bruising, petechiae and mucosal haemorrhage, such as epistaxis and gum bleeding. Blast cell infiltration of tissues can cause hepatosplenomegaly, lymphadenopathy, skin rashes and gum hypertrophy. ALL, in particular, has a predilection for the CNS, testes and thymus.

Investigations

- FBC shows the presence of cytopaenias. Some patients may have a high white cell count owing to the presence of blasts in the peripheral blood.
- The coagulation screen demonstrates that the presence of blasts in the blood can trigger DIC, which is recognised by the presenting feature of acute promyelocytic leukaemia, a type of AML.
- The blood film may show circulating blast cells. Dysplastic features in blood cells suggest evolution from myelodysplasia.
- A bone marrow biopsy should be performed.
- Cytogenetic analysis is usually performed on marrow cells and provides prognostic information.
- The use of immunophenotyping of primitive cells to determine blast cell lineage has largely replaced immunocytochemistry in all but the most difficult cases.
- All children undergo lumbar puncture at diagnosis to obtain a sample of the CSF, which is examined for leukaemia cells.

Management – supportive care

All patients fit for intensive chemotherapy require the insertion of a tunnelled central venous catheter to administer chemotherapy; other drugs such as antiemetics, antibiotics or antifungal agents; and blood products. The line can also be used for phlebotomy. Patients with high white cell counts, significant organ infiltration or high serum urate levels are at risk of developing hyperkalaemia, hyperuricaemia and acute renal failure on commencing chemotherapy (the 'tumour lysis syndrome'). This can be avoided by intravenous hydration and the use of allopurinol (a xanthine oxidase inhibitor) prior to chemotherapy. All patients require the prompt treatment of infections. Antiviral and antifungal agents are used to prevent infection. Patients receive specific prophylaxis against *Pneumocystis carinii (jiroveci)*, which causes pneumonia in immunosuppressed patients. Side effects of treatment include potentially life-threatening neutropaenic sepsis, nausea and vomiting, hair loss, and infertility.

Cytotoxic therapy

Intensive treatment begins with induction chemotherapy, in which combinations of drugs are used to induce *morphological remission*, defined as the presence of <5% blasts in a normocellular marrow. Consolidation chemotherapy is then required to eliminate the hidden leukaemic cell population. In AML, patients usually undergo four cycles of chemotherapy at 3–4-week intervals. In childhood ALL, following consolidation, maintenance treatment is given to boys for 3 years and to girls for 2 years. Children with high-risk ALL and all patients with CNS disease require CNS-directed therapy, as standard chemotherapy cannot effectively cross the blood–brain barrier. High-dose intravenous methotrexate and intrathecal injections of chemotherapy are commonly used. Cranial irradiation can also be used in children with ALL with CNS disease at presentation.

Older patients who are not fit for intensive treatment can be given non-intensive chemotherapy to control the disease. Patients who are not fit for non-intensive chemotherapy can be managed with transfusion support and hydroxycarbamide to control the white cell count.

Prognosis

ALL in children between the ages of 1 and 9 years has an excellent cure rate with chemotherapy alone. Poor-risk groups include infants; those with a high white cell count at presentation; those with poor-risk cytogenetics such as t(9,22) (the Philadelphia chromosome); and those with poor early response to treatment, which can now be identified through the monitoring of minimal residual disease (MRD). MRD represents the number of leukaemia cells that can be detected by laboratory techniques with a sensitivity of 1 in 10 (i.e. that are able to detect 1 leukaemia cell in 10 000 marrow cells).

The outcome of AML in adults depends largely on the age of the patients, the cytogenetic abnormalities present in their leukaemia cells, and their responses to induction.

Patients with AML over the age of 60 years have a worse outlook, which partly reflects the higher proportion of cases with high-risk cytogenetics, resistant disease and a history of evolution from myelodysplasia.

Allogeneic transplantation

Allogeneic stem cell transplantation involves the harvesting of stem cells from a donor who may be a human leukocyte antigen (HLA)–matched sibling or, if no sibling match is available, a matched unrelated donor (MUD). Myeloablative conditioning (chemotherapy with/without total body irradiation) is given, and the donor stem cells are then infused. The patient is at risk of severe infections that may be life threatening. Once engraftment occurs, graft-versus-host disease (GvHD) can develop. Donor T-cells in the graft attack the host's cells, causing inflammation, which can affect several different organs.

In some diseases, reduced-intensity allogeneic transplants are performed in older patients. Immunosuppressive rather than myeloablative conditioning is used, and success depends on optimising the graft-versus-leukaemia effect – that is, donor T-cells in the graft attacking the neoplastic cells remaining in the host.

In paediatric ALL, allogeneic transplantation in first remission is only considered in very-high-risk disease. Early relapse in the marrow will require re-induction and serious consideration of an allogeneic transplant.

Patients with high-risk AML are considered for allogeneic stem cell transplantation in first remission if they have a HLA-identical sibling. Standard-risk patients may be offered an allograft as part of a clinical trial. Patients who relapse following chemotherapy are also eligible for allogeneic transplantation, with long-term disease-free survival rates of 30–40%. Myeloablative allogeneic transplant carries a transplant-related mortality of approximately 20%, risk of developing acute and chronic GvHD, and an increased risk of secondary cancers, especially if total body irradiation is used in conditioning.

Myelodysplastic syndromes (MDSs)

MDSs are a group of clonal stem cell disorders characterised by dysplasia and ineffective haematopoiesis in one or more of the major myeloid cell lines. MDS occurs predominantly in older individuals, with a median age of presentation of 70 years. MDS may arise *de novo*, or can develop following exposure to alkylating agents and/or radiotherapy.

The majority of patients present with symptoms related to their low blood counts (anaemia, thrombocytopaenia or neutropaenia). Blood cells with dysplastic features may be seen on the blood film. The marrow is dysplastic and usually hypercellular or normocellular; the cytopaenias result from ineffective haematopoiesis. Cytogenetic analysis of marrow cells is important as karyotype affects the prognosis of the disorder. Cytogenetic abnormalities can be divided into good-risk, intermediate-risk and poor-risk abnormalities.

Overall prognosis is dependent on age, percentage of bone marrow blasts, karyotype and number of cytopaenias.

Aplastic anaemia (AA)

AA is characterised by diminished or absent haemopoietic precursors in the bone marrow, most often due to injury to the pluripotent stem cell. AA is a rare condition, with an incidence in Europe of approximately 2 per million per year. Both congenital and acquired forms exist.

The condition has a biphasic age distribution, with peaks between the ages of 10 and 25 years and over the age of 60 years. Patients present with symptoms related to their cytopaenias, and commonly have pancytopaenia, macrocytosis and reticulocytopaenia with a hypocellular marrow. Cytogenetic abnormalities are only found in a small proportion of cases. The clinical severity of the disease can be classified according to the blood count and marrow cellularity.

Patients with non-severe AA require transfusion support. Immunosuppressive therapy with horse or rabbit antithymocyte globulin (ATG), in combination with ciclosporin, is used if the patient becomes transfusion dependent.

Young patients with severe or very severe AA are eligible for allografting if they have an HLA-identical sibling. If no matched sibling is available, a trial of immunosuppressive treatment is given, and a matched unrelated donor (MUD) transplant is considered if immunosuppression fails to improve counts. Patients over the age of 40 years are given immunosuppressive therapy prior to the consideration of transplant.

Chronic myeloproliferative disorders (MPDs)

The classical MPDs are polycythaemia rubra vera (PRV), essential thrombocythaemia (ET) and idiopathic myelofibrosis (IMF). They are clonal stem cell disorders characterised by proliferation in the marrow of one or more of the myeloid lineages. Patients have raised blood counts and may have a palpable spleen. All MPDs can progress to marrow failure as a result of myelofibrosis, or can undergo clonal evolution and transform to acute leukaemia.

Almost all patients with PRV have an acquired point mutation. Untreated PRV carries a high risk of thrombosis. Isolated erythrocytosis can be treated with venesection, aiming for a haematocrit of 0.45. If the platelet or white cell count is also raised, hydroxycarbamide is used to control the counts.

ET presents with thrombocytosis. High-risk patients (over the age of 60 years, previous thrombotic event, platelet count $>1000 \times 10^9$/l) require treatment with hydroxycarbamide. Low-dose aspirin is also given once the platelet count begins to fall (patients may be haemorrhagic with very high platelet counts).

IMF may initially present with raised counts and a hypercellular marrow. However, over time, the marrow becomes progressively hypocellular and fibrotic. The liver and spleen may enlarge significantly to compensate for the marrow failure (extramedullary haemopoiesis). Many patients eventually require transfusion support.

Lymphomas

The lymphomas are a heterogeneous group of diseases caused by malignant lymphocytes that usually accumulate in lymph nodes, causing lymphadenopathy, but may enter the peripheral blood or infiltrate organs. Lymphomas are histologically subdivided into non-Hodgkin lymphoma (NHL) and Hodgkin lymphoma.

Hodgkin lymphoma

The WHO histological classification divides Hodgkin lymphomas into two disease entities:

- Nodular lymphocyte–predominant Hodgkin lymphoma (NLPHL).
- Classical Hodgkin lymphoma (CHL).

NLPHL

NLPHL is characterised histologically by neoplastic B-cells (known as 'lymphocytic and histiocytic' or 'L&H' cells) residing in a meshwork of follicular dendritic cells and reactive lymphocytes. The neoplastic cells are atypical variants of the Reed–Sternberg (RS) cells seen in CHL (see the following text), and they harbour damaged immunoglobulin genes.

NLPHL usually presents in relatively young men aged 30–50 years, with localised peripheral lymphadenopathy. Surgical excision, combined with involved field radiotherapy (if excision is not complete), is usually successful in controlling localised disease in the long term.

CHL

In CHL, neoplastic B-cells (RS cells) sit among inflammatory cells such as eosinophils, plasma cells, reactive lymphocytes and histiocytes. RS cells are large cells with abundant cytoplasm and a bi-lobed nucleus. They harbour immunoglobulin gene rearrangements and demonstrate characteristic staining patterns with immunohistochemical stains. CHL can be subtyped based on the histological appearance of the lymph node (Table 20A.8).

CHL has a bimodal age distribution, with a peak at 15–35 years and a second peak in later life. About 75% of cases involve cervical lymph nodes, and the disease spreads contiguously. B symptoms (see Table 20A.9) may be present, and confer a worse prognosis. CT is used to determine the extent of disease at diagnosis, and staging is based on the Ann Arbor staging system with Cotswold modifications (see Table 20A.10).

Table 20A.8 Histological subtypes of CHL.

Nodular sclerosis.
Mixed cellularity.
Lymphocyte depleted.
Lymphocyte rich.

Table 20A.9 B symptoms.

Recurrent drenching night sweats during the previous 1 month.

Unexplained, persistent or recurrent fever (>38°C) during the previous 1 month.

Unexplained weight loss of >10% body weight during the previous 6 months.

Table 20A.10 Cotswold revision of the Ann Arbor staging system.

Stage I	Involvement of a single lymph node region or lymphoid structure.
Stage II	Involvement of two or more lymph node regions on the same side of the diaphragm.
Stage III	Involvement of lymph node regions or structures on both sides of the diaphragm.
Stage IV	Involvement of extranodal site(s) beyond those designated E.

A = absence of B symptoms; B = B symptoms present; X = bulky disease; E = involvement of a single extranodal site, contiguous or proximal to the known nodal site of disease.

Treatment

Localised disease (stages I and IIA) can be categorised as favourable or unfavourable based on prognostic factors at diagnosis – such as age, number of nodal regions involved, presence of B symptoms and the presence of bulky mediastinal disease. Both favourable and unfavourable early stage disease is treated with three to four cycles of combination chemotherapy.

Advanced disease (stages IIB, III and IV) requires six to eight cycles of combination chemotherapy. Consolidation radiotherapy is used for patients with bulky disease at diagnosis. Positron emission tomography (PET)/CT following two cycles of chemotherapy may be useful in identifying patients who require more intensive primary treatment.

Relapsed disease is usually salvageable with chemotherapy, especially if the duration of the first remission is long. Autologous stem cell transplantation is considered for patients who relapse within 3 years of treatment and those with primary resistant disease. Non-myeloablative allogeneic stem cell transplantation may be an option for patients who relapse following an autograft.

NHL

NHL encompasses many histological subtypes that vary in clinical aggressiveness and prognosis. The WHO histological classification broadly divides NHL into the B-cell and T-cell neoplasms, and takes into account the immunophenotype of the neoplastic cell, the site of origin of the tumour and its clinical aggressiveness.

The majority of patients present with nodal disease, with or without B symptoms. Extranodal involvement is less common. Lymph node biopsy is required to identify the histological subtype, and the disease is staged using CT and bone marrow biopsy. The staging system used is the same as that described for Hodgkin lymphoma.

The most common mature B-cell neoplasms are diffuse large B-cell NHL (DLBCL) and follicular NHL, which together make up 50% of all NHL. DLBCL is an aggressive lymphoma with different morphological variants. Prognosis is assessed at diagnosis using the International Prognostic Index (IPI), which takes into account factors such as age, stage, performance score, serum lactate dehydrogenase (LDH) and extranodal involvement. The 5-year survival in patients with a low IPI score is 83%, as compared to 32% for those with a high score.

Treatment of stage II, III or IV DLBCL is with CHOP chemotherapy (cyclophosphamide, doxorubicin, vincristine, prednisolone) combined with rituximab. Rituximab is a monoclonal antibody that targets the CD20 surface marker found on B-cells.

Follicular NHL is an indolent B-cell NHL. Most patients present with stage III and IV disease, but do not require treatment if they are asymptomatic. Once symptoms appear, CVP-R (cyclophosphamide, vincristine and prednisolone with rituximab) can be used as first-line treatment, and has approval from NICE. NICE guidance issued in 2008 allows the use of combination chemotherapy plus rituximab to induce remission in patients with relapsed stage III or IV disease, and also allows rituximab monotherapy to be used to maintain remission.

The mature T-cell and natural killer cell neoplasms make up only a small proportion of NHL, and most are clinically aggressive, requiring intensive chemotherapy. In general, they respond less well to chemotherapy than aggressive B-cell NHL, and therefore autologous stem cell transplantation is often considered in first remission.

20B   HAEMOSTASIS

Overview of normal haemostasis

Haemostasis refers to the process whereby blood coagulation and clot breakdown are initiated and terminated in a highly regulated manner. The traditional model of the coagulation cascade has been superseded by the concept of 'coagulation network' (Figure 20B.1). This newer model recognises the central role of tissue factor in the initiation of coagulation.

In vivo clot formation involves a complex interaction between the vascular endothelium, platelets, von Willebrand factor (vWF) and coagulation factors. This interaction leads to the generation of thrombin and the formation of a stable fibrin clot. To prevent inappropriate extension of the clot, the process is controlled by naturally occurring anticoagulants and the fibrinolytic system. Cellular models of coagulation demonstrate that the interaction between tissue factor and factor VII is of primary importance in the initiation of coagulation, and that many of the coagulation reactions occur on the surface of cells, particularly platelets (Figure 20B.2).

Normally, the coagulant and anticoagulant components of the process are in perfect balance. Bleeding or thrombosis may occur when this balance is disturbed.

Inherited bleeding disorders

Haemophilia A

Haemophilia A is an X-linked recessive bleeding disorder characterised by a low or absent level of factor VIII coagulant

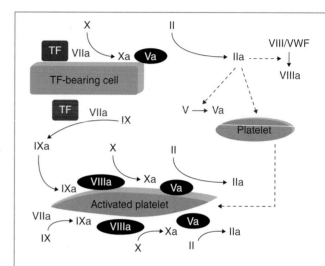

Figure 20B.2 Cellular model of haemostasis.

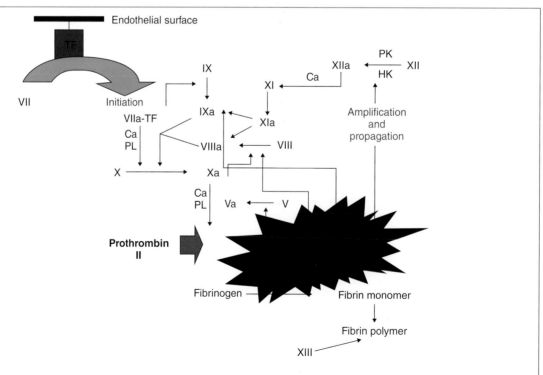

Figure 20B.1 The coagulation network. The Roman numerals refer to the various factors.

activity (FVIII:C) in the plasma. The worldwide incidence of haemophilia A is estimated at 1 in 5000 male births. It is caused by mutation in the FVIII gene, which disrupts the production of FVIII, an essential component of the coagulation system. The majority of patients are males who have a family history of the disorder. Up to one-third of cases result from spontaneous mutation. The FVIII gene is located on the long arm of the X chromosome.

Haemophilia B

Haemophilia B is caused by mutation of the FIX gene on the X chromosome, resulting in low or absent levels of FIX in the plasma. Haemophilia B is less common than haemophilia A (1 in 25 000 males worldwide), but it has the same mode of inheritance, and is clinically indistinguishable from haemophilia A.

The clinical severity of haemophilia directly correlates with the baseline FVIII or IX level in the blood (Table 20B.1).

A child with severe haemophilia classically presents with unexplained severe bruising or bleeding when he or she first begins to mobilise. Moderate and mild haemophilia may not be diagnosed until later in childhood, or even in adulthood. The main weight-bearing joints (ankles, knees and elbows) are commonly affected in severe haemophilia, although bleeding can occur into any joint. Recurrent or poorly treated haemarthroses may lead to progressive joint deformity and disability (Figure 20B.3). Muscle bleeding can occur at any site, but most commonly presents in the load-bearing muscles of the thighs, calves, buttocks and posterior abdominal walls. Although uncommon, spontaneous intracranial haemorrhage occurs more frequently in patients with severe haemophilia than in the general population, and was a significant cause of death in the past. Oropharyngeal bleeding is also uncommon, but is potentially life threatening, since extension through the soft tissues of the floor of the mouth may compromise the airway.

Laboratory diagnosis

- Coagulation screen shows a prolonged activated partial thromboplastin time (APTT), with a normal prothrombin time and fibrinogen.
- Factor assays demonstrate a low or absent level of FVIII or IX, with other factor assays normal.
- Normal thrombin time.
- Normal vWF level.

Treatment

All patients with moderate or severe haemophilia are registered at a Haemophilia Comprehensive Care Centre, where there is a multidisciplinary team approach to their care. Patients are provided with green haemorrhagic states cards, which detail their diagnoses and the types of treatment they require for bleeding episodes. The cards also provide the contact details of the haemophilia specialists involved in their care.

Bleeding episodes into muscles and joints require bed rest, immobilisation of the affected joint or muscle, factor replacement and physiotherapy input. Patients with mild haemophilia A may be given DDAVP (1-deamino-8-D-arginine vasopressin, a synthetic analogue of vasopressin), rather than factor replacement (Table 20B.2).

Minor bleeding, particularly mucosal bleeding, often responds to antifibrinolytic agents such as tranexamic acid.

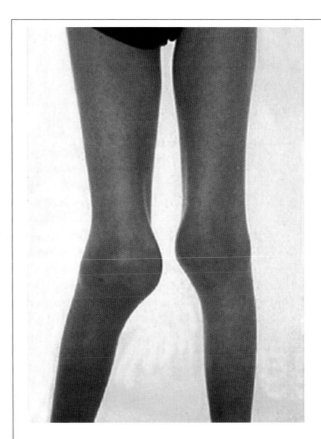

Figure 20B.3 Haemophiliac arthropathy.

Table 20B.1 Clinical features of haemophilia A and B.

Severity of haemophilia	FVIII/IX concentration	Clinical features
Severe	<1%	Spontaneous bleeding episodes, predominantly into joints or muscles
Moderate	1–5%	Some spontaneous bleeding, bleeding after minor trauma
Mild	>5%	Bleeding after surgery and trauma

Table 20B.2 DDAVP.

DDAVP can be given intravenously, subcutaneously or intranasally.

It stimulates the release of FVIII and vWF from vascular endothelial cells. FVIII levels peak 30–60 min post-infusion, but the length of response varies between patients.

Side effects include flushing, headache, water retention, hyponatraemia, seizures and myocardial infarction.

To minimise some of these side effects, all patients should be fluid restricted to 1 litre for 24 hours after treatment.

The drug is contraindicated in pregnancy, in children under the age of 2 years and in those with a history of epilepsy. The drug should also be used with caution in the elderly.

The response to DDAVP diminishes with successive infusions (tachyphylaxis), and hence repeated infusions to treat a single bleeding episode are not recommended.

Tranexamic acid is a synthetic amino acid that inhibits fibrinolysis by binding to the lysine-binding site on plasmin, thereby preventing the substrate fibrin from binding. It should be used with caution in patients with a history of ischaemic heart disease or stroke, and in patients at high risk of thrombosis.

Most female carriers of haemophilia have normal coagulation factor levels, or have levels at the low end of the normal range. A small minority have lower FVIII or FIX levels, requiring haemostatic cover prior to surgery.

In the UK, the majority of patients with severe haemophilia begin regular factor replacement two to three times a week after they have their first major bleed. The aim of prophylaxis is to prevent spontaneous bleeding episodes by maintaining the plasma factor concentration at >1%. The availability of factor concentrates in the UK and the use of prophylaxis means that many patients with severe haemophilia develop little or no arthropathy nowadays. Many patients can now lead an active life, with normal educational and employment opportunities.

Patients with moderate or mild haemophilia do not require prophylaxis, and receive 'on demand' treatment only (factor replacement to treat bleeds when they occur).

The development of recombinant products

Over the past 50 years, there have been significant advances in the development of safer and more effective treatments for haemophilia. The legacy of virus infection of haemophiliacs from blood products during the 1980s has been a driving factor in the development of recombinant products (products not manufactured from donated blood).

Variant Creutzfeldt–Jakob disease (vCJD) was first recognised in 1996, and is thought to be caused by dietary exposure to the bovine spongiform encephalopathy (BSE) agent that infects cattle. The infectious agent is abnormal prion protein. To minimise the potential risk of transmission through blood products, a number of precautionary measures have been introduced.

In addition to these measures, for public health purposes, all patients who have received UK plasma between 1980 and 2001 are considered to be at risk of vCJD. Therefore, they cannot donate blood, organs or other tissues. Also, following some invasive procedures, the surgical instruments used on these individuals may not be used for other patients.

Management of haemophilia patients undergoing dental surgery

Patients should inform their dental practitioners if they suffer from bleeding disorders, and they should carry their green haemorrhagic states cards. Close liaison is required with a haemophilia centre, since patients will require haemostatic treatment pre- and postoperatively. DDAVP infusion can be used preoperatively for mild haemophiliacs. Patients with moderate and severe haemophilia require FVIII/IX replacement prior to surgery, with monitoring of factor levels to ensure that an adequate factor concentration has been achieved to cover the procedure. Factor levels are taken immediately prior to factor infusion (trough level) and 15 min after infusion (post-level).

During surgery, an atraumatic technique is important, with close attention paid to securing local haemostasis. Oral tranexamic acid or tranexamic acid mouthwash can be used postoperatively to reduce postoperative bleeding. The principles of managing haemophilia patients undergoing dental surgery are summarised in Table 20B.3.

von Willebrand disease

von Willebrand disease (vWD) is the most common inherited bleeding disorder, affecting up to 1% of the UK population. The classifications of the disease are shown in Tables 20B.4 and 20B.5.

Table 20B.3 Management of haemophilia patients undergoing dental surgery.

Close liaison with haemophilia centres.

Preoperative infusion of haemostatic product, with close monitoring of plasma factor levels.

Perioperative use of atraumatic technique; secure local haemostasis.

Postoperative use of tranexamic acid.

Table 20B.4 Primary classification of vWD.

	Type of vWF deficiency	vWF protein function
Type 1	Quantitative partial deficiency	Normal
Type 2	Qualitative functional deficiency	Abnormal
Type 3	Quantitative complete deficiency	Undetectable

Table 20B.5 Classification of type 2 vWD.

Subtype	Platelet-binding function	FVIII-binding capacity	Multimer analysis
2A	Decreased	Normal	Absent multimers
2B	Increased affinity for glycoprotein 1b	Normal	Usually reduced or absent
2M	Decreased	Normal	Normal and occasionally ultra-large forms
2N	Normal	Markedly reduced	Normal

The primary defect common to all variants is the deficiency of vWF functional activity, causing impaired haemostasis. The abnormality is either quantitative (i.e. a reduced level of vWF) or qualitative (i.e. an abnormal function of vWF). vWF has two main functions:

- It acts as the carrier molecule for FVIII in the circulation, preventing degradation of FVIII (which explains why some patients with vWD who have low levels of vWF also have low FVIII levels).
- It promotes platelet adhesion to damaged vascular endothelium, and therefore has a role in primary haemostasis.

Enhanced release of vWF can be stimulated by vasopressin (which explains why DDAVP is used in the treatment of vWD), pregnancy, hyperthyroidism, stress, exercise, acute inflammation and malignancy. Neonates have a raised vWF level, which only falls to adult levels by 6 months of age. Thus, type 1 vWD cannot be reliably diagnosed in children under the age of 6 months, and repeat tests are needed when they are older.

The vWF gene is located on chromosome 12 and is an extremely large gene. The genotypic basis of the disorder is not yet fully established. Multiple causative mutations have been identified. In some patients with type 1 vWD, the genetic defect appears to lie outside the vWF gene itself.

Clinical features

Patients have a variable bleeding phenotype and may have a positive family history of bleeding. Type 1 and 2 vWD commonly present with easy bruising, mucosal bleeding (epistaxis, menorrhagia, gastrointestinal bleeding) and post-surgical or post-traumatic bleeding. Type 3 vWD presents with joint and muscle bleeds, in a similar fashion to severe haemophilia. Unlike haemophilia, small vessel bleeding also occurs.

Laboratory diagnosis

- FBC: thrombocytopaenia may be seen in type 2B vWD.
- Coagulation screen: a prolongation of the APTT may occur.
- FVIII levels may be reduced.
- The vWD screen assesses the amount of vWF in plasma (vWF:ag), and its function.

vWF function can be assessed by:

- In the FVIII binding capacity test, an FVIII assay is performed initially; if reduced, vWF is assayed.

- FVIII binding capacity is measured via an enzyme-linked immunosorbent assay (ELISA).
- In the platelet-dependent function test (ristocetin cofactor activity, or 'RiCof'), dilutions of patient plasma are tested for their ability to promote platelet agglutination in the presence of the antibiotic ristocetin.

Treatment

Milder bleeding phenotypes can be managed with local haemostatic measures in combination with antifibrinolytic agents. Patients with type 1 vWD respond to DDAVP. Patients with type 2 and 3 vWD require treatment with intermediate-purity FVIII concentrates, which contain both FVIII and VWF. These are plasma-derived products that are virus inactivated. Monitoring of treatment is required using trough and 15-min post-infusion levels. Depending on the type of vWD, determination of vWF:ag levels, FVIII levels and functional assays may be required during monitoring.

The management of patients with vWD undergoing dental surgery follows the same broad principles as outlined earlier for haemophilia patients.

Acquired vWD

Rarely, patients with no family history of bleeding and no prior bleeding problems can present with bleeding symptoms identical to those with hereditary vWD.

Pathological mechanisms include autoantibody formation, adsorption of vWF onto cells, disintegration of vWF by shear stress within the circulation, increased proteolysis of vWF and reduced synthesis of vWF.

Rare inherited coagulation disorders

The rare inherited coagulation disorders are autosomal recessive conditions with a low prevalence, varying between 1 in 500 000 and 1 in 2 million. The disorders are prevalent in populations in which consanguineous marriages are common. FXIII and FX deficiencies, and occasionally afibrinogenaemia, are associated with a severe bleeding phenotype, and may present with umbilical stump bleeding or bleeding into the CNS.

Table 20B.6 The inherited platelet disorders.
Inherited thrombocytopaenias.
Severe disorders of platelet function (e.g. Glanzmann's thrombasthenia, Wiskott–Aldrich syndrome).
Disorders of receptors and signal transduction pathways.
Abnormalities of platelet granules (e.g. storage pool disorders).
Disorders of phospholipid exposure.

Table 20B.7 Acquired disorders of coagulation.
Liver disease.
DIC.
Massive blood loss.
Acquired haemophilia.
Vitamin K deficiency.

Inherited platelet disorders

Inherited platelet disorders are rare, and they encompass disorders affecting platelet number and/or function (Table 20B.6). Severe disorders of platelet function present in early childhood with severe mucosal bleeding – such as CNS or umbilical stump bleeding, or bruising on handling. Milder disorders present later in life with bleeding following a haemostatic challenge such as dental extractions.

Glanzmann's thrombasthenia is a severe disorder characterised by a deficiency or functional defect of platelet glycoprotein (GP) IIb/IIIa, which mediates aggregation of activated platelets. Patients can be managed with antifibrinolytics. Platelet transfusion is usually avoided, as it can stimulate the formation of HLA antibodies, resulting in platelet refractoriness. Recombinant FVIIa is licensed for use in patients who develop platelet refractoriness.

Acquired disorders of haemostasis

Acquired coagulation disorders are listed in Table 20B.7. In DIC, the release of procoagulant material into the circulation triggers widespread activation of coagulation, leading to the consumption of clotting factors and platelets, and intravascular fibrin deposition. Patients may present acutely with a bleeding diathesis or, less commonly, with microthrombosis. Occasionally, the condition runs a more chronic course. Laboratory tests show a prolonged PT, APTT and thrombin time, low fibrinogen, raised D-dimers and thrombocytopaenia. A large number of conditions are associated with DIC, including sepsis, trauma, malignancy and obstetric complications.

Acquired haemophilia is a rare condition in which an autoantibody (inhibitor) directed against FVIII develops, which can cause severe bleeding. The condition usually presents in the elderly, and may be idiopathic or secondary to an underlying autoimmune condition or malignancy. Occasionally, it occurs in young women in the post-partum period. Extensive bruising, mucosal haemorrhage and bleeding into the muscles may occur. The APTT is prolonged and, following incubation of the sample for 1 hour at 37°C, a 50:50 mix with normal plasma fails to correct the APTT by >50%, indicating the presence of an inhibitor. FVIII levels are low, and the inhibitor can be quantified. Significant bleeding is treated with FVIII inhibitor–bypassing agent or recombinant FVIIa. Immunosuppression is also commenced to eradicate the inhibitor.

Vitamin K deficiency is commonly seen in newborns. At birth, infants have low levels of vitamin K–dependent clotting factors. Vitamin K levels can fall further in the first few days of life, particularly if the infant is breastfed, as breast milk contains very little vitamin K. Liver immaturity and an inability to synthesise vitamin K due to lack of gut flora also contribute to the deficiency. Bleeding may develop (haemorrhagic disease of the newborn) from any site, and intracranial haemorrhage is a potential complication. Bleeding can be prevented by the prophylactic administration of vitamin K after birth.

Acquired platelet disorders

Tables 20B.8 and 20B.9 list some of the common acquired causes of thrombocytopaenia and platelet dysfunction.

Acute idiopathic thrombocytopaenic purpura (ITP) in children can develop following a virus infection. Autoantibodies form that attach to the platelets and cause them to be removed early from the circulation by the spleen. The child is well, with a short history of purpura and petechiae and an isolated thrombocytopaenia. In the majority of cases, the condition is self-limiting. Therefore, if the child has only minor bleeding, no intervention is required, even if the platelet count is $<10 \times 10^9$/l. If the child has significant mucosal haemorrhage, treatment can be given to raise the platelet count. Intravenous immunoglobulin will raise the platelet count transiently. If the platelet count is not improving after 6–8 weeks, a bone marrow biopsy is required to confirm the diagnosis before commencing steroids.

Adult ITP may be idiopathic, or can be associated with other autoimmune conditions, HIV and malignancy. The diagnosis is one of exclusion. A bone marrow aspirate shows plentiful megakaryocytes, indicating normal platelet production. If the platelet count is $>30 \times 10^9$/l, no treatment is required. If the platelet count is lower or the patient has significant mucosal bleeding, patients are usually given high-dose prednisolone as first-line treatment to suppress autoantibody production.

TTP classically presents with MAHA, thrombocytopaenia, fever, fluctuating neurological signs and renal impairment, although, in many cases, only MAHA and thrombocytopaenia are seen. Platelet microthrombi form, particularly in renal and cerebral vessels. Urgent treatment in the form of daily plasma

Table 20B.8 Acquired causes of thrombocytopaenia.

Bone marrow failure – haemopoietic stem cell disorder, marrow infiltration.

Drugs (e.g. cytotoxics).

Infection – viruses, malaria.

Increased consumption of platelets.

- Immune (e.g. idiopathic thrombocytopaenic purpura (ITP), heparin-induced thrombocytopaenia, other drugs such as gold, penicillins, quinine).
- Non-immune (e.g. TTP, DIC).

Abnormal distribution of platelets – pooling within an enlarged spleen.

Dilutional (e.g. massive transfusion).

Table 20B.9 Acquired disorders of platelet function.

Drugs (e.g. antiplatelet agents).

Myeloproliferative disorders.

Paraproteinaemia.

Uraemia.

Table 20B.10 BCSH recommendations for patients requiring invasive procedures in the community who are stably anticoagulated with International Normalised Ratios (INRs) between 2 and 4.

Warfarin should not be discontinued, because the risk of serious embolic complications associated with temporary cessation of warfarin outweighs the risk of significant bleeding.

Check INR 72 hours prior to surgery.

Table 20B.11 Other key BCSH recommendations.

Patients on warfarin requiring non-invasive dental procedures such as prosthodontics, scaling/polishing and some conservation work (fillings, crowns and bridges) do not require measurement of the INR preoperatively.

Patients on warfarin with unstable INRs, suffering from co-existing medical problems such as liver disease, renal disease, and thrombocytopaenia, or who are also on antiplatelet agents, should be managed in hospital settings.

Bleeding may be reduced by the use of local measures to secure haemostasis. Local measures may include the use of oxidised cellulose ('Surgicel') or collagen sponges and sutures. Tranexamic acid mouthwash is also effective, but is not easily available in the community in the UK.

Avoid the use of NSAIDs and COX II inhibitors.

exchange is required to remove the autoantibody and to replace the deficient protease. The condition may be associated with pregnancy, infection, drugs such as ciclosporin and autoimmune disorders. There is clinical overlap between TTP and haemolytic–uraemic syndrome (HUS), which tends to occur in children, often following infective diarrhoea. HUS is associated with more overt renal involvement but fewer neurological signs as compared to TTP.

Antiplatelet agents are associated with platelet dysfunction. Aspirin works by inhibiting platelet cyclooxygenase (COX), an enzyme needed for the synthesis of thromboxane A2, which is important in platelet activation. Clopidogrel is an antagonist for the $P2Y_{12}$ platelet receptor. Normally, adenosine diphosphate (ADP) released from platelet granules binds to the G-protein-linked $P2Y_{12}$ receptor, triggering platelet activation. ADP is prevented from binding in the presence of clopidogrel, and platelet activation does not occur.

Warfarin and dental surgery

Over the past two decades, there has been a significant rise in the number of patients receiving long-term anticoagulation with warfarin. Multiple indications for long-term anticoagulation have become accepted, including recurrent venous thromboembolism, prosthetic cardiac valves and stroke prevention in atrial fibrillation. A wide variation exists in warfarin dosage requirements between individuals, owing to genetic and environmental factors. Genetic mutations that reduce the rate of warfarin metabolism can increase sensitivity to warfarin.

Changes in diet, liver disease and concomitant medication also affect warfarin requirements. Anticoagulated patients undergoing invasive procedures need careful management of their anticoagulation to balance the risk of bleeding against that of thromboembolism if warfarin is reduced or omitted.

Potentially invasive dental procedures that may take place in the community include local anaesthesia, extractions (single and multiple), minor oral surgery, periodontal surgery, biopsies and subgingival scaling. Patients on oral anticoagulation undergoing such procedures present a challenge to the primary care team, and different approaches to their management have been considered. In 2007, the British Committee for Standards in Haematology (BCSH) published their guidelines, outlining a consensus approach (see Tables 20B.10 and 20B.11).

Mechanism of action of warfarin

The vitamin K–dependent coagulation factors II, VII, IX and X are synthesised in the liver. Dietary vitamin K is reduced by enzymes in the liver (epoxide reductase and quinone reductase) to a hydroquinone form. Hydroquinone is required to add glutamic acid residues to FII, FVII, FIX and FX (γ-carboxylation). Warfarin acts as a competitive inhibitor of vitamin K, binding to epoxide reductase and quinone reductase, leading to a deficiency in hydroquinone. γ-Carboxylation no longer occurs, resulting in the formation of PIVKAs (proteins induced by vitamin K absence), which cannot function as coagulation factors. An anticoagulant effect is thereby produced.

Warfarin and bleeding risk

The risk of bleeding on warfarin varies between published studies. The intensity of anticoagulation and age appear to correlate consistently with bleeding risk. Other risk factors include hypertension, history of gastrointestinal bleeding, previous cerebrovascular accident and recent initiation of anticoagulation.

The risk of bleeding following dental surgery

A meta-analysis by Wahl reviewed >2000 dental surgical procedures in 774 patients on continuous warfarin with INRs of up to 4. Over half of the patients underwent single, multiple and full-mouth extractions. Although some patients had minor oozing, requiring local haemostatic measures, >98% of patients had no serious bleeding problems.

Data from five randomised controlled trials showed no statistically significant difference in bleeding rates between those who continued and those who temporarily stopped warfarin prior to surgery. The data also suggest that, if patients continue oral anticoagulation prior to dental surgery, and local haemostatic measures are used, serious bleeding is rare.

The risk of discontinuing anticoagulation prior to surgery

The meta-analysis by Wahl demonstrated that, although the risk of thromboembolic events in patients who temporarily stopped warfarin prior to dental surgery was small, the complications were potentially serious. Four out of 493 patients undergoing >500 dental procedures had fatal thromboembolic events.

There has been a marked change in the management of warfarinised patients in dental practice. Most patients are treated without discontinuation of warfarin, provided that the INR is ≤4.

Current recommendations for the management of warfarinised patients in dental practice are given in the *British National Formulary*.

Direct Oral Anticoagulants (DOACs)

DOACs have emerged as a commonly used alternative to warfarin in patients who require anticoagulation, and are approved for both the treatment of venous thrombosis and for stroke prevention in patients with atrial fibrillation. There are two main groups of DOACs: thrombin inhibitors (e.g. Dabigatran) and factor Xa inhibitors (e.g. Rivaroxaban, Apixaban, Edoxaban).

DOACs have a much more specific anticoagulant effect as compared to warfarin, and are administered using a standard dose, requiring no routine laboratory monitoring. There are few drug and dietary interactions. The advantages also include a rapid onset of action and rapid clearance (if renal function normal). When DOACs first became available, there were no reversal agents for use when bleeding occurred; however, an antidote for Dabigatran is now available, and a Xa inhibitor antidote is under development.

DOACs and dental surgery

A pragmatic approach to dental surgery has been advocated in patients receiving DOACs, using the lessons learnt from managing patients on warfarin. Hence, other than the lack of the requirement for pre-operative INR testing, the dental management for patients taking DOACs is the same as would be the case for a patient taking warfarin, considering he or she has a stable INR with readings consistently less than 4.0. For dental procedures associated with a particularly high risk of bleeding, omission of the DOAC dose on the morning of the procedure is suggested.

20C TRANSFUSION MEDICINE

Introduction

Transfusion medicine continues to expand as a speciality, encompassing immunology, microbiology, stem cell work and transplantation. The safety of blood transfusion remains at the forefront of public awareness following several cases of virus transmission via blood in the 1980s. The discovery of new pathogens that may be transmitted through blood has brought new challenges, both in ensuring the safety of the blood supply and in developing new methods of pathogen detection. Haemovigilance schemes have highlighted how errors in transfusion occur, resulting in the introduction of measures to prevent the transfusion of incorrect blood components.

Blood group systems

A blood group system includes two or more red cell antigens produced either from allelic genes at a single genetic locus, or from genes at two or three closely linked loci. A red cell antigen is a protein or carbohydrate structure on the surface of the red cell that is detected by a specific alloantibody. There are 29 known blood group systems currently recognised by the International Society for Blood Transfusion. The two most important human blood group systems are the ABO and Rhesus blood group systems.

The ABO blood group system

The ABO blood group system was instituted in 1901. A and B antigens are expressed on all body tissues, and their expression is governed by the A and B genes on chromosome 9 and the H gene on chromosome 19. Antibodies to A and B antigens are naturally occurring IgM antibodies, which form at 3–6 months of age. Table 20C.1 illustrates the red cell antigens and the corresponding serum antibodies in the ABO blood group system. Table 20C.2 indicates the frequency of the ABO blood groups in the UK.

The ABO antibodies are extremely potent at activating complement. Transfusion of ABO-incompatible blood can result in an acute haemolytic transfusion reaction, with severe clinical consequences.

Table 20C.1 The ABO blood group system.

Blood group	Antigen on red cell	Antibody in serum
A	A	Anti-B
B	B	Anti-A
O	None	Anti-A,B
AB	A and B	None

Table 20C.2 Frequency of ABO blood groups in the UK.

Blood group	Percentage of UK population
A	43
B	9
O	45
AB	3

The Rhesus (Rh) blood group system

The Rh blood group system is a complex system of 45 antigens, of which five are clinically relevant (D, C, c, E, e). The D antigen is the main antigen; 85% of the UK population have the D antigen on the surface of their red cells, and are therefore 'D antigen–positive' (or 'Rh D–positive'). The remaining 15% of the population lack the D antigen on their cells, and are therefore termed 'Rh D–negative'. Rh D–negative individuals are capable of making immune anti-D on exposure to D-positive cells. Exposure may occur through blood transfusion, but more commonly occurs through pregnancy. Immune anti-D can cause haemolysis of foetal red cells in future pregnancies where the foetus is Rh D–positive (see the section titled 'Alloantibodies in pregnancy').

Red cell antibodies

Antibodies may be produced in individuals who are exposed to red cell antigens that are not expressed on their own red cells (Landsteiner's law). This can occur following the transfusion of blood components where the donated cells express antigens not found on the recipient's red cells. Antibodies can also form during pregnancy. Mixing of blood between the mother and foetus can expose the mother to 'foreign' foetal red cell antigens, resulting in maternal antibody formation. Antibodies can also be 'naturally occurring', as is the case with the ABO antibodies described in the ABO blood group system.

Alloantibody production

When the immune system of an individual is first exposed to an antigen that it does not recognise, it produces IgM antibody in low levels. Antibody production may take months to occur. This is known as a 'primary immune response'. If no further exposure to the antigen occurs, the IgM titre falls to undetectable levels. Further exposure to the same antigen results in rapid production (within days) of IgG alloantibody in large quantities. This is the 'secondary immune response'.

Antibodies that are capable of causing red cell destruction *in vivo* are termed 'clinically significant' antibodies. Red cell destruction may be intravascular or extravascular. If an individual who requires a blood transfusion is found to have a clinically significant alloantibody in his or her serum, this must be considered, and the appropriate blood provided.

Alloantibodies in pregnancy

During pregnancy, sensitising events may result in foetomaternal haemorrhage (FMH). FMH may also occur silently, or following delivery. Mixing of blood between an Rh D–negative mother and an Rh D–positive foetus can stimulate IgG anti-D production in the mother. During subsequent pregnancies, if the woman is again carrying an Rh D–positive foetus, maternal anti-D is able to cross the placenta and cause haemolysis of the foetal red cells, leading to foetal anaemia. This is known as 'haemolytic disease of the newborn' (HDN), and, if severe, may require intrauterine transfusion (IUT) of red cells. In an attempt to try and reduce the incidence of maternal anti-D alloimmunisation, NICE introduced guidelines in 2002 recommending that all non-sensitised Rh D–negative women be given routine intramuscular anti-D prophylaxis during pregnancy.

To prevent anti-D alloimmunisation through blood transfusion, BCSH guidelines recommend that all red cell and platelet transfusions be Rh D identical.

Blood components

There are over 1.5 million blood donors in the UK. Approximately 450 ml of whole blood is collected from each donor. The donation is then spun and separated into components (red cells, platelets and plasma). All cellular components undergo filtration to remove white blood cells. This process is known as 'leukodepletion', and was introduced in 1999 as a precaution against vCJD transmission. The risk of transmission of other infections carried by white blood cells, such as cytomegalovirus and human T lymphotropic virus (HTLV), is also reduced by the filtering process.

High-titre testing

Group O products can contain high-titres of anti-A and anti-B, and, rarely, passive transfusion of these antibodies can cause acute haemolysis of the recipient's red cells. The risk of haemolysis is higher if large volumes of plasma are transfused, or if children who are not group O receive group O products (children have a smaller plasma volume, and therefore may be less able to dilute out the antibodies). The National Blood Service (NBS) tests all donations for the presence of high-titre anti-A and anti-B.

Hospital pre-transfusion testing

Red cell or 'packed cell' transfusion may be given to correct anaemia or replace blood loss. All hospital patients requiring transfusion have a blood sample ('group and save') sent to the hospital transfusion laboratory. The transfusion laboratory performs several tests on the 'group and save' sample:

- The patient's ABO and Rh D groups are determined.
- An antibody screen is performed to try and detect any alloantibodies present in the patient's serum. If alloantibodies are detected, further tests are required to identify the antibodies.
- All results are checked against any tests performed on the patient in the past.
- If the patient requires a red cell transfusion, then ABO and Rh D–compatible red cells are selected for transfusion. If the patient is found to have alloantibodies in his or her serum, this must be considered, and the appropriate blood selected.

Selecting ABO-compatible blood

BCSH guidelines emphasise that, when selecting red cells for transfusion, the component of choice should be ABO identical. If ABO-identical blood is not available, then ABO-compatible blood can be given.

Once selected, blood is then crossmatched, either electronically or serologically, to exclude incompatibility between the donor and recipient. Serological crossmatch involves mixing the patient's serum (containing any antibodies) with red cells from the donor unit and looking for evidence of red cell agglutination. The development of red cell agglutination suggests that an alloantibody in the patient's serum has reacted against an antigen on the red cells, agglutinating them.

Once the appropriate blood has been selected and crossmatched, each unit can be transfused over approximately 90 min (faster if the patient is bleeding). If further transfusions are required, a fresh 'group and save' sample is often needed, to ensure that no new antibodies have formed following transfusion.

Haemovigilance in the UK

The Serious Hazards of Transfusion (SHOT) scheme is an anonymised national reporting scheme that collects data on all adverse events, including near-miss events, related to the transfusion of blood products. It was launched in 1996, and publishes an annual report that contains recommendations aimed at improving the safety of transfusion. SHOT collects data on adverse events occurring at all stages in the 'transfusion chain' – from the collection of blood samples to laboratory errors and the collection and administration of units.

Minimising errors in blood transfusion

ABO incompatibility is the cause of most fatal transfusion reactions, and it usually occurs following a clerical error or a mistake in patient identification. Table 20C.3 highlights some simple measures that can reduce such errors.

'Right blood, right patient'

The 'bedside check', performed at the point of administration, is the last opportunity to identify if an error has been made at any previous stage of the transfusion chain. Table 20C.4 highlights how a 'bedside check' is performed.

Platelets

An adult therapeutic dose of platelets can be obtained by one of two methods:

- Single-donor apheresis.
- Derived from four whole-blood donations ('recovered' platelets or 'buffy coat' platelets).

Platelets are suspended in plasma or platelet suspension medium, and each unit has a volume of 200–300 ml. Platelets are stored at room temperature, and have a 5-day shelf life. They can be transfused over 30 min. Platelet transfusion is indicated for the prevention and treatment of haemorrhage in patients with thrombocytopaenia or platelet function defects. Crossmatching is not required; however, since platelets express ABO antigens, and the units contain small amounts of red cell stroma (which may cause D sensitisation), platelet units should be ABO and Rh D – compatible with the recipient.

Table 20C.3 Four simple steps to taking a blood specimen.

1. Positively identify the patient. Ask the patient to state his or her name and date of birth, *and* check the patient's wristband. For outpatients, check the patient's notes or appointment card.
2. If you have the correct patient, take the blood specimen.
3. Label the tubes at the chair or bedside. For a 'group and save' specimen, the label must be handwritten.
4. Double-check the label against the wristband, notes or appointment card.

Table 20C.4 The bedside check.

The patient should be asked to identify himself/herself (unless unconscious).

The information on the unit should be checked against the patient's wristband.

The expiry date of the unit must be checked.

Fresh frozen plasma

Fresh frozen plasma (FFP) is rich in coagulation factors. FFP is frozen within 8 hours of collection to minimise the loss of labile coagulation factors, and it can be stored for up to 2 years at –30°C. FFP does not require crossmatching, but should be ABO-compatible with the recipient's blood group. As there is very little red cell stroma in FFP, it does not need to be Rh D–compatible.

At present, owing to the potential transmission of vCJD through blood products, all plasma for fractionation is obtained from the USA. In the UK, children born after 1 January, 1996, will not have been exposed to BSE through their diet, and are therefore given non-UK-sourced plasma to prevent potential exposure to vCJD through plasma. As the risk of virus transmission is higher in the USA as compared to the UK, all USA-sourced plasma undergoes virus inactivation procedures.

Indications for FFP

According to the 2004 BCSH guidelines on the use of FFP, cryoprecipitate and cryosupernatant, FFP can be given to replace coagulation factors in clinical situations such as massive transfusion and DIC with bleeding. In addition, patients with liver disease who are bleeding or who need to undergo an invasive procedure may require FFP.

FFP is not used in most single coagulation factor deficiencies, since factor concentrates are available. FFP should only be used to replace single coagulation factor deficiencies where no fractionated product is available.

FFP is not recommended for warfarin reversal. The method used to reverse anticoagulation depends on several factors – including patient comorbidities, the presence and severity of bleeding, the degree of overanticoagulation and the urgency at which the INR needs to be lowered. Warfarin should be omitted, and the administration of oral or intravenous vitamin K may be required. In life- or limb-threatening haemorrhage, a prothrombin complex concentrate (PCC) should be given in addition to intravenous vitamin K to reverse anticoagulation immediately. PCCs contain high concentrations of vitamin K–dependent clotting factors, and are therefore more reliable at reversing warfarin than FFP.

Cryoprecipitate

If FFP is frozen at –60°C, thawed and then spun, cryoprecipitate forms, which is rich in fibrinogen. Five single units of cryoprecipitate, each with a volume of 20–40 ml, are combined to form one pooled unit. A standard adult dose is two pooled units. Cryoprecipitate may be indicated in clinical situations where the plasma fibrinogen is below 1 g/l, such as in DIC with bleeding. As with FFP, there is no requirement for crossmatch, but the units should be ABO compatible with the recipient.

Risks of transfusion

Transfusion of blood products always carries a degree of risk to the recipient. Transfusion of an incorrect blood component, allergic or immune reactions to blood components and transfusion-transmitted infection form the majority of potential complications.

Transfusion reactions can vary from mild to severe, and may be classified as follows:

- Transfusion-transmitted infections.
- Febrile non-haemolytic transfusion reactions.
- Acute haemolytic transfusion reactions.
- Delayed haemolytic transfusion reactions.
- Allergic reactions.
- Transfusion-related acute lung injury.
- Transfusion-associated graft-versus-host disease.
- Post-transfusion purpura.

Preventing transfusion reactions

Unnecessary transfusions can be avoided by ensuring that blood is only given to patients when clinically indicated. The use of clear protocols to ensure correct patient identification at blood sampling, laboratory processing and blood product administration can also reduce the incidence of transfusion of incorrect blood components. In addition, in certain circumstances, alternatives to blood transfusion may be appropriate.

Alternatives to blood transfusion

Transfusion triggers may help guide decisions on when it is appropriate to consider transfusion, although the needs of an individual patient must always be considered. Particularly in surgical practice, there are several measures that may help to reduce the need for blood transfusion.

Preoperative assessment provides an opportunity to optimise a patient's Hb prior to surgery. Dietary advice, haematinics or erythropoietin can be used to correct anaemia. Decisions regarding discontinuation of anticoagulant or antiplatelet agents preoperatively can also be made.

During surgery, positioning of the patient by the anaesthetist can help limit blood loss. A variety of surgical measures – such as ultrasound scalpels, diathermy, fibrin sealant and haemostatic swabs – may also be used. Pharmacological agents that help in reducing bleeding include fibrin glue, tranexamic acid, aprotinin and recombinant factor VII. In addition, cell salvage may be used during certain types of operations. *Cell salvage* is the process by which blood shed during or after surgery is collected, filtered, washed and reinfused into the patient. Blood may be collected during surgery, and then returned to the patient either intraoperatively or postoperatively. Red cells can also be collected from wound drains postoperatively and reinfused.

FURTHER READING

Available from: http://www.sdcep.org.uk/published-guidance/anticoagulants-and-antiplatelets.

Available from: http://www.b-s-h.org.uk/guidelines/guidelines/management-of-patients-on-oral-anticoagulants-requiring-dental-surgery/.

MULTIPLE CHOICE QUESTIONS

1. Macrocytic anaemia is typically found in:
   a) Iron deficiency.
   b) Lead poisoning.
   c) B_{12} deficiency.
   d) Blood loss.
   e) Anaemia of chronic disease.
   Answer = C

2. Which of the following is *not* a cause of iron deficiency?
   a) Chronic blood loss.
   b) Coeliac disease.
   c) Menorrhagia.
   d) Poor dietary intake of iron.
   e) Pernicious anaemia.
   Answer = E

3. A 50-year-old man presents to the accident and emergency department with severe gastrointestinal bleeding. He is on warfarin, and the INR is 11. Which one of the following is best for rapid and complete reversal of his INR?
   a) Prothrombin complex concentrates plus intravenous vitamin K.
   b) Fresh frozen plasma plus intravenous vitamin K.
   c) Intravenous vitamin K.
   d) Oral vitamin K.
   e) Intramuscular vitamin K.
   Answer = A

4. How quickly does the administration of intravenous vitamin K usually lead to INR reversal in a patient receiving warfarin?
   a) 15 minutes.
   b) 1 hour.
   c) 24 hours.
   d) 4–6 hours.
   e) 10–12 hours.
   Answer = D

5. Blasts are typically seen in the blood in the following:
    a) Myeloma.
    b) Chronic lymphocytic leukaemia.
    c) Acute myeloid leukaemia.
    d) B_{12} deficiency.
    e) Liver disease.
    Answer = C

6. A 72-year-old patient requires two dental extractions. He is on warfarin for atrial fibrillation, and the INR is 2.5. Which of the following is correct?
    a) Perform the extractions in hospital.
    b) Stop the warfarin for 2 days prior to the extractions.
    c) Proceed with the extractions.
    d) Stop warfarin and give heparin before the extractions.
    e) Give vitamin K prior to the extractions.
    Answer = C

7. A low factor IX is found in:
    a) Haemophilia B.
    b) Haemophilia A.
    c) von Willebrand disease.
    d) Thrombocytopenia.
    e) Dabigatran therapy.
    Answer = A

8. Which of the following statements about dabigatran is correct?
    a) Used for anticoagulation in prosthetic heart valves.
    b) An antidote for rapid reversal is available.
    c) Reduces vitamin K–dependent clotting factors.
    d) Is a factor Xa inhibitor.
    e) Is mainly cleared via the liver.
    Answer = B

9. A positive DAT is typically found in:
    a) HS.
    b) SCD.
    c) AIHA.
    d) Anaemia of chronic disease.
    e) Myeloma.
    Answer = C

10. A low serum ferritin is typically found in:
    a) Iron deficiency anaemia.
    b) Liver disease.
    c) Thalassaemia.
    d) B_{12} deficiency.
    e) Folate deficiency.
    Answer = A

CHAPTER 21
Medical emergencies

M Greenwood

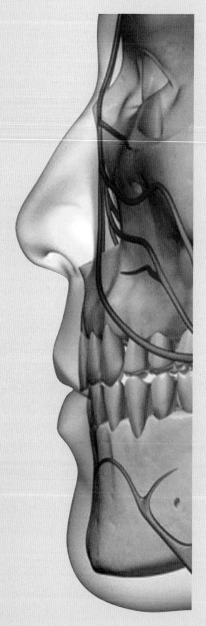

Key topics

- Medical emergencies in dental practice.
- Management of medical emergencies in dental practice.

Learning objectives

- To understand and recognise the presentation of medical emergencies that may occur in dental practice.
- To know the initial management of medical emergencies that can occur in dental practice.

Essentials of Human Disease in Dentistry, Second Edition. Mark Greenwood.
© 2018 John Wiley & Sons Ltd. Published 2018 by John Wiley & Sons Ltd.
Companion website: www.wiley.com/go/greenwood/human-disease-in-dentistry

Introduction

A thorough history should draw the practitioner's attention to potential medical emergencies that could occur, and therefore facilitate taking appropriate steps to prevent them from happening. One example might be the prompt treatment of a diabetic patient at a predictable time, thereby preventing hypoglycaemia.

The General Dental Council (GDC) requires registrants to undertake 10 hours of Continuing Professional Development (CPD) on the management of medical emergencies, once every 5 years. In addition, they recommend that practice scenarios be carried out on a regular basis, as well as Basic Life Support (and, increasingly, Immediate Life Support) training. Dental procedures can jeopardise the airway, which must therefore be adequately protected. Patients with pre-existing medical conditions such as asthma or angina will usually be taking prescription medications, and the practitioner should always check that these are readily available and have been taken on the day of treatment. Patients who have asthma attacks and have not brought their normal medication with them will not be helped significantly by oxygen alone (due to bronchoconstriction). They must bring their inhaler(s) with them, and the inhalers must also be available in the emergency drug box. The drugs to be included in an emergency box for the dental surgery are shown in Table 21.1.

In the history, it is important to enquire about known allergies or adverse reactions to medication, so that these can be avoided.

In all emergency situations, the basic principles of resuscitation should be remembered, and the 'ABCDE approach' to the sick patient used in all cases (discussed in the following text). Key points in the management of medical emergencies are listed in Table 21.2. All medical emergencies and near misses should be documented.

Table 21.1 Contents of the emergency drug box (completeness and expiry dates to be checked regularly).

- Adrenaline (epinephrine, 1 in 1000 solution)
- Aspirin (300 mg)
- GlucoGel®
- Glucagon (1 mg)
- Midazolam buccal solution (10 mg)
- Glyceryl trinitrate (GTN) tablets/spray
- Oxygen CD size cylinder
- Salbutamol

Optional items

- Flumazenil
- Chlorphenamine (10–20 mg)
- Glucose intravenous infusion (20%/50%)
- Hydrocortisone injection (100 mg)

Table 21.2 Factors to consider in the management of medical emergencies.

Conduct emergency drills, so that everyone knows their roles.

Keep emergency phone numbers at hand.

Check emergency kit regularly to ensure it is up to date.

Work to *prevent* emergencies as far as possible.

Ensure that patients always have their medications with them (e.g. a GTN spray for angina), or ensure that it is available in the emergency kit.

The ABCDE approach to the sick patient

All sick patients should be managed using the ABCDE approach. Here is a summary of the approach:

- *A* = Airway.
- *B* = Breathing.
- *C* = Circulation.
- *D* = Disability.
- *E* = Exposure.

The *airway* should be opened by using a head tilt/chin lift method, or by using a jaw thrust method to push the mandible forward (see Figures 21.1 and 21.2). The latter should be used in cases of known or suspected cervical spine injury, or in cases of cervical spine fusion or immobility.

Breathing should be checked by the look–listen–feel method for 10 seconds.

The concept of checking for *circulation* is not mandatory for dental practitioners, as the sign to start resuscitation is the absence of breathing, or the presence of the so-called 'agonal gasp breathing'. If competent, at the same time as checking for breathing, a central pulse such as the carotid pulse can be checked.

Disability refers to the neurological status of the patient, and this can be checked using the 'AVPU method', summarised as follows:

- *A* = *Alert* – Is the patient responsive?
- *V* = *Voice* – Does the patient respond to verbal stimuli?
- *P* = *Pain* – Does the patient respond to a painful stimulus?
- *U* = *Unresponsive*.

Exposure refers to the appropriate exposing of a part of the patient's body for a defined purpose. One example might be the application of chest pads of an automated external defibrillator (AED). Other purposes include examining for a rash in an allergic reaction and examining for traumatic injuries.

When using the ABCDE approach, it is important to remember not to move on to the next stage before the previous stage has been completed. For example, there is no point in moving from the airway stage until the airway has been adequately opened, as the other aspects will ultimately be futile. Likewise, it is important to return if necessary to the start of the process if circumstances change.

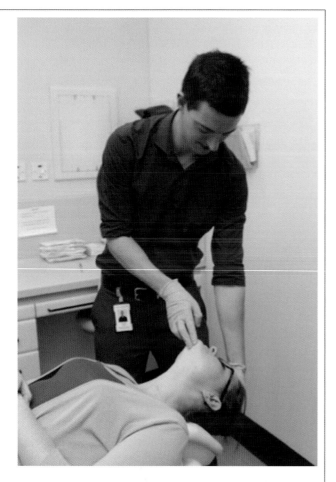

Figure 21.1 The head tilt/chin lift method of opening the airway.

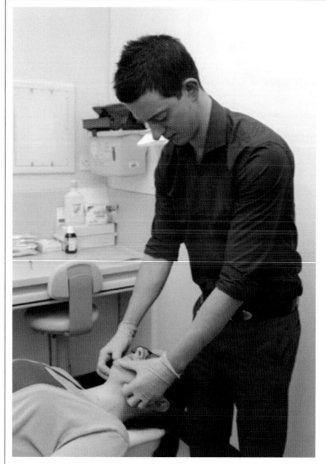

Figure 21.2 The jaw thrust method of opening the airway. When done correctly, the cervical spine will not move.

Table 21.3 Management of collapse of unknown cause.
Lie the patient flat and raise his or her legs.
Maintain the airway and administer oxygen (15 litres per minute via a non-rebreathe mask (see Figure 21.3).
If no pulse is palpable – cardiac arrest – institute cardiopulmonary resuscitation (CPR).
If a pulse is palpable, assume hypoglycaemia and treat by intramuscular glucagon if unconscious. If there is no risk to the airway, i.e. the patient is conscious, oral glucose may be given.
Get help.

The collapsed patient

The most common cause of loss of consciousness in dental practice is vasovagal syncope (fainting). If recovery is not rapid after appropriate treatment, other possibilities should be considered, such as myocardial infarction (MI), bradycardia, heart block, stroke, hypoglycaemia or anaphylaxis. If the cause of collapse is uncertain, the steps outlined in Table 21.3 should be followed in a patient who may or may not have lost consciousness.

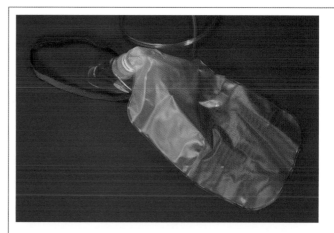

Figure 21.3 A non-rebreathe mask to facilitate oxygen delivery at as high a concentration as possible.

Fainting (vasovagal syncope)

Fainting is the most common medical emergency seen in dental practice. Pain and anxiety are predisposing factors.

Signs and symptoms

The patient may:

- Feel nauseated, with cold, clammy skin.
- Notice a visual disturbance, together with a feeling of dizziness.
- Have a pulse initially rapid and weak, becoming slow on recovery.
- Lose consciousness.

Management

- Before the patient loses consciousness, the possibility of hypoglycaemia should be borne in mind and a glucose drink may be helpful.
- Lay the patient flat, so that the legs are higher than the head (and heart).
- Loosen any tight clothing around the neck.
- Recovery is usually rapid; as the patient regains consciousness, his or her body may occasionally jerk in a manner resembling a fit.
- Prolonged unconsciousness should lead to consideration of other causes of collapse.

Chest pain

Most patients who experience chest pain of cardiac origin in the dental environment are likely to have a previous history of cardiac disease. Again, the history is important, as is recognising the risk factors for cardiovascular disease (Chapter 5, titled 'Cardiovascular disorders').

It is important for patients who use medication to control angina to have this with them, or to ensure that it is readily available in the emergency kit in case they need it. Likewise, it is important for the patients to have taken their normal medications.

Some features make the pain unlikely to be cardiac in origin, such as: pains that, however, severe last less than 30 seconds; stabbing pains; well-localised left submammary pain; and pains that continually vary in location. A chest pain that is made better by stopping exercise is more likely to be cardiac in origin than one that is not related. Pleuritic pain is sharp and made worse on inspiration – for example, following pulmonary embolism.

Oesophagitis may cause a retrosternal pain that is worse on bending or lying down. Oesophageal pain, as with cardiac pain, may be relieved by sublingual nitrates – for example, GTN.

Hyperventilation may produce chest pain. Gall bladder and pancreatic pain may also mimic cardiac pain. Musculoskeletal pain is often accompanied by tenderness to palpation in the affected region. A summary of the main possible causes of chest pain is listed in Table 21.4.

Clearly, it is important to exclude angina and MI when a patient complains of chest pain.

Table 21.4 A differential diagnosis of chest pain.
Angina.
MI.
Pleuritic (e.g. pulmonary embolism).
Musculoskeletal.
Oesophageal reflux.
Hyperventilation.

Signs and symptoms

- The pain of angina and MI may be very similar, comprising a crushing central chest pain (like a tight band around the chest) radiating to the left arm (usually) or mandible.
- Angina is usually relieved by the patient's medication, which in most cases will be a GTN spray. The pain of angina usually lasts for <3 min if GTN is used.
- MI is often accompanied by other symptoms such as sweating, nausea and palpitations, and is not relieved by GTN.
- There may be breathlessness and vomiting.
- Occasionally, a patient may lose consciousness.

Management

- A calm and reassuring manner from the practitioner is important.
- If the patient has a history of angina, get the patient to use his or her normal medication – there should be a rapid response (within a few minutes) if the cause is angina. GTN should be part of the emergency drug box in case patients do not have their own medications with them.
- If MI is suspected, summon help at an early stage, and administer 300 mg aspirin to be chewed (if not contraindicated).
- The patient will be most comfortable in a sitting position.
- Ensure that the airway is maintained, and administer a 50/50 mix of nitrous oxide and oxygen, which has analgesic and anxiolytic effects, or 15 litres per minute oxygen.

A patient who has had a MI may be given one of the so-called 'clot busting' agents, such as streptokinase. There are strict criteria regarding the types of patients in whom this medication should be used, since widespread bleeding may result. As a consequence of this, a patient who has undergone recent surgery should be excluded. More recent management advances include immediate angioplasty, in situations where the necessary facilities and expertise are available.

The diabetic patient

A history of recurrent hypoglycaemic episodes and markedly varying blood glucose levels means that a patient attending for dental treatment is much more likely to develop hypoglycaemia. It is wise to treat diabetic patients first in the morning, ensuring that they have had their normal antidiabetic medication and something to eat prior to attending the surgery.

Hypoglycaemia is much more likely to be encountered in dental practice than hyperglycaemia, since the former has a more rapid onset. Principally seen in diabetics, hypoglycaemia may be seen in very anxious patients who have starved themselves for whatever reason prior to attending the dental treatment session. Diabetic control may be adversely affected by oral sepsis, leading to increased risk of complications.

Diabetic emergencies

If hypoglycaemia occurs, glucose should be given orally – as tablets, syrup or sugary drinks – if the patient can cooperate. For those patients who are not able to cooperate, glucose is also available as an oral gel in a dispenser (e.g. GlucoGel^R). If these measures are impossible or ineffective – for example, in an uncooperative, semi-conscious or comatose patient – the usual treatment of first choice is glucagon (1 mg/ml injection) 1 mg, intramuscular or subcutaneous. Patients who do not respond to glucagon, or who have been hypoglycaemic for some time and may have exhausted their supplies of liver glycogen, will require up to 50 ml of intravenous glucose solution. Clearly, patients who have reached this stage should be managed under medical supervision, and are unlikely to be seen in dental practice.

Signs and symptoms

- Uncharacteristic aggression.
- Drowsiness.
- Moist skin.
- Rapid, full pulse.
- Low blood sugar.

Management

- Lie the patient flat.
- If the patient is conscious, give oral glucose (four lumps of sugar) or GlucoGel®.
- If the patient is unconscious, give 1 mg of glucagon intramuscularly. (Glucagon is more easily administered than intravenous glucose.)
- Get medical help.

The mainstay of hyperglycaemia treatment is intravenous rehydration, which requires medical intervention and is beyond the scope of this discussion.

Hypersensitivity reactions – anaphylaxis

Anaphylaxis is a type I severe hypersensitivity reaction (see Chapter 4, titled 'Immunological disease'). In dentistry, the most common cause is penicillin or latex, but NSAIDs can also cause this. Rarely, local anaesthetics may be responsible.

Signs and symptoms

- Facial flushing/pallor/cyanosis/oedema.
- Skin cold and clammy.
- Urticaria (itchy rash), oedema.
- Wheezing/laryngospasm.
- Tachycardia, hypotension.

Management

- Lie the patient flat.
- Administer 0.5 ml of 1:1000 adrenaline intramuscularly, and repeat at 5-min intervals as necessary. Adrenaline has both α and β effects. It reverses peripheral vasodilatation and reduces oedema. β Activity dilates the airway, increases the force of myocardial contraction, and also suppresses histamine and leukotriene release. Adverse effects from adrenaline are rare when appropriate doses are given intramuscularly.
- Ensure the airway is clear, and administer 100% oxygen.

'Second-line' drugs – not required to be administered by dental practitioners

- 10–20 mg chlorphenamine (antihistamine) intravenously (if competent).
- 100 mg of hydrocortisone sodium succinate intravenously, which helps to reduce oedema and stabilises mast cells (if competent).
- An inhaled β$_2$-agonist can be useful to facilitate bronchodilation.
- Arrange for hospital admission, as there may be a rebound attack.

Chlorphenamine and hydrocortisone need not be given by non-medical first responders. If the practitioner is confident in drug administration, it will do no harm to administer these drugs. Whatever the status of the resuscitator, adrenaline must be given (the preferred injection site is shown in Figure 21.4, but the deltoid muscle may also be used).

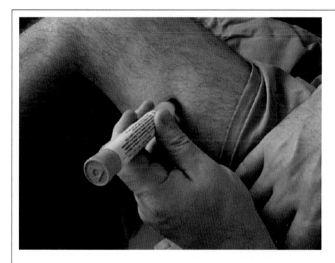

Figure 21.4 Preferred injection site – anterolateral thigh.

Many patients with a history of anaphylactic reactions will carry an 'EpiPen', which contains 300 µg of epinephrine.

Angioedema

Angioedema is triggered when mast cells release histamine and other chemicals (essentially vasoactive peptides) into the blood, producing rapid swelling. From a medical perspective, angioedema is life-threatening if the swelling produced compromises the airway. It may be precipitated by substances such as latex, as well as by drugs – including penicillin, NSAIDs and ACE inhibitors (e.g. captopril and lisinopril). There is a hereditary component to angioedema.

Swelling of the skin occurs, especially around the eyes and lips, but also in the throat and on the extremities. Laryngeal oedema and bronchospasm lead to the same clinical situation as anaphylaxis. In cases of severe angioedema, patients may be prescribed the steroid prednisolone. Acute allergic oedema of this type can develop alone, or may be associated with anaphylactic reactions.

Hereditary angioedema (HANE) is caused by continued complement activation, resulting from a deficiency of the inhibitor of the enzyme C1 esterase. The inheritance is usually autosomal dominant, and may not present until adult life. C1 esterase inhibitor concentrates are available to supplement the deficiency. Such supplements should be administered prior to dental treatment if such treatment has, in the past, triggered the onset of angioedema.

Fits

The nature of the fits (seizures), their frequency and degree of control, including the type of medication used, are all important factors to be elicited.

Signs and symptoms

The signs and symptoms of fits vary widely, depending on the underlying cause. An obvious fit is easily recognised.

Management

- In most cases, the main aim is to prevent patients from injuring themselves during fits episodes.
- If a fits episode has stopped and the patient is in the immediate aftermath ('post-ictal phase'), he or she should be placed in the recovery position.
- If the convulsions are ongoing, buccal administration of midazolam buccal solution (10 mg) should be carried out after 5 minutes of continuous seizure.
- The possibility of the patient's airway becoming occluded should always be kept in mind, and the airway must therefore be protected.

It may be appropriate to abort dental treatment if a patient suffers a fits episode during treatment.

Cardiac arrest

Cardiac arrest is denoted by the absence of a pulse and breathing.

Possible causes of cardiac arrest

- MI.
- Choking.
- Bleeding.
- Drug overdose.
- Hypoxia.

Signs and symptoms

- The patient loses consciousness.
- There is no respiration or pulse.

Management

Basic life support (BLS) implies that no equipment is employed other than a protective airway device. It has been suggested that cardiopulmonary resuscitation (CPR) can be performed effectively in the dental chair, but it is important that this is confirmed in each case.

Interruptions to chest compression in resuscitation are common, and are associated with a reduced chance of survival. The ideal situation is to be able to deliver continuous chest compressions while giving ventilations independently. This is only possible, however, when an advanced airway is placed. Chest-compression-only CPR is another way to increase the number of compressions, but is only effective for a period of about 5 min. For this reason, this technique is not recommended as standard management. The principle that compression-only CPR works upon is that, during the first few minutes after a non-asphyxial cardiac arrest, the blood oxygen content remains high, and, therefore, ventilation is less important than chest compression at this stage.

Rescuers are now taught to place the heel of their one hand in the centre of the chest (sternum), with the other hand on top. The chest should be compressed at a rate of about 100/min.

The basic algorithm for adult basic life support is given in Figure 21.5.

In guidelines published by the Resuscitation Council (UK), the concept of checking for 'signs of a circulation' was introduced. This change from previous regulations was made because it had been found that checking the carotid pulse to diagnose cardiac arrest could be unreliable, sometimes even when attempted by healthcare professionals. In the current guidelines, an absence of breathing is the main sign of cardiac arrest. Also highlighted is the need to identify agonal gasps (in addition to the absence of breathing) as a sign to commence CPR.

In the new guidelines, it is still stressed that, before resuscitation attempts are made, the environment should be ensured to be safe.

Use of defibrillation

Ventricular fibrillation (VF) is the most common cause of cardiac arrest. It is a rapid and chaotic rhythm. As a result, the heart is unable to contract, and thus unable to sustain its function as a pump.

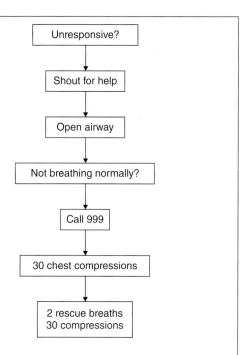

Figure 21.5 The adult basic life support algorithm (Resuscitation Council, UK).

'Defibrillation' is a term that refers to the termination of fibrillation. It is achieved by administering a controlled electrical shock to the heart that may restore an organised rhythm, enabling the heart to contract effectively. It is now well recognised that early defibrillation is important. The only effective treatment for VF is defibrillation, and the sooner the shock is given, the greater the chance of survival.

The provision of defibrillation has been made easier by the development of AEDs. AEDs are sophisticated, reliable and safe computerised devices that use voice and visual prompts to guide rescuers, and are suitable for use by healthcare professionals as well as lay people. The devices analyse the victim's rhythm, determine the need for a shock and then deliver a shock. The AED algorithm is given in Figure 21.6.

Pacemakers

Pacemakers are used to treat certain types of arrhythmias, one example being bradycardia. Some devices used in dentistry can interfere with the normal functioning of pacemakers. Such devices include some types of ultrasonic scalers, electroanalgesic devices, electrocautery devices and electronic apex locaters. It is important that the relevant literature supplied by the manufacturers of such devices be consulted.

If a patient with a pacemaker develops bradycardia, all electrical equipment should be switched off, and the patient placed supine with the legs raised. Immediate medical assistance should be summoned.

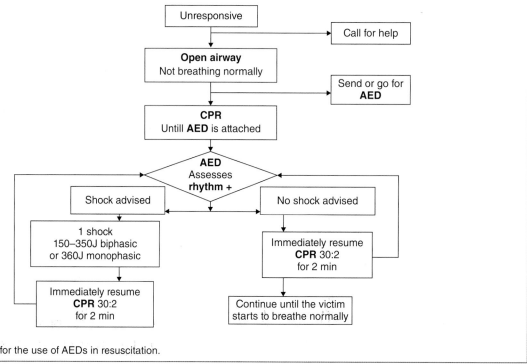

Figure 21.6 Algorithm for the use of AEDs in resuscitation.

Asthma

It is important to get an idea of the severity of the condition, which will usually come from the history. Important facts to ascertain are the effectiveness of medication, precipitating factors, hospital admissions due to asthma and the use of systemic steroids.

It is important that asthmatic patients bring their usual inhalers/medication with them to dental appointments. If the inhaler has not been brought, it must be in the emergency kit, or treatment should be deferred. If the asthma is in a particularly severe phase, elective treatment may be best postponed. Drugs that may be prescribed by dental practitioners, particularly NSAIDs, may worsen asthma, and are therefore best avoided.

Signs and symptoms

- The patient is breathless with an expiratory wheeze, and may be using the accessory muscles of respiration.
- The patient will usually be tachycardic. Bradycardia is a worrying sign.

Management

- A calm and reassuring manner from the practitioner is important.
- The patient will be most comfortable in a sitting position.
- The patient should use his or her normal asthma medication.
- Oxygen should be administered.
- Further inhalation should be via a spacer device filled with 12 actuations of the inhaler.
- If the attack does not respond rapidly when using only the patient's usual medication, he or she should be admitted to the hospital.

The use of a spacer device improves delivery of the patient's own inhaler contents. The method described in the *British National Formulary* is to apply the mouthpiece of the inhaler to the underside of a paper cup, through which a hole has been cut. If the open end of the cup is placed against the mouth and nose, aerosol delivery should be improved.

Hyperventilation

Hyperventilation is a more common emergency than is often thought. When hyperventilation persists, it is extremely distressing to the patient. Anxiety is the principal precipitating factor.

Signs and symptoms

- The patient may feel weak and light-headed or dizzy.
- They may complain of paraesthesia (e.g. in the hands), or complain of muscle pain.
- They may have palpitations and chest pain, and indeed are sometimes convinced that they are having an MI.
- Carpopedal spasm may occur if hyperventilation is prolonged (Figure 21.7).

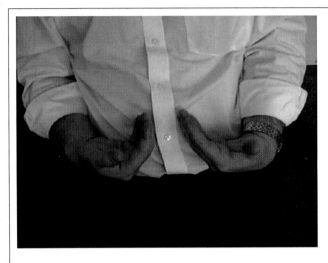

Figure 21.7 The position of the hands in carpal spasm.

Management

- Clearly, a calm and sympathetic approach by the practitioner is important.
- The diagnosis is not always as obvious as it may seem.
- When other causes for the symptoms have been excluded, the patient should be encouraged to rebreathe their own exhaled air, so as to increase the amount of carbon dioxide being inhaled. Hyperventilation leads to carbon dioxide being 'washed out' of the body, thus producing an alkalosis. Rebreathing exhaled air returns the situation to normal. This is achieved by breathing in and out of a paper bag held over the mouth and nose. A spacer device can be used for rebreathing exhaled air with the end blocked off where the inhaler would normally be placed.

Choking

A foreign body may lead to either mild or severe airway obstruction. Signs and symptoms that aid in differentiation are listed in Table 21.5, which is taken from the Resuscitation Council (UK) guidelines. In the conscious victim, it is useful to ask the question 'Are you choking?'.

An algorithm for the management of choking patients has been published by the Resuscitation Council (UK). This is shown in Figure 21.8. The back blows shown in the algorithm are given by standing to the side of the victim and slightly behind. The chest should be supported with one hand, and the victim should lean well forward, so that, when the obstruction is dislodged, it is expelled from the mouth, rather than passed further down the airway. Up to five sharp blows should be given between the shoulder blades with the heel of the other hand. After each back blow, a check should be made to see if the obstruction has been relieved.

If the back blows fail to relieve the obstruction, up to five abdominal thrusts should be given. The method is as follows:

- Stand behind the victim, put both arms around the upper part of his or her abdomen, and lean the victim forward.
- The rescuer's fist should be clenched and placed between the umbilicus and the lower end of the sternum.
- The clenched fist should be grasped with the other hand and pulled sharply inwards and upwards.
- This should be repeated up to five times.

Table 21.5 Choking – signs and symptoms.

General signs of choking

- Attack occurs while the victim is eating/has misplaced dental instrument/restoration.
- Victim may clutch his or her neck.

Signs of mild airway obstruction

Response to the question 'Are you choking?'

- Victim speaks and answers 'YES'.

Other signs

- Victim is able to speak, cough and breathe.

Signs of severe airway obstruction

Response to the question 'Are you choking?'

- Victim unable to speak.
- Victim may respond by nodding.

Other signs

- Victim is unable to breathe.
- Breathing sounds wheezy.
- Attempts at coughing are silent.
- Victim may be unconscious.

- If the obstruction is not relieved, an alternating pattern of five back blows with five abdominal thrusts should be used.

Other aspects of the management of inhaled foreign bodies are discussed in Chapter 6, titled 'Respiratory disorders'.

Adrenal crisis

Adrenal crisis may result from adrenocortical hypofunction, leading to hypotension, shock and death. It may be precipitated by stress induced by trauma, surgery or infection.

Adrenocortical hypofunction may be primary or secondary. An example of primary hypotension is Addison's disease (see Chapter 12, titled 'Dermatology and mucosal lesions'), in which there are circulating autoantibodies to the adrenal cortex. This results in atrophy and failure of secretion of hydrocortisone and aldosterone. Tuberculous destruction of the adrenal glands will produce the same effect.

Secondary hypoadrenocorticism results from adrenocortical hypofunction, owing to ACTH deficiency. This happens due to the suppression of adrenocortical function following the use of systemic corticosteroids.

The use of supplemental steroids prior to dental surgery in patients at risk of an adrenal crisis is a contentious issue. The rationale for steroid supplementation is as follows. A normal physiological response to trauma is to increase corticosteroid production in response to stress. If this response is absent, hypotension, collapse and death will occur. The hypothalamo–pituitary–adrenal axis will fail to function if either the pituitary or adrenal cortex ceases to function for the reasons mentioned in the preceding text. This happens in secondary hypoadrenocorticism, since administration of corticosteroids leads to negative feedback to the hypothalamus, causing decreased ACTH production and adrenocortical atrophy. This atrophy

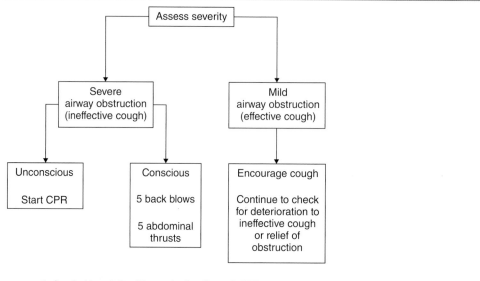

Figure 21.8 Algorithm for the management of a choking victim (Resuscitation Council, UK).

means that an endogenous steroid boost cannot be produced in response to stress.

Studies have suggested that dental surgery may not require supplementation. However, more invasive procedures, such as third molar surgery, may still require cover. It is wise, if supplementary steroids have not been used, to monitor the blood pressure of patients taking steroids. If the diastolic pressure falls by >25%, then an intravenous steroid injection (100 mg of hydrocortisone) is indicated. Patients who may require supplementation are those who are currently taking corticosteroids or have done so in the last month. A supplement may also be required if steroid therapy has been used for >1 month in the previous year. If the patient is receiving the equivalent of 20 mg of prednisolone daily, then extra supplementation is not likely to be required.

Signs and symptoms

- The patient loses consciousness.
- The patient has a rapid, weak or impalpable pulse.
- The patient's blood pressure falls rapidly.

Management

- Lie the patient flat.
- Ensure a clear airway and administer oxygen, 15 litres per minute, via a non-rebreathe mask.
- Call an ambulance or dial the hospital emergency number.
- Administer 200 mg (at least) of hydrocortisone sodium succinate intravenously (if competent).

Local anaesthetics emergencies

Allergy to local anaesthetics is rare, but should be managed similar to any other case of anaphylaxis. When taken in the context of the number of local anaesthetics administered, complication rates are low, but can occur. The signs and symptoms cover the whole range of allergies up to those of anaphylaxis.

Fainting in association with the injection of local anaesthetics is rather more common, and can usually be avoided by administering local anaesthetics while the patient is supine. Intravascular injection of local anaesthetics can be avoided by the use of an aspirating syringe. An intravascular injection may induce agitation, drowsiness or confusion, with fits and, ultimately, loss of consciousness.

Cardiovascular problems in association with local anaesthetics

The most common symptoms to be precipitated are palpitations, which will subside naturally with time. An MI may rarely be precipitated in a susceptible patient.

It is possible for interactions with antihypertensive drugs to precipitate hypotension. It is important in these circumstances to ensure that the airway remains clear, and that the patient is reassured. Medical assistance should be sought. Hypertension should likewise be managed with medical assistance.

In any circumstances in which a cardiovascular event is precipitated, treatment should be deferred for another occasion (see also Chapter 14, titled 'Pain and anxiety control').

Temporary facial palsy or diplopia

Complications such as these arise from the local anaesthetics agent tracking towards the facial nerve or the orbital contents. The patient should be reassured, since the effects wear off as the effects of the local anaesthetics diminish. If the temporal and zygomatic branches of the facial nerve are involved, it is important to protect the cornea, and an eye patch is indicated as a temporary measure.

Stroke

Stroke is discussed in detail in Chapter 9 (titled 'Neurology and special senses'). It is unlikely that a patient will have a stroke in dental surgery; nevertheless, it is still possible. Signs and symptoms vary according to the area of the brain affected.

There may be loss of consciousness, and/or weakness of the limb(s) on one side of the body. The side of the face may be weak; if so, this will be an upper motor neurone lesion, and therefore the forehead will not be affected on that side.

The dental surgeon's role, if such an event occurred, would be to first recognise (or suspect) the possibility. There is an ongoing public education programme regarding early stroke recognition using the acronym 'FAST', denoting:
- *F*ace drooping.
- *A*rm weakness.
- *S*peech difficulty.
- *T*ime to call emergency services.

Initial management would involve employing the ABCDE approach, and avoidance of aspiration of secretions as part of this, as well as calling for emergency help. Clearly, ongoing management would be the province of the specialist.

Needle breakage

Needle breakages are rare with modern needles. When they do happen, they often occur at the hub of the needle, and are more common with needles of smaller diameter. If this event does occur, the needle should be retrieved immediately if possible using fine artery forceps. This is only possible if the needle is not inserted to the hub while the injection is given, and, for this reason, the needle should not be inserted to this degree on any occasion.

If immediate retrieval is not possible, the patient should be informed about what has happened and referred immediately to the local maxillofacial unit. It is important for medicolegal reasons that the incident be accurately and clearly documented.

Sedation emergencies

Sedation emergencies are usually avoidable by careful technique, but may relate to overdose or hypoxia, or both. Either of these situations may lead to a respiratory arrest if not addressed, and the patient will be obviously cyanosed. During any dental treatment, the vital signs should be observed, but this is particularly important during sedation, when they should be formally monitored.

Management

- Do not give any further sedation agent.
- Open and maintain the airway and give oxygen.
- Ventilate the patient.
- If an overdose is suspected, consider the use of the reversal agent flumazenil (a benzodiazepine antagonist).

Emergencies arising from impaired haemostasis

It is important that any potential problems with haemostasis be uncovered in the medical history, so that it can be anticipated and prevented. Despite this, however, haemorrhage may occur postoperatively in dental patients, and may be classified as *primary* (bleeding at the time of surgery) or *reactionary* (bleeding a few hours after surgery). Reactionary haemorrhage is often attributable to the effects of vasoconstrictor-containing local anaesthetics wearing off. Secondary haemorrhage is that which occurs a few days after the operative procedure, and is usually attributable to infection. Further details on the management of patients with impaired haemostasis are given in Chapter 20 (titled 'Haematology').

SUMMARY

Medical emergencies occurring in dental practice can be alarming. A thorough history should be taken, so that possible emergencies can be anticipated to some extent.

Having a good working knowledge of how to manage emergencies is mandatory for all practising clinicians.

FURTHER READING

British National Formulary. Available from: bnf.org.

Resuscitation Council, UK. Available from: www.resus.org.uk.

MULTIPLE CHOICE QUESTIONS

1. In anaphylaxis, the correct initial dose of adrenaline to be administered intramuscularly is:
   a) 0.5 mg, 1:10 000.
   b) 1 mg, 1:10 000.
   c) 1.25 mg, 1:1000.
   d) 1 mg, 1:1000.
   e) 1.5 mg, 1:1000.
   Answer = D

2. In a patient who is choking owing to severe airway obstruction, which of the following is *not* true?
   a) The patient should be encouraged to cough.
   b) If the patient is unconscious, CPR should be started.
   c) If the patient is conscious, five back blows should be alternated with five abdominal thrusts.
   d) The patient will have an ineffective cough.
   e) The patient may be unable to speak.
   Answer = A

3. Which of the following drugs is *not* currently recommended for including in the emergency drug box as a required medication in dentistry?
   a) Aspirin 300 mg.
   b) Glucagon 1 mg.
   c) Glucagon 10 mg.
   d) Salbutamol inhaler.
   e) GTN tablets/spray.
   Answer = C

4. In a hyperventilating patient, which of the following is true?
   a) If hyperventilation persists, the partial pressure of carbon dioxide in the blood will increase.
   b) If hyperventilation persists, the partial pressure of carbon dioxide in the blood will remain unaltered.
   c) If hyperventilation persists, the partial pressure of carbon dioxide in the blood will decrease.

d) If hyperventilation persists, the blood pH will reflect acidosis.

e) If hyperventilation persists, the blood pH will remain unchanged.

Answer = C

5. Regarding cardiac arrest, which of the following is true?
   a) Most paediatric cardiac arrests fundamentally occur secondary to cardiac dysfunction.
   b) Most paediatric cardiac arrests will require defibrillation.
   c) Most adult cardiac arrests will not require defibrillation.
   d) Asystole is the commonest cardiac arrest arrhythmia in adults.
   e) A reversible underlying aetiological factor in a pulseless electrical activity (PEA) arrest is hypoxia.

Answer = E

6. After what length of time should a patient who has an epileptic seizure be given benzodiazepine?
   a) 1 minute.
   b) 2 minutes.
   c) 3 minutes.
   d) 4 minutes.
   e) 5 minutes.

Answer = E

7. The correct flow rate of oxygen to be given to a patient who needs it is:
   a) 2 litres per minute.
   b) 5 litres per minute.
   c) 10 litres per minute.
   d) 15 litres per minute.
   e) 20 litres per minute.

Answer = D

8. A patient is described as being hypoglycaemic if his or her blood glucose level falls to:
   a) 4 mmol per litre.
   b) 6 mmol per litre.
   c) 8 mmol per litre.
   d) 10 mmol per litre.
   e) 12 mmol per litre.

Answer = A

9. The first stage in CPR for an adult patient (after the area has been declared safe and an arrest has been confirmed) is:
   a) 2 rescue breaths.
   b) 5 rescue breaths.
   c) 5 chest compressions.
   d) 15 chest compressions.
   e) 30 chest compressions.

Answer = E

10. In the UK, the in-hospital telephone number to call in the event of a cardiac arrest is:
    a) 999.
    b) 2222.
    c) 3333.
    d) 4444.
    e) 5555.

Answer = B

Appendix: normal reference ranges

There is variation between laboratories regarding normal reference ranges, but the following are the indicative values:

Basic haematology values		
Haemoglobin	Men	130–180 g/l
	Women	115–160 g/l
Mean cell volume (MCV)		76–96 fl
Platelets		150–400 × 10⁹/l
White cells		4–11 × 10⁹/l
Neutrophils		40–75%
Lymphocytes		20–45%
Eosinophils		1–6%
Urea and electrolytes (U and E)		
Sodium		135–145 mmol/l
Potassium		3.5–5 mmol/l
Creatinine		70–150 μmol/l
Urea		2.5–6.7 mmol/l
Calcium		2.12–2.65 mmol/l
Albumin		35–50 g/l
Proteins		60–80 g/l
Liver function tests (LFTs)		
Bilirubin		3–17 μmol/l
Alanine aminotransferase (ALT)		3–35 U/l
Aspartate transaminase (AST)		3–35 U/l
Alkaline phosphatase		30–300 U/l
Other		
C-reactive protein (CRP)		<10 mg/l
Erythrocyte sedimentation rate (ESR)		0–6 mm in 1 hour normal
		>20 mm in 1 hour abnormal

Essentials of Human Disease in Dentistry, Second Edition. Mark Greenwood.
© 2018 John Wiley & Sons Ltd. Published 2018 by John Wiley & Sons Ltd.
Companion website: www.wiley.com/go/greenwood/human-disease-in-dentistry

Index

Note: Page numbers in *italic* refer to figures, those in **bold** to tables.

Essentials of Human Disease in Dentistry, Second Edition. Mark Greenwood.
© 2018 John Wiley & Sons Ltd. Published 2018 by John Wiley & Sons Ltd.
Companion website: www.wiley.com/go/greenwood/human-disease-in-dentistry